TEXTBOOK OF

GLOBAL CHILD HEALTH

Deepak M. Kamat, MD, PhD, FAAP
Philip R. Fischer, MD, FAAP

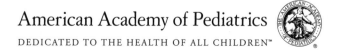

American Academy of Pediatrics
DEDICATED TO THE HEALTH OF ALL CHILDREN™

American Academy of Pediatrics Department of Marketing and Publications Staff

Maureen DeRosa, MPA, Director, Department of Marketing and Publications

Mark Grimes, Director, Division of Product Development

Jennifer McDonald, Manager, Online Content

Carrie Peters, Editorial Assistant

Sandi King, MS, Director, Division of Publishing and Production Services

Theresa Wiener, Manager, Publications Production and Manufacturing

Jason Crase, Editorial Specialist

Peg Mulcahy, Manager, Graphic Design and Production

Kevin Tuley, Director, Division of Marketing and Sales

Linda Smessaert, Manager, Clinical and Professional Publications Marketing

Library of Congress Control Number: 2010909673

ISBN: 978-1-58110-523-0

eISBN: 978-1-58110-524-7

MA0573

The recommendations in this publication do not indicate an exclusive course of treatment or serve as a standard of medical care. Variations, taking into account individual circumstances, may be appropriate.

Every effort has been made to ensure that the drug selection and dosage set forth in this text are in accordance with the current recommendations and practice at the time of publication. It is the responsibility of the health care provider to check the package insert of each drug for any change in indications and dosage and for added warnings and precautions.

The mention of product names in this publication is for informational purposes only and does not imply endorsement by the American Academy of Pediatrics.

The publishers have made every effort to trace the copyright holders for borrowed material. If they have inadvertently overlooked any, they will be pleased to make the necessary arrangements at the first opportunity.

Printed in the United States of America.

9-300/1011

1 2 3 4 5 6 7 8 9 10

■ CONTRIBUTORS

Jocelyn Y. Ang, MD, FAAP
Assistant Professor
Division of Infectious Diseases
Carman and Ann Adams Department
 of Pediatrics
Wayne State University
Children's Hospital of Michigan
Detroit, MI

Victor Balaban, PhD
Travelers' Health and Animal
 Importation Branch
Division of Global Migration and
 Quarantine
Centers for Disease Control and
 Prevention (CDC)
Atlanta, GA

Elizabeth D. Barnett, MD
Professor of Pediatrics
Boston University School of Medicine
Maxwell Finland Laboratory for
 Infectious Diseases
Boston Medical Center
Boston, MA

Zulfiqar A. Bhutta, MD, PhD, FAAP
Noordin Noormahomed Endowed
 Professor
Founding Chair, Division of Women and
 Child Health
Aga Khan University
Karachi, Pakistan

**David R. Boulware, MD, MPH,
 CTropMed**
Assistant Professor
Associate Director of Global Health
Infectious Disease and International
 Medicine
Department of Medicine
University of Minnesota
Minneapolis, MN

Michael U. Callaghan, MD
Assistant Professor
Division of Hematology and Oncology
Carman and Ann Adams Department
 of Pediatrics
Wayne State University School of
 Medicine
Children's Hospital of Michigan
Detroit, MI

John C. Christenson, MD, FAAP
Director, Ryan White Center for Pediatric
 Infectious Disease
Director, Pediatric Travel Medicine Clinic
Professor of Clinical Pediatrics
Indiana University School of Medicine
Riley Hospital for Children at Indiana
 University Health
Indianapolis, IN

Elaine G. Cox, MD, FAAP
Associate Professor of Pediatrics
Ryan White Center for Pediatric
 Infectious Diseases
Indiana University School of Medicine
Associate Medical Director, Infection
 Control
Director, Pediatric HIV/AIDS Program
Riley Hospital for Children
Indianapolis, IN

Sachin N. Desai, MD
Associate Research Scientist
International Vaccine Institute
Seoul, Korea

Ruth A. Etzel, MD, PhD, FAAP
Adjunct Professor
Department of Environmental and
 Occupational Health
George Washington University School of
 Public Health and Health Services
The George Washington University
Washington, DC

Michelle Falk, MA
Center for Advanced Study of Language
University of Maryland
College Park, MD

Philip R. Fischer, MD, FAAP
Consultant, Travel and Tropical
 Medicine Clinic
Professor of Pediatrics
Mayo Clinic
Rochester, MN

David Fox II, MD
Professor
Amoud University
Borama, Somaliland

Corryn Greenwood, MD, FAAP
Fellow, Neonatal-Perinatal Medicine
Cincinnati Children's Hospital
   Medical Center
Cincinnati, OH

Peter J. Hammer, JD, PhD
Professor of Law and Director
Damon J. Keith Center for Civil Rights
Wayne State University Law School
Detroit, MI

Britteny M. Howell, MA
Department of Anthropology
University of Kentucky
Lexington, KY

Gregory Juckett, MD, MPH
Professor of Family Medicine
Director, West Virginia University
   International Travel Clinic
West Virginia University
Morgantown, WV

Linda M. Kaljee, PhD
Pediatric Prevention Research Center
Carman and Ann Adams Department
   of Pediatrics
Wayne State University School of
   Medicine
Detroit, MI

Deepak M. Kamat, MD, PhD, FAAP
Professor
Vice Chair of Education
Carman and Ann Adams Department
   of Pediatrics
Childrens Hospital of Michigan
Wayne State University
Detroit, MI

Karin Karlsson, RD
Laurel Regional Hospital
Laurel, MD
Prince George's Hospital Center
Cheverly, MD

Ambika Mathur, PhD
Associate Dean, the Graduate School
Professor of Pediatrics
Director, MD/PhD Program
Wayne State University School
   of Medicine
Detroit, MI

James T. McElligott, MD, MSCR
Assistant Professor
Department of Pediatrics
Medical University of South Carolina
Charleston, SC

**Margaret Nakakeeto-Kijjambu,
   MBChB, MMed**
Consultant Paediatrician/Neonatologist
Director, Kampala Children's Hospital
   Limited
Director, Childhealth International
Mulago Hospital
Kampala, Uganda

Dena Nazer, MD, FAAP
Assistant Professor of Pediatrics
Wayne State University
Medical Director, Child Protection Center
Children's Hospital of Michigan
Detroit, MI

Linda S. Nield, MD, FAAP
Associate Professor of Pediatrics
Pediatrics Residency Program Director
West Virginia University School
   of Medicine
Morgantown, WV

Cliff O'Callahan, MD, PhD, FAAP
Associate Professor
University of Connecticut
Farmington, CT
Pediatric Faculty, Family Practice Group
Director of Nurseries, Middlesex Hospital
Middletown, CT

Barbara Oettgen, MD, MPH, FAAP
Assistant Professor, Pediatrics
Wayne State University School
   of Medicine
Children's Hospital of Michigan
Detroit, MI

Vincent J. Palusci, MD, MS, FAAP
Professor of Pediatrics
Department of Pediatrics
New York University Medical Center
New York, NY

Clydette Powell, MD, MPH, FAAP
Associate Professor of Pediatrics (adjunct),
 Department of Pediatrics
Attending Staff, Division of Child
 Neurology
The George Washington University
 School of Medicine
Washington, DC

Chokechai Rongkavilit, MD
Associate Professor
Division of Infectious Diseases
Carman and Ann Adams Department
 of Pediatrics
Wayne State University
Children's Hospital of Michigan
Detroit, MI

David Sleet, PhD, FAAHB
Associate Director for Science
Division of Unintentional Injury
 Prevention
National Center for Injury Prevention
 and Control
Centers for Disease Control and
 Prevention (CDC)
Atlanta, GA

Tina Slusher, MD, FAAP
Associate Professor of Pediatrics
Division of Global Health
University of Minnesota
Pediatric Intensive Care
Hennepin County Medical Center
Minneapolis, MN

Bonita Stanton, MD, FAAP
Professor and Schotanus Family Endowed
 Chair of Pediatrics
Pediatrician-in-Chief
Carman and Ann Adams Department
 of Pediatrics
Wayne State University School of
 Medicine
Children's Hospital of Michigan
Detroit, MI

Andrea P. Summer, MD, MSCR, FAAP
Department of Pediatrics
Medical University of South Carolina
Charleston, SC

Michael A. Tolle, MD, MPH
Associate Director
Botswana-Baylor Children's Clinical
 Centre of Excellence
Gaborone, Botswana
Assistant Professor, Pediatrics
Retrovirology and Global Health
Baylor College of Medicine
Texas Children's Hospital
Houston, TX

Yvonne Vaucher, MD, MPH
Director, Infant Special Care Follow-Up
 Program
Clinical Professor of Pediatrics
University of California San Diego
San Diego, CA
Neonatal-Perinatal Consultant
Makerere University
Kampala, Uganda

Lisa M. Vaughn, PhD
Associate Professor, Pediatrics
General and Community Pediatrics
Emergency Medicine
Cincinnati Children's Hospital Medical
 Center
University of Cincinnati College
 of Medicine
Cincinnati, OH

Carol Cohen Weitzman, MD, FAAP
Associate Professor of Pediatrics and
 Child Study Center
Director, Section of Developmental-
 Behavioral Pediatrics
Yale University School of Medicine
New Haven, CT

Jennifer R. Wies, PhD
Assistant Professor of Anthropology
Department of Anthropology, Sociology,
 and Social Work
Eastern Kentucky University
Richmond, KY

Aisha K. Yousafzai, PhD
Assistant Professor
Department of Paediatrics and
 Child Health
Division of Women and Child Health
Aga Kahn University
Karachi, Pakistan

■ REVIEWERS

Carol D. Berkowitz, MD, FAAP
Professor of Clinical Pediatrics
David Geffen School of Medicine
University of California Los Angeles
(UCLA)
Executive Vice Chair
Department of Pediatrics
Harbor-UCLA Medical Center
Torrance, CA

Sanjay Chawla, MD, FAAP
Assistant Professor of Pediatrics
Wayne State University
Associate Fellowship Program Director
Neonatal-Perinatal Medicine
Children's Hospital of Michigan, Hutzel
Women's Hospital
Detroit, MI

Cindy Howard, MD, MPHTM
Associate Professor of Pediatrics
University of Minnesota
Minneapolis, MN

W. Charles Huskins, MD, MSc
Consultant, Pediatric Infectious Diseases
Mayo Clinic
Rochester, MN

Jonette Keri, MD, PhD
Associate Professor of Dermatology and
Cutaneous Surgery
University of Miami
Miller School of Medicine
Chief, Dermatology Service
Miami VA Hospital
Miami, FL

Eric McGrath, MD
Assistant Professor of Pediatrics
Carman and Ann Adams Department
of Pediatrics
Division of Infectious Diseases
Children's Hospital of Michigan
Wayne State University School of
Medicine
Detroit, MI

Tarissa Mitchell, MD, FAAP
Medical Officer
Immigrant, Refugee, and Migrant
Health Branch
Division of Global Migration and
Quarantine
Centers for Disease Control and
Prevention (CDC)
Instructor, Department of Pediatrics
Emory University School of Medicine
Atlanta, GA

Karen Olness, MD, FAAP
Professor of Pediatrics
Global Health and Diseases
Case Western Reserve University
Cleveland, OH

J. Routt Reigart, MD, FAAP
Professor of Pediatrics
Medical University of South Carolina
Charleston, SC

Mary Allen Staat, MD, MPH, FAAP
Associate Professor of Pediatrics
Division of Infectious Diseases
Director, International Adoption Center
Cincinnati Children's Hospital
Medical Center
Cincinnati, OH

Patricia F. Walker, MD, DTM&H
HealthPartners Center for International
Health and Travel Medicine Clinics
Associate Program Director, Global
Health Pathway
Associate Professor, Division of Infectious
Disease and International Medicine
Department of Medicine
University of Minnesota
Minneapolis, MN

■ TABLE OF CONTENTS

■ FOREWORD

Even with great strides in the battle worldwide against several childhood diseases, the fact is that children across the globe continue to struggle with life-threatening illnesses, with more than 7 million preschool-aged children dying every year. Pediatric health care professionals in resource-rich countries are stepping up to this challenge, spending time, energy, and money in combating these illnesses of global child health. To be effective globally, a pediatric health care practitioner must gain knowledge and skills necessary to serve across cultural and national boundaries. And so we offer the *American Academy of Pediatrics Textbook of Global Child Health.*

In this, the first book of its kind, we begin by presenting foundational information to build understanding of disease, health, medicine, culture, law, and the environment. In the second section of the textbook, we provide information for health care practitioners in preparing families traveling with children. Finally, in the third section, we discuss health and illness in tangible ways to guide the practice of pediatrics in resource-limited regions of the planet.

We are grateful to the American Academy of Pediatrics (AAP) for leadership in and support of the field of global child health. We are pleased that this textbook can serve health care practitioners in conjunction with other AAP publications, such as *Working in International Child Health,* 2nd Edition (2008), and *Atlas of Pediatrics in the Tropics and Resource-Limited Settings* (2009). We are thrilled to have the participation of 40 stellar authors from around the world. These authors also served as reviewers of chapters. Finally, we are grateful for the expertise and assistance of peer reviewers who provided excellent suggestions to further strengthen the text.

Our goal, however, was never to simply provide a textbook but to see this book used as a resource to inspire, educate, and empower readers throughout the world. The Nobel Laureate Gabriela Mistral said, "Many things we need can wait. The child cannot. Now is the time his bones are formed, his mind developed. To him we cannot say tomorrow, his name is today." Let us seize the opportunity today to work together to improve the health of the children of the world.

Deepak M. Kamat, MD, PhD, FAAP
Philip R. Fischer, MD, FAAP

Understanding Principles of Global Child Health

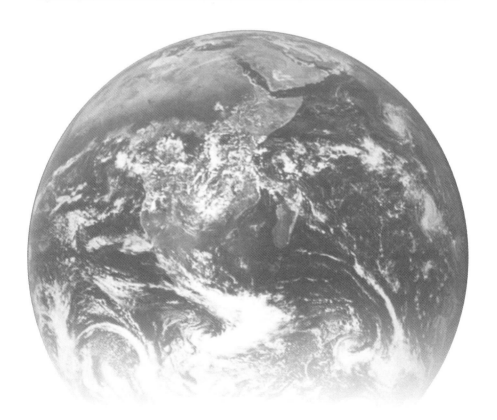

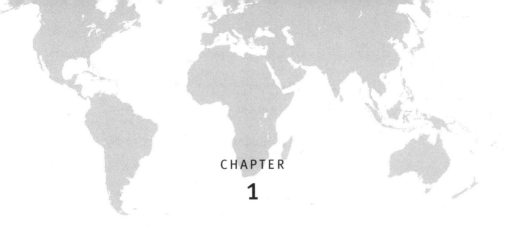

The Reality of Child Mortality

Barbara Oettgen, MD, MPH, FAAP
Ambika Mathur, PhD

"We have an opportunity to focus global attention on what should be obvious: every mother, and every child, counts. They count because we value every human life. The evidence is clear that healthy mothers and children are the bedrock of healthy and prosperous communities and nations."
— *Dr LEE Jong-wook, former World Health Organization Director-General*

■ CURRENT STATUS OF CHILD MORTALITY

A shocking reality of global child health is the sheer magnitude of child mortality. As of 2009, it is estimated that every year, 8.1 million children die before their fifth birthday—the equivalent of 22,000 children dying every day.[1] More than one third of children die before the age of 1 month. However, global statistics fail to describe the great inequality of childhood mortality rates from country to country. Most child deaths are increasingly concentrated in 60 developing countries with Africa and Asia representing a combined 93% of the deaths (Figure 1-1).[2-4] Sub-Saharan Africa continues to have the highest mortality rate (129 per 1,000 live births), which is double that of other developing regions and 20 times more than developed countries.[1]

Figure 1-1. 60 Priority Countries for Child Survival Targeted by Countdown to 2015

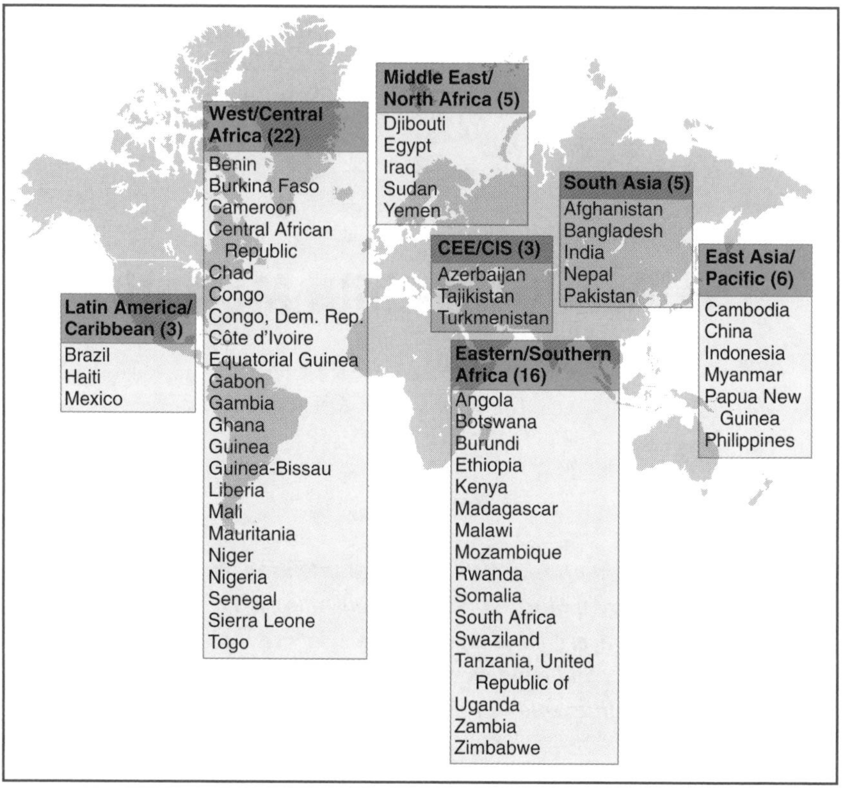

West/Central Africa (22)
Benin
Burkina Faso
Cameroon
Central African
  Republic
Chad
Congo
Congo, Dem. Rep.
Côte d'Ivoire
Equatorial Guinea
Gabon
Gambia
Ghana
Guinea
Guinea-Bissau
Liberia
Mali
Mauritania
Niger
Nigeria
Senegal
Sierra Leone
Togo

Middle East/ North Africa (5)
Djibouti
Egypt
Iraq
Sudan
Yemen

South Asia (5)
Afghanistan
Bangladesh
India
Nepal
Pakistan

CEE/CIS (3)
Azerbaijan
Tajikistan
Turkmenistan

East Asia/ Pacific (6)
Cambodia
China
Indonesia
Myanmar
Papua New
  Guinea
Philippines

Latin America/ Caribbean (3)
Brazil
Haiti
Mexico

Eastern/Southern Africa (16)
Angola
Botswana
Burundi
Ethiopia
Kenya
Madagascar
Malawi
Mozambique
Rwanda
Somalia
South Africa
Swaziland
Tanzania, United
  Republic of
Uganda
Zambia
Zimbabwe

From United Nations Children's Fund. *The State of the World's Children 2008: Child Survival.* New York, NY: United Nations Children's Fund; 2007:16

Accurate data of child mortality are difficult to obtain consistently, especially from developing countries. Therefore, in 2001, the World Health Organization (WHO) and United Nations Children's Fund (UNICEF) launched a joint venture called Child Health Epidemiology Research Group (CHERG) to obtain better estimates on causes of childhood mortality, especially in countries and regions that are unable to collect their own data. The primary causes of global child mortality are shown in Figure 1-2 and include neonatal causes, acute respiratory infection (ARI), diarrhea, malaria, measles, and HIV. Globally, the number one cause of child death is ARI.[2]

There is regional variation in childhood death patterns. Sub-Saharan Africa is one of the regions with the highest child mortality; on average, 1 in 6 children dies before the age of 5 years and mortality rates have only decreased by 14% since 1990.[2,3] Malaria is the primary killer of children younger than 5 years in this region and while infectious diseases account for 64% of deaths globally, they are responsible for 81% of the

Figure 1-2. Global Distribution of Cause-Specific Mortality Among Children Younger Than 5 Years

Undernutrition is implicated in up to 50% of all deaths of children younger than 5 years.

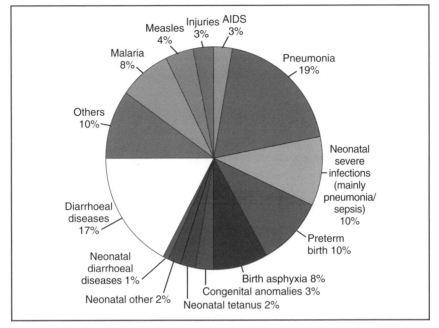

From United Nations Children's Fund. *The State of the World's Children 2008: Child Survival.* New York, NY: United Nations Children's Fund; 2007:8

deaths in Africa. More than half of deaths caused by infections can be ascribed to 5 pathogens—*Plasmodium falciparum, Streptococcus pneumoniae,* rotavirus, measles, and *Haemophilus influenza* type b (Hib).[5]

Another significant factor in childhood mortality is malnutrition, contributing to 50% of deaths in this age group.[2] War, poverty, lack of education, and the indirect effects of the HIV epidemic have also contributed significantly to child mortality across the globe. Clearly, the current status of child health is unacceptable, morally and ethically.

■ MILLENNIUM DEVELOPMENT GOALS FOR 2015

In 2000, at the UN Millennium Summit, 189 governments and at least 23 international organizations convened to adopt a uniform worldwide set of 8 goals—Millennium Development Goals (MDGs)—to promote continued progress toward improving global public health (Table 1-1). Several of these goals pertain to child health. Millennium Development Goal 4 sets the goal to decrease the mortality of children younger than 5 years to 5 million per year by 2015. Essentially, successful implementation of MDG 4 will decrease deaths by two thirds of the levels seen in

Table 1-1. Health and the Millennium Development Goals

GOAL	HEALTH TARGETS	HEALTH INDICATORS
GOAL 1 **Eradicate extreme poverty and hunger**	**Target 2** Halve, between 1990 and 2015, the proportion of people who suffer from hunger	Prevalence of underweight children under five Proportion of population below minimum level of dietary energy consumption
GOAL 4 **Reduce child mortality**	**Target 5** Reduce by two thirds, between 1990 and 2015, the under-five mortality rate	Under-five mortality rate Infant mortality rate Proportion of one-year-olds immunized against measles
GOAL 5 **Improve maternal health**	**Target 6** Reduce by three quarters, between 1990 and 2015, the maternal mortality ratio	Maternal mortality ratio Proportion of births attended by skilled health personnel
GOAL 6 **Combat HIV and AIDS, malaria and other diseases**	**Target 7** Halt and begin to reverse, by 2015, the spread of HIV and AIDS	HIV prevalence among pregnant women aged 15–24 Condom use rate of the contraceptive prevalence rate Ratio of school attendance of orphans to school attendance of non-orphans aged 10–14
	Target 8 Halt and begin to reverse, by 2015, the incidence of malaria and other major diseases	Prevalence and death rates associated with malaria Proportion of population in malaria-risk areas using effective malaria prevention and treatment measures Prevalence and death rates associated with tuberculosis Proportion of tuberculosis cases detected and cured under Directly Observed Treatment Short-Course (DOTS)

Table 1-1. Health and the Millennium Development Goals, continued		
GOAL	HEALTH TARGETS	HEALTH INDICATORS
GOAL 7 Ensure environmental sustainability	Target 10 Halve, by 2015, the proportion of people without sustainable access to safe drinking water and basic sanitation	Proportion of population using an improved water source, urban and rural
	Target 10 By 2020, achieve a significant improvement in the lives of at least 100 million slum dwellers	Proportion of population using improved sanitation, urban and rural
GOAL 8 Develop a global partnership for development	Target 17 In cooperation with pharmaceutical companies, provide access to affordable essential drugs in developing countries	Proportion of population with access to affordable essential drugs on a sustainable basis

Adapted from World Health Organization. *Health and the Millennium Development Goals*. Geneva, Switzerland: World Health Organization; 2005:11.

1990 (13 million). Other MDGs will indirectly improve child mortality rates. For example, MDG 5 is aimed at reducing maternal mortality by three fourths (which will affect neonatal mortality), and MDG 6 strives to reverse the spread of HIV/AIDS and malaria. Other MDGs include halving poverty and hunger (MDG 1), achieving universal primary education (MDG 2), creating gender equality in education (MDG 3), and halving the proportion of people without access to safe water (MDG 7).[2,6]

■ THE EVOLUTION OF GLOBAL CHILD HEALTH

A variety of public health approaches already had marked success at reducing child mortality rates by 50% from 1960 through 1999.[7] Mass immunization campaigns conducted in the 1950s through the 1970s resulted in eradicating smallpox and reducing other vaccine-preventable diseases. The Expanded Program on Immunization (EPI) established in 1974 allowed for continued strides in improving worldwide vaccination status among children—from a baseline of 5% in 1974 to a current rate of 75%. The UNICEF GOBI (growth monitoring for undernutrition, oral rehydration, breastfeeding, and immunization) program, instituted in 1982, expanded the focus of public health programs from solely immunizations to include other important interventions. There began a growing awareness and interest in improving the primary care infrastructure to better disseminate a greater number of interventions that positively affected child health.[2]

The Integrated Management of Childhood Illness (IMCI) program was created in the mid-1990s.[2] In this program, local-level caseworkers were identified in rural and urban communities and trained to provide health education and support to families for a variety of maternal and childhood diseases and conditions. The IMCI program was initially created as a facility-based program using case management with a defined set of evidence-based guidelines for sick children. It was eventually expanded to include interventions that could be performed in the household, in the community, or by referral. Such a change required making improvements to case management and health systems, as well as family and community services, including health education in growth promotion and development, disease prevention, care, and compliance with the advice of health workers.

The IMCI program has faced many challenges over the years. First initiated in 1996 in Tanzania and Uganda, it expanded over the last 10 years to include more than 100 countries. The IMCI program did not initially address neonatal mortality but subsequently evolved to include interventions to decrease neonatal mortality as well as mortality caused by the HIV epidemic. The IMCI program requires continued refinement to address the needs of various regions and faces challenges in countries with the weakest health services and the highest mortality rates.[2] The IMCI program costs are similar to or lower than conventional case management.[8]

Evaluation of the IMCI program has been positive and negative. Studies have demonstrated that training of IMCI workers improved quality of care, and in countries with low health care use at baseline, the IMCI program improved numbers of people seeking care.[9] For example, in Bangladesh, 19% of sick children in an IMCI area were taken to a health worker versus 9% in a non-IMCI area.[10]

Adoption of all IMCI program aspects (facility-based services, case management, and family and community health services) is not complete, even in countries with the most effective implementation. While these countries have well-trained community health workers, changes in their health systems and family health practices have been slow. Therefore, because the complete program is not fully implemented but rather only adopted piecemeal by various regions, it is difficult to state with accuracy whether it is truly successful. Encouraging reports from Tanzania show a 13% decrease in mortality following IMCI implementation; however, no change was seen in Brazil or Peru.

Evaluators note that one of the significant problems associated with IMCI implementation has been high staff turnover, which makes it difficult to achieve a sustained effect. The staffing problem has been a greater issue among facility-based staff (who could be moved from the area) than with staff who are local community women, demonstrating that it may be preferential to increase participation of local workers. The future success of the IMCI program requires that regions work from the top down (strengthening the health service system) and also from the bottom up (mobilizing the community to use those services).[9]

■ MAJOR CAUSES OF CHILD MORTALITY

Improvements in global child public health require improvements in primary care infrastructure for women, newborns, and children, allowing for the successful dissemination of interventions known to be effective for the major causes of maternal, newborn, and child mortality. The following 3 recurrent themes emerge in the description of progress addressing the major causes of child mortality:

1. A need to strengthen and improve community-based services for a greater effect on diseases (ie, ARI, diarrhea, malaria)
2. A need to address the inequities of how effective interventions are being disseminated
3. A need to address the HIV epidemic, which has caused such severe disruption in economies and human capital and has made it difficult to move forward with child survival goals

Acute Respiratory Infection

Acute respiratory infection is associated with 19% or 2 million childhood deaths every year—a number greater than deaths from AIDS, malaria, and measles combined. Worldwide statistics show that ARI is the number one killer of children younger than 5 years.[11,12] If one factors in neonatal deaths from sepsis and pneumonia, this figure inches closer to 3 million children dying from ARI each year (29%). More than half of these deaths occurred in South Asia and sub-Saharan Africa. While actual data on the etiology remain scarce, it is likely that the pathogens are the same as those seen in industrialized countries—Hib, *S pneumoniae* (pneumococcus), staphylococcal infections, and respiratory syncytial virus. One approach in the fight against ARI is early detection and prompt treatment. It is essential to educate and encourage families to seek care early in the course of respiratory illness; the IMCI program is an ideal conduit for education and treatment.

First, families can be taught to observe respiratory rates and chest wall appearance (eg, in-drawing), and then IMCI workers can be trained to refer or institute prompt treatment. However, Multiple Indicator Cluster Surveys (a tool used by UNICEF to assess interventions) indicate that only 25% to 30% of caregivers recognize fast breathing or breathing difficulty and that only 57% of caregivers worldwide seek care. This number is even lower in sub-Saharan Africa (40%).[2] Unfortunately, when last studied in 2006, the rate of care-seeking had not changed appreciably over the preceding 6 years (2000–2006), underscoring the need to improve the community-based services that promote education, assessment, and selective antibiotic use after detection. UNICEF estimates that effective case management could decrease pneumonia mortality by 37% or 700,000 lives annually. IMCI workers can also encourage breastfeeding, improved nutrition (including increased zinc intake), and hand washing.[2]

Expanded use of Hib and pneumococcal vaccines is predicted to decrease mortality rates associated with ARI by 1 million deaths.[13,14] Hib vaccination has been shown to be very effective in Kenya where the incidence of Hib disease decreased to 12% of its baseline level in children younger than 5 years over the first 3 years it was distributed there.[15] In 2000, the Global Alliance for Vaccines and Immunisation (GAVI) began financially supporting Hib vaccination in 72 of the poorest countries. Countries apply for GAVI funding based on a financial plan, vaccine introduction plan, and a 5-year national vaccine strategy. Initially, uptake of Hib vaccine was very slow. When the Hib initiative was launched in 2005 to accelerate introduction of the Hib vaccine there was a sharp increase in the number of eligible countries using the Hib vaccine.[14] By the end of 2007, 80% of eligible African and American countries were using the Hib vaccine. However, pockets of need remain. Only 1 in 9 countries in the Southeast Asia region regularly use the Hib vaccine.[16]

These numbers translate to about 22% of the world's birth cohort being vaccinated against Hib. Inequities in the use of Hib vaccine remain and are related to a nation's poverty status. Thus, while only 51% of lower/middle-income* countries (not GAVI eligible) have the

---

*Over the past several decades, multiple terms have been used to describe comparatively different economic conditions in countries, including *first world* and *third world,* *developed* and *developing,* *industrialized* and *nonindustrialized,* and *Northern* and *Southern.* We have elected to use *higher income, middle income,* and *lower income* to describe these differences, recognizing that each of these dichotomies is limited in its ability to describe the much larger variation between countries, as well as to avoid hierarchical terminology that assumes that Western and industrialized nations are the pinnacle of development.

Hib vaccine, 86% of upper-middle-income countries and 92% of higher-income countries are in active distribution.[16]

The Pneumococcal Vaccines Accelerated Development and Introduction Plan (PneumoADIP) was established to encourage use of the pneumococcal vaccine.[13] The WHO recommends using any available and approved pneumococcal vaccine in children because studies to date, even in developing countries, show a substantial effect on the incidence of pneumonia and the child mortality rate associated with pneumonia.[17,18]

PneumoADIP provides technical and financial assistance to establish surveillance networks for pneumococcal disease, as well as to complete vaccine efficacy and cost-effectiveness studies. This information will allow public health professionals to make more informed decisions about the potential effect of vaccination as well as alert practitioners about local strains of pneumococcus and antibiotic resistance. Currently, pneumococcal vaccine is not in widespread use, which is likely because of its significant cost.

Diarrhea

Diarrhea is responsible for 18% (1.7 million) of child deaths worldwide.[19,20] CHERG estimates that the majority of deaths (73%) occur in only 15 developing countries, mostly located in Africa and Southeast Asia.[21] Fortunately, significant strides were made in diarrhea control over the last 15 years. One of the leading success stories in public health is the use of oral rehydration therapy (ORT) as a key element in the fight against diarrhea. Deaths due to diarrhea have decreased by two thirds since 1980 and diarrhea is no longer the number one cause of death.[22]

The etiology of diarrhea can be viral (rotavirus being the most common), bacterial, or parasitic.[19,20] The primary approaches to controlling diarrhea remain education, ORT with oral rehydration solutions, and continued feeding. The ultimate goal in the fight against diarrhea is improved sanitation and a safer water supply (MDG 7).[19,20]

Oral rehydration solutions have evolved over time and now are composed of a lower salt concentration than previously recommended in the 1980s and 1990s. Overall, about one third of children receive the recommended treatment for diarrhea (increased fluids and continued feeding) with the highest rates (61%) in East Asia and the Pacific (except China); the lowest rates (31%) are in sub-Saharan Africa.

As with ARI, little progress in coverage was observed in the 2000 to 2006 period.[19,20] Inequities in treatment occur depending on the socio-economic status—children are 1.5 times as likely to receive treatment in households with higher income levels. There are also urban-rural inequities; those in urban settings are more likely to receive treatment than those in rural areas (43% vs 34%).[19,20]

Other important mechanisms to control diarrhea include hand washing, increased breastfeeding, and micronutrient supplementation, especially with vitamin A and zinc. Hand washing is estimated to decrease the rate of diarrheal illness by 30%, thus saving almost 500,000 lives.[23] In a study done in Pakistan, families in the low-income neighborhood of Karachi were taught about hand washing; in these houses, a 53% reduction of diarrhea was noticed in children younger than 15 years and a 39% reduction in children younger than 1 year.[24]

Because rotavirus infection is the leading cause of severe-acute diarrhea worldwide, accounting for 40% of diarrheal hospitalizations, an important consideration is the use of an effective rotavirus vaccine.[25] GAVI can provide monetary assistance to low-income countries to introduce the rotavirus vaccine, especially in regions where the rotavirus vaccine was shown to be effective, such as in the Americas and Europe.[25] Trials to determine the efficacy of the rotavirus vaccine in Africa and Asia are ongoing.[25,26]

Human Immunodeficiency Virus

Children are affected directly and indirectly by the HIV/AIDS epidemic. Children not only contract HIV, but they are adversely affected when they live with family members, especially parents or other caregivers, who are infected. These children may be left responsible for heading households and earning wages to support their family. Children lose access to education, health care, and adequate food supplies in the many communities where teachers, health care workers, and farmers are infected with HIV. It is estimated that more than 16 million children worldwide have lost at least one parent to HIV.[27–29] This HIV epidemic dealt a severe blow to progress with child mortality, not only directly because of deaths of children but also because of the necessity of redirecting resources to deal with HIV and its fallout. The resulting economic disruption of countries further contributes to malnutrition and poor health among the children in affected communities.

Sub-Saharan Africa is still the most severely affected region. Of the 33 million people infected with HIV, two thirds live in sub-Saharan Africa (22.5 million), including the majority of the 2.5 million children infected with HIV (Figure 1-3). In heavily affected areas of southern Africa, such as Botswana and Zimbabwe, HIV accounts for one third of all deaths among children younger than 5 years. Countries with high HIV prevalence report life expectancy levels at or below the levels of

Figure 1-3. Global Prevalence of HIV, 2009: 33.3 Million People Living With HIV

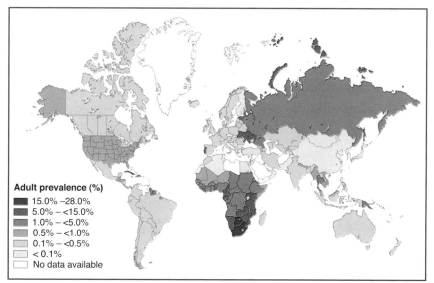

Adult prevalence (%)
- 15.0% –28.0%
- 5.0% – <15.0%
- 1.0% – <5.0%
- 0.5% – <1.0%
- 0.1% – <0.5%
- < 0.1%
- No data available

From Joint United Nations Programme on HIV/AIDS (UNAIDS). Global Report. *UNAIDS Report on the Global AIDS Epidemic 2010.* 2010;23. http://www.unaids.org/globalreport/documents/20101123_GlobalReport_full_en.pdf. Accessed June 27, 2011

the 1950s (Figure 1-4). Fortunately, the percentage of adults with HIV has plateaued since 2000.[28] In 14 out of 17 African countries with good survey data, the percentage of pregnant women with HIV reportedly decreased. This decrease is attributed primarily to access to anti-HIV medications.[28] Unfortunately, females are disproportionately infected, increasing the risk of bearing infected children (Figure 1-5).

In contrast with adult data, surveillance data for children with HIV are sparse. However, from reports that are available, it appears that HIV infections in children peaked in 2000 and deaths caused by HIV peaked in 2003, probably because of the stabilization of HIV-infected women, as well as the increase of effective perinatal transmission prevention programs.[28] The majority of children infected with HIV (90%) acquire the infection perinatally or through breastfeeding. Unfortunately, HIV-positive mothers are not regularly receiving proper anti-HIV medications during pregnancy or at the time of delivery. Without perinatal medicines, the risk of HIV transmission from mother to child is 15% to 30% and with prolonged breastfeeding, the transmission rate can be as high as 45%.[30,31] However, progress has been made. Between 2004 and 2009, the number of HIV-positive women who were evaluated to receive antiretroviral prophylaxis increased from 9% to 51%.[29]

Figure 1-4. Life Expectancy at Birth, Selected Regions, 1950–1955 to 2005–2010

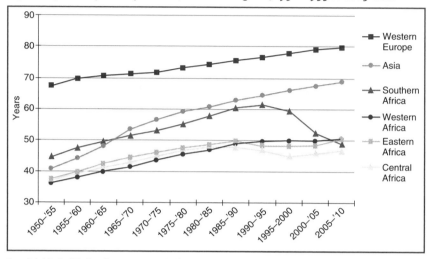

From Joint United Nations Programme on HIV/AIDS. *08 Report on the Global AIDS Epidemic.* 2008;45. http://www.unaids.org/en/KnowledgeCentre/HIVData/GlobalReport/2008/2008_Global_report.asp. Accessed June 13, 2011. Source: Population Division of the Department of Economic and Social Affairs of the United Nations Secretariat, World Population Prospects: The 2006 Revision.

Figure 1-5. Trends in Women Living With HIV: Proportion of People 15 Years and Older Living With HIV Who Are Women, 1990–2009

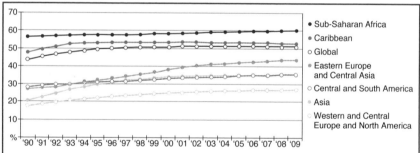

From Joint United Nations Programme on HIV/AIDS (UNAIDS). Global Report. *UNAIDS Report on the Global AIDS Epidemic 2010.* 2010;25. http://www.unaids.org/globalreport/documents/20101123_GlobalReport_full_en.pdf. Accessed June 27, 2011

Inadequate access to perinatal screening may be one of the barriers. Overall, only 26% of pregnant women were tested for HIV in antenatal clinics; however, in some high-prevalence regions, such as South Africa, as many as 95% of pregnant women were tested.[29] In southern Africa, once women were known to be HIV positive, 80% of them received retroviral prophylaxis. Where there is political will, change is possible. In Botswana, a country in which the government put a high priority on screening programs, the rate of perinatal transmission dropped to 4%.[32]

The president of Botswana declared that all women in antenatal clinics would be screened unless they refused, and subsequently the screening rate of women jumped to 90%. In stark contrast, the number of infants receiving prophylaxis who were born to HIV-positive mothers is not as successful with a coverage rate increase of only 12% to 20% from 2005 to 2007.[28] One reason is the difficulty in providing children with antiretroviral treatment (ART) in appropriate and affordable pediatric formulations. The proportion of mothers and infants receiving newer and more effective regimens also need improvement.[29]

While the use of ART is increasing, there is still a great need to increase access to older children; from 2005 to 2007 the number of children who received ART increased 2.6-fold, but only 10% of children with HIV were receiving medicines (198,000 of 2 million children).[28] In comparison with adults, children are only one third as likely to receive ART. There has been a strong push to treat infants as early as possible because mortality can be significantly reduced; without treatment, about 50% of children infected by HIV from their mothers will die before their second birthday. Breastfeeding by HIV-positive mothers is also controversial, but the recommendation remains that infants should be breastfed because it is considered the safest alternative even though there is a 10% to 20% transmission rate. Because there is still no treatment to prevent transmission from breastfeeding, the recommendation in developing countries is exclusive breastfeeding followed by early weaning.[33]

While HIV infection in newborns and infants remains a concern, the group becoming infected at the highest rate is 15- to 24-year-olds because of their risky behaviors, including unprotected sex and drug abuse. The HIV epidemic faces tremendous hurdles for reversal until the rate of new infection decreases, especially in the 15- to 24-year-old age group. Education is a critical first step toward achieving risk reduction in this population.[28]

The 4 priority areas for HIV/AIDS include
1. Prevent mother-to-child transmission.
2. Provide treatment to HIV-infected children.
3. Prevent infection in the 15- to 24-year-old age group.
4. Protect and support children affected by HIV.[27]

Measles

The quest to decrease measles morbidity and mortality has, so far, occurred in 3 phases.

Phase 1: Measles cases decreased from 135 million (and 6 million deaths) in the 1960s to 1.9 million deaths in 1987. This decrease was largely because of the EPI, which promoted one dose of measles vaccine at 9 months of age.

Phase 2: The increased immunity of populations that received 2 doses of a measles vaccine was recognized. Industrialized countries, as well as other countries in the Americas, began giving a second dose of measles vaccine in the 1990s.

Phase 3: Immunization efforts against measles were significantly increased in 45 countries, which accounted for 90% of the measles morbidity. The strategies employed include

1. Achieve 90% coverage with the first dose of measles vaccine.
2. Increase the second dose of measles vaccine opportunities (because it is known that the one dose at 9 months only confers immunity to about 85% of children).
3. Use accurate surveillance.
4. Aggressively manage the onset of new measles cases, including the administration of vitamin A.[34]

Increased immunization rates through supplementary immunization and catch-up activities are decreasing mortality from this disease.

Immunization activity was spearheaded by the Measles Initiative, formed in 2001 as a collaboration of the Red Cross, Centers for Disease Control and Prevention, UNICEF, and WHO with support from GAVI and the International Finance Facility for Immunization.[34] The Measles Initiative helps countries implement WHO/UNICEF recommendations. The coverage rate of measles vaccine increased from 70% in the 1980s to 82% in 2007.[35] With these worldwide initiatives, there was a 74% reduction in measles deaths since 2000 and a 66% reduction in measles cases (Figure 1-6).[35] In 2005, 89% of the 192 member countries of UNICEF were offering a second measles vaccine. Vitamin A supplementation is also believed to be a significant factor in reducing measles cases.[35] Africa was extremely successful in controlling measles from 2001 to 2008, with an increase in single-dose vaccination from 57% to 73%. There has been a subsequent 93% decrease in the numbers of measles cases (from approximately 500,000 to 30,000) and a 90% decrease in deaths associated with measles.[36] Most other regions also saw a significant decline since 1999, except in Europe and the Americas where immunization rates were already relatively high and measles rates were already low.

The next goal is to achieve 90% vaccine coverage globally by 2010 with a 90% reduction in measles-associated deaths. This strategy will be to

• Increase immunization activities in large countries with low rates, such as Pakistan, India, and Indonesia.

Figure 1-6. Estimated Number of Measles Deaths Worldwide, 2000–2007

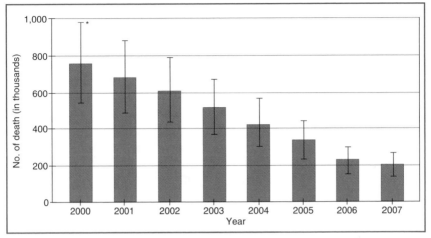

*95% uncertainty interval. Based on Monte Carlo simulations that account for uncertainty in key input variables (ie, vaccination coverage and case-fatality ratios).

From Centers for Disease Control and Prevention. Progress in global measles control and mortality reduction, 2000–2007. *MMWR Morb Mortal Wkly Rep.* 2008;57(48):1303–1306

- Sustain current activities of immunizing at least 90% of children by 9 months of age.
- Continue supplementary activities every 2 to 4 years.
- Have good field surveillance.[34,35]

Malaria

Millennium Development Goal 6 is a defined goal to halt and reverse the spread of malaria by 2015. This goal is proving difficult to achieve because of drug resistance, mosquito resistance to pesticides, and lack of drug availability. Annually, 1 million deaths are ascribed to malaria, of which 90% are children younger than 5 years mostly living in sub-Saharan Africa. This equates to one child dying of malaria every 30 seconds. Malaria is the number one killer of children in the sub-Saharan region, exceeding the number of children who die from ARI. Malaria also causes significant morbidity; recurring infections can cause chronic anemia and impaired growth and development. Perinatal infection also leads to low birth weight.[37,38] Nearly all deaths due to malaria are caused by infection with *P falciparum.*[5]

Evidence of political will to decrease disease from malaria was demonstrated in 2000 when 44 African leaders signed the Abuja Declaration to cut malaria deaths in half by 2010.[39] Increasing attention to the fight against malaria is also reflected in the activities of the Global Fund to Fight AIDS, Tuberculosis and Malaria, as well as the World Bank Booster Program for Malaria Control in Africa and the US President's Malaria Initiative.

Multipronged programs that encourage early detection and prompt treatment, use of insecticide-treated bed nets (ITNs), and targeted spraying have been very successful.[39] One example of such a multipronged program is the Roll Back Malaria partnership (collaboration of the World Bank, UNICEF, President's Malaria Initiative, and the Global Fund to Fight AIDS, Tuberculosis and Malaria).

Families are encouraged to seek early care for their febrile ill-appearing child by medical workers or IMCI staff who are able to provide prompt and early treatment based on clinical findings.[37,38] Unfortunately, as with care for pneumonia and diarrhea, trends in early treatment of malaria show stagnation, pointing to problems with integrated community-based treatment and the need to strengthen that system. Furthermore, challenges such as resistance of *P falciparum* have arisen, resulting in the WHO recommendation to treat patients with artemisinin-combination therapies in certain regions of the world. Although artemisinin therapies are about 10 times as expensive as other therapies and there is a supply shortage, the number of countries purchasing and promoting these effective medicines has increased dramatically since 2005. Funding to purchase these medications and the medication supply itself also increased since 2005.[37,38]

Preventive intermittent treatment during pregnancy in endemic areas (2 doses of an antimalarial drug in the second and third trimester) is another element in the fight against malaria. This treatment has considerably reduced the number of women with anemia as well as the incidence of placental malarial infection and low birth weight.[40]

Use of ITNs as another form of prevention has increased greatly. If used regularly, ITNs are shown to decrease mortality in children by 20%.[41] The use of ITNs associated with a decrease in mortality rates is shown to be sustainable over time.[42] Bed nets not only protect the individual using the net but also those individuals in close proximity because of the insecticidal or repellent effects of the ITNs.[43] In sub-Saharan Africa, use of ITNs rose from 2% in 2000 to 20% in 2006. It is estimated that about 150 million ITNs were distributed thus far, which is enough to cover approximately 40% of the at-risk population.[37,38]

An innovative and highly effective approach is to combine ITN distribution programs with other interventions such as immunization.[44,45] In 2005, ITNs were distributed as an adjunct to a polio campaign in Niger. Two million ITNs were distributed in this manner, increasing ownership from 6% to 70%. Encouragingly, this strategy did not decrease polio vaccine intake.[46] However, there is still a great need for progress. In 2003, a survey revealed that only 6.7% of households in sub-Saharan Africa possessed an ITN, which translates to 16.7 million ITNs. It is estimated that 130 to 264 million nets are still needed to reach the targeted 80% coverage rate.[47]

Neonatal Causes

Newborn Care

Progress has been made in reducing the mortality rate among children younger than 5 years, with rates decreasing by 33% since 1980. However, mortality rates have only dropped by one fourth among neonates and causes of neonatal death have become proportionally more prominent.[48] The primary causes of neonatal death are infection (36%), preterm birth (28%), and asphyxia (23%) (Figure 1-7).

It is essential to address neonatal causes of mortality if the MDGs are to be achieved. Every year 3.6 million neonates die within the first 28 days of life (41% of all deaths of children younger than 5 years).[49] Three quarters of neonatal deaths occur in the first week of life and 25% to 45% occur in the first 24 hours of life (Figure 1-8).[7] Two thirds of these deaths are concentrated in Africa and Southeast Asia where the neonatal mortality rate (NMR) is approximately 41 per 1,000 live births, compared with 3 per 1,000 live births in industrialized countries (Figure 1-9).[7]

Figure 1-7. Global Distribution of Neonatal Deaths by Direct Cause (2000)

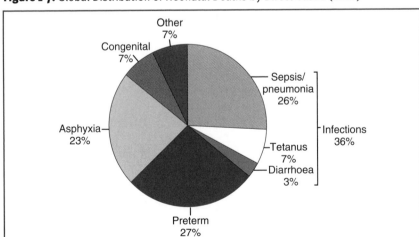

From Lawn JE, Cousens S, Zupan J, for the Lancet Neonatal Survival Steering Team. 4 million neonatal deaths: when? Where? Why? *Lancet.* 2005;365(9462):891–900, with permission from Elsevier.

Figure 1-8. Daily Risk of Death During the First Month of Life Based on Analysis of 47 Demographic and Health Surveys Data Sets (1995–2003) With 10,048 Neonatal Deaths

Deaths in first 24 h recorded as occurring on day 0, or possibly day 1, depending on interpretation of question and coding of response. Preference for reporting certain days (7, 14, 21, and 30) is apparent.

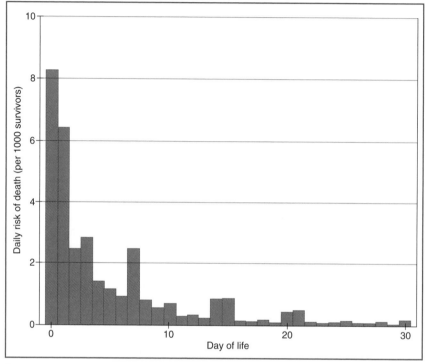

From Lawn JE, Cousens S, Zupan J, for the Lancet Neonatal Survival Steering Team. 4 million neonatal deaths: when? Where? Why? *Lancet.* 2005;365(9462):891–900, with permission from Elsevier.

Success in decreasing NMRs in low-income countries can be achieved without access to advanced technology. Even in developed countries, the biggest declines in NMR occurred before the advent of the neonatal intensive care unit (NICU). In England, the NMR fell from 30 per 1,000 live births in 1940 to 10 per 1,000 live births in 1975, mostly because of free antenatal care and improved care during labor.[50] In some regions, a concerted effort to address neonatal mortality has been fruitful. For example, there was a 50% decrease in the NMR in Latin America.[7] Honduras, Indonesia, Moldova, Sri Lanka, and Vietnam also showed improvements. The NMR in Sri Lanka in 1950 was approximately 50 deaths per 1,000 live births. These numbers declined to about 10 per 1,000 live births by 1990 even though the first NICU was not established until the mid-1980s (at which time the NMR had already fallen below 20 deaths per 1,000 live births).

Figure 1-9. Most Neonatal Deaths Occur in Sub-Saharan Africa and Asia, Where Neonatal Mortality Rates Are Highest

Neonatal mortality rate (per 1,000 live births), by region, 2009

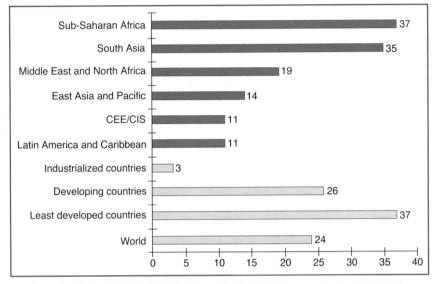

Data from United Nations Children's Fund. *The State of the World's Children 2011.* New York, NY: United Nations Children's Fund; 2011

From United Nations Children's Fund. Child info: Monitoring the Situation of Children and Women. Statistics by Area/Newborn Care. http://www.childinfo.org/newborncare.html. Accessed July 25, 2011

The success in Sri Lanka was attributed to an investment in the primary care infrastructure, ensuring that there was an extensive network of midwives who could provide outreach antenatal care so there was almost 100% coverage in 1999.[50] Significant progress can also be achieved with simple community interventions that are performed by community health workers, including family education for breastfeeding promotion, clean cord care, and thermal care. Using these simple measures, Darmstadt et al predict that neonatal deaths could decrease by 18% to 37%.[51]

Maternal Care

The lack of improvement in neonatal mortality in Africa is certainly linked to the minimal progress in maternal mortality reduction.[49] There is an urgent need to improve women's health in pregnancy, especially nutrition. Maternal malnutrition-associated low birth weight reportedly accounts for 60% to 80% of neonatal deaths.[7] Care for mother and baby should be provided at and immediately after delivery and should extend to baby care for at least the first few weeks following birth. To achieve the desired MDGs, significant funding must be provided for more technical interventions, such as skilled maternal care and immediate neonatal care, emergency obstetric care, and emergency neonatal care.[51] Table 1-2 shows the decrease in NMRs when skilled birth attendants are available. If a mother dies during delivery or shortly after, there is a much greater risk of subsequent neonatal death. A study conducted in Afghanistan showed that of live infants born to women who died during delivery or shortly after, 74% of the infants subsequently died.[52] Millennium Development Goal 5 recommends reducing maternal mortality by three fourths from 1990 to 2009, but little progress has been made toward achieving this target.

The global inequalities in maternal health are also stark. The lifetime risk of maternal death in a developing country is 300 times that of an industrialized country. In Sweden there is a 1 in 17,400 chance of dying during delivery, while in Sierra Leone the chance of dying is 1 in 8.[52] Most of the approximate 500,000 maternal deaths occur in South Asia (35%) and sub-Saharan Africa (49%).[52] Maternal and newborn mortality can be addressed with the following priorities[52]:

1. Access to family planning
2. Quality antenatal care
3. Prevention of HIV transmission
4. Basic preventive care, such as tetanus immunization, ITNs, and ORT
5. Access to safe water

Table 1-2. Place of Birth and Skilled Attendance at Childbirth by Degree of Neonatal Mortality				
	MORTALITY SETTING			
	NMR >45	NMR 30–45	NMR 15–29	NMR <15
Numbers of neonatal deaths (1000s) (number of countries)	1147 (18)	1759 (39)	838 (40)	254 (95)
Institutional delivery, median coverage (IQR)*	33% (16–49)	48% (18–78)	65% (51–91)	98% (95–99)
Skilled attendance at birth, median coverage (IQR)*	41% (22–44)	50% (27–77)	85% (62–96)	99% (95–100)
Traditional birth attendants present, median coverage (IQR)	20% (18–25; 7 countries)	18% (8–37; 21 countries)	9% (1–31; 16 countries)	9% (9–41; 3 countries)

*Based on WHO/UNICEF estimates for around year 2000 for 192 countries.

From Lawn JE, Cousens S, Zupan J, for the Lancet Neonatal Survival Steering Team. 4 million neonatal deaths: when? Where? Why? *Lancet.* 2005;365(9462):891–900, with permission from Elsevier.

6. Access to skilled health personnel at delivery
7. Emergency obstetric care
8. Postnatal visits
9. Maternal nutrition

Ideally, local and federal governments as well as global child health programs should move forward with a seamless, integrated continuous health system for mothers to neonates to children. The past approach was to implement discrete programs; today there is need for political will, locally and regionally, to creatively flesh out programs in communities and beyond.[53]

> "Poor health care is a weapon of mass destruction. Poor education is a weapon of mass destruction. Discrimination is a weapon of mass destruction. Let us abolish such weapons of mass destruction here at home."
> — Dennis Kucinich

Equally important is the need to empower women. If women are not accorded better status, it will be more difficult to make progress with child health.[2] Programs to facilitate the goals of MDG 2 (universal education) and MDG 3 (gender equality and empowering women) must be moved forward because enhancing a woman's ability to participate in important decision-making translates into taking better care of her children. Women must be empowered at home, in the community, and in politics to achieve these goals.[2]

Education plays a significant role in increasing empowerment. Less-educated caregivers are less likely to know when to access care appropriately. Educated women are better able to earn an income and invest in their children's health care, nutrition, and education. They are also more likely to participate in community life and advocate for improvements.[2] Educated mothers are more likely to seek health care for themselves and have a skilled birth attendant. They are more likely to delay marriage and avoid pregnancy while they are very young and thus avoid the increased risks associated with teen pregnancy.[52] In Bangladesh it is shown that a child's chance of survival increases by 20% if the mother has a primary education. A child's chance of survival increases to 80% if the mother has a secondary education.[2] Unfortunately, as of 2007, there was still an estimated 101 million children without primary education, mostly in South Asia (35 million) and sub-Saharan Africa (46 million).[52] While this is an improvement over the 115 million lacking education in 2002, there is still need for significant strides to provide more children with basic education.

Women face illiteracy and social-cultural practices that prevent them from leaving their homes to access health services. Twenty percent of girls in South Asia and sub-Saharan Africa do not attend school and an alarming two thirds of illiterate adults are women.[52] In many countries, women report that they do not make decisions about health for themselves or their children—their husbands do. This is particularly true in sub-Saharan Africa where 75% of women in Burkina Faso, Mali, and Nigeria reported that their husbands make the decisions about their health.[2] The same husband-directed care was reported by 50% of women in Bangladesh and Nepal.[52]

Training women as community health workers has made considerable inroads in surmounting some of these barriers. There is a doorstep program in Bangladesh in which health workers are able to provide care by going to the homes of women who are not allowed to access health services outside the home.[2] In Pakistan, immunization rates for tetanus in women increased by 30% after Lady Health Workers were able to do home visits and provide vaccines to women who were reluctant to receive them from male vaccinators.[2]

Malnutrition

The goal of MDG 1 is to reduce the proportion of people who suffer from hunger by half by 2015.[2] Malnutrition is estimated to contribute to at least half of all child deaths and contribute to significant morbidity due to prenatal malnutrition (eg, iodine deficiency causing devastating neurologic problems) and postnatal malnutrition (eg, iron deficiency leading to learning problems).[2] Reduced immunity is a major consequence of malnutrition.[2] Diseases associated with maternal and child undernutrition (including stunting, wasting, and deficiencies of essential vitamins) are of high prevalence in middle- and low-income countries; it is estimated that stunting, wasting, and intrauterine growth retardation (IUGR) account for 2.2 million deaths annually for children younger than 5 years and significantly contribute to the disease burden of children.[54] Suboptimal breastfeeding alone accounts for 1.4 million deaths. Putting these data together, 22% of deaths and 11% of disease burden can be attributed globally to low birth weight and IUGR.[54]

Maternal nutrition is important for pregnancy outcome; women with short stature (possibly due to malnutrition) are at increased risk for needing assistance with delivery which is often not available, placing mother and baby at risk. While maternal undernutrition does not seem to affect breast milk composition, there may be micronutrient deficiencies.[54] If a baby is born at term with intrauterine growth restriction and a birth weight of 1,500 to 1,999 g, that baby is 8 times more likely to die, usually with complications from birth asphyxia or sepsis. If the birth weight is 2,000 to 2,499 g, the baby is 2.8 times as likely to die. Globally, the prevalence of underweight births is 20% with south-central Asia (at 33%) and eastern Africa (at 28%) being particular problem spots.[54] These regions also have the highest rates of stunting and wasting (Table 1-3). Thirty six countries account for 90% of stunted children worldwide.[54] Table 1-4 shows the increased odds ratio for mortality as affected by poorer growth measurements for some of the most common causes of death. The same socioeconomic inequalities hold true for malnutrition as for other diseases; children from poor families have approximately twice the likelihood of being stunted as children from wealthier families.

Malnutrition may not be apparent as it is not always manifested in low weight. Deficiencies in vitamin A, zinc, iron, and iodine can all contribute to a weakened immune system. Vitamin A deficiency is responsible for 0.6 million deaths in the first 6 months of life and contributes to deaths from diarrhea and measles.[54] Vitamin A also causes significant morbidity secondary to xerophthalmia, causing corneal scarring and blindness. Xerophthalmia is the most common preventable cause of blindness in children in the developing world. Zinc deficiency is related to increased risk of death from diarrhea, malaria, and pneumonia and accounts for 0.4 million deaths annually.[54] Iron and iodine, while not significant factors in childhood death, do cause significant morbidity, with iron deficiency affecting cognitive development and behavior in children.[54] The Maternal and Child Undernutrition Study Group reviewed available interventions that positively affect malnutrition. Its report suggests that the following interventions could be helpful: iron and folate supplementation to pregnant women, vitamin A supplementation in the neonatal period and infancy, preventive zinc supplementation, and universal iodized salt. This group estimates that implementation of these interventions could decrease stunting by 36% and mortality of children from birth to 3 years of age by 25%.[23]

The recommendation for child-feeding practices is exclusive breastfeeding for the first 6 months and subsequent continued breastfeeding until the age of 2 years; however, in Asia, Africa, and Latin America the rate of exclusive breastfeeding is quite low—47% to 57% of infants younger than 2 months, and 25% to 31% between the ages of 6 and 11 months.[54] Only 6% of infants in Africa and 10% in Asia are exclusively breastfed.[54] There is increased risk of mortality from diarrhea and pneumonia with relation to the degree of breastfeeding, highlighting the extraordinary protective effect of breastfeeding and the need for breastfeeding promotion and education by community health workers.

Table 1-3. Childhood Stunting, Severe Wasting, and Underweight Estimates and Numbers Affected in 2005 Based on World Health Organization Child Growth Standards by United Nations Regions and Subregions

	CHILDREN <5 YEARS IN MILLIONS*	PERCENTAGE STUNTED (95% CI)	NUMBER STUNTED IN MILLIONS (95% CI)	PERCENTAGE SEVERELY WASTED (95% CI)	NUMBER SEVERELY WASTED IN MILLIONS (95% CI)	PERCENTAGE UNDERWEIGHT (95% CI)	NUMBER UNDERWEIGHT IN MILLIONS (95% CI)
Africa	141·914	40·1 (36·8-43·4)	56·9 (52·2-61·6)	3·9 (2·2-5·7)	5·6 (3·0-8·0)	21·9 (19·8-24·0)	31·1 (28·1-34·0)
Eastern	48·807	50·0 (42·3-57·9)	24·4 (20·7-28·3)	3·6 (1·5-8·4)	1·8 (0·7-4·1)	28·0 (23·6-32·9)	13·7 (11·5-16·1)
Middle	20·197	41·5 (38·3-44·8)	8·4 (7·7-9·1)	5·0 (2·0-12·0)	1·0 (0·4-2·4)	22·5 (19·2-26·1)	4·5 (3·9-5·3)
Northern	22·171	24·5 (17·3-33·9)	5·4 (3·8-7·5)	3·3 (1·2-8·9)	0·7 (0·3-2·0)	6·8 (2·8-15·3)	1·5 (0·6-3·4)
Southern	6·075	30·2 (25·4-35·6)	1·8 (1·5-2·2)	2·7 (1·0-6·8)	0·2 (0·06-0·4)	11·4 (8·0-15·7)	0·7 (0·5-1·0)
Western	44·663	37·7 (33·5-42·1)	16·8 (15·0-18·8)	4·3 (1·8-9·6)	1·9 (0·8-4·3)	23·9 (21·0-26·9)	10·7 (9·4-12·0)
Asia	356·879	31·3 (27·5-35·1)	111·6 (98·1-125·1)	3·7 (1·2-6·2)	13·3 (4·4-22·3)	22·0 (18·5-25·6)	78·6 (65·9-91·3)
Eastern	95·070	14·5 (13·5-15·5)	13·7 (12·8-14·7)	0·7 (0·3-1·6)	0·7 (0·3-1·6)	5·1 (4·8-5·4)	4·8 (4·5-5·1)
South-central	181·481	40·7 (34·2-47·7)	73·8 (62·0-86·5)	5·7 (2·4-12·8)	10·3 (4·4-23·3)	33·1 (26·6-40·3)	60·1 (48·3-73·0)
Southeastern	54·970	34·3 (26·5-43·5)	18·9 (14·5-23·9)	3·6 (1·4-8·8)	2·0 (0·8-4·9)	20·7 (17·2-24·6)	11·4 (9·5-13·5)
Western	25·358	20·6 (10·0-38·8)	5·2 (2·5-9·8)	1·6 (0·4-5·8)	0·4 (0·1-1·5)	8·9 (2·8-24·2)	2·2 (0·7-6·1)

Table 1-3. Childhood Stunting, Severe Wasting, and Underweight Estimates and Numbers Affected in 2005 Based on World Health Organization Child Growth Standards by United Nations Regions and Subregions, continued

	CHILDREN <5 YEARS IN MILLIONS*	PERCENTAGE STUNTED (95% CI)	NUMBER STUNTED IN MILLIONS (95% CI)	PERCENTAGE SEVERELY WASTED (95% CI)	NUMBER SEVERELY WASTED IN MILLIONS (95% CI)	PERCENTAGE UNDERWEIGHT (95% CI)	NUMBER UNDERWEIGHT IN MILLIONS (95% CI)
Latin American	56·936	16·1 (9·4-22·8)	9·2 (5·3-13·0)	0·6 (0·2-1·0)	0·3 (0·1-0·6)	4·8 (3·1-6·4)	2·7 (1·8-3·7)
Caribbean	3·657	8·2 (3·9-16·7)	0·3 (0·1-0·6)	1·0 (0·4-2·5)	0·03 (0·01-0·9)	5·1 (2·7-9·6)	0·2 (0·1-0·4)
Central America	16·161	23·1(13·9-36·4)	3·7 (2·5-5·9)	0·6 (0·2-1·7)	0·1 (0·04-0·3)	6·2 (3·4-11·0)	1·0 (0·5-1·8)
South America	37·118	13·8 (6·9-26·3)	5·1 (2·6-9·8)	0·6 (0·2-1·6)	0·2 (0·07-0·6)	4·1 (2·5-6·7)	1·5 (0·9-2·5)
All developing countries	555·729	32·0 (29·3-34·6)	177·7 (162·9-192·5)	3·5 (1·8-5·1)	19·3 (10·0-28·6)	20·2 (17·9-22·6)	112·4 (99·3-125·5)

Stunting=height-for-age less than −2 SD; Severe wasting=weight-for-length or weight-for-height less than −3 SD; Underweight=weight-for-age less than −2 SD.

*UN Department of Economic and Social Affairs, Population Division. World Population Prospects, the 2004 revision. New York: United Nations, 2005

From Black RE, Allen LH, Bhutta ZA, et al. Maternal and child undernutrition: global and regional exposures and health consequences. *Lancet.* 2008;371(9608):243–260, with permission from Elsevier.

Table 1-4. Odds Ratio for Mortality By Weight-for-Age			
	<-3 (95% CI)	-3 TO <-2 (95% CI)	-2 TO <-1 (95% CI)	MORE THAN -1
WEIGHT-FOR-AGE (Z SCORE)			
Overall*	9·7 (5·2-17·9)	2·5 (1·8-3·6)	1·8 (1·2-2·7)	1·0
Diarrhoea*	9·5 (5·5-16·5)	3·4 (2·7-4·4)	2·1 (1·6-2·7)	1·0
Pneumonia*	6·4 (3·9-10·4)	1·3 (0·9-2·0)	1·2 (0·7-1·9)	1·0
Malaria†	1·6 (1·0-2·7)	1·2 (0·5-3·5)	0·8 (0·2-3·2)	1·0
Measles‡	6·4 (4·6-9·1)	2·3 (1·7-3·2)	1·3 (1·1-1·5)	1·0
HEIGHT-FOR-AGE (Z SCORE)			
Overall*	4·1 (2·6-6·4)	1·6 (1·3-2·2)	1·2 (0·9-1·5)	1·0
Diarrhoea*	4·6 (2·7-8·1)	1·6 (1·1-2·5)	1·2 (0·9-1·7)	1·0
Pneumonia*	3·2 (1·5-6·7)	1·3 (0·9-2·1)	1 (0·6-1·6)	1·0
Malaria†	2·1 (0·9-4·9)	1·0 (0·4-2·4)	0·7 (0·5-0·9)	1·0
Measles‡	2·8 (1·4-5·8)	1·7 (0·8-3·6)	0·7 (0·5-0·9)	1·0
WEIGHT-FOR-HEIGHT (Z SCORE)			
Overall*	9·4 (5·3-16·8)	3·0 (2·0-4·5)	1·5 (1·2-1·9)	1·0
Diarrhoea*	6·3 (2·7-14·7)	2·9 (1·8-4·5)	1·2 (0·7-1·9)	1·0
Pneumonia*	8·7 (4·8-15·6)	4·2 (3·2-5·5)	1·6 (1·1-2·4)	1·0
Malaria†	2·3 (1·6-3·2)	3·0 (1·0-8·9)	0·9 (0·3-2·6)	1·0
Measles‡	6·0 (4·3-8·2)	3·7 (2·5-5·5)	1·8 (0·9-2·6)	1·0

*Ghana, Senegal, Guinea Bissau, the Philippines, India, Nepal, Bangladesh, Pakistan.
†Ghana, Senegal, and Guinea Bissau.
‡Nepal, Ghana, Senegal, Guinea Bissau, and the Philippines.

From Black RE, Allen LH, Bhutta ZA, et al. Maternal and child undernutrition: global and regional exposures and health consequences. *Lancet.* 2008;371(9608):243–260, with permission form Elsevier.

Immunizations

Immunizations are among the single most cost-effective public health interventions that exist. Of the 10 million annual deaths of children younger than 5 years, approximately 2 million are caused by vaccine-preventable diseases (Figure 1-10). Significant strides in immunizing children were made over the past 40 years. Polio is almost completely eradicated (Figure 1-11).[55–57] Starting with the EPI in 1974, the coverage

Figure 1-10. Percentage of Deaths From Vaccine-Preventable Diseases* Among Children Younger Than 5 Years, by Disease, Worldwide, 2002*

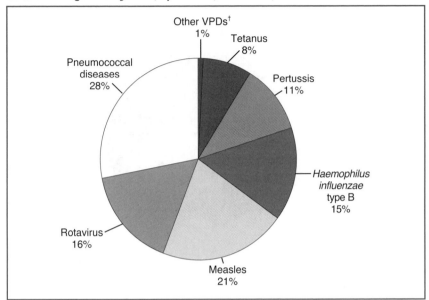

*An estimated 2.5 million deaths worldwide (of a total of 10.5 million for this age group) are caused by diseases for which vaccines are currently available.

†Diphtheria, hepatitis B, Japanese encephalitis, meningococcal disease, poliomyelitis, and yellow fever. (In older age groups, approximately 600,000 hepatitis B deaths are preventable by routine immunization.)

From Centers for Disease Control and Prevention. Vaccine preventable deaths and the Global Immunization Vision and Strategy, 2006–2015. *MMWR Morb Mortal Wkly Rep.* 2006;55(18):511–515

for diphtheria, pertussis, and tetanus (DPT3) increased from 20% in 1974 to 81% in 2007. However, approximately 23 million children were still not immunized with DPT3, particularly in India and some countries in Africa.[55–57] There is also a slow expansion in the number of vaccines recommended for global distribution; hepatitis B was added in 1992 and Hib vaccine in 1998.[58] In 2005, the WHO and UNICEF created the Global Immunization Vision and Strategy (GIVS) to address the problem of vaccine distribution to children who need them.[58] It addresses the following 4 areas[58]:

- Improving immunization coverage by trying to ensure at least 4 immunization contacts per child and expanding programs to immunize people of all ages
- Introducing new vaccines and technologies
- Integrating immunizations into other health interventions
- Creating global partnerships to finance immunizations

Figure 1-11. Of the World's 23.2 Million Children Not Immunized With Diphtheria, Pertussis, and Tetanus (DPT3), 16.2 Million Live in 10 Countries

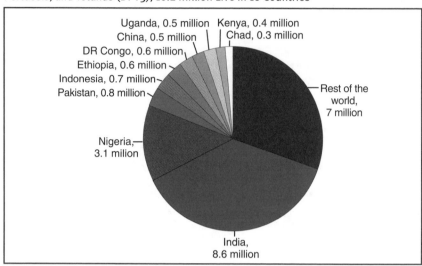

From United Nations Children's Fund. Statistics by area: child survival and health: current status: DPT3 immunization coverage, 2009. http://www.childinfo.org/immunization_status.html. Accessed June 13, 2011

Strategies to increase routine vaccination coverage are encouraged. Reaching Every District is an example of such a strategy; it includes supervision, regular outreach, community links with service delivery, and better planning of vaccine delivery based on data.[58] Unfortunately, long-term funding issues remain a challenge. Programs such as GAVI help increase support for vaccines. GAVI is a public-private partnership created in 1999 to enable the poorest countries to provide vaccines. Countries with DPT3 coverage below 80% and a national income less than $1,000 per head, per year, are eligible to apply.[59] By the end of 2005, GAVI helped 73 countries with financing for vaccines. An assessment of the program in 2004 examined DPT3 coverage rates from 1999 to 2004 after countries received GAVI funding. The results demonstrated that GAVI significantly affected countries with less than 65% coverage at baseline.[59] Accelerated introduction of Hib vaccine over the last 4 years gives hope of success for the introduction of other vaccines such as those for rotavirus and pneumococcus.[55-57]

War

Armed conflict has a profound effect on children and their health. It is estimated that 90% of deaths during a war are civilian and half of those civilian deaths are children.[60] About 2 million children died in the last 10 years due to war; 6 million more suffered a disability, and many more (estimated at or greater than 20 million) were forced to flee from their homes and become refugees.[60] Children are forced to become child soldiers, endure rape, and undergo unimaginable psychological stress. Unfortunately, war affects countries in poverty. Of the 10 countries with the highest younger-than-5 mortality rate, 7 were involved in conflict. War leads to fewer resources to improve child health and decreases the availability of health care and immunizations.[60]

Poverty

Millennium Development Goal 1 addresses poverty—eradicate extreme poverty, and cut in half the numbers of people whose income is less than $1 per day. Many diseases would not have such a stronghold if there was less poverty. Those children born in impoverished nations have a much greater risk of dying; the chance of dying before the age of 5 years is almost 90 times greater in Sierra Leone than in Sweden.[2] To have a lasting effect on child mortality, economic inequalities exemplified by the fact that the world's 225 richest people have a combined wealth equivalent to the annual income of the poorest 2.5 billion people, must be addressed.[61]

> "This indifference—by politicians, policy makers, donors, research funders, and civil society—is a betrayal of our collective hope for a stronger and more just society, one that values every life no matter how young or hidden from public view that life might be. It signifies an unbalanced world in which only those with money, military strength, and political leverage determine what counts and who counts. As health professionals, we should not accept this pervasive disrespect for human life."[62]
> —Richard Horton

■ CURRENT STATUS OF MILLENIUM DEVELOPMENT GOALS

The Countdown to 2015 group was formed to track MDG progress globally and to assess access to proven interventions by all people, including marginalized populations such as the poor and uneducated. Its most recent publication, *Countdown to 2015 Decade Report (2000–2010)*, is sobering.[49] Some progress has been made with an overall reduction in mortality of 90 deaths per 1,000 live births (1990) to 60 deaths per 1,000 live births (2009).[1] The average rate of child mortality reduction has also improved since the 1990s from 1.4% per year (1990–2000) to 2.8% per year (2000–2009).[1] However, only 19 of 68 priority countries are on track to reach MDG 4 and while many countries have made great progress, the rate is insufficient to reach MDG 4.[49]

Africa, where half of all maternal and child deaths occur and the HIV epidemic increases the burden on many nations, continues to be one of the most problematic regions. In fact, 12 countries in Africa are experiencing a worsening of younger-than-5 mortality rates.

The most recent coverage levels for effective interventions in the 68 priority countdown countries are shown in Figure 1-12, including 79% for measles vaccination, 54% for a skilled birth attendant, 86% for 2 doses of vitamin A, 34% for exclusive breastfeeding, 27% for antibiotics for pneumonia, and 19% for ITNs.[49] There is a significant lack of contraceptive services, skilled birth attendants, and adequate newborn management.[62] Coverage of interventions that can be scheduled (eg, antenatal care, immunizations, ITN, vitamin A supplementation) is

Figure 1-12. Median Coverage for Effective Maternal, Newborn, and Child Interventions in 68 Countdown Countries

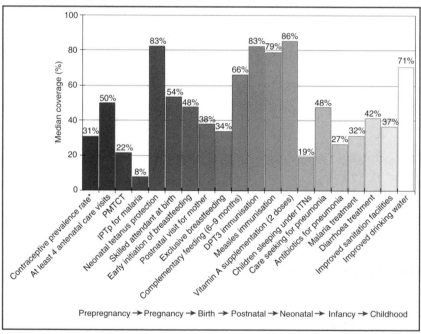

Data are most recent available estimates since 2000.

Abbreviations: PMTCT, prevention of maternal-to-child transmission of HIV; IPTp, intermittent preventive treatment for malaria; DPT3, diphtheria, pertussis, and tetanus; ITNs, insecticide-treated bed nets.

*Target coverage rate is not 100%.

From Bhutta ZA, Chopra M, Axelson H, et al. Countdown to 2015 decade report (2000–10): taking stock of maternal, newborn, and child survival. *Lancet.* 2010;375(9730):2032–2044, with permission from Elsevier.

improving.[49,62–65] However, the coverage for interventions that require clinical skills or that must be available at all hours (ie, skilled care during child birth; treatment of kids for pneumonia, diarrhea, and malaria) remains low.[49] The result is uneven care, with mothers getting antenatal care but incomplete care around the time of delivery; children are given immunizations but have inadequate access to skilled care during the newborn period or for childhood diseases such as pneumonia, malaria, and diarrhea.[1,62,63] Mothers are not consistently receiving proven interventions with their scheduled prenatal care, such as preventive intermittent treatment for malaria or medicine to prevent HIV transmission.[64]

In addition, inequities continue between and within countries. While the median rate of care-seeking for pneumonia in the 68 countdown countries was 48%, Korea's rate was greater than 90% while Chad's was about 10% (in 2004).[49] Within countries, the poorest continue to receive less than the rich and urban patients have better access to health care than rural populations. Figure 1-13 demonstrates the wide span of coverage of interventions between the poorest and the wealthiest in 38

Figure 1-13. Average Coverage Levels of Selected Interventions in the Poorest and Richest Wealth Quintiles of 38 Countdown Countries

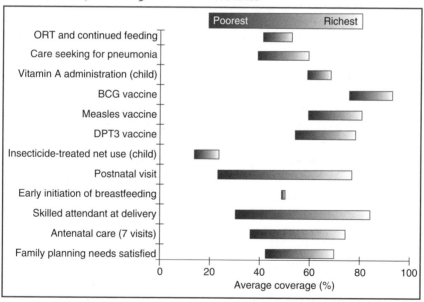

Long bars correspond to greater magnitude of inequalities than do short bars. Postnatal care indicator refers to postnatal care for all newborn infants.

Abbreviations: ORT, oral rehydration therapy; DTP3, diphtheria, pertussis, and tetanus.

From Bhutta ZA, Chopra M, Axelson H, et al. Countdown to 2015 decade report (2000–10): taking stock of maternal, newborn, and child survival. *Lancet.* 2010;375(9730):2032–2044, with permission form Elsevier.

countdown countries.[49] The disturbing trend over the last 2 decades is that more countries increased the disparity between poor and rich than decreased it.[1] Gender discrimination and low levels of education also contribute to inequities within countries, masked by countrywide statistics. Children of educated mothers are more likely to survive. In China and India girls have a higher mortality than boys.[1]

While many of these inequity findings suggest insurmountable odds, the experience in Brazil proves otherwise. There has been a 5% annual reduction (ahead of target) in child deaths and a drop of stunting from 19.9% (1990) to 7.1% (2006). This tremendous progress is attributed to a number of economic and health interventions accompanied by a committed political agenda.

An examination of funding shows that while there has been a 64% increase since 2003, programs are still underfunded overall.[63] Four new priorities have been identified.[63]

- A strengthening of health systems—it is not sufficient to simply provide a country with an initial start-up for several projects; the systems, infrastructure, supplies, planning, management, and supervision need to be improved on a continuing basis after the initial start.
- An awareness that the HIV epidemic and war have a huge effect on health and improvement of efforts to address this effect.
- A continued effort to integrate 2 or more interventions, such as immunizations and ITNs, or linking programs to prevent mother-to-child HIV transmission to antenatal, perinatal, and postnatal care.
- Development of better and more data.

There is reason for optimism—13,000 fewer children are dying every day than in 1990 and the rate of decline in child deaths has doubled.[4] Also, several poor countries are showing that they can move forward and have moved forward. Nepal, Laos, Bangladesh, and Bolivia all reduced their mortality of children younger than 5 years by half since 1990.[63] Tanzania also demonstrated gains in child survival by decreasing its younger-than-5 mortality rate from 140 to 82 from 1990 to 2004; the changes that Tanzania implemented included doubling its public health expenditure, decentralizing financing to districts, and increasing coverage of programs such as IMCI, ITNs, vitamin A supplementation, immunization, and exclusive breastfeeding.[66] These types of interventions have led to progress in mortality reduction in other countries as well.[1] There are also several new alliances promoting child health; for example, the International Health Partnership, the Global Campaign for the Health MDGs, the Catalytic Initiative to Save a Million Lives, and a Health 8 group of global health leaders.[63]

*"If access to health care is considered a human right, who is
considered human enough to have that right?"*
— *Paul Farmer*

■ NEXT STEPS

Younger-than-5 mortality rates must be decreased by 8% per year to
achieve MDG 4. Some countries, such as Bangladesh, Brazil, Egypt,
Indonesia, Mexico, Nepal, and the Philippines, are making good
progress.[9] More attention needs to be focused on the 68 countries
where child mortality is the highest. The Child Survival series and the
Neonatal Child Survival series published in the *Lancet* in 2003 and 2005
argue that 60% to 70% of child deaths can be affordably prevented using
already existing proven effective interventions, including those found
in Figure 1-12.[1-5,7,50,51]

Health systems must be improved to effectively distribute these effective interventions across the continuum of maternal, newborn, and
pediatric care. Shortages in personnel are certainly a stumbling block
for implementation—only 22% of the 68 countdown countries had
adequate personnel who were often distributed unevenly geographically.
However, countries are starting to increase the scope of services provided
by their community-based health workers (IMCI). From 2008 to 2010,
the number of countries allowing community health workers to treat
pneumonia increased from 18 to 29.[49]

*"Children and mothers are dying because those who have the
power to prevent their deaths choose not to act."[62]*
— *Richard Horton*

■ NECESSARY RESOURCES

Adequate progress toward MDG 4 will not occur without attention
to health systems and improved infrastructure. Political leadership
is required to create and implement quality policies, adequately and
equitably fund implementation of those policies, and manage health
workers. Tanzania is an example of a country that achieved significant
success because the leadership made a commitment to improving infrastructure. It was able to increase its capacity by doubling spending on
health and expanding coverage of key interventions despite the huge
challenges of HIV and a high fertility rate.[62]

In a policy analysis conducted by the Countdown to 2015 working
group, it was shown that among the 68 priority countries, there was a

wide variation in the components required to improve infrastructure, including substantial gaps in policy adoption, which could make it difficult to achieve significant progress in a short period.[67] There are 3 possible barriers that might hinder policy uptake.

Commercial interests. Policies that affect trade or financial sectors seem to be the hardest to adopt; for example, policies on marketing breast milk substitutes. An International Code of Marketing Breast-milk Substitutes currently exists but is being challenged in court by commercial interests.

Professional interests. Giving increased responsibility to lower-level workers is often met with resistance by higher levels. For example, resistance may be encountered when giving nurse midwives more responsibility to perform lifesaving tasks or having community health workers manage pneumonia. There needs to be better dialogue and understanding among professionals and local health workers, as well as better review of what is considered safe and unsafe.

Product availability. Products that help children's health should be freely available. However, important products, such as appropriate formulations to provide zinc supplements for children with diarrhea, are not marketed. Thus, to effectively implement policies, strong global and national commitments, adequate financial resources, and intensive technical support are required. Hib vaccination was quickly implemented in several countries because of the availability of these resources, but this progress cannot be sustained unless good practices, good systems, and commitment are in place. Success is not solely dependent on large financial commitments. For example, Sri Lanka improved outcomes through systems and implementation without a large expenditure of funds.[67]

■ FINANCING

In 2007, the level of overseas development aid for maternal, newborn, and child health was about $4.1 billion, which is a 16% increase over 2006 and almost double that in 2003.[49] However, the need for such assistance is probably closer to $11 billion annually for high-priority countries to achieve all MDGs.[68]

The major funding comes from individual countries (bilateral donors), as well as the World Bank, UNICEF, GAVI alliance, and the Global Fund to Fight AIDS, Tuberculosis and Malaria (multilateral funders). The preferred method of funding was through projects even though the route with the broadest effect would be budget or infrastructure support. However, as with coverage of interventions, there are inequities among countries. While most of the priority countries saw an increase in funding, there were still 16 countries that saw a decrease in assistance by an average of 22%. Another problem with funding is that it can be erratic and variable from year to year, making it difficult for countries to plan and move forward with strategic initiatives.[69]

Investing money in health programs makes considerable sense. Research by the Copenhagen Consensus Center (a group of Nobel-laureate economists who evaluate information about the costs and benefits of different solutions to world problems) studied vitamin A and zinc supplementation. It found that if $60 million is spent on providing vitamin A to children in sub-Saharan Africa and South Asia, the annual benefits resulting from decreased morbidity and mortality would yield $1 billion.[70]

There are programs that contribute other types of unique funding, such as the Grand Challenges in Global Health initiative of the Gates Foundation ($450 million, with additional funding from the Wellcome Trust [$27 million] and the Canadian Institutes of Health [$4.5 million]), which contributed funds in 43 grants.[71] However, these grants and funds do not address health care delivery systems but rather innovative challenges, such as giving single-dose vaccines shortly after birth, developing vaccines that do not require refrigeration or are needle free, creating new vaccines, controlling insects that transmit disease, improving nutrition through plant engineering technology to make all nutrients available through a single staple plant, improving drug treatment of infectious diseases, and improving health status measurements. This is significant progress considering that previously only 10% of the world's medical research focused on new ways to address the diseases of the poor.[71] The improvements in technology will undoubtedly contribute to decreasing mortality rates in the future.

■ KEY POINTS

- *Statistics*
  - Global child mortality has substantially declined over the last 25 years, but continued progress is still needed to achieve MDG 4.
  - It should be unacceptable that almost 9 million children younger than 5 years die every year—most from preventable causes.
- *Interventions*. The knowledge and tools to further decrease child mortality and morbidity exist.
  - Maternal and neonatal care
  - Strengthening community-based services such as the IMCI program
  - Addressing the HIV epidemic
  - Immunization, ITNs

- *Political will.* More leaders and their governments are needed to embrace MDG 4 and put into place the infrastructure and programs that work.
- *Equity.* Infrastructure improvements must reach all people equitably— not only from one region to another but also within a country's borders.
- *Financing.* The most impoverished nations
  — Require continued and increased financial assistance.
  — Require long-term financial commitment so there is no threat of nonrenewal, allowing countries to make long-term changes in infrastructure and keep trained staff.

We cannot afford to sit on the sidelines and be content with the status quo. We need to be a loud voice for our children, for if we care for them in a fair and equitable manner, we will pave the way to a more just society.

"It is health that is real wealth and not pieces of gold and silver."
— Mohandas Gandhi

■ REFERENCES

1. You D, Jones G, Hill K, Wardlaw T, Chopra M. Levels and trends in child mortality, 1990–2009. *Lancet.* 2010;376:931–933
2. United Nations Children's Fund. *The State of the World's Children 2008. Child Survival.* UNICEF; 2007:1–25. http://www.unicef.org/sowc08. Accessed June 9, 2011
3. Black RE, Morris SS, Bryce J. Where and why are 10 million children dying every year? *Lancet.* 2003;361:2226–2234
4. United Nations Children's Fund. Child Mortality-Overview. http://www.childinfo.org/mortality.html. Accessed December 7, 2009
5. Elliott SR, Beeson JG. Estimating the burden of global mortality in children aged < 5 years by pathogen-specific causes. *Clin Infect Dis.* 2008;46;1794–1795
6. United Nations Children's Fund. Millennium Development Goals. http://www.childinfo.org/mdg.html. Accessed June 29, 2009
7. Lawn JE, Cousens S, Zupan J, for the Lancet Neonatal Survival Steering Team. 4 million neonatal deaths: When? Where? Why? *Lancet.* 2005;365:891–900
8. Armstrong Schallenberg JRM et al. Effectiveness and cost of facility-based Integrated Management of Childhood Illness (IMCI) in Tanzania. *Lancet.* 2004;364:1583–1594
9. Ellis M, Allen S. Towards Millennium Development Goal four. *Arch Dis Child.* 2006;91:728–730
10. El Arifeen S, Blum LS, Haque DME, et al. Integrated Management of Childhood Illness (IMCI) in Bangladesh: early findings from a cluster-randomised study. *Lancet.* 2004;364:1595–1602
11. United Nations Children's Fund. Pneumonia: the Challenge. http://www.childinfo.org/pneumonia_challenge.html. Accessed June 23, 2009
12. United Nations Children's Fund. Pneumonia: Progress. http://www.childinfo.org/pneumonia_progress.html. Accessed June 23, 2009

13. Pollard A. Pneumococcal disease in the developing world: current state of vaccine programs. Presented at: Pediatric Academic Societies and Asian Society for Pediatric Research; May 4, 2008; Honolulu, HI

14. Cohen AL. Accelerating introduction of Hib vaccine worldwide. Presented at: Pediatric Academic Societies and Asian Society for Pediatric Research; May 4, 2008; Honolulu, HI

15. Cowgill KD, et al. Effectiveness of *Haemophilus influenzae* type b conjugate vaccine introduction into routine childhood immunization in Kenya. *JAMA*. 2006;296:671–678

16. Centers for Disease Control and Prevention. Progress toward introduction of the *Haemophilus influenzae* type b vaccine in low-income countries—worldwide, 2004–2007. *MMWR*. 2008;57(6):148–151

17. World Health Organization. Pneumococcal conjugate vaccine for childhood immunization—WHO position paper. *Wkly Epidemiolog Rec*. 2007;82:93–104

18. Cutts FT, et al. Efficacy of nine-valent pneumococcal conjugate vaccine against pneumonia and invasive pneumococcal disease in The Gambia: randomized, double-blind, placebo-controlled trial. *Lancet*. 2005;365:1139–1146

19. United Nations Children's Fund. Diarrhea: the challenge. http://www.childinfo.org/709.html. Accessed July 6, 2009

20. United Nations Children's Fund. Diarrhea: progress. http://www.childinfo.org/709_progress.html. Accessed July 6, 2009

21. Boschi-Pinto C, Velebit L, Shibuya K. Estimating child mortality due to diarrhea in developing countries. *Bull WHO*. 2008;86:710–717

22. Victora CG, Bryce J, Fontaine O, Monasch R. Reducing deaths from diarrhoea through oral rehydration therapy. *Bull WHO*. 2000;78:1246–1255

23. Bhutta ZA, Ahmed T, Black RE, et al. Maternal and child undernutrition 3: what works? Interventions for maternal and child undernutrition and survival. *Lancet*. 2008;371:417–440

24. Luby SP, Agboatwalla M, Painter J, Altaf A, Billhimer WL, Hoekstra RM. Effect of intensive handwashing promotion on childhood diarrhea in high-risk communities in Pakistan. *JAMA*. 2004;291:2547–2554

25. Centers for Disease Control and Prevention. Rotavirus surveillance—worldwide, 2001–2008. *MMWR*. 2008;57(46):1255–1257

26. Glass RI, Bresee JS, Turcios R, Fischer TK, Parashar UD, Steele AD. Rotavirus vaccine: targeting the developing world. *J Infec Dis*. 2005:192(Suppl 1):S160–S166

27. United Nations Children's Fund. HIV/AIDS. http://www.childinfo.org/hiv_aids.html. Accessed October 16, 2009

28. Joint United Nations Programme on HIV/AIDS. *2008 Report on the Global AIDS Epidemic*. http://www.unaids.org/en/KnowledgeCentre/HIVData/GlobalReport/2008/2008_Global_report.asp. Accessed October 16, 2009

29. Joint United Nations Programme on HIV/AIDS. *Children and Orphans*. 2008. http://www.unaids.org/en/PolicyAndPractice/KeyPopulations/ChildandOrphans/default.asp. Accessed May 2008

30. De Cock KM, et al. Prevention of mother to child HIV transmission in resource-poor countries: translating research into policy and practice. *JAMA*. 2000;283(9):1175–1182

31. Guay LA, et al. Intrapartum and neonatal single-dose nevirapine compared with zid-ovudine for prevention of mother-to-child transmission of HIV-1 in Kampala, Uganda: HIVNET 012 randomized trial. *Lancet*. 1999;354:795–802

32. Donnelly J. Saving the babies: a victory for Africa. *Boston Globe*. August 27, 2007. www.boston.com/yourlife/health/children/articles/2007/08/27/saving_the_babies_a_vistory_in_africa. Accessed October 16, 2009

33. Effect of breast feeding on infant and child mortality due to infectious diseases in less developed countries; a pooled analysis. *Lancet.* 2000;355(9202):451–455

34. Wolfson LJ, Strebel PM, Gacic-Dobo M, Hoekstra EJ, McFarland JW, Hersh BS, for the Measles Initiative. Has the 2005 measles mortality reduction goal been achieved? A natural history modeling study. *Lancet.* 2007;369:191–200

35. Centers for Disease Control and Prevention. Progress in global measles control and mortality reduction, 2000–2007. *MMWR.* 2008;57(48):1303–1306

36. Centers for Disease Control and Prevention. Progress toward measles control—African region, 2001–2008. *MMWR.* 2009;58(37):1036–1041

37. United Nations Children's Fund. Malaria: the challenge. http://www.childinfo.org/malaria.html. Accessed June 23, 2009

38. United Nations Children's Fund. Malaria: progress. http://www.childinfo.org/malaria_progress.html. Accessed July 6, 2009

39. Centers for Disease Control and Prevention. World malaria day—April 25, 2008. *MMWR.* 2008;57(16):436

40. Verhoeff FH, Brabin BJ, Chimsuku L, Kazembe P, Russell WB, Broadhead RL. An evaluation of the effects of intermittent sulfadoxine-pyrimethamine treatment in pregnancy on parasite clearance and risk of low birthweight in rural Malawi. *Ann Trop Med Parasitol.* 1998;92(2):141–150

41. Fegan GW, Noor AM, Akhwale WS, Cousens S, Snow R. Effect of expanded insecticide-treated bednet coverage on child survival in rural Kenya: a longitudinal study. *Lancet.* 2007;370(9592):1035–1039

42. Lindblade KA, et al. Sustainability of reductions in malaria transmission and infant mortality in western Kenya with use of insecticide-treated bednets. *JAMA.* 2004;291:2571–2580

43. Gu W, Novak RJ. Predicting the impact of insecticide-treated bed nets on malaria transmission: the devil is in the detail. *Mal J.* 2009;8:256

44. Centers for Disease Control and Prevention. Baseline data from the Nyando Integrated Child Health and Education Project—Kenya, 2007. *MMWR.* 2007;56(42):1109–1113

45. Grabowsky M, Nobiya T, Selaniko J. Sustained high coverage of insecticide-treated bednets through combined catch-up and keep-up strategies. *Trop Med Int Health.* 2007;12(7):815–822

46. Centers for Disease Control and Prevention. Distribution of insecticide-treated bednets during a polio immunization campaign—Niger, 2005. *MMWR.* 2006;55(33):913–916

47. Miller JM, Korenromp EL, Nahlen BL, Steketee RW. Estimating the number of insecticide-treated nets required by African households to reach continent-wide malaria coverage targets. *JAMA.* 2007;297:2241–2250

48. United Nations Children's Fund. Newborn care: the challenge. http://www.childinfo.org/newborncare.html. Accessed July 6, 2009

49. Bhutta Z, et al. Countdown to 2015 decade report (2000–10): taking stock of maternal, newborn, and child survival. *Lancet.* 2010;375:2032–2044

50. Martines J, Paul VK, Bhutta ZA, et al. Neonatal survival: a call for action. *Lancet.* 2005;365:1189–1197

51. Darmstadt GL, Bhutta ZA, Cousens S, Adam T, Walker N, deBernis L, for the Lancet Neonatal Survival Steering Team. Evidence-based, cost-effective interventions: how many newborn babies can we save? *Lancet.* 2005;365:977–988

52. United Nations Children's Fund. *The State of the World's Children 2009: Maternal and Newborn Health.* UNICEF; December 2008:1–154

53. Freedman LP, Graham WJ, Brazier E, et al. Practical lessons from global safe mother-hood initiatives: time for a new focus on implementation. *Lancet.* 2007;370:1383–1391

54. Black RE, et al. Maternal and child undernutrition 1: maternal and child under-nutrition: global and regional exposures and health consequences. *Lancet.* 2008;371:243–260

55. United Nations Children's Fund. Immunization summary. http://www.childinfo.org/immunization.html. Accessed July 6, 2009

56. United Nations Children's Fund. Trends in immunization coverage. http://www.childinfo.org/immunization_trends.html. Accessed June 29, 2009

57. United Nations Children's Fund. Immunization current status. http://www.childinfo.org/immunization_status.html. Accessed July 6, 2009.

58. Centers for Disease Control and Prevention. Vaccine preventable deaths and the Global Immunization Vision and Strategy, 2006–2015. *MMWR.* 2006;55(18):511–515

59. Lu C, Michaud CM, Gakidou E, Khan K, Murray CJ. Effect of the Global Alliance for Vaccines and Immunizations on diphtheria, tetanus, and pertussis vaccine coverage: an independent assessment. *Lancet.* 2006;368:1088–1095

60. United Nations Children's Fund. Children in conflict and emergencies. http://www.unicef.org/protection/index_armedconflict.html. Accessed May 15, 2008

61. Worldwatch Institute. Matters of scale: spending priorities. *World Watch Magazine.* 1999;12(1). http://www.worldwatch.org/node/764. Accessed May 9, 2008

62. Horton R. Countdown to 2015: a report card on maternal, newborn, and child survival. *Lancet.* 2008;371:1217–1219

63. Salama P, Lawn J, Bryce J, et al. Making the countdown count. *Lancet.* 2008;371:1219–1221

64. Countdown Coverage Writing Group. Countdown to 2015 for maternal, newborn, and child survival: the 2008 report on tracking coverage of interventions. *Lancet.* 2008;371:1247–1258

65. United Nations Children's Fund. Countdown to 2015. http://www.childinfo.org/countdown.html. Accessed June 29, 2009

66. Masanja H, et al. Child survival gains in Tanzania: analysis of data from demographic and health surveys. *Lancet.* 2008;371:1276–1283

67. Countdown Working Group on Health Policy and Health Systems. Assessment of the health system and policy environment as a critical component to tracking intervention coverage for maternal, newborn, and child health. *Lancet.* 2008;371:1284–1293

68. Powell-Jackson T, Borghi J, Mueller DH, Patouillard E, Mills A. Countdown to 2015: tracking donor assistance to maternal, newborn, and child health. *Lancet.* 2006;368:1077–1087

69. Greco G, Powell-Jackson T, Borghi J, Mills A. Countdown to 2015: assessment of donor assistance to maternal, newborn, and child health between 2003 and 2006. *Lancet.* 2008;371:1268–1275

70. Lomborg B. *Wall Street Journal.* May 22, 2008

71. Litzow J, Bauchner H. The grand challenges of the Gates Foundation: what impact on global child health? *J R Soc Med.* 2006;99:171–174

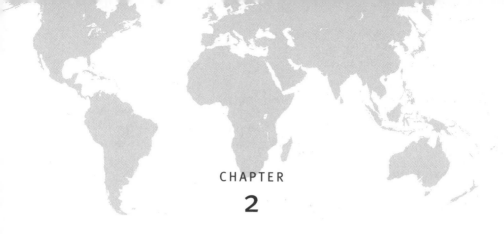

Poverty, Politics, War, and Health

Linda M. Kaljee, PhD
Bonita Stanton, MD, FAAP

■ INTRODUCTION

Pediatric training, like most medical education, primarily focuses on the biomedical causes, cures, and preventive modalities of disease that affect child health and well-being. Medical missions by small groups of pediatricians and other health professionals from lower-, middle-, and higher-income countries historically focused on curative, biomedical approaches. Such missions accomplish much good for the children they serve and for the medical teams involved.[1] Increasingly, pediatricians and students of child health are becoming interested in approaches reaching a wider spectrum of the population and whose effects are sustainable. Pediatricians in the United States, Canada, and other higher-income nations seek to partner with their colleagues in middle- and lower-income nations to bring about fundamental change in child health across the globe. Numerous national and pediatric organizations, including the Federation of Pediatric Organizations (www.fopo.org), the umbrella organization for 7 major pediatric associations in the United States and Canada, are actively involved in global child health as part of their core missions and strategic plans.

Critical to understanding child health dynamics across the globe is to appreciate the integrated roles of culture, economics, and politics on the well-being of children and families. Indeed, much of the health disparity between and within nations can be attributed to the intersection of the biological basis of diseases and the sociocultural and political economic context in which a child develops and matures. Pediatricians and child health specialists who wish to work toward the achievement of improved child health within diverse populations across the world must be aware of these issues and their actions guided by this understanding.

■ DEFINING CHILDHOOD AND ADOLESCENCE

The World Health Organization (WHO) defines *children* as 0 to 9 years of age and *adolescents* as 10 to 19 years of age. However, childhood and adolescence are age-based social constructions that vary historically and across cultures.[2–4] Concepts about child development and parenting are based in social and cultural contexts and may be strongly associated with values and ideals in relation to religion, kinship, and social and familial obligations.[5–9]

Not so long ago in the United States and Western Europe (and still in many societies today), children grew into adulthood with little of the transitional period demarcated in Western medicine and social sciences as adolescence.[8] This period of development emerged in the United States and Europe in the late 19th century as a part of industrialization and globalization as young people worked independently outside of an agrarian economy, stayed in school longer, and delayed marriage.[3]

A majority of mid-20th century research on childhood development and psychology was based in a Western-focused conceptualization of development categories. Such research normalized the Western models for childhood development, parenting, and even the clinical manifestations of disease.[10] However, in the last 20 years, more attention to psychology, anthropology, child development, education, and pediatric literature led to a recognition of the need to describe and understand the variations of childhood and adolescence across time and cultures, and also to develop methodologies that improve cross-cultural research with children.[11]

■ EFFECT OF SOCIOCULTURAL, POLITICAL, AND ECONOMIC ISSUES ON GLOBAL CHILD HEALTH

Poverty and Resource Disparities

Tran lives with her husband on a small island in the South China Sea. Her husband is a fisherman and is away from home 2 to 3 weeks a month. During the rainy season, access to the mainland is often difficult. One afternoon, Tran's 3-year old daughter begins acting fretful and develops a fever and very loose watery diarrhea. The trip to the hospital on the mainland is about 45 minutes, but Tran is concerned because the water is very rough with heavy rains. Her husband is out fishing despite the conditions. She thinks she might be able to borrow money from her sister if she does go to the hospital. Tran treats her daughter with soupy rice and tea made from leaves she grows in her garden. Her mother taught her how to treat diarrhea with these leaves. Her daughter's condition only worsens as she begins vomiting and having large watery stools every half hour. Tran goes to the pharmacy where she obtains an antibiotic and oral rehydration therapy. However, her daughter cannot keep the liquids in her body and eventually is unable to take the fluids. She is no longer crying tears and is not responsive. She dies later that same evening.

An estimated 8.1 million children younger than 5 years die every year.[1] A majority of these children would survive if they had access to existing interventions. Seventy-five percent of these deaths occur in Africa and Southeast Asia.[12,13] The major causes of these deaths are pneumonia, diarrheal diseases, and malaria. More than 20 million children are severely malnourished; 30% of childhood mortality for those younger than 5 years is associated with undernutrition.[13]

Economic conditions and the distribution of resources within and among communities, regions, and nations have significant direct and indirect effects on the health of children of all ages. It is not possible to address global health without acknowledging the relationship between income and child health and well-being.

An examination of data presented in the annual United Nations Children's Fund (UNICEF) *State of the World's Children* report illustrates the parallel courses between economic and health disparities (www.unicef.org/publications/index.html). (Also see www.gapminder. org for information on country-specific economic conditions and health disparity.) For example, *The State of the World's Children 2008: Child Survival*[14] reports that children younger than 5 years experience a mortality rate of 6 per 1,000 live births in countries with a gross national income (GNI) per capita greater than or equal to $37,000. In countries with a per capita GNI of less than $2,000, children younger than 5 years experience a rate of 79 deaths per 1,000 live births. However, this relationship between income and childhood mortality is not absolute. For example, among the 11 nations with a younger-than-5 mortality rate greater than 200 children per 1,000 live births, 3 have an annual GNI per capita greater than $800 while the remaining 8 have an annual GNI per capita less than $800. Also, among those nations with a GNI per capita less than $800, 36 report child mortality rates of less than 200 per 1,000 live births. Bangladesh and South Africa have a younger-than-5 mortality rate of 69 per 1,000 live births; yet, the annual per capita GNI of Bangladesh is $480 and of South Africa is $48,282. Similarly, Eritrea and Algeria, with GNIs of $200 and $33,351, respectively, have younger-than-5 mortality rates of 74 per 1,000 live births. These figures illustrate that while poverty and wealth are important, there are by no means simple correlations between countrywide income and child survival.

Resource disparities and distribution of wealth within countries also contributes to child mortality within lower-, middle-, and higher-income nations. Among countries in sub-Saharan Africa, with a younger-than-5 mortality rate of 160 per 1,000 live births, the poorest 40% of the population controls only 13% of the wealth, while the wealthiest 20% controls 55% of the wealth. In South Asia, where the per capita GNI of $777 is marginally lower than that of sub-Saharan Africa ($851), the poorest 40% of the population controls 19% of the resources, while the wealthiest 20% controls 46% of the wealth. The South Asian younger-than-5 mortality rate of 83 per 1,000 live births is roughly half the rate of sub-Saharan Africa and close to the global median of 72 per 1,000 live births.[14] These data suggest that more equitable distribution of even limited resources can affect child health.

Research suggests that income inequality (calculated as a ratio of the amount of income to the top 20% of households to the amount of income to the lowest 20% of households) in high-income countries also has significant negative effects on child health and social and educational well-being. Among 21 high-income nations, the United States ranks first in income inequality, and evidence suggests that within the United States those regions and states with greater inequality show higher rates for poor health outcomes including low birth weight and infant mortality.[15]

Access to Health Care

Prana lives in Kolkata with her husband and 4 children. Her husband works as a laborer. Prana heard from her neighbors and saw a flyer posted in the common area of her housing about a campaign taking place over the next 2 weeks to ensure that all children are immunized against polio. Vaccination will take place at a local site within a 5-minute walk from her residence. Prana's husband heard from some men with whom he works that the vaccine might be unsafe and cause infertility in their children. Although Prana knows that her children are not vaccinated against polio and she would like for them to receive the vaccine, she is reluctant to go against her husband's decision. She decides not to participate in the campaign.

Related to poverty and inequitable access to resources is the issue of access to health care. Access to health care is mediated by multiple factors including social, political, and economic conditions that can affect availability of care, particularly for poor or marginalized populations. While health care costs and lack of adequate numbers of health providers are the most obvious barriers to households obtaining health care for children, other barriers include language, social or legal status, gender inequalities, isolation or distance to travel to health facilities, traditional beliefs about disease etiologies, and distrust of the existing health system, as well as the disruption of health services from civil unrest and war. Evidence suggests that households with higher incomes are more likely to seek health care for their children and also receive higher care quality. Meanwhile, children in the poorest households are at greatest risk for disease because of malnutrition, poor sanitation, and indoor pollutants yet are the least likely to receive adequate health care.[16] Inequities in health care include high-cost procedures for small numbers of patients, medical programs that may discourage those in greatest need from accessing services, and disparities between local community members' perceptions of needed and desired programs and programming that is evidence-based and supported by the scientific and medical community.[17,18]

There are significant differences among countries and regions in terms of number of available skilled health workers (eg, doctors, nurses, midwives). In the European region there are 78 nurses or midwives and 32 doctors for a population of 10,000. In Southeast Asia there are 12 nurses or midwives and 5 doctors, and in Africa there are 11 nurses or midwives and 2 doctors for a population of 10,000. In 2005, lower-income countries spent an estimated 4% of total public expenditures on health care, compared with 16% in higher-income countries. As a consequence, lower-income countries pay a significantly greater proportion of private health care spending out of pocket. In lower- and lower/middle-income countries, an estimated 90% of private health costs are out of pocket, compared with 39% in higher-income countries.[19] On the positive side, between 2003 and 2006 there was an increase by approximately 40% in donor-assistant financing for maternal, newborn, and child health.[20]

In 1974 the WHO established the Expanded Program on Immunization (EPI). At that time fewer than 5% of children living in lower-income countries were receiving vaccines, which were readily available in higher-income countries. Today, through the EPI, it is estimated that 80% of infants and children worldwide receive available vaccines against tetanus, pertussis, measles, diphtheria, and polio. In addition, *Haemophilus influenzae* type b, rubella, and mumps vaccines were recently added to the EPI schedule in some countries. It is estimated that 3 million children's lives are saved annually as a result of EPI.[21]

Despite such significant accomplishments in vaccine coverage, there remain countries and populations with limited or no access to EPI because of warfare, political instability, and social and economic isolation.[22] In addition, traditional beliefs can affect use of immunization programs. For example, worldviews that incorporate beliefs about balancing hot and cold elements within the body to maintain health can contribute to refusal to use certain vaccines as well as other Western medicines. In Vietnam, Western medicines, including vaccines and antibiotics, are considered hot. Infants and children are perceived as vulnerable to these hot elements, which can cause them illness or delay their development.[23] Thus, parents may not want their child to receive a vaccine that entails multiple doses or may not complete a full course of antibiotics to minimize the effects of the hot elements.

Access to health care can also affect children when parents or other caregivers or providers are unable to access care for themselves. Most notable in this respect is a woman's access to prenatal and antenatal care, as well as voluntary and accessible birth control. Access to health care during and after pregnancy can help improve a woman's nutritional status, provide access to tetanus toxoid immunization, and decrease risks for HIV and other sexually transmitted infections, malaria, and tuberculosis.[24] Access to and communication with health care resources during pregnancy can also increase the likelihood of a household's participation in childhood immunization programs. Research in Pakistan and Indonesia indicates that a woman's immunization for tetanus during pregnancy and her knowledge of the disease increased chances that her children received EPI immunizations.[25,26]

Human immunodeficiency virus/AIDS and access to antiretroviral therapy (ART) directly and indirectly affect child health. In 2007, only 31% of persons eligible to receive ART living in lower- and middle-income countries were receiving therapy.[27] A woman's access to ART during pregnancy and delivery significantly decreases risks for her child. In addition, the death of one or both parents due to HIV/AIDS has left approximately 15 million children younger than 18 orphaned worldwide. While many children are incorporated into other relatives' households, others become homeless or institutionalized. For all of these children, the effects of parental loss due to HIV/AIDS can include stigmatization, grief, and psychological and emotional distress.[28,29]

Homelessness

Nguyen has worked selling postcards, books, souvenirs, and various sundries to tourists since he was 9 years old. Now, at the age of 15, he lives in a one-room rental space with his 18-year-old brother. His mother lives outside the city. Nguyen works every day from early morning until late in the evening. On some days he is "lucky" and makes several dollars, but most days he does not sell any postcards or just one or two. His diet primarily consists of noodles purchased from small snack stands on the street. When Nguyen is sick he seeks advice from some of the women who also sell to tourists. However, he does not have the ability to receive care through public or private clinics. Throughout his years selling on the street he is approached by men willing to pay him as much as $100 for sex. He knows other young men who participate in these sexual exchanges and is tempted to accept the offers when he has gone a long time with little or no money.

An estimated 100 to 200 million children and adolescents worldwide live in shelters or on the street.[3] Children and adolescents can become homeless as a result of their parents' loss of income, work, or housing; extreme poverty; natural disasters; warfare; becoming orphaned due to HIV/AIDS; or voluntarily leaving their residence. Brazil, which has the highest number of street children in Latin America, also has the greatest income inequality in the region.[30]

Some children live on the street to earn money for themselves or their family. Others want to escape overcrowded housing, family disapproval, or abusive conditions.[31] In lower- and middle-income countries, generally more boys than girls live on the street, although these numbers are more equal in higher-income countries. Street children may have no contact with their families, may have some regular contact with family, or may be part of a family that has no permanent home.

Children living on the street are frequently represented as threats to social order. Their living conditions and associated poor health are normalized as the expected results of street life.[32] While living or working on the street can contribute to an increased likelihood of drug use and sexual and reproductive health issues, it is problematic to disassociate many other nutritional and health concerns among street children from those of all children living in extreme poverty.[30,33]

Child Labor

As previously discussed, conceptualization of childhood development and obligations are culturally constructed. The role of children as workers within families and their contributions to household income varies significantly between cultures and higher- and lower/middle-income countries. In many societies in Africa and Asia, children are expected to contribute to the household and are raised to feel a lifelong obligation to support their parents and maintain their lineage. Within agrarian societies, children at early ages take on a range of chores, and work is a significant part of socialization and is not conceived as a violation of a child's rights. For example, in Kenya, an estimated 10% of children between the ages of 5 and 15 years are engaged in work. Even though a majority of these children are contributing to family farm labor, these children can still be exposed to conditions that can negatively affect their well-being.[34] In Bangladesh, an estimated 19% of children between the ages of 5 and 14 years are in the labor force. While poverty and insufficient household income are reasons the children work, cultural perceptions of the children's role in the household and that children should not be idle contribute to rates of child labor.[35]

Child labor is of mounting concern as children are exposed to increasingly urbanized and industrialized settings.[4] Children often work in non-organized, informal work sectors (eg, selling on the streets) that lack regulations for safety or health. In middle- and lower-income countries children also work in factories, mines, and domestic service. These children are exposed to dangerous chemicals and machinery and are frequently exploited and abused.[36] Children's levels of maturity and experience to judge hazardous conditions make them more vulnerable to work-related health risks. Children's biological and developmental characteristics can increase their risks in relation to carcinogenic and other toxic substances.[37] In the most extreme cases, children and adolescents from rural regions are sold and forced to work in manufacturing facilities, providing businesses with labor at little cost in an increasingly competitive global market.[3]

Child Prostitution

Liu ning works at a "massage parlor" 6 evenings a week. This massage parlor, like many in the city, is set up to provide sexual services for local and traveling businessmen. Liu ning is now 17 years old and has worked at the parlor for about a year. Liu ning traveled to the city from the countryside where her parents have a small farm. Her father has a respiratory illness and is often unable to work.

Liu ning came to the city to work as a waitress but was only able to find part-time work that paid poorly. One of the girls at the rooming house where Liu was staying introduced her to work at the massage parlor. The girls working at the massage parlor are Liu's age and younger, but an older woman *oversees the operation. Liu ning was reluctant at first but was convinced to work for "just a short time" to make as much as $500 a month. Like most Chinese children, Liu ning feels an obligation to repay her parents for the debt she owes for her birth and upbringing.*

Liu ning has sexual relationships with about 10 men a week. Five or 6 of her clients are regulars, but most of them only come for one visit. Liu ning feels shame when she engages in sex with these men, as they are often verbally abusive to her and occasionally physically abusive. Liu ning was told about using condoms when she started working at the parlor, but her regular clients and some of the one-time clients pay her extra to not use them.

The sex work industry throughout the world is closely associated with multiple social, economic, and political changes and therefore the accuracy of statistics and information about the industry is uncertain and transient. Sex work is illegal in most countries and workers and clients are frequently marginalized. Sex work throughout the world is associated with organized crime and gangs, government corruption, and human trafficking. Regardless of the legal status of the industry, sex tourism brings money into lower- and middle-income countries and therefore is often "overlooked" by national and local government authorities.

Globally, the sex work industry generates approximately US $20 billion per year with a quarter of that from child workers.[39] In 4 Asian countries (Malaysia, Thailand, Indonesia, and the Philippines), the sex industry is estimated to account for between 2% and 14% of the gross domestic product.[40] The main users of this sex industry are local men. The vastness of this industry is built on multiple sociocultural factors including gender inequality, sexual stigma, and constructions of masculinity, as well as such economic factors as rural-to-urban migration and lack of accessible well-paid legal employment for the large populations of young people.[40-42]

Throughout Asia as well as much of the world, sex work often starts at an early age. Data suggest that in some regions of Asia the prime age for entering into sex work is 12 to 16 years. One study indicates between 30% and 35% of sex workers in the Mekong Delta region are 12 to 17 years old.[36] In a rapid assessment study of 74 sex work establishments in Vietnam, 37% of the workers were younger than 18 years.[43] Research in China indicates that many establishment-based (eg, massage parlors, karaoke bars) female sex workers are young, have little education, and come from rural areas.[44] In poor Kenyan rural coastal regions, it is estimated that 30% of girls (some as young as 12) and young women are engaged in some form of casual sex work.[45]

While a majority of sex workers are female, young men also engage in the sex work industry. These young men are a particularly vulnerable population because of social and cultural taboos in many countries with regard to men having sex with men. These taboos create barriers to identifying and providing services for these young men.[40]

In addition to children and adolescents engaged in sex work within their own countries, the trafficking of youth between countries results in forced engagement in sex work, physical abuse, and isolation from resources. In many instances, these youth or their parents are told that they will be working as domestics or in some other industry.[46] At least 1 million children, with estimates as high as 10 million, are forced into the sex work industry annually.[39]

Gender, Ethnic, and Racial Inequalities

Margarita came to the United States from a village in El Salvador at the age of 14 years to live with her aunt in an East Coast city. Margarita started school but found it very difficult and quit after about 6 months to work with her aunt cleaning office buildings. Margarita met Carlos, who was 20 years old, had his green card, and worked a steady construction job. Margarita and Carlos moved in together when they learned that Margarita was pregnant. They plan to get married as soon as Carlos becomes a US citizen. Margarita's urban neighborhood started to undergo many changes and housing costs went up throughout the area. Margarita and Carlos were forced to move out of their apartment when it was bought to be redeveloped as condominiums. They moved outside of the city into a neighborhood where few people speak Spanish. Margarita needs to find a doctor to provide care during her pregnancy but is delaying because of her fears of language barriers, questions about her legal status, and concerns about the costs.

Ethnicity, race, and gender are social categories that are constructed and reconstructed across time and place. These categories are often naturalized as biological distinctions, thus providing an authenticity to the existing social order.[47] The characteristics of ethnicity, race, and gender further become imbedded within a society's structural and knowledge systems.[48]

Many of the consequences of inequality on child well-being are inseparable from those associated with poverty. Inequality affects children's access to education, housing, and adequate nutrition. Furthermore, inequalities and associated discriminations and recriminations can significantly compound issues such as health care access,[49,50] the negotiations between traditional and biomedical worldviews, and child health outcomes. Analysis of the US National Survey of Children's

Health from 2003 to 2004 indicates Latino(a) respondents were significantly more likely to be uninsured (21% versus 6% for white Americans) and less likely to have a regular source for child health care (61% versus 90%). Other disparities between majority white American respondents and Latino(a), African American, First Nation, and Asian respondents included poor health outcomes (eg, higher rates of asthma) and lack of access to health facilities (eg, problems obtaining specialty care).[51] In other research with US farmworkers, of whom 87% are Latino(a), data indicate that these workers' children were 2 times more likely to be uninsured than other low-income US children.[52]

Constructed gender roles and responsibilities can significantly affect child and adolescent well-being. In some cultures, as girls reach puberty they may be perceived as sexually vulnerable and consequently married at a young age. In many countries in South Asia and Africa, more than 50% of girls are married before the age of 18 years. Between 1998 and 2007 in Bangladesh, 64% of 20- to 24-year-old women respondents on national and international surveys were married prior to becoming 18 years old.[53] These young women experience pressure to produce children soon after marriage, resulting in low contraceptive use and high fertility. As a result, Bangladeshi women 15 to 19 years of age experience higher rates of mortality than young men of the same age.[54] In this instance, gender constructs intersect with high levels of poverty to increase these adolescent women's vulnerabilities to risks associated with early and multiple pregnancies.

Other health outcomes in relation to social inequalities for children and adolescents can include psychological distress and associated syndromes, increased risks for sexually transmitted infections (ie, young women's abilities to negotiate condom use), and increased likelihood of incarceration.[55–57] Furthermore, the construction of ethnic categories can lead to violence, civil unrest, and warfare, and the consequential effects of these conditions on children and their families.

War and Civil Unrest

Iqbal is 16 years old and a soldier in his nation's army. He has not seen his parents for the 3 years he has been in the army. His family is very poor. When the army passed through his village on the way to war, he was told he would earn a lot of money, which would be sent to his parents. He has not seen the money and has not heard from his parents so he does not know if they received it. He no longer wants to fight, but he is in another country and does not know how he could return home. Lately he has been alone on the night watch and spends much of the night crying.

All governments, regardless of the governing model, profoundly determine child health outcomes in their own nation through direct and indirect actions, active and passive decisions, and policies, whether or not they specifically speak to child health. The effects of war and disruptions of life during periods of civil unrest profoundly affect the well-being of children living in those nations engaged in war or those areas under political, economic, and social chaos during regional conflicts. These periods of extreme violence and volatility negatively affect every facet of childhood development and health.

Since the end of World War II, an estimated 250 major wars have taken the lives of 23 million people. Prior to World War I, an estimated 90% to 95% of direct war casualties were soldiers; in World War II this ratio dropped precipitously to 50%. In modern day wars, civilians account for approximately 90% of the casualties, with women and children accounting for 75% of these deaths.[58]

In modern time, wars (defined as armed combat with more than 1,000 casualties) are consistently prevalent, with most occurring within the boundaries of a nation.[59] For example, in the year 1996 there were 30 major armed conflicts, all of which were internal.[60] The first decade of the 21st century hosted more than 3-dozen wars, most of which are also internal conflicts. Over the last 2 decades an estimated 4 million children were killed as a consequence of war.[58,61] Many of these conflicts lasted longer than a decade, resulting in entire generations of children whose developmental trajectory from infancy through young adulthood was shaped by war.[62] For example, Angola has been engaged in civil combat for nearly 3 decades.[63]

Direct mortality figures account for only a portion of the total negative effect of war on children. In 1996 the United Nations commissioned a report addressing the full consequences of war on children entitled *Promotion and Protection of the Rights of Children: Impact of Armed Conflict on Children*.[62] This document identifies and discusses 8 broad areas in which war negatively affects virtually all aspects of child well-being and development. In addition, children in military families face unique challenges during times of war whether or not they live in a country in which the conflict is being waged.

Disruption of Basic Child Health Pediatric Care and Services

War disrupts services essential for child well-being. Food and water supplies are interrupted, resulting in inadequate amounts and unsafe products; immunization programs are crippled; and health care providers may be unavailable. Most contemporary wars are occurring in lower-income nations, placing children with preexisting malnutrition or other health conditions in particularly vulnerable situations. Diarrheal and respiratory diseases are responsible for the majority of childhood deaths during wartime, as they are in most developing countries regardless of the present conflict.[62] Tuberculosis and malaria are likely to reemerge even in countries where they were previously controlled. Studies in Angola demonstrate direct relationships between combat and rising rates of under-immunization and malnutrition. Normal food production was severely disrupted and immunization programs were paralyzed, with greater effects in areas of the country most affected by war.[63] Child mortality rates increased nearly 50% during the Bangladesh war of independence, and Uganda immunization rates plummeted from more than 70% to less than 10% during wartime.[62]

Health facilities that provide preventive and curative services to children, including services to disabled children, may be destroyed by war, abandoned because of a lack of available personnel, or co-opted to provide for military needs. Reproductive health services, including family planning, prenatal and antenatal care, and testing and treatments for sexually transmitted infections, will often be curtailed because of limited health care providers and resources.[64] In the 1970s and 1980s, during the Khmer Rouge period in Cambodia, only about 30 physicians remained in the country.[62]

The range of psychological assaults and potential disruption to identity formation, which children experience living through wars, are limitless, including post-traumatic stress disorder (PTSD), anxiety, depression, and behavioral problems. The response of an individual child to these exposures is widely variable, but children of both genders, regardless of age, may be affected.[65]

Gunfire, Land Mines, and Unexploded Ordnance

Global data addressing exact causes of death among child war victims are not readily available. However, a study conducted among Croatian children between the ages of birth and 19 years who died as a result of weapon-related injury before, during, or after the civil war provides insight. Seventeen percent of all childhood injury-related deaths were directly caused by war operations; 82% of weapon-related deaths were caused by firearms and 18% by explosive devices.[62]

Whether this ratio of firearms to land mine–related deaths applies to other countries is unknown; what is known is that the morbidity and mortality resulting from land mines is substantial. An estimated 110 million land mines contaminate at least 68 countries. Land mines and other unexploded ordnance are indiscriminate, exploding when triggered by friend or foe, child or adult, human or animal. All continents are affected, although Africa may be the most afflicted. Angola alone has an estimated 10 million land mines and as of 1996 housed more than 70,000 amputees, including 8,000 children, as a result of land mine explosions.[62] Chechnya experienced nearly 1,400 land mine explosions in 2000 and 2001; one quarter of the victims was children. Almost one third of the children were injured while playing where the explosives lay, and in some cases curious children tampered with them.[66] Butterfly mines used extensively by the former USSR are brightly colored and appear to have wings. As populations become more accustomed to the presence of mines, they incorporate them into their daily lives. In Chechnya, children used mines as wheels for toy trucks and to play games.[62]

Children and adults set off explosive devices while engaged in economic activities such as cultivating fields and foresting.[66] The affected individuals carrying out these activities are often among the poorest in the nation. Although antipersonnel mines are not designed to kill, children are more likely to die. In Cambodia approximately 20% of childhood mine injuries result in death. For those who survive, adult or child, the economic consequences are significant, with more than 60% of families of mine victims in debt in one study. It was estimated that clearing mines takes 100-fold longer than deploying and a $3 mine may require $1,000 to remove. Because most of the nations with land mines have severely constrained resources, national funds for their removal are often not available.[62]

Refugee Status

During times of conflict families may feel that they have no option but to flee or send their children to safer locations. It is estimated that there are 23 million refugees worldwide, of whom approximately 40% are children younger than 18 years. In many instances, these children are not accompanied by parents or other adult guardians. Persons in flight are highly vulnerable during the escape, while in a refugee camp in their own or another country, and even when they successfully reach asylum. Children in refugee situations may experience PTSD, grief, loss, and separation anxiety. Diseases such as cholera and measles may sweep through the refugee camps, particularly where immunization programs were greatly disrupted. Girls in particular may be vulnerable to rape and sexual abuse within these camps.[67]

Multiple models for working with refugee children have evolved over the years. Such models include those that focus on the individual and a more biomedical or therapeutic approach, and those based in a theory of sociocultural re-adaptation in which a safe and structured environment is established for children.[68]

Destruction of the Environment and Chemical Toxins

War and conflict devastate natural environments, which in turn threatens the well-being of adults and children living in these regions. During the Gulf War, Kuwaiti oil wells were purposefully set on fire and crude oil spilled into waterways. During the 1970s and 1980s in Cambodia, 35% of the forest cover was destroyed. During the years of conflict in Angola, 90% of the wildlife was eradicated.[69]

During the Vietnam-American War, 77 million liters of herbicides, including nearly 50 million liters of Agent Orange/dioxin, were released over 2.6 million acres of forests and countryside.[70] Dioxins are stable and their half-life within the human body is from 7 to 11 years. Because of this stability, they are cumulative in the environment; therefore, the higher on the food chain, the greater the dioxin concentration. Short-term effects of dioxins on humans include skin lesions and altered liver function. Long-term exposure compromises the immune system and affects development of the nervous, endocrine, and reproductive systems.[71] While negative health outcomes from exposure during the war are accepted, research continues to document potential effects from current exposure in regions affected during the war. Recent studies found elevated amounts of a dioxin consistent with exposure to Agent Orange in areas where the chemical was sprayed during the 1960s and 1970s.[72]

A meta-analysis of 22 studies indicates that parental exposure to Agent Orange appears to be associated with a range of birth defects among children born to US and Vietnamese veterans and Vietnamese nationals, with the magnitude of the association increasing with degree of exposure.[70] In addition to the exposures of the Vietnamese people, young soldiers from the United States were exposed to Agent Orange. The US Department of Veterans Affairs currently recognizes association between multiple diseases and exposure including Hodgkin disease, multiple myeloma, non-Hodgkin lymphoma, prostate cancer,[73] and multiple respiratory cancers and soft-tissue sarcomas. In addition, Veterans Affairs provides benefits to children born with spina bifida to female veterans exposed to Agent Orange.[74]

Child Soldiers

At any given time an estimated 250,000 to 300,000 children younger than 18 years are serving as soldiers.[75] They may be forcibly recruited, be sold into armed service by their parents, or feel that they have no other option for self-protection or protection of their families. Child soldiers may be used as messengers, martyrs, guards, foragers, or sexual servants. Given the developmental stage of these young adolescents, they are especially vulnerable to the pressures of group ideology, romantic illusions of martyrdom, and failure to appreciate the danger of violent situations.[2] Their reentry into society is typically not negotiated during cease-fire agreements and does not take into account the violence they suffered, witnessed, or perpetrated. They may have lost their families or they may not be welcomed by their families, especially if they are girls who were raped or who served in a sexual capacity. A study among Nepali child soldiers found high rates of depression and PTSD.[62]

Gender-Based Violence

Rape and other forms of gender-based violence, unlike murder and torture, are not widely recognized as war crimes. Adolescents (generally girls but also boys) are particularly at risk. The fine line between rape and sex for food or for survival during war underscores the importance of zero tolerance for gender-based violence. Rape also occurs frequently in detainment camps, not uncommonly by international soldiers and security personnel.

Educational Needs

Schooling is important for the age-appropriate transfer of knowledge to the child as well as to maintain a sense of routine during disruptions of war and conflict. However, schooling will generally be anything but normal during wartime, with a loss of teachers to enlistment, draft, or displacement; possible attacks on or appropriation of school buildings for military purposes; an unstable student body with migration and population movement; and a lack of reliable resources (eg, schoolbooks, school supplies, water, electricity). Even when classes are held, difficulties can exist in terms of abilities of students and teachers to concentrate on learning.

Deployment and Children

Families are profoundly affected when one or both parents are deployed. Deployment is associated with higher divorce rates and spousal violence. Evidence from the aftermath of the Persian Gulf War suggests that rates of child abuse increase in military families during times of stress.[76,77]

■ THE ROLE OF PEDIATRICS AND CHILD HEALTH SPECIALISTS

The examples in this chapter provide a brief overview of the many political, economic, and sociocultural factors with devastating implications for global child well-being. Two overarching concerns are poverty and inequitable distribution of resources within and among countries, and gender, ethnic, and racial inequalities. Economic decision-making and priority setting are deeply entwined within politics and health care, whether at a local, national, or global level. It is essential that pediatricians be part of the political process to guide decisions about distribution of much-needed resources.

Such advocacy must be well-informed and consistent with other child welfare advocacy. However, pediatricians have unique roles in these efforts. First, evidence-based programs are important in industrialized countries; they are critical in lower- and middle-income countries.[78] Pediatricians can help guide policy makers in such approaches.[53,78] There are a vast number of reviews and meta-analyses of programs addressing high-impact issues in lower-income countries. For example, Bhutta and colleagues[79] published a comprehensive review that examined 186 studies, including 64 community-based studies. Although the authors found significant gaps in the literature, they were able to identify several groups of intervention approaches for which there is credible evidence of high impact on important outcomes. Likewise, the Cochrane Collaboration conducted intervention reviews on 26 topics of importance in lower- and middle-income countries including nutritional interventions, education interventions, perinatal-neonatal survival interventions, and tobacco cessation programs.[80]

When pediatricians are invited to work in other settings or are asked to help develop programs in new settings, it is their responsibility to be well versed in the outcomes literature addressing the programs in which they will be involved. Obtaining these reviews and becoming familiar with successful programs (and program components) as well as unsuccessful programs will allow the visiting pediatrician to contribute to the host country rather than simply take away experience.

At the same time it is important to recognize that change comes slowly and often programs in place that are not evidence based (or are even contrary to the existing evidence base) have their own history and reason for existence within a community. Equally important for physicians are health outcomes that are epidemiologically important but for which no evidence base exists or is only for countries with a very different socioeconomic and health structure. In such situations the pediatrician may share with the hosts in the developing country the data that do exist and possibly work with the hosts to develop an intervention trial.

Many of the issues discussed in this chapter are difficult to research, and limited baseline information is available about the extent of effects on child health and well-being. For example, child prostitution is illegal and often well hidden. There remains insufficient data on the number of children involved, as well as the morbidity and mortality rates associated with these exploitative practices.[39,81] Pediatricians and other health professionals can contribute through collaborative efforts with local organizations to develop, implement, and evaluate intervention programming. At a national and international level, pediatricians can advocate for stronger policies addressing the exploitation of these children and work for more funding to increase knowledge about the health status of these children to develop more targeted and effective programs.[39]

War, civil disorder, and other conflicts present multiple challenges for intervention. Pediatricians have uniquely important roles in sustaining services through these political actions by supporting combat-free immunization days (in which they may participate if they are in the country); supporting group efforts such as the World Food Programme, which seeks to establish reliable food chains; and working as long-term volunteers in refugee camps with established groups such as Doctors Without Borders.

Pediatricians can play a key role in protecting children from land mines by working with schools, parents, and children in countries where land mines and unexploded ordnance remain. Pediatricians can teach them how to recognize these devices, regard them as serious weapons, and discourage their use as toys. Pediatricians can also support international political action prohibiting the use of land mines and creating funds to clear mines, such as the UN Voluntary Trust Fund for Assistance in Mine Action.[62]

Pediatricians can work to rejoin children with their nuclear or extended families. UNICEF developed emergency kits to facilitate the work of volunteer relief workers; pediatricians planning to work in such settings should be familiar with these kits to ensure that their well-intended actions are actually helping. Likewise, if pediatricians are in a situation to advise families living in combat zones about evacuation of children, parents should be encouraged to do so with care and knowledge of the proposed routes and detailed documentation of persons responsible for conveyance and reception of the children to avoid risks of child trafficking.[62]

Pediatricians, whether working in regions of conflict or attending to the needs of children in safe-haven or refugee settings, can help youth who lived in war-torn nations by doing the following:

- Assist parents in reconstructing their social networks and in rebuilding a secure home life.
- Encourage youth to be involved in normal school routines and where possible, in community-building efforts.
- Integrate psychological support for the child and parent in routine clinical and preventive care.
- Avoid questioning youth about painful memories while at the same time inviting them to discuss issues that might be disturbing them.
- Be knowledgeable about local accessible mental health services to offer the family and youth if needed.

Pediatricians should serve as champions for continued education and be knowledgeable about existing resources. For example, relief agencies have long known of the importance of continued schooling. UNICEF; United Nations Educational, Scientific and Cultural Organization; and others developed teacher's emergency packs to aid teachers in delivering education during the first few months of war while more sustainable strategies for education are developed. In refugee situations, pediatricians should attempt to find out where children can receive education to guide families, as often refugees will not be permitted to attend public school in host countries. Pediatricians may also play an advocacy role reminding local government and donor agencies that in addition to reconstructing the physical infrastructure, resources must be focused on teacher recruitment, retention, and training.[62]

Pediatricians can help by offering to speak to military personnel about their responsibilities to civilian women and children and to support measures designed to encourage the reporting and treatment of rape as a war crime. Pediatricians can work with international efforts to identify rape and exploitation of children as specific war crimes.[67] As long as leaders in the global society condone this action through their silence, it will continue unabated. Pediatricians can play a critical role in this regard. Further, they can and should provide reproductive and psychological support to victims of gender-based crimes.[64] Pediatricians may also be in a position to advocate for the special educational and mental health needs of former child soldiers. Pediatricians should join international efforts, whether at home or abroad, to prohibit the use of soldiers younger than 18 years.

It is likely that wherever a pediatrician practices, he or she will have patients whose family was deployed. Being aware of the deployment status, openly acknowledging and inquiring about the possible stresses facing the family (including the children), and being aware of local services to address concerns are important services to these families and their children.

The UNICEF *The State of the World's Children 2008: Child Survival* identifies 7 broad precepts regarding improved global health. These precepts contain economic implications and can serve as useful guides to pediatricians working abroad. Although a visiting pediatrician will generally not be in the position to develop entirely new systems, he or she can help make a difference, regardless of the size and cost of the health plan, by following these guiding precepts:

1. Focus on countries and communities with the highest mortality rates.
2. Package essential services to improve coverage and efficacy.
3. Actively engage the community to develop programs that will be sustained after the pediatrician leaves.
4. Provide a continuum of care linking communities to health care facilities.
5. Develop a strategic, result-oriented approach to health care in which maternal, infant, and child care are central.
6. Recognize the importance of political partnerships and the need to incorporate sustained financing into program development.
7. Work collaboratively with other health partners.

■ KEY POINTS

- As pediatricians from higher-, middle-, and lower-income countries partner to address global child health issues, the dynamic intersection of biological, sociocultural, and political-economic factors needs to be recognized and addressed through education, research, and practice.
- While poverty and the associated lack of basic resources for children and their families are integrally related to childhood morbidity and mortality, broader sociopolitical and economic conditions across and within countries can compound or ameliorate poor health outcomes. Social constructs of ethnicity, race, and gender lead to social and economic inequalities for large portions of the global population, affecting children's access to safe housing, education, adequate nutrition, and health care services. These inequalities can result in psychological distress and associated syndromes and lead to violence, civil unrest, and warfare and the consequential effects of these conditions on children and families.

- Access to pediatric, prenatal, and antenatal health care is affected by a range of factors including costs of services, number of trained providers, distance to available services and lack of transportation, language barriers, gender and ethnic inequalities, disparate health belief systems, distrust of government services, and disruptions to services during times of economic-political instability, civil unrest, and war.
- Through the WHO EPI, an estimated 80% of children worldwide receive available vaccines against tetanus, pertussis, measles, diphtheria, and polio. Lack of access to health care for women and children in some regions of the world continues to hinder the delivery of these basic lifesaving preventive measures.
- Multiple sociocultural and political-economic conditions result in homelessness and child labor. Children may be homeless and living with their family, or they may be street children living independently all or part of the time. These children have less access to health care services and are vulnerable to physical and sexual violence, substance abuse, and poor nutrition.
- Globally, the sex work industry generates approximately US $20 billion dollars per year, with one quarter of that from child workers. These children and adolescents are at a high risk for substance abuse, exposure to sexually transmitted infections and HIV, and victimization from physical and sexual violence.
- Modern warfare results in the disproportionate death of women and children, as 90% of war mortalities are civilian and 75% of those deaths are women and children.
- Children suffer a multitude of health-related negative outcomes associated with war and civil unrest during and after conflict.
  - Exposure to land mines and unexploded ordnance can result in death and severe injury.
  - Chemical warfare can result in birth defects through parents' exposure and continued concentration in soil and food sources.
  - In some countries, children are at risk of being conscripted as soldiers and girls and young women raped.
  - Children may become refugees and have inadequate access to food, water, education, and health care services.
  - Children suffer from emotional and psychological sequelae from their direct experiences with war as well as indirect experiences through the deployment, injury, or death of a parent.

- Pediatricians can serve in many roles to positively affect global child health.
  - Advocate for children's rights and access to health care.
  - Participate in research and practice that increase the number of evidence-based programs in middle- and lower-income countries.
  - Collaborate and volunteer with local non-governmental organizations and governments in developing and implanting interventions directed at vulnerable children (eg, those living on the street, engaged in sex work, engaged in political actions) to decrease risks such as exposure to land minds and ordnance, labor exploitation, and human trafficking.

■ REFERENCES

1. Ross RD, Delius R, Weinstein S, Rosenkrantz ER, Palaez de Pichardo N, Madera F. Forming a consortium to promote pediatric cardiac care in a developing country. *J Pediatr.* In press

2. Caldwell JC, Caldwell P, Caldwell BK, et al. The construction of adolescence in a changing world: implication for sexuality, reproduction, and marriage. *Stud Fam Plann.* 1998;29(2):137–153

3. Dehne KL, Riedner G. Adolescence: a dynamic concept. *Reprod Health Matters.* 2001;9(17):11–15

4. Myers WE. The right rights? Child labor in a globalizing world. *Ann Am Acad Pol Soc Sci.* 2001;575:38–55

5. Keats DM. Cross-cultural studies in child development in Asian contexts. *Cross-cultural Research.* 2000;34:339–352

6. Super CM, Harkness S. The developmental niche: a conceptualization at the interface of child and culture. *Int J Behav Dev.* 1986;9:545–570

7. Martin D. The meaning of children in Hong Kong. In: Tremayne S, ed. *Managing Reproductive Life: Cross-Cultural Themes in Sexuality and Fertility.* New York, NY: Berghanh; 2001:157–174

8. Boyden J. Some reflections on scientific conceptualisations of childhood and youth. In: Tremayne S, ed. *Managing Reproductive Life: Cross-Cultural Themes in Sexuality and Fertility.* New York, NY: Berghanh; 2001:175–193

9. Hollos M The cultural construction of childhood: changing conceptions among the Pare of Northern Tanzania. *Childhood.* 2002;9(2):167–182

10. Daley TC. The need for cross-cultural research on the pervasive developmental disorders. *Transcult Psychiatry.* 2002;39(4):531–550

11. Schousboe I. Local and global perspectives on the everyday lives of children. *Cultur Divers Ethnic Minor Psychol.* 2005;11(2):207–225

12. World Health Organization. Ten Facts on Global Burden of Disease. 2008. http://www.who.int/features/factfiles/global_burden/facts/en/index.html. Accessed December 4, 2008

13. World Health Organization. Ten Facts on Child Health. 2008. http://www.who.int/features/childhealth2/en/index.htm. Accessed December 4, 2008

14. United Nations Children's Fund. *State of the World's Children 2008.* Oxford, UK: Oxford University Press; 2008. http://www.unicef.org/sowc08. Accessed June 27, 2011

15. Pickett KE, Wilkinson RG. Child wellbeing and income inequality in rich societies: ecological cross sectional study. *BMJ.* 2007;335:1080–1088

16. World Health Organization. *Commission on Social Determinants of Health.* Geneva, Switzerland: World Health Organization; 2007. http://www.who.int/child_adolescent_health/news/archive/2007/29_10/en/print.html. Accessed January 30, 2009

17. Deaton A. Is world poverty falling? *Finance Dev.* 39(2): 4–7

18. Fiscella K, Franks P, Gold MR, Clancy CM. Inequality in quality: addressing socioeconomic, racial, and ethnic disparities in health care. *JAMA.* 2000;283:2579–2584

19. World Health Organization. *World Health Statistics 2008.* Geneva, Switzerland: World Health Organization; 2008

20. Greco G, Powell-Jackson T, Borghi J, Mills A. Countdown to 2015: assessment of donor assistance to maternal, newborn, and child health between 2003 and 2006. *Lancet.* 2008;371:1269

21. World Health Organization. Regional office for the Western Pacific. Expanded programme on immunisation. http://www.wpro.who.int/sites/epi. Accessed February 4, 2009

22. Azzam H, Kaljee LM. Vaccines and women: cultural and structural issues for acceptability. In. Murthy P, Lanford CL, eds. *Women's Global Health and Human Rights.* Sudbury, MA: Jones and Bartlett; 2010:311–328

23. Kaljee L, Thiem V, von Seidlein L, et al. Healthcare utilization for diarrhea and dysentery in actual and hypothetical cases, Nha Tran, Viet Nam: options and choises. *J Health Popul Nutr.* 2004;22:139–149

24. World Health Organization. *Antenatal Care in Developing Countries: Promises, Achievements, and Missed Opportunities. An Analysis of Trends, Levels, and Differentials 1990 to 2001.* Geneva, Switzerland: World Health Organization; 2003

25. Siddiqi N, Khan A, Nisar N, Siddiqi AF. Assessment of EPI (expanded programme of immunisation) vaccine coverage in a peri-urban slum. *J Pak Med Assoc.* 2007; 57(8):391–395

26. Roosihermiatie B, Nishyama M, Nakae K. Factors associated with TT (tetanus toxoid) immunization among pregnant women in Saparua, Maluku, Indonsia. *Southeast Asian J Trop Med Public Health.* 2000;31(1):91–95

27. World Health Organization. *Towards Universal Access. Scaling up Priority HIV/AIDS Interventions in the Health Sectors.* Geneva, Switzerland: World Health Organization; 2008. http://www.who.int/hiv/mediacentre/2008progressreport/en. Accessed February 4, 2009

28. Li X, Kaljee L, Zhang L, et al. Psychosocial consequences for children experiencing parental loss due to HIV/AIDS in Henan City. *AIDS Care.* In press

29. Andrews G, Skinner D, Zuma K. Epidemiology of health and vulnerability among children orphaned and made vulnerable by HIV/AIDS in sub-Saharan Africa. *AIDS Care.* 2006;18(3):269–276

30. Scanlon TJ, Tomkins A, Lynch MA, Scanlon F. Street children in Latin America. *Br J Med.* 1998;316(7144):1596–1600

31. World Health Organization. *Working with Street Children: A Training Package of Substance Use, Reproductive and Sexual Health including HIV/AIDS and STDs.* Geneva, Switzerland: World Health Organization

32. Bernat CJ. Children and the politics of violence in Haitian context: statis violence, scarcity and street child agency in Port-au-Prince. *Crit Anthropol.* 1999;19:121–140

33. Van Beers H. A plea for a child-centered approach in research with street children. *Childhood*. 1996;3(2):195–201

34. Ministry of Health, Kenya. *National Profile: The Status of Children's Environmental Health*. 2004

35. Amin S, Quayes MS, Rives J. Poverty and other determinants of child labor in Bangladesh. *South Econ J*. 2004;70(4):876–892

36. United Nations Children's Fund. Child protection from violence, exploitation, and abuse. http://www.unicef.org/protection/index_childlabour.html. Accessed February 2, 2009

37. World Health Organization. Child labour and adolescent workers. *The Global Occupational Health Network Newsletter*. Summer 2005;9

38. Barboza D. China says abusive child labor ring is exposed. *The New York Times*. http://www.nytimes.com/2008/05/01/world/asia/01china.html. Accessed February 2, 2009

39. Willis BM, Levy BS. Child prostitution: global health burden, research needs, and interventions. *Lancet*. 2002;359(9315):1417–1422

40. World Health Organization. *STIs/HIV: Sex Work in Asia*. Geneva, Switzerland: World Health Organization; 2001

41. Li X, Stanton B, Fang X, et al. HIV/STD risk behaviors and perceptions among rural-to-urban migrants in China. *AIDS Educ Prev*. 2004;16(6):538–556

42. Brown TL. *Sex Slaves: The Trafficking of Women in Asia*. London, England: Virago; 2000

43. Duong LB. *Viet Nam Children in Prostitution in Hanoi, Hai Phong, Ho Chi Minh City and Can Tho: A Rapid Assessment*. Bangkok, Thailand: International Labour Organization, International Programme on the Elimination of Child Labour; 2002

44. Hong Y, Li X. Behavioral studies of female sex workers in China: a literature review and recommendations for future research. *AIDS Behav*. 2008;12(4):623–636

45. United Nations Children's Fund. Poverty drives Kenyan girls into sex work. http://www.unicef.org/protection/kenya_46571.html. Accessed February 6, 2009

46. United Nations Children's Fund. Rescuing victims of child sex trafficking in the United Kingdom. http://www.unicef.org/protection/uk_46977.html. Accessed February 6, 2009

47. Di Leonardo M. *The Varieties of Ethnic Experience: Kinship, Class, and Gender Among California Italian-Americans*. Ithaca, NY: Cornell University; 1984

48. Brodkin K. *Sisters and Wives: The Past and Future of Sexual Equality*. Urbana, IL: University of Illinois Press; 1982

49. Horton S. Different subjects: the healthcare system's participation in the differential construction of the cultural citizenships of Cuban refugees and Mexican migrants. *Med Anthropol Q*. 2004;18(4):472–489

50. Spitzer D. In visible bodies: minority women, nurses, time, and the new economy of care. *Med Anthropol Q*. 2004;18(4):490–508

51. Flores G, Tomany-Korman SC. Racial and ethnic disparities in medical and dental health, access to care, and use of services in US children. *Pediatrics*. 2008;121(2):e286–e298

52. Rodriguez RL, Elliott MN, Vestal KD, Suttorp MJ, Schuster MA. Determinants of health insurance status for children of Latino immigrant and other US farm workers: findings from the National Agricultural Workers Survey. *Arch Pediatr Adolesc Med*. 2008;162(12):1175–1180

53. United Nations Children's Fund. *State of the World's Children 2008*. Oxford, UK: Oxford University Press; 2008

54. Rashad SF. *Durbolota* (weakness), *chinta rog* (worry illness), and poverty: explanations of white discharge among married adolescent women in an urban slum in Dhaka, Bangladesh. *Med Anthropol Q.* 2007;21(1):108–132

55. Brondolo E, Brady ver Halen N, Pencille M, Beatty D, Contrada RJ. Coping with racism: a selective review of the literature and a theoretical and methodological critique. *J Behav Med.* 2009;32(1): 64–88

56. Nemoto T, Iwamoto M, Colby D, et al. HIV related risk behaviors among female sex workers in Ho Chi Minh City, Vietnam. *AIDS Educ Prev.* 2008;20(5):435–453

57. Golembeski C, Fullilove R. Criminal (in)justices in the city and its associated health consequences. *Am J Public Health.* 2005;95(10):1701–1706

58. World Revolution Organization. Global issues overview: peace, war and conflict. http://worldrevolution.org/.../globalissuesoverview/overview2/PeaceNew.htm. Accessed February 16, 2009

59. International Committee of the Red Cross. *Child and War: International Review of the Red Cross.* No. 844. 2001;1163–1173

60. Smith C, Henrickson D. *Transformation of Warfare and Conflict in the Late Twentieth Century.* London, England: Center for Defense Studies, Kings' College; 1996

61. United Nations Children's Fund. *State of the World's Children.* Oxford, UK: Oxford University Press; 1996

62. Machel Ga. *Promotion and Protection of the Rights of Children: Impact of Armed Conflict on Children.* New York, NY: United Nations; 1996

63. Agadjanian V, Prata N. Civil war and child health: regional and ethnic dimensions of child immunization and malnutrition in Angola. *Soc Sci Med.* 2003;56:2515–2527.

64. World Health Organization. *Reproductive Health During Conflict and Displacement: A Guide for Program Managers.* Geneva, Switzerland: World Health Organization

65. Joshi PT, O'Donnell DA. Consequences of child exposure to war and terrorism. *Clin Child Fam Psycho Rev.* 2003;6(4):276–292

66. Bilukha OO, Brennan M, Anderson M, Tsitsaev Z, Murtazaeva E, Ibragimov R. Seen but not heard: injuries and deaths from landmines and unexploded ordinance in Chechnya 1994–2005. *Prehosp Disaster Med.* 2007;22:507–512

67. Black M. Girls and war: an extra vulnerability. *People Planet.* 1998;7(3):24–25

68. Davies M, Webb E. Promoting the psychological well-being of refugee children. *Clin Child Psychol Psychiatry.* 2000;5:541–556

69. United Nations. No conflict too remote to affect local environment. http://www.un.org/News/Press/docs/2004/sgsm9573.doc.htm. Accessed February 5, 2009

70. Ngo AD, Taylor R, Roberts CL, Nguyen TV. Association between Agent Orange and birth defects: systematic review and meta-analysis. *Int J Epidemiol.* 2006;35(5):1220–1230

71. World Health Organization. Dioxins and their effects on human health. http://www.who.int/mediacentre/factsheets/fs225/en. Accessed February 5, 2009

72. Schecter A, Quynh HT, Papke O, Tung KC, Constable JD. Agent Orange, dioxins and other chemicals of concern in Vietnam: update 2006. *J Occup Environ Med.* 2006;48(4):408–413

73. Chamie K, DeVere White RW, Lee D, Ok JH, Ellison LM. Agent Orange exposure, Vietnam War veterans, and the risk of prostate cancer. *Cancer.* 2008;113(9):2464–2470

74. United States Department of Veterans' Affairs. Agent Orange-Herbicide Exposure. http://www/vba/va/gov/bin/21/benefits/Herbicide/#bm03. Accessed February 5, 2009

75. Kohrt BA, Jordans MJ, Tol WA, et al. Comparison of mental health between former child soldiers and children never conscripted by armed groups in Nepal. *JAMA.* 2008;300:691–702

76. Ursano RJ, Norwod AE. *Emotional Aftermath of the Persian Gulf War: Veterans, Families, Communities, and Nations.* Washington, DC: American Psychiatric Press; 1996

77. Rentz ED, Marshall SW, Loomis D, Casteel C, Martin SL, Gibbs DA. Effect of deployment on the occurrence of child maltreatment in military and nonmilitary families. *Am J Epidem.* 2007;165:1199–1206

78. Siddiqi S, Haq IU, Ghaffar A, Akhtar T, Mahaini R. Pakistan's maternal and child health policy: analysis, lessons and the way forward. *Health Policy.* 2004;69:117–130

79. Bhutta ZA, Darmstadt GI, Hasan BS, Haws RA. Community-based interventions for improving perinatal and neonatal health in developing countries. A review of the evidence. *Pediatrics.* 2005;115(2 Suppl):519–617

80. Doyle J, Waters E, Yach D, et al. Global priority setting for Cochrane systematic reviews of health promotion and public health research. *J Epidemiol Commun Health.* 2005;59:193–197

81. Walker KE. Exploitation of children and young people through prostitution. *J Child Health Care.* 2002;6(3):182–188

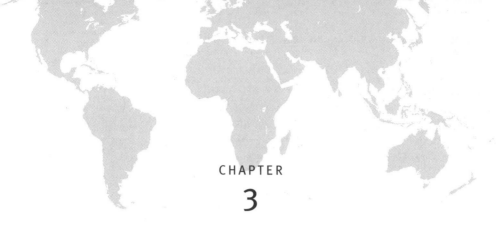

CHAPTER

3

Medical Anthropology

Jennifer R. Wies, PhD (corresponding author)
Britteny M. Howell, MA
Michelle Falk, MA

■ INTRODUCTION

Practices related to maintaining health or treating illness are grounded in a culture's belief system, which provides a framework for understanding and explaining illnesses, diseases, symptoms, causes, and treatments. This chapter explores the discipline of medical anthropology and provides cross-cultural examples of ethnomedical systems and the accompanying illness causation theories, diagnosis processes, and treatment beliefs. As partners in pediatric health care, medical anthropologists provide insight into the cultural context of health and healing and facilitate the incorporation of cross-cultural knowledge in medical education and health services research.[1]

■ ANTHROPOLOGY

Anthropology is broadly defined as the holistic study of humans, past and present. Anthropologists focus on culture as it exists throughout all levels and domains of societies throughout the world. Furthermore, Whyte states, "Anthropologists pride themselves on trying to elucidate other worldviews, showing that they are logical in their own terms if we just put aside our own preconceptions."[2] Therefore, a principle aim of the discipline of anthropology is to describe varying ways of life without devaluing the cultural differences found among societies.

Anthropologists use qualitative and quantitative methodologies to study the concept of culture. The primary qualitative methodology in anthropology is participant observation, wherein the anthropologist participates in everyday, community activities and observes the quotidian activities of the culture invisible to the casual observer.[3] The goal of participant observation is to gain an in-depth understanding of the study population and the power structures that affect a culture.

Culture

Within anthropology, a widely referenced definition of culture "is that complex whole which includes knowledge, belief, art, morals, law, custom, and any other capabilities and habits acquired by man as a member of society."[4] Culture includes the behaviors and ideas we take for granted in everyday life, from following traffic signals, to the language one speaks, to recognizing national symbols, such as the bald eagle in the United States. Culture encompasses our daily lives, consciously and unconsciously. It is not static; it is constantly responding to economic, political, and social forces.

Culture includes the traditions and customs that form and guide the beliefs and behaviors of people exposed to them. It is not biological, as individuals are not born knowing what actions are considered appropriate in their society. Culture is learned through communication and observation in the process of enculturation, wherein children and adults learn the norms, values, beliefs, customs, and traditions that govern behavior in society. Additionally, all cultures have health care systems. It is within the purview of cultural anthropology and, more specifically, medical anthropology to discover the epidemiology, health perceptions, definitions of illness and disease, role of the curer, and appropriate medical treatment within and across cultures.

■ MEDICAL ANTHROPOLOGY

Medical anthropology is the anthropologic study of health, illness, and healing across the range of human societies and over the course of the human experience.[5] It is centered on how different cultures explain the causes of illness, the types of treatment they deem acceptable, and to whom they turn for treatment.[6] The anthropologic study of health care systems and "primitive medicine" was pioneered in the 1940s by Erwin H. Ackerknecht. In these early days of anthropologic study, much of the literature was published in medical journals rather than anthropologic publications. The term *medical anthropology* came into use in 1963 with Norman Scotch's article, "Medical Anthropology," in the *Biennial Review of Anthropology*.[7]

Medical anthropology is the "application of anthropological theories and methods to questions of health, illness, medicine, and healing."[8] By focusing on the intersection of culture and health, medical anthropologists bring with them the qualitative methodologic experience indicative of anthropology and a commitment to exploring health, medicine, or healing in a cultural context. Medical anthropology builds on the theoretical bodies of anthropologic literature by "becoming a powerful tool for reassessing what is taken as natural and normal in connection with the human body."[9]

Additionally, medical anthropology places the body, as the center of health and illness, in the midst of the greater political, economic, and social webs of power in society. Heggenhougen asserts that "the gaze of medical anthropologists must also be critically inclusive and set on a whole range of social, political, and economic, as well as cultural facts."[10] In other words, he believes medical anthropology must use a holistic and multifaceted approach while maintaining critical reflexivity. This includes constantly assessing notions of class, race, gender, and age to better understand health, culture, and social situations. Thus, by critically analyzing illness in particular cultural settings, medical anthropology scrutinizes medical systems and health-related cultural understandings.[11] Moreover, medical anthropologists have focused their gaze on child and adolescent health across cultures.[12-14]

Health, Disease, and Illness

A guiding principle in medical anthropology is that health, disease, and illness are culturally defined. The World Health Organization defines health as "a state of complete physical, mental, and social well-being and not merely the absence of disease or infirmity."[15] A *disease* is a health threat that is externally verifiable, often through a clinical or scientific process.[16] It can be genetic in origin or caused by bacterial, viral, fungal, or parasitic agents, or other pathogens. Alternatively, *illness* is a condition of poor health felt by the individual—a perception.[6] Therefore, it is possible to become ill without a disease or have a disease without being ill. This nuance is important to consider when developing therapies, treatments, and healing prescriptions for patients of diverse cultural backgrounds. Overcoming cultural dissonance that exists among individuals from divergent medical systems is possible, as examples in this chapter will demonstrate.

■ CULTURE AND ETHNOMEDICAL SYSTEMS: BRIDGING BELIEF AND UNDERSTANDING

A medical system encompasses the "cultural beliefs and practices that are learned and shared by a group of people."[8] *Ethnomedicine* is defined as "culturally constructed medical systems."[8] Both definitions rely on the notion that a medical system is a product of the culture in which it exists. The central focus in ethnomedical approaches to studying healing is to understand the "group's conceptualizations of illness, its causes and cures, the role of healers, and the relationship between concepts of disease and cosmology."[17] The ethnomedical approach focuses on understanding how medical systems are constructed cross-culturally, how they are similar and different cross-culturally, and ways in which they reflect cultural norms and values. For example, spiritualism in Mexico is as culturally based as biomedicine because each system is specific to the culture's beliefs. The biomedical belief in prescription drugs is a cultural construct based on the metaphor that the body is a machine, while another culture might believe that the body is an extension of the natural environment and logically rely on herbal treatment. Since a fundamental theoretical foundation of medical anthropology is that all medical systems are bound by cultural beliefs, a disciplinary priority is to examine biomedicine as a form of ethnomedicine alongside all other medical systems.[18] All ethnomedical systems have a theory of illness causation or etiology, mechanisms for diagnosing the cause of illness, and norms for prescribing appropriate, diagnosis-based therapy.[8]

Etiology

All ethnomedical systems provide a framework for understanding the cause of disease and illness. There are 3 primary etiologic theories: naturalistic, personalistic, and emotionalistic.[19,20] Originally created to aid in the cross-cultural comparisons of non-Western medical systems, cultural etiologies of disease and illness help us understand the potential options for diagnosis and treatment.

Naturalistic Disease Theory

Naturalistic disease theories explain disease through scientifically identified agents. Health is accomplished through equilibrium and balance. Within this framework, diseases are thought to derive from natural forces, mainly causing an imbalance of bodily elements. This imbalance may be caused by cold, heat, wind, and dampness.[19] Because of the causes attributed to disease and illness in naturalistic theories, a specialist in symptomatic treatment is required for healing. Preventive measures can generally be described as "things not to do," such as abstaining from smoking or drinking. Hippocrates' humoral system of health, which revolves around the balance of 4 bodily liquids, is considered a naturalistic disease framework. Belief in the humoral system is centralized in Asia, Latin American, and parts of the Middle East. Additionally, Western biomedicine is considered an ethnomedical system that uses the naturalistic disease theory characterized by externally testable variables observed and measured within controlled conditions.

Personalistic Disease Theory

Personalistic disease theory explains disease and illness as caused by the active or purposeful intervention of an agent. That agent may be human (eg, witch, sorcerer), nonhuman, or supernatural. Individuals are victims of personalistic disease for reasons known only to them. Consequently, personalistic disease etiology remains at the individual, not population, level. Personalistic disease theory situates poor health as the result of individual behavior, wherein the victim acted in such a way as to cause the illness.

Emotionalistic Disease Theory

According to Foster and Anderson,[20] there exists a third disease theory in which emotional states are thought to cause disease and illness; this is referred to as emotionalistic disease theory. In this framework, intense anger, jealousy, shame, grief, fright, and other extreme emotions result in poor health. Symptoms are psychological and physical in nature, as someone may report disassociation from daily life, persistent lethargy, and other withdrawal symptoms. In addition, individuals report loss of appetite, sudden weight loss, and insomnia. Healers include shamans, household members, and other culturally appropriate community members.

Diagnosis and Treatment in Cross-cultural Perspective: Culture-Bound Syndromes

To illustrate the variety of options available when health is situated within diverse ethnomedical systems, the following examples of culture-bound syndromes unravel the mechanisms for diagnosing and treating disease and illness cross-culturally. Culture-bound syndromes are illnesses specific to a particular society or cultural tradition and treated in a specific way.[21] The following examples illustrate the complexity of maintaining good health in an ever-increasingly globalized world where individuals and households experience health and wellness through multiple etiologic lenses. In the course of medical care, a patient may or may not describe an ethnomedical belief system with causal or etiologic information. Indeed, a patient may begin to describe poor health conditions by explaining the culturally appropriate mode of treatment or therapy, which will in turn assist the medical provider with framing the individual's course of care. Therefore, the examples also provide cultural information that sheds light on pathways to culturally appropriate and complementary treatment and therapy options for the practicing biomedical physician.

Nervios

Nervios, or nerves, is an emotionalistic disease found throughout Latin America and the Mediterranean. Nervios attacks include shaking, feelings of heat or pressure in the chest, difficulty moving limbs, feelings of the mind "going blank," and loss of consciousness (Table 3-1).

ILLNESS	SYMPTOMS	POSSIBLE CAUSES
Nervios	Shaking, feelings of heat/pressure in the chest, difficulty moving limbs, mind "going blank," loss of consciousness, heartache, extreme sadness, feelings of despair and loss, anger	Biomedical explanation includes anxiety, depression, panic attacks stemming from low social or socioeconomic status.
Brain Fag	Visual (blinded by light) or auditory sensory disturbance, impairment of intellectual activity, emotional disturbances, inability to read, inability to understand or recall what is being read, head and neck pain, fatigue	Pressure for group achievement in schools but individual personality, motivation, emotion, stimulant use, and sleep deprivation may be factors.
Susto	Appetite and weight loss, distraction, lethargy, diarrhea, vomiting, fever, sleeplessness, crying	Believed by locals to be caused by the loss of the soul through sudden fright; no agreed-on biomedical explanation
Latah	Overreacting to stimulus, dropping objects, shouting inappropriate words, displaying violent body movements, mimicking, assuming a defensive posture	Believed by locals to be caused by the loss of the soul through sudden fright; biomedical explanation includes social factors such as marginality, disorder, transcendence.
Mal'Uocchiu	Yawning, hiccups, eye twitches, nervous tension, mental confusion, depression, headaches, stomach cramps, exhaustion	Internal evil power caused by envy, jealousy, and anger that emanates through a person's eyes causing illness; no agreed-on biomedical explanation

Table 3-1. Summary of Culture-Bound Illnesses

Symptoms result from a slow buildup stemming from the problems one experiences in life, especially concerning household and financial issues, culminating in an acute attack. Nervios attacks afflict adults and children. Children experience heartache, extreme sadness, and feelings of despair and loss that may lead to acts of anger. Reports indicate that nervios can result in children harming themselves or attempting suicide.

Nervios attacks are more likely to occur in children coping with a parent that has migrated, often to the United States. Children experience frustration, lack of control, and feelings of abandonment as their parents, particularly their fathers, migrate for work.[22] Nervios often persists in children even after their households are reunited, a result of the constant uncertainty inherent in today's globalized world. The social, political, and economic status of Latinos and Latino Americans reveals a widespread "sense of hopelessness, helplessness, and lack of control,"[23] often experienced disproportionately by women,[24] that manifests as nervios.

Nervios is an example that illustrates the concept of social suffering that "results from what political, economic, and institutional power does to people and, reciprocally, from how these forms of power themselves influence responses to social problems."[25] Through ethnographic research with individuals afflicted by nervios, we are able to connect the illness to the transnational migrant work networks that result from global economic inequalities. Thus, the illness, while experienced by individuals, is also bound to populations most affected by larger, structural factors.[26]

Brain Fag

Brain fag syndrome was first described by Prince[27] among Nigerian students. The name *brain fag* is derived from his patients describing the cause of their illness as fatigue of the brain from extensive brain work. Symptoms generally arise during periods of intense reading or studying or following periods of intense study.[27,28] The syndrome has the following 4 classes of symptoms: sensory disturbances, impairment of intellectual activity, emotional disturbances, and somatic complaints. Intellectual impairment manifests itself as an inability to read, grasp content, or recall what was just read. Sensory disturbances are chiefly visual but sometimes auditory. The patient's vision is often altered in a way he finds difficult to describe, sometimes using the phrase "blinded by a light." Most commonly, patients complain of head and neck pain as well as a general weakness of the body and easy fatigability. Emotional effects are the least stressed but could be expressed as depressive symptoms[27] (Table 3-1).

Onset is usually gradual with somatic symptoms arising prior to intellectual impairment. It is seen particularly among Western Africans in non-African educational systems where success is measured by individual achievement. West African societies are collectivist and often measure success by the achievements of the group. Genetics, intelligence, or parental literacy are not thought to be directly related to the eitiology.[27] Instead, this syndrome may have a multifactorial etiology including personality, motivation and emotion, stimulant use, and sleep deprivation.[28]

Susto

Susto is a fright illness believed to cause soul loss after a person experiences a fearful situation or a sudden, loud disturbance. It is similar to nervios, though distinct in its acuteness.[29] Commonly found in Latin America and Latin American immigrant populations, symptoms include loss of appetite, weight loss, distraction, and lethargy,[30] as well as diarrhea, vomiting, fever, sleeplessness, and crying in children[31] (Table 3-1). In children, susto is often cured by their mothers, an elder female, or shamans called curanderos who perform rituals that call the soul back to the body and aim to restore the psychological and spiritual balance of the patient.[32] Mothers with children suffering from susto report that biomedical physicians cannot cure the disease because the cause of susto is not pathological; therefore, very few children are taken to a biomedical doctor's office.[31]

In addition, susto sufferers have higher rates of morbidity and mortality than control groups.[30] Individuals who suffer from susto are at great risk for suffering from poor mental health.[29] Interestingly, individuals with susto do not meet the biomedical criteria for depression, as was commonly thought, although individuals with depression are likely to report previous experience with susto (and nervios). It is hypothesized that individuals use the culture-bound syndrome of susto to express psychological distress and seek assistance in an effort to curtail the likelihood that the illness escalates to depression.[29]

Latah

Latah is characterized by the sufferer's unusual startle response to fright; the individual appears to be overreacting to the stimulus by dropping objects, shouting inappropriate words, displaying violent body movements, mimicking, or assuming a defensive posture (Table 3-1). Latah is reported primarily among populations in Malaysia and is also found in Myanmar, Thailand, the Philippines, Siberia, southwestern Africa, and Japan.[33] In Malaysia, sudden fright is believed to make a person susceptible to the intrusion of supernatural forces and is known to be an involuntary response. It is often associated with local witchcraft beliefs, shamanism, and the idea that the individual can gain religious insight and power through a "loss of self."[34] In all parts of the world where an exaggerated startle response is culturally defined, locals believe fright can cause soul loss that may lead to the invasion of evil spirits. Curative practices are aimed at expelling evil spirits as well as recalling the victim's soul back to the body. Children are especially vulnerable to latah as they are thought to startle more easily.

Anthropologists attribute this startle reaction to a number of social factors, such as marginality, disorder, and transcendence. Kenny (1985) states that latah is an appropriate way for people to express their socially marginal position to others.[34] Shamans express their ability to initiate contact with the supernatural, while socially marginal people are able to express their marginality and distress while publicly acknowledging the situation; others may express latah as a way to engage in socially unacceptable behaviors such as ribald language, jokes, and mimicry.

Mal'Uocchiu

One of the most well-known examples of personalistic disease is evil eye. Many cultures throughout the world believe in evil eye, but it is concentrated in the circum-Mediterranean region.[35] Evil eye is known as mal'uocchiu among Sicilian Canadians, mal ojo in Latin America, vaskania in Greece, and mal occhio in Italy. It involves envy and an aggressor's desire (explicit or implicit) to have something in the victim's possession (eg, items, emotions, beauty). Women, babies, and small children are particularly susceptible to evil eye. Evil eye can be inflicted intentionally and unintentionally. It is generally believed to be an internal evil power that emanates through a person's eyes, causing illness, and anyone can be capable of casting evil eye. Treatment is usually performed by a supernatural healer who chants secret prayers and incantations while performing anointment rituals.[36]

Among Sicilian Canadians, mal'uocchiu victims are thought to be in a state of disequilibrium. Their internal strength exceeded or fell below a particular level because of a physical disability or previous exposure, making them susceptible. Children are believed to be particularly vulnerable because they have not yet developed the internal strength to prevent illness. Informants disclosed that mal'uocchiu begins with presymptomatic processes such as uncontrollable yawning, hiccups, and eye twitches. Within a day of exposure, symptoms include nervous tension, mental confusion, depression, headaches, stomach cramps, and exhaustion[37] (Table 3-1). Intentionally caused symptoms usually appear within 3 to 5 days after the person is afflicted. Although the symptoms are the same as an unintentional affliction, they are much more severe and longer lasting. Intentional cases do not run a natural course and severe cases can lead to mental disorders, paralysis, or death.[37]

With an understanding of ethnomedical systems and etiologies, the examples in this chapter illustrate that various symptoms are interpreted and explained in different ways by people with diverse cultural worldviews. The diversity of symptoms that individuals express is indeed linked to their beliefs of the illness causation and is subsequently connected to their diagnosis. Thus, familiarizing oneself with the possibilities for causation models and diagnosis options necessarily leads to reflections concerning treatment and therapy. For example, nervios is categorized as an emotionalistic disease caused by mental distress, but the diagnostic symptoms of weight loss and diarrhea are 2 commonly accepted health problems within a biomedical system.

■ APPLYING MEDICAL ANTHROPOLOGY TO CHILD HEALTH

Due to globalization, acculturation, and the increase in biomedical training worldwide, cultural groups often believe in multiple disease theory systems. Believing in and practicing multiple disease causation theories is referred to as *pluralistic health care practices,* as Pelto and Pelto[38] assert.

> *In most areas where traditional care predominated in the 1940s and 1950s, there is now widespread acceptance of many aspects of cosmopolitan medicine, often without any apparent sharp reduction in traditional beliefs and healing practices. Studies in Asia, Africa, and Latin America have shown that families utilize both indigenous and cosmopolitan health care resources, sometimes serially, sometimes simultaneously.*

Therefore, the challenges for the biomedical clinician are to seek an understanding of a person's disease causation theory, validate the reality of that belief, and seek mutually acceptable modes of therapy and treatment.[39] Medical anthropologists partner with biomedical practitioners, indigenous healers, and health care institutions around the world to incorporate the cultural diversity of health and healing beliefs. The partnership between medical anthropologists and medical educators is leading to improvements in the quality of health care through an "anthropology devoted to helping health practitioners do their work better."[40]

Medical Education: Incorporating Cross-cultural Content to Enhance Patient Care

A result of this collaborative research with medical practitioners is the introduction of the culture concept and various ethnomedical systems in the medical curricula to reflect the plurality on health care practices worldwide. Institutions commonly require medical and nursing students to complete introductory anthropology or medical anthropology courses to increase exposure to diverse cultures. Additionally, the Accreditation Council for Graduate Medical Education has mandated cross-cultural education in medical training.

In medical education, books such as Anne Fadiman's *The Spirit Catches You and You Fall Down: A Hmong Child, Her American Doctors, and the Collision of Two Cultures*[41] and Emily Benedek's *Beyond the Four Corners of the World: A Navajo Woman's Journey*[42] describe the tensions and misunderstandings between indigenous Hmong cultural beliefs and Western biomedical culture. Both texts present compelling arguments for cultural competency, sensitivity, and humility in providing health care. Effective cross-cultural medical education uses anthropologic understandings of the vitality of culture and focuses on the acquisition of skills, such as knowledge of various disease etiologies, diagnosis models, and treatment options, to develop collaborative relationships between the clinician and the patient to develop mutually acceptable treatment plans.

Furthermore, medical anthropologists have worked to ensure that medical education does not place culture as a protagonist when different notions of health and healing collide, which could lead one to blame culture as you would any other character for disastrous and tragic outcomes. Medical anthropology serves to remind us that "'Culture' is not a 'thing,' somewhere 'out there,' that books are 'about.' It is a process of making meanings, making social relations, and making the world that we inhabit, in which all of us are engaged—when we read and teach, or when we diagnose and treat...."[43]

Improving the Pediatric Health Care Delivery System

Medical anthropologists are also concerned with improving children's health services research by examining the "structure, processes, and outcomes of health services for children for the ultimate purpose of improving the health and well-being of children."[44]

Specifically, research exposing communication dissonance between providers and the patient or household members is a focus of medical anthropology. Foundational to this body of literature is the notion that improved communication, at all levels, is a vehicle for enhancing the delivery of health services. This research demonstrates that as a result of increased trust and disclosure, communication between providers and household members improves the quality of care and outcomes for the pediatric patient.[45] Furthermore, medical anthropology research has illustrated that it is important for communication in the clinical setting to meet the patient's satisfaction, which leads to more positive pediatric patient outcomes.[46–48]

Therefore, medical anthropologists facilitate efforts to include the patient and family in diagnosis, creating treatment plans, decision-making, and evaluating medical programs.[49–51] A pediatrician who understands the concepts and practices of different cultures will be better at communicating with the patient and her household and improving health outcomes.[52] Similarly, pediatricians that reflexively recognize their health care system as one that is culturally constructed will be better positioned to assist their patients in negotiating possible cultural divides.[53,54]

Through the lens of medical anthropology, this chapter focused on the intersection of culture and health. Medical anthropologists study culture to understand the ways that cultural groups diagnose and treat illness and disease. When unpacked, the relationship between culture and health can provide valuable insight into factors that differently affect the health of populations living in a culture, structural factors that affect some cultural populations disproportionately, and ways health care providers can improve their sensitivity to cultural difference to provide effective health interventions. Threads of culture connect populations by weaving different historical, political, and economic experiences. Medical anthropologists, with their commitment to understanding variety and difference and to placing concepts and social situations in a holistic framework, are uniquely qualified to unpack these variables in ways that makes them useful for pediatric practice and research.

■ KEY POINTS

- Anthropologists study *culture,* defined as behaviors, ideas, and processes that guide everyday life.
- Medical anthropologists examine the relationship between culture and health, illness, and healing.
- All cultures possess an ethnomedical belief system that includes theories of illness causation, mechanisms for diagnosing cause of illness, and norms for prescribing appropriate, diagnosis-based therapy.

- Culture-bound syndromes, such as nervios, are often treated with pluralistic medical systems and therefore require health care practitioners to negotiate mutually agreeable, collaborative treatment plans.
- Medical anthropologists apply their cross-cultural research to enhance medical education and strengthen health services to improve pediatric care and outcomes across the globe.

■ REFERENCES

1. Sobo EJ. Prevention and healing in the household: the importance of socio-cultural context. In: Sobo EJ, Kurtin PS, eds. *Child Health Services Research: Applications, Innovations, and Insights.* San Francisco, CA: Jossey-Bass; 2003:67–119

2. Whyte SR. Constructing epilepsy: images and contexts in East Africa. In: Ingstad B, Whyte SR, eds. *Disability and Culture.* Berkeley, CA: University of California Press; 1995:226–245

3. Burawoy M, ed. *Ethnography Unbound: Power and Resistance in the Modern Metropolis.* Berkely, CA: University of California Press; 1991

4. Tylor EB. *Primitive Culture: Researches Into the Development of Mythology, Philosophy, Religion, Art, and Custom.* London, England: J Murray: Harper & Row; 1871

5. Janzen JM. *The Social Fabric of Health: An Introduction to Medical Anthropology.* Boston, MA: McGraw Hill; 2002

6. Helman C. *Culture, Health, and Illness: An Introduction for Health Professionals.* 3rd ed. Oxford, UK: Butterworth-Heinemann; 1994

7. Scotch N. Medical anthropology. *Biennial Review of Anthropology.* 1963;3:30–68

8. Brown PJ, Barrett RL, Padilla MB. Medical anthropology: an introduction to the fields. In: Brown PJ, ed. *Understanding and Applying Medical Anthropology.* Mountain View, CA: Mayfield Publishing Co; 1998:10–19

9. Lindenbaum S, Lock M, eds. *Knowledge, Power, and Practice: The Anthropology of Medicine and Everyday Life.* Berkeley, CA: University of California Press; 1993

10. Heggenhougen HK. More than just "interesting!": anthropology, health and human rights. *Soc Sci Med.* 2000;50:1171–1175

11. Good B. *Medicine, Rationality, and Experience: An Anthropological Perspective.* Cambridge, MA: Cambridge University Press; 1994

12. Scheper-Hughes N, ed. *Child Survival: Anthropological Perspectives on the Treatment and Maltreatment of Children.* Boston, MA: Kluwer Academic Publishers; 1987

13. Panter-Brick C. Street children, human rights, and public health: a critique and future directions. *Ann Rev Anthropol.* 2002;31:147–171

14. Scheper-Hughes N, Sargent CF, eds. *Small Wars: The Cultural Politics of Childhood.* Berkeley, CA: University of California Press; 1998

15. World Health Organization. *Constitution of the World Health Organization.* Geneva, Switzerland: World Health Organization; 1946

16. Hahn RA. The state of federal health statistics on racial and ethnic groups. In: Brown PJ, ed. *Understanding and Applying Medical Anthropology.* Mountain View, CA: Mayfield Publishing; 1998:261–266

17. Rubel AJ, Hass MR. Ethnomedicine. In: Sargent CF, Johnson TM, eds. *Medical Anthropology: Contemporary Theory and Method.* Rev ed. Westport, CT: Praeger; 1996:113–130

18. Rhodes LA. Studying biomedicine as a cultural system. In: Sargent CF, Johnson TM, eds. *Medical Anthropology: Contemporary Theory and Method.* Rev ed. Westport, CT: Praeger; 1996:165–180

19. Foster G. Disease etiologies in non-Western medical systems. *Am Anthropol.* 1976;78:773–782

20. Foster G, Anderson B. *Medical Anthropology.* New York, NY: McGraw Hill; 1978

21. Hughes CC. Culture-bound or construct-bound? In: Simons RC, Hughes CC, eds. *The Culture-Bound Syndromes: Folk Illnesses of Psychiatric and Anthropological Interest.* Boston, MA: D. Reidel Publishing Co; 1985:3–24

22. Pribilsky J. Nervios and 'modern childhood': migration and shifting contexts of child life in the Ecuadorian Andes. *Childhood.* 2001;8:251–273

23. DeLaCancela V, Guarnaccia PJ, Carillo JE. Psychosocial distress among Latinos: a critical analysis of ataques de nervios. *Humanity Society.* 1986;10:431–557

24. Baer RD, Weller SC, Alba Gd, et al. A cross-cultural approach to the study of the folk illness nervios. *Cult Med Psychiatry.* 2003;27:315–337

25. Kleinman A, Das V, Lock MM, eds. *Social Suffering.* Berkeley, CA: University of California Press; 1997

26. Guarnaccia PJ, Lewis-Fernandez, Roberto M, Rivera M. Toward a Puerto Rican popular nosology: nervios and ataque de nervios. *Cult Med Psychiatry.* 2003;27:339–366

27. Prince R. The "brain fag" syndrome in Nigerian students. *J Mental Sci.* 1960;106: 559–569

28. Morakinyo O. A psychophysical theory of a psychiatric illness (the brain fag syndrome) associated with study among Africans. *J Nerv Ment Dis.* 1980;168:84–89

29. Weller SC, Baer RD, Garcia GdA, Javier SR, Ana L. Susto and nervios: expressions for stress and depression. *Cult Med Psychiatry.* 2008;32:406–420

30. Rubel AJ, O'Nell CW, Collado-Ardon R. *Susto: A Folk Illness.* Berkley, CA: University of Califonia Press; 1991

31. Baer R, Bustillo M. Susto and mal de ojo among Florida farmworkers: emic and etic perspectives. *Med Anthropol Q.* 1993;7:90–100

32. Trotter R. Folk medicine in the southwest: myths and medieval facts. *Postgrad Med.* 1985;78:167–179

33. Simons RC. The resolution of the Latah paradox. In: Simons R, Hughes CC, eds. *The Culture-Bound Syndromes: Folk Illnesses of Psychiatric and Anthropological Interest.* Boston, MA: D. Reidel Publishing Co; 1985:43–62

34. Kenny MG. Paradox lost: the Latah problem revisited. In: Simons RC, Hughes CC, eds. *The Culture-Bound Syndromes: Folk Illnesses of Psychiatric and Anthropological Interest.* Boston, MA: D. Reidel Publishing Company; 1985:63–76

35. Winkelman M. *Culture and Health: Applying Medical Anthropology.* San Francisco, CA: Jossey-Bass; 2009

36. Lykiardopoulos A. The evil eye: towards an exhaustive study. *Folklore.* 1981;92:221–230

37. Migliore S. Evil eye or delusions: on the "consistency" of folk models. *Med Anthropol Q.* 1983;14:4–9

38. Pelto P, Pelto G. Studying knowledge, culture and behavior in applied medical anthropology. *Med Anthropol Q.* 1997;11(2):147–163

39. Foulks E. Comment on Foster's "Disease etiologies in non-Western medical systems". *Am Anthropol.* 1978;80:660–661

40. Chrisman NJ, Johnson TM. Clinically applied anthropology. In: Sargent CF, Johnson TM, eds. *Medical Anthropology: Contemporary Theory and Method.* Rev ed. Westport, CT: Praeger; 1996:88–109

41. Fadiman A. *The Spirit Catches You and You Fall Down: Hmong Child, Her American Doctors, and the Collision of Two Cultures.* New York, NY: Farrar, Straus, and Giroux; 1997

42. Benedek E. *Beyond the Four Corners of the World: A Navajo Woman's Journey.* New York, NY: Random House; 1995

43. Taylor JS. Confronting "culture" in medicine's "culture of no culture". *Acad Med.* 2003;78:555–559

44. Kurtin PS. An introduction to applied child health services research: connecting knowledge and action. In: Sobo EJ, Kurtin PS, eds. *Child Health Services Research: Applications, Innovations, and Insights.* San Francisco, CA: Jossey-Bass; 2003:3–24

45. Prussing E, Sobo EJ, Walker E, Dennis K, Kurtin P. Communicating with pediatricians about complementary/alternative medicine: perspectives from parents of children with Down syndrome. *Ambul Pediatr.* 2004;4:488–494

46. Eisenberg J. Sociologic influences on medical decision making by clinicians. *Ann Intern Med.* 1979;90:957–964

47. Stewart M, Brown J, Boon H, Galajda J, Meredith L, Sangster M. Evidence on patient-doctor communication. *Cancer Prev Control.* 1999;3:25–30

48. Smedley BD, Stith AY, Nelson AR, eds. *Unequal Treatment: Confronting Racial and Ethnic Disparities in Health Care.* Washington, DC: National Academy Press; 2003

49. Britto M, DeVellis R, Hornung R, DeFriese G, Atherton H, Slap G. Health care preferences and priorities of adolescents with chronic illnesses. *Pediatrics.* 2004;114:1272–1280

50. Vaughn L, Forbes J, Howell B. Enhancing home visitation programs: input from a participatory evaluation using Photovoice. *Infants Young Child.* 2009;22:132–145

51. Wade S, Michaud L, Maines T. Putting the pieces together: preliminary efficacy of a family problem-solving intervention for children with traumatic brain injury. *J Head Trauma Rehabil.* 2006;21:57–67

52. Carillo J, Green A, Betancourt J. Cross-cultural primary care: a patient-based approach. *Ann Intern Med.* 1999;130:829–834

53. Sobo EJ, Seid M. Cultural issues in health services delivery: what kind of "competence" is needed? *Ann Behav Sci Med Ed.* 2003;9:97–100

54. Sobo EJ, Kurtin P. Variation in physicians' definitions of the competent parent and other barriers to guideline adherence: the case of pediatric minor head injury management. *Soc Sci Med.* 2003;56:2479–2491

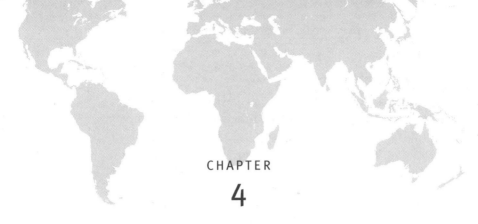

Cultural Sensitivity, Awareness, and Competency in Pediatric Practice

Lisa M. Vaughn, PhD

■ INTRODUCTION

There is a significant need for culturally competent health care services to address existing health disparities for minority children and mend fragmented systems of care in which some receive better services than others; however, cultural competency is difficult to achieve with families and children. Culture itself is translated through parents, family, and community members. Therefore, pediatricians may not see a family's cultural differences because they are not physically apparent (eg, belief systems, religion, socioeconomic status). In addition, if children are primarily raised in one culture and their parents in another, the children may have a differing cultural presentation than their parents.

Pediatricians may not understand the culture of some families and children because they maintain stereotypical views of particular culturally different groups. Ultimately, if caregivers do not feel understood or do not feel involved in their children's health care, the result may be that families are marginalized from the health care system, do not function as good advocates for their children, and engage in poor medical adherence to their children's treatment. Complex global changes in demographic diversity, cultural health beliefs, decreased health equity, pediatric practice abroad, and relevant policies and standards demand cultural sensitivity, awareness, and competence in pediatric practice.

■ CHANGING DEMOGRAPHICS

We are an increasingly diverse society with an explosion of social, linguistic, religious, and cultural differences. The startling rate of globalization is due to advances in economic and geopolitical activity, telecommunications, and transportation. Worldwide, there are changes in the composition of populations with increases in foreign-born children and families from diverse nations. In the United States, it is estimated that by 2020, close to half of school-aged Americans will be of a racial or ethnic minority group.[1] This diversity is further complicated by increases in the number of internationally adopted children in Europe and the United States as well as the growing numbers of multicultural families in which parents come from different backgrounds (eg, nationality, religion, race, ethnicity) and children display hybridization and alternation between 2 or more cultures.

These growing diverse communities have varied health beliefs, values, and practices, as well as diverse social factors that affect their lives. Countries like the United States, Canada, Australia, and Britain have large Southeast and East Asian communities. Large immigrant communities like these, and like existing African and Caribbean communities in Britain, can lead to an increased perception of cultural distance within societies. In addition, growing multicultural societies create culture shock and opportunities for intercultural adjustment. These phenomena do not only affect immigrants adjusting to new cultures but also people within society who interact with these diverse communities in their daily lives.

Along with foreign-born families to societies worldwide, linguistic diversity is on the rise. There are an estimated 5,000 to 6,000 different languages spoken worldwide. In the United States, there are more than 329 languages spoken, with 32 million people speaking a language other than English at home.[2] Eight-hundred seventy-four million people across 16 countries speak Mandarin Chinese—the most spoken language in the world—as a native language. Hindi is the next most spoken language in the world, with approximately 366 million people across 17 countries. Following is 341 million people speaking English in 104 countries and approximately 322 million to 358 million native Spanish speakers across 43 countries.[3] It is clear that there are many multicultural nations with multiple languages spoken daily requiring increased health services resources.

■ CULTURAL HEALTH BELIEFS

Cultural backgrounds significantly affect people's beliefs and attributions about health, illness, and medical care in ways that have important implications for health care professionals.[4-6] African Americans in the United States are likely to make external attributions related to the will of God, destiny, and the power of prayer.[7] On the other hand, there is evidence that white Americans are likely to attribute disease to individual behavior and perceive treatment as mechanistic and unrelated to religion, family, or other systems.[4,8]

The varied belief systems that exist across cultural groups differ in multiple factors, including disease models, perceptions of providers, specific disorders and diagnoses, and the use of unique treatments and health care practices. Some traditional cultures attribute a soul to all natural objects including human beings. These cultures may perceive illness as stemming from moral and theologic thought, with the ultimate cause of illness being disharmony in the relationship between the sick person and another being.[9] Individuals of the Mixtec culture in Mexico believe that illness can occur through exposure to disruptive forces, including extreme temperature, negative social relationships and interactions, or evil spiritual entities.[10] Helman suggests that people attribute causes of illness to factors within 1 of 4 spheres.[11]

1. Factors within individuals themselves (ie, bad habits or negative emotional states)
2. Factors within the natural environment (ie, pollution and germs)
3. Factors associated with others or the social world (ie, interpersonal stress, medical facilities, and actions of others)
4. Supernatural factors (God, destiny, and indigenous beliefs such as witchcraft or voodoo)[11]

Differences in causal attribution translate to differences in perceived cures. Because Westerners tend to attribute illness to individual or environmental factors, they typically believe that illness can be treated without reference to family, community, or deities. People from nonindustrialized countries often attribute illness externally to social factors or the will of God or the supernatural and, as such, are likely to have a much different perception of what is an appropriate or effective treatment.

A British study by Furnham demonstrates the wide variety of health-related beliefs that exist across cultural groups. In the study, religiosity, age, political beliefs, and comfort with alternative medicine were all significantly associated with beliefs about health and illness.[12] Older participants emphasized external causes for illness, and religious individuals tended to believe in supernatural causes. Across cultures, even greater differences were found in health beliefs and attributions. With comparisons across Britain and African countries (South Africa and Uganda), Furnham found that British participants regarded fatalistic factors as unimportant, and African participants sometimes attributed illness to "evil others." Despite the differences there were also similarities; African and British participants identified social stressors as factors associated with illness.[4] A more recent study examined health beliefs in British Caucasians and British Gujarati Indian immigrants and found little difference in health-related attributions associated with social and environmental factors. However, British Gujarati Indian immigrants were more likely to incorporate supernatural explanations for illness.[13]

■ HEALTH EQUITY

Families and children worldwide face stark realities of health disparities and commiserate lack of health equity. In general, there are widening disparities in health and human rights worldwide and simultaneously patient populations are becoming increasingly more vulnerable (advancing age, growing diversity, higher burden of chronic illness, and socioeconomic decline[14]). The big problems in global health are defined as HIV/AIDS, malnutrition, lack of access to medical care, and lack of adequate resources.[15]

There is much less research on health disparities in ethnic minority youths in the United States and worldwide. Relatively few studies address whether minority youths receive important procedures and are prescribed intensive treatments at the same rate as majority youths. However, there is some evidence that disparities exist in this area. For example, US data indicate that the ethnicity of children with asthma is associated with physicians not adhering to national care guidelines,[16] minority adolescents receiving fewer services,[17] racial or ethnic differences in the probability of children receiving prescription medications,[18] and US Latino children receiving lower quality health care, including fewer laboratory tests, radiographic examinations, and prescriptions for nebulizers after asthma-related hospitalizations.[19]

The American Academy of Pediatrics (AAP) Committee on Pediatric Research specifically called for more research on racial, ethnic, and socioeconomic disparities in treatment and clinical outcomes for minority youths.[20] In fact, there is minimal existing literature on disparities in treatment or care for children with type 1 diabetes.

To fully understand the severity of health disparities and increase health equity globally, there must be joint consideration of race and ethnicity combined with social class and culture. Many social and contextual factors affect how patients view their illness and this may affect how and if the treatment regimen is followed (medical adherence). In addition, health and well-being are increasingly recognized as contextually based, composed of a complex set of factors (eg, poverty; air pollution; racism; inadequate housing and income inequalities; other social, economic, and physical environment factors) that contribute to the disproportionate burden of disease experienced by marginalized communities.[21] Globally, pediatricians must practice cultural competence so that these global health disparities are addressed, thereby increasing health equity worldwide.

■ GLOBAL PEDIATRICS

With amplified internationalization and globalization and simultaneous world population growth and migration, the world has become a smaller place. As such, pediatric trainees and physicians across the United States have traveled and experienced more of the world than most other generations. In addition, educational institutions and organizations have a growing interest in addressing global health challenges and disparities,[22] which takes pediatricians increasingly into non-US settings. The proliferation of study-abroad programs, international travel, incorporation of global health content into medical curricula, medical training occurring outside of the birth country, and international humanitarian efforts[23–28] all require the practice of cultural competency in a different cultural context than at home.

Cultural sensitivity, awareness, and competence in pediatric practice are needed anywhere in the world, and lessons learned abroad about culturally effective health care can be applied at home and vice versa.[29] As early as 1969, an editorial in *JAMA: The Journal of the American Medical Association* encouraged young US doctors to spend time working in a developing country to practice "better medicine at home and abroad."[30] Supporting the notion of global pediatrics, the American Board of Pediatrics is collaborating with other countries to establish the Global Pediatric Education Consortium, a working group to share the tasks of developing common standards for postgraduate training.[31]

■ POLICIES AND STANDARDS OF CULTURAL COMPETENCE

To clearly appreciate policies and standards of cultural competence, we must understand the nuances in the meanings of cultural diversity, sensitivity, and awareness. *Cultural diversity* reflects the myriad of cultural differences with culture broadly defined. *Cultural sensitivity* is the knowledge that cultural similarities and differences exist. *Cultural awareness* is being conscious of cultural similarities and differences.

Cultural competence can be defined at individual and organizational levels. At the individual level, cultural competence requires personal growth through firsthand knowledge, effective interactions with people from various cultural groups, and an examination of one's own biases. Organizationally, cultural competence is a set of values, behaviors, attitudes, policies, and practices that enable staff to work with multicultural populations.[32]

In medicine, cultural competence has been described as "a set of congruent behaviors, knowledge, attitudes, and policies that come together in a group of healthcare professionals that enables effective work in cross-cultural situations. It combines the tenets of patient/family-centered care with an understanding of the social and cultural influences that affect the quality of medical services and treatment."[33] Being culturally competent requires that health care professionals strive to acquire knowledge, skills, attitudes, awareness, and experience in the pursuit of lifelong development of cultural competence.

Primarily because of the recognition of health disparities for racial and ethnic minorities, the term *cultural competence* began appearing in medical literature in the early 1990s. The Institute of Medicine report, *Unequal Treatment: Confronting Racial and Ethnic Disparities in Health Care,* published in 2002, continued to highlight these disparities and included many studies that provided evidence for the lower quality of care that people of color often receive.[34] Eventually, the report's study committee determined that health care professionals would have to receive cross-cultural training to eradicate health disparities. Other reports from professional nursing organizations, public health entities, and other health profession bodies consistently identify the essential requirements of a culturally competent workforce.[35]

The AAP uses the term *culturally effective pediatric care* to describe cultural competence. According to the AAP, culturally effective pediatric care refers to "the delivery of care within the context of appropriate physician knowledge, understanding, and appreciation of all cultural distinctions leading to optimal health outcomes."[36] Culturally effective pediatric care is preferred over cultural competence because outcomes of the physician and patient/family interaction are considered. The AAP further recognizes the complexities of the term *culture* and includes all distinct attributes of population groups within its definition as well as the importance of traditional aspects of culture. The AAP emphasizes barriers to accessing care and how these barriers may relate to low levels of health literacy or particular health care needs of population groups. The AAP maintains a Web site, Health Equity, dedicated to understanding and combating health disparities and thus promoting health equity through the implementation of culturally effective pediatric care.[37]

In undergraduate and graduate medical education, the Accreditation Council for Graduate Medical Education and Association of American Medical Colleges cite the importance of cultural competence. However, systematic efforts to integrate cultural competence training into curricula for medical and health professional students have been lacking.[38]

The United Nations Convention on the Rights of the Child was passed by the UN General Assembly in 1989.[39] Containing 54 core articles, it defines basic human rights applicable to all children. It was ratified by all countries except Somalia and the United States. There are 4 core articles with related principles that apply to pediatric health care settings globally.

Article 2. Every child has the right to equal respect for all the rights in the convention (non-discrimination)

Article 6. The right to life and optimal development (fundamental right to life, survival, and development)

Article 12. The right to be listened to and be taken seriously (respect for the views of the child)

Article 16. The right to privacy and respect for confidentiality (devotion to the best interests of the child)

In addition, the US Office of Minority Health (OMH) established national standards for culturally and linguistically appropriate services (CLAS) in health care.[40] The OMH CLAS standards were designed to promote health services as more responsive to all patients and consumers and ultimately improve the health of all Americans and contribute to the elimination of racial and ethnic health disparities. Standards 1 through 7 of the 14 CLAS standards indicate cultural competence in direct care to include client respect, staff recruitment and training, and language access. Standards 8 through 14 call for organizational support of policies, structure, and processes so that the first 7 standards can be successfully implemented.

■ CULTURE AND HEALTH

Health is defined broadly to include physical, mental, social, and spiritual well-being; this definition is similar to the one offered by the World Health Organization (WHO). The breadth of the definition emphasizes an inextricable link between health and culture. The definition of culture eludes most, perhaps because of the complexity of the concept and the many disparate definitions previously suggested. There is lack of consensus about the meaning of culture and yet the notion seems to permeate so many aspects of our lives, including personal tastes, manners, beliefs, values, worldviews, and actions. Although culture is usually thought of as national identity, the scope has broadened to include many aspects of social difference including, but not limited to, race, ethnicity, gender, social class, religion, and sexuality. Even though much of culture in the nationalistic sense is tangible and visual (eg, food, clothing, housing, rituals), many elements cannot be seen, such as socioeconomic status, religion, and sexual orientation.

A broader definition of culture is an integrated pattern of learned beliefs and behaviors that are shared among groups. These beliefs and behaviors include thoughts, communication styles, ways of interacting, views of roles and relationships, values, practices, and customs.[41,42] We are all culturally different given our different family backgrounds, religions, occupations, disabilities, gender, socioeconomic status, and sexual orientation. Beyond race and ethnicity, we all are part of and influenced by multiple cultures. Each of us is a multicultural individual with many sets of cultures in different contexts, which may or may not coincide.[43]

Traditionally, culture has been considered the purview of anthropologists. In the medical field, the concept of culture is often oversimplified to refer to language, and cultural clashes are viewed as problems solved simply by an interpreter. Neutralization of cultural differences have also been attempted using mandatory diversity training in many organizations, during which employees purportedly learn to embrace the more superficial aspects of culture and celebrate multiculturalism.[43] It is important to remember that one size does not fit all. All cultures cannot be defined and understood in the same way because culture is a combination of many different elements, such as history, economic activity, and religion. However, the overarching characteristics seem to be that culture, in general, is shared, reflects an interaction between humans and their environment, and is carried over across generations and time periods.[44]

Two models offer theoretical frameworks highlighting the importance of the relationship between culture and health. Figure 4-1 depicts the cultural and social determinants of health and shows the complexity of many interrelated factors. This model suggests that there are multiple influences of culture on health and health outcomes.

Figure 4-1. Cultural and Social Determinants of Health

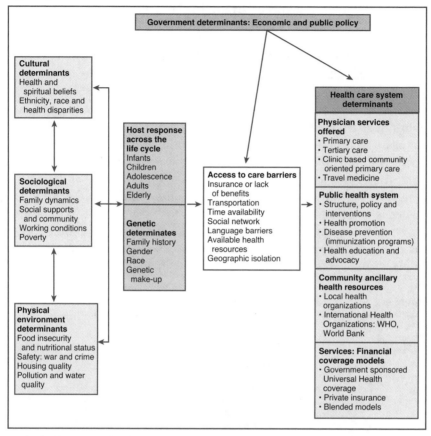

Reprinted with permission from Philip Diller, MD. The Christ Hospital University of Cincinnati Family Medicine Training Program.

A second model describes 6 cultural variables that differ among cultural groups and determine personal health traditions.[45] *Environmental control* refers to a society's traditional medical practices, which can have a direct effect on environmental factors. *Biological variations* determine basic physical characteristics of a society, such as stature or skin color. People in a society develop their own ideas surrounding health due to their *social organization*. It is this environment that also presents barriers to receiving health care, such as poverty and unemployment. *Communication* may explain another kind of barrier—language and nonverbal behavior—that comes between people and quality health care. Complications may arise from differences in what people consider appropriate personal and public *space*. Finally, because different cultural groups have different perceptions of *time,* these groups will subsequently entertain different thoughts on health care and illness prevention (Figure 4-2).

Aspects of Culture Affecting Pediatric Practice in a Global Context

As described earlier in this chapter, cultural influences on health attributions, beliefs, and practices are well recognized. However, across the globe, there have been paradigmatic shifts in the goals of and approach to health and the definition of health itself. First, the goal of medicine has changed from simply being an eradication of illness to prevention of disease and promotion of health through the adoption of a healthy lifestyle. The definition of health has changed to include social and mental well-being. With the expansion of this definition, there is a corresponding focus on social and behavioral sciences to explain the roots of health problems.[46] This underscores the importance of context via community-based approaches and the important role that sociocultural, behavioral, and environmental factors play in health such as poverty, social support,

Figure 4-2. Six Cultural Variables Related to Health

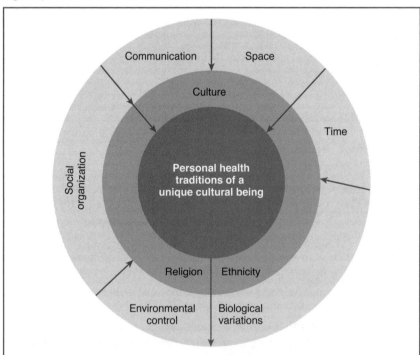

Adapted from Potter PA, Perry AG. *Fundamentals of Nursing.* 3rd ed. St. Louis, MO: Mosby-Year Book; 1993, with permission from Elsevier.

medical adherence or compliance with treatment regimen, resilience, acculturation, immigration, and even shared water sources. In addition, there is more consideration of culturally sensitive approaches to health care as well as indigenous and alternative forms of healing as legitimate forms of treatment. Particular aspects of culture have a major effect on pediatric practice including immigration and acculturation, poverty, and culture-bound syndromes.

Immigration and Acculturation

Immigration profoundly affects health. Immigrants are exposed to a host of conditions that may make them more susceptible to illness. Many diseases are simply endemic to the country of origin and stress because of economic hardship; disrupted family and social networks will only exacerbate illness. In the country of arrival, immigrants frequently work in low-paying jobs, face poverty, lack health insurance, have limited access to health care and social services, and have communication difficulties because of language differences. Immigration can take a toll on children in particular, as they are forced to adjust to an unfamiliar environment during formative years. Immigrant children can have infectious diseases that Western pediatricians are not used to diagnosing and treating. In addition, immigrant children often lack adequate immunization. The psychosocial factors of immigration may impose additional stressors on immigrant children (eg, disparities in social, economic, and professional status from the family's country of origin). Immigrant children may experience ongoing mental health issues because of relocation and potential atrocities experienced in their home country as well as adaptation issues with school and peer groups. Like their parents, immigrant children may lack a larger social support network of family and friends, which was present in their country of origin.[47]

Immigrants can be further disadvantaged when it comes to receiving health care. They may not be able to afford quality health care or a means of getting to a hospital; language and cultural barriers complicate the process even more, possibly making the immigrant feel uncomfortable or discriminated against. Immigrants may simply lack the knowledge of a new and complex health care system and what services are available to them. Foreign-born immigrants are twice as likely to lack health insurance as those born in the United States.[48] Recent immigrants to the United States have less contact in general and less timely contact with the health care system[49] and are more likely to have infectious diseases, especially tuberculosis, hepatitis B, and parasitic infections, as compared with US natives.[50–53]

Not only can immigrants suffer from a loss of social support, but they can also be negatively affected by *acculturation*—the process of adapting to a new environment. Acculturative stress occurs as immigrants lose touch with self-identifying constants, values, and social institutions of their former homeland, and can lead to depression and other mental disorders. Acculturation can have negative implications for children and their parents/family who experience uncertainty about the future, along with heightened levels of anxiety. These tensions may contribute to family dysfunction, which can manifest as strict and authoritarian child-rearing practices, including harsh disciplinary methods and possible severe, physical abuse.[46,54-56] Additionally, in households in which both parents work, children may be left unsupervised or neglected and, in some cases, left behind in their native country. These circumstances can increase conflicts surrounding relationships, gender roles, and respect issues.[54]

Although acculturation is experienced differently by everyone, Berry identified 5 general features of the process.[57] First, there is the stress that comes as a result of having to deal with 2 cultures simultaneously. Immigrants then evaluate the task of acculturation and determine whether it will be more or less challenging for them. Individuals also tend to employ coping strategies to aid in the adjustment, especially if the adjustment is deemed difficult. The fourth feature of acculturation encompasses various physiological and psychological responses to cultural adjustment. And finally, Berry identifies the possibility of long-term adaptation to the new culture, depending on the success of the process.

Culture-Bound Syndromes

There are physical and mental illnesses that are unique to particular cultures, directly influenced by cultural belief systems. The *Diagnostic and Statistical Manual of Mental Disorders* of the American Psychiatric Association defines such illnesses not recognized by Western medicine as *culture-bound*. For example, dhat is an illness that afflicts Indian males and involves an intense fear of losing semen; its symptoms include fatigue, depression, and suicidal inclinations.[58] In Latin America, mal de ojo (evil eye) refers to the illness experienced by a child when they are surveyed admiringly by a more powerful adult. According to Latin American culture, children who have experienced mal de ojo are fussy, cannot sleep, and may even have seizures. Treatment for evil eye can include physical contact or touch from the perpetrator, typically on the head, or prayer and ritual with an egg.[59]

Cultural ideals of beauty can also be the culprit for illnesses such as eating disorders. Eating disorders span physical and mental boundaries of cultural health and, especially in highly industrialized societies, incidence continues to rise.[58] Although in some cultures being stout and plump is associated with good health and prosperity (certain historical periods celebrated voluptuous women—consider the Rubenesque woman), the cultural ideal of women being thin and fit has increased in popularity.[58,60,61] In the Western world, especially among young women, the cultural notion of thinness as the ideal body image makes it clear that culture definitely influences attitudes toward body size and shape and eating behaviors.[60]

Physical ailments caused by stress or emotional distress (somatization) are common, especially in collectivistic societies, perhaps because people avoid expressing psychological complaints to families and friends.[58] A person suffering from depression or anxiety might use somatization as a culturally sanctioned way to signal distress.[62] Recognizing that there are culture-bound syndromes and that the expression and formation differs culturally paves the way for practicing culturally sensitive medicine and psychotherapy. Otherwise, misdiagnosis can occur when ethnic and cultural differences are not considered.

■ APPROACHES TO CULTURAL SENSITIVITY, AWARENESS, AND COMPETENCY RELEVANT FOR PEDIATRICS

The need for culturally sensitive, culturally aware, and culturally competent approaches to medical care has become more important as recognition of the overwhelming link between cultural beliefs and health beliefs and outcomes increases. Many global health care institutions incorporate linguistic competence into their services and employ interpreters and translators to manage linguistic diversity for their patients. However, being linguistically competent is not the same as being culturally competent. For example, although a site may have interpreters available for patients, the site may still impose a Western biomedical values-based health care environment (eg, lack of religious accommodations such as nondenominational spaces for prayer or not observing certain feeding practices and dietary mandates).

There are many cited approaches to cultural competence within medicine. The majority of approaches include culture-specific information with enhancements to communication and assessment skills. Many of these techniques and strategies have similarities and can be classified into the following 4 main categories of culturally competent approaches to health and healing:

1. Collaborative approaches
2. Personality approaches
3. Assessment techniques
4. Partnership/empowerment strategies[43]

A more holistic model that pediatricians can use in a global context with culturally different populations is intercultural adjustment as proposed by Vaughn and Phillips.[63] Their model includes 3 facets for which the individual is responsible.

1. Ability for reflection and self-awareness (intrapersonal competence)
2. Relationships with others (interpersonal competence)
3. Ability to take information about others gathered through these interactions and apply it to cultural groups (cultural competence)

Intrapersonal competence refers to the cultivation of self-understanding and self-discovery. A person who achieves intrapersonal competence recognizes her own judgments and biases and the human tendency to want to categorize people and use generalizations to make better sense of the world. Intrapersonal competence also infers a kind of flexibility in thinking, an ease in assimilating new schemas and ideas into one's existing bank of knowledge. The Matsumoto et al "psychological engine of adjustment" is a helpful framework for thinking about intrapersonal competence.[64] It involves the psychological characteristics of

- *Emotion regulation*—the ability to monitor and manage one's emotions, experiences, and expressions
- *Openness*—the ability to incorporate new experiences, emotions, and thoughts
- *Flexibility*—the ability to incorporate new experiences, schemas, and ways of thinking
- *Critical thinking*—the ability to think outside the box

The second component of the Vaughn and Phillips model is interpersonal competence. As the name suggests, this kind of competence has to do with an individual's relationship to other people. An interpersonally competent person is able to relate to others with a background different than his own. Bochner[65] empirically confirmed that poor interpersonal skills have adverse effects in intercultural situations. Interpersonally, people prefer others that they perceive as similar to themselves, which is known as the *similarity-attraction hypothesis*.[66] This makes interpersonal competence difficult to achieve because we might not put the energy or time into interpersonal relationships with people whom we perceive as different.

Finally, there is cultural competence, which combines intrapersonal and interpersonal competence in the application of knowledge about your own and others' cultures. Betancourt et al present cultural competence via 3 points of intervention, which connect communication with health outcomes—organizational, structural, and clinical.[67] At the organizational level, cultural competence encompasses policies, procedures, and systems that are aligned with the target population served. At this level, there should be diversity in leadership and the workforce that reflects the racial and ethnic diversity of the general population. The structural level of cultural competence involves quality service and access to the target population, which means having appropriate interpreters to address oral and written language and comprehension. The structural level also includes compliance and access to health care providers. The clinical level emphasizes the mutually productive interaction between health care professionals and families within the larger community. Culturally competent interventions at this level are marked by acceptance, appreciation, respect, exploration, and integration of sociocultural differences between the provider and family. The Purnell model of cultural competence[68] offers a systematic framework for assessing 4 macro aspects of culture—global society, community, family, and the person—and 12 microcultural domains and their concepts—overview/heritage, communication, family roles and organization, workforce issues, bio-cultural ecology, high-risk behaviors, nutrition, pregnancy and childbearing practices, death rituals, spirituality, health care practices and health care practitioners, and unknown phenomena of culture that grows with greater cultural competence, practices, and characteristics of the individual or target group.

Given the complex interplay of psychological, social, physical, and spiritual influences within culture, providers may become overwhelmed and disempowered given the complex, multifaceted, and often misunderstood needs of children. Pediatricians may need to address and advocate for the family or child in many nontraditional ways for medical care to be effective. As such, it is helpful if providers are informed of more creative approaches that do not rely on traditional approaches of changing the persons involved but instead focus on different ways to manage the system as a whole. Several nontraditional approaches to pediatric care across cultures include the life domains approach, cultural brokers, and lay health workers.

The *life domains approach* stresses the importance of examining the many different facets of a given culture to better understand that culture's relationship to health beliefs and practices.[69] Using this strategy, health care professionals may choose to investigate the many things that comprise a cultural identity, including language, daily living habits, education, work, intimate relations, child rearing, and special celebrations.

Because physicians often lack time to do a thorough cultural assessment or go to the depth that may be necessary with some families or patients, other intermediaries such as cultural brokers and lay health workers should be considered. *Cultural brokers* are patient advocates who can help bridge the gap between physician and patient by working to understand the patient's background and facilitating a successful health outcome.[70] *Lay health workers*—often termed promotores in Latino communities—are members of the community who provide basic public health services to disadvantaged people. Because lay health workers are embedded in the very community in which they serve, it is easy for them to adopt the perspective of their patients.[71] There is good evidence that these types of models work because they are culturally appropriate and integrated into communities.[72] In fact, the WHO describes qualities of a 21st century "5-star doctor" to be community oriented, reconciling individual and community needs, and initiating actions on behalf of the community.[73]

■ PRACTITIONER GROWTH IN CULTURAL SENSITIVITY, AWARENESS, AND COMPETENCY

Development of cultural sensitivity, awareness, and competency is a lifelong and incremental process. One does not achieve cultural competency by taking a particular class or serving abroad. Rather, pediatricians must develop an orientation of critical consciousness and social justice[74] that "places medicine in a social, cultural, and historical context," recognizes societal problems, and works toward achieving contextually appropriate solutions. As such, all children across the globe, regardless of background, are treated fairly and receive high-quality pediatric care. Such an orientation combines the best aspects of physician professionalism, humanism, and compassion with cultural openness and humility.

To truly appreciate culture, physicians must go deeper than an "Epcot Center approach,"[43,75] which focuses on food, dances, and customs and minimizes more serious issues like health disparities and

racism. Practicing or studying abroad, particularly in developing countries, certainly exposes various social contexts of enormous health and
economic disparities, but this is not enough. Physicians need to make
a personal commitment to culturally responsive practice and growth
throughout their career. To continue growth in cultural sensitivity,
awareness, and competence, physicians must strive to attain what
McPhatter terms "enlightened consciousness, a grounded knowledge
base, and cumulative skill proficiency."[76]

Enlightened consciousness requires a shift in primary worldview—
"this essential transformation begins with a shifting of consciousness
and awareness of just how endemic and narrow one's socialization
has been."[76]

A grounded knowledge base consists of critical analysis and reflection to reframe one's existing knowledge base and incorporate a
multicultural framework.

Finally, cumulative skill proficiency assumes that cultural skills can be
learned through systematic and motivated efforts such that all children,
regardless of cultural background (eg, nationality, race/ethnicity, poverty,
religion) and context (at home or abroad), experience compassionate,
accepting, and equal pediatric care.

■ KEY POINTS

- Complex global changes require cultural sensitivity, awareness, and
  competence in pediatric practice.
- Demographic diversity, cultural health beliefs, decreased health
  equity, pediatric practice abroad, and relevant policies and standards
  contribute to the need for proficiency in culturally responsive
  pediatric practice.
- Culture and health are broadly defined and include multiple and
  complex factors.
- Particular aspects of culture have a major effect on pediatric
  practice including immigration and acculturation, poverty, and
  culture-bound syndromes.
- There are many cited approaches to cultural competence within
  medicine; more global and creative models include intercultural
  adjustment and nontraditional approaches to pediatric care.
- Practitioners can achieve growth in cultural awareness, sensitivity, and
  competence through consistent efforts at an enlightened consciousness, a grounded knowledge base, and cumulative skill proficiency.

■ REFERENCES

1. US Census Bureau. *Projections of the Total Resident Population by 5-Year Age Groups, Race, and Hispanic Origin with Special Age Categories*. Washington, DC: Population Projections Program, Population Divison, US Census Bureau; 2000. http://www.census.gov/population/projections/nation/summary/np-t4-e.txt. Accessed December 7, 2006

2. Anderson LM, Scrimshaw SC, Fullilove MT, Fielding JT, Normand J, the Task Force on Community Preventive Services. Culturally competent healthcare systems: a systematic review. *Am J Prev Med*. 2003;24(3S):68–79

3. Gordon RG, Grimes BF, eds. *Ethnologue: Languages of the World*. 15th ed. Dallas, TX: Summer Institute of Linguistics; 2005

4. Furnham A, Akande D, Baguma P. Beliefs about health and illness in three countries: Britain, South Africa and Uganda. *Psychol Health Med*. 1999;4(2):189–201

5. Kleinman A. Concepts and a model for the comparison of medical systems as cultural systems. In: Currer C, Stacey M, eds. *Concepts of Health, Illness, and Disease: A Comparative Perspective*. Oxford, UK: Berg Publishing; 1986:29–47

6. Murguia A, Peterson RA, Zea MC. Use and implications of ethnomedical health care approaches among Central American immigrants. *Health Soc Work*. 2003;28(1):43–51

7. Klonoff E, Landrine H. Belief in healing powers of prayer: prevalence and health correlates for African-Americans. *West J Black Stud*. 1996;20(4):207–210

8. Landrine H, Klonoff A. Cultural and health-related schemas: a review and proposal for interdisciplinary integration. *Health Psychol*. 1992;11(4):267–276

9. Kinsley DR. *Health, Healing, and Religion: A Cross-Cultural Perspective*. Upper Saddle River, NJ: Prentice Hall; 1996

10. Bade B. Alive and well: generating alternatives to biomedical health care by Mixtec migrant families in California. In: Fox J, Rivera-Algado G, eds. *Indigenous Mexican Migrants in the United States*. La Jolla, CA: University of California-San Diego, Center for US-Mexican Studies; 2004:205–247

11. Helman C. *Culture, Health and Illness*. 4th ed. London, England: Arnold; 2001

12. Furnham A. Explaining health and illness: lay perceptions on current and future health, the causes of illness, and the nature of recovery. *Soc Sci Med*. 1994;39(5): 715–725

13. Jobanputra R, Furnham A. British Gujarati Indian immigrants' and British Caucasians' beliefs about heath and illness. *Int J Soc Psychiatry*. 2005;51(4):350–364

14. Ezzati M, Friedman AB, Kulkarni SC, Murray CJL. The reversal of fortunes: trends in county mortality and cross-county mortality disparities in the United States. *PLoS Med*. 2008;5(4):e66

15. Vamus H, Klausner R, Zerhouni E, Acharya T, Daar AS, Singer PA. Grand challenges in global health. *Science*. 2003;302:398–399

16. Ortega AN, Gergen PJ, Paltiel AD, Bauchner H, Belanger KD, Leaderer BP. Impact of site of care, race, and Hispanic ethnicity on medication use for childhood asthma *Pediatrics*. 2002;109:1–6

17. Elster A, Jarosik J, VanGeest J, Fleming M. Racial and ethnic disparities in health care for adolescents: a systematic review of the literature. *Arch Pediatr Adolesc Med*. 2003;157:867–874

18. Hahn BA. Children's health: racial and ethnic differences in the prescription of medications. *Pediatrics*. 1995;95:727–732

19. Flores G, Fuentes-Afflick E, Barbot O, et al. The health of Latino children: urgent priorities, unanswered questions, and a research agenda. *JAMA*. 2002;288:82–90

20. American Academy of Pediatrics Committee on Pediatric Research. Race/ethnicity, gender, socioeconomic status -research exploring their effects on child health: a subject review. *Pediatrics.* 2000;105:1349–1351

21. Israel B, Schulz A, Parker E, Becker A. Community-based participatory research: policy recommendations for promoting a partnership approach in health research. *Educ Health.* 2001;14(2):182–197

22. Crump JA, Sugarman J, Working Group on Ethics Guidelines for Global Health Training (WEIGHT). Global health training: ethics and best practice guidelines for training experiences in global health. *Am J Trop Med.* 2010;83:1178–1182.

23. McAlister CC, Orr K. A student's plea for global health studies in the medical school curriculum. *Clin Invest Med.* 2006;29:185–186

24. Drain PK, Primack A, Hunt D, Fawzi WW, Holmes KK, Gardner P. Global health in medical education: a call for more training and opportunities. *Acad Med.* 2007;82:226–230

25. Drain PK, Holmes KK, Skeff KM, Hall TL, Gardner P. Global health training and international clinical rotations during residency: current status, needs, and opportunities. *Acad Med.* 2009;84:320–325

26. Shah SK, Wu T. The medical student global health experience: professionalism and ethical implications. *J Med Ethics.* 2008;34:375–378

27. Shah SK, Nodell B, Montano SM, Behrens C, Zunt JR. Clinical research and global health: mentoring the next generation of health care students. *Glob Public Health.* 2010;14:1–13

28. Kanter SL. Global health is more important in a smaller world. *Acad Med.* 2008;83: 115–116

29. Castillo J, Goldenhar LM, Baker RC, Kahn RS, DeWitt TG. Reflective practice and competencies in global health training: lesson for serving diverse patient populations. *J Grad Med Educ.* 2010;2:449–455

30. Overseas medical aid. *JAMA.* 1969;209:1521–1522

31. Stockman I, Ham HP. Global standards for postgraduate training in general pediatrics: the international pediatric community considers a vision. *J Pediatr.* 2010;156:693–694

32. Pérez MA, Luquis RR. *Cultural Competence in Health Education and Health Promotion.* San Francisco, CA: Jossey-Bass; 2008

33. Association of American Medical Colleges. http://www.aamc.org/meded/tacct/culturalcomped.pdf. 2005

34. Institute of Medicine. *Unequal Treatment: Confronting Racial and Ethnic Disparities in Health Care.* 2002

35. Doutrich D, Storey M. Education and practice: dynamic partners for improving cultural competence in public health. *Fam Commun Health.* 2004;27(4):298–307

36. American Academy of Pediatrics Committee on Pediatric Workforce. Ensuring culturally effective pediatric care: implications for education and health policy. *Pediatrics.* 2004;114(6):1677–1685

37. American Academy of Pediatrics. Community Pediatrics: Health Equity. http://www.aap.org/commpeds/resources/health_equity.html

38. Purden M. Cultural considerations in interprofessional education and practice. *J Interprof Care.* 2005;19(Suppl 1):224–234

39. United Nations Children's Fund. Convention on the rights of the child http://www.unicef.org/crc. Accessed March 5, 2008

40. Office of Minority Health. *National Standards for Culturally and Linguistically Appropriate Services in Health Care: Final Report.* Washington, DC: US Department of Health and Human Services; 2001

41. Donini-Lenhoff FG, Hedrick HL. Increasing awareness and implementation of cultural competence principles in health professions education. *J Allied Health.* 2000;29(4):241–245

42. Robins LS, Fantone JC, Hermann J, Alexander GL, Zweifler AJ. Improving cultural awareness and sensitivity training in medical school. *Acad Med.* 1998 Oct;73(10 Suppl):S31–S34

43. Vaughn LM. Families and cultural competency: where are we? *Fam Commun Health.* 2009;32(3)

44. Triandis HC. Culture and psychology: a history of the study of their relationship. In: Kitayama S, Cohen D, eds. *Handbook of Cultural Psychology.* New York, NY: The Guilford Press; 2007:59–76

45. Giger JN, Davidhizar RE. *Transcultural Nursing: Assessment and Intervention.* 2nd ed. St. Louis, MO: Mosby; 1995

46. Berry JW, Poortinga YH, Segall MH, Dasen PR. *Cross-Cultural Psychology: Research and Applications.* 2nd ed. Cambridge, UK: Cambridge University Press; 2002

47. American Academy of Pediatrics Committee on Community Health Services. Providing care for immigrant, homeless, and migrant children. *Pediatrics.* 2005;115(4):1095–1100

48. Thamer M, Richard C, Casebeer AW, Ray NF. Health insurance coverage among foreign-born US residents: the impact of race, ethnicity, and length of residence. *Am J Public Health.* 1997;87(1):96–102

49. Leclere FB, Jensen L, Biddlecom AE. Health care utilization, family context, and adaptation among immigrants to the United States. *J Health Soc Behav.* 1994;35(4):370–384

50. Hernandez DJ, Charney E, eds. *From Generation to Generation: The Health and Well-Being of Children in Immigrant Families.* Washington, DC: National Academy Press; 1998

51. Liu Z, Shilkret KL, Tranotti J, Freund CG, Finelli L. Distinct trends in tuberculosis morbidity among foreign-born and US-born persons in New Jersey, 1986 through 1995. *Am J Public Health.* 1998;88(7):1064–1067

52. Centers for Disease Control and Prevention. Screening for hepatitis B virus infection among refugees arriving in the United States, 1979–1991. *MMWR Morb Mortal Wkly Rep.* 1991;40(45):784–786

53. Gavagan T, Brodyaga L. Medical care for immigrants and refugees. *Am Fam Physician.* 1998;57(5):1061–1068

54. Thomas TN. Acculturative stress in the adjustment of immigrant families. *J Soc Distress Homeless.* 1995;4(2):131–142

55. Warheit GJ, Vega WA, Auth J, Meinhardt K. Mexican-American immigration and mental health: a comparative analysis of psychosocial stress and dysfunction. In: Vega WA, Miranda MR, eds. *Stress and Hispanic Mental Health: Relating Research to Service Delivery.* Rockville, MD: National Institute of Mental Health; 1985:76–109

56. Smart JF, Smart DW. Acculturative stress: the experience of the Hispanic immigrant. *Couns Psychol.* 1995;23:25–42

57. Berry JW. Immigration, acculturation and adaptation. *Appl Psychol Int Rev.* 1997;46: 5–68

58. Gardiner HW, Kosmitzki C. *Lives Across Cultures: Cross-Cultural Human Development.* 4th ed. Boston, MA: Pearson Allyn & Bacon; 2008

59. Spector RE. *Cultural Diversity in Health & Illness.* 6th ed. Upper Saddle River, NJ: Prentice Hall; 2004

60. Adams PJ, Katz RC, Beauchamp K, Cohen E, Zavis D. Body dissatisfaction, eating disorders, and depression: a developmental perspective. *J Child Fam Stud.* 1993;2(1):37–46
61. Crawford M, Unger R. *Women and Gender: A Feminist Psychology.* 4th ed. Boston, MA: McGraw-Hill; 2004
62. Draguns JG. Applications of cross-cultural psychology in the field of mental health. In: Brislin RW, ed. *Applied Cross-Cultural Psychology.* Newbury Park, CA: Sage; 1990:302–324
63. Vaughn LM, Phillips R. Intercultural adjustment for cultural competence in shared context: "the company we keep." *Int J Interdiscip Soc Sci.* 2009;3(11):1–12
64. Matsumoto D, LeRoux J, Ratzlaff C, et al. Development and validation of a measure of intercultural adjustment potential in Japanese sojourners: the Intercultural Adjustment Potential Scale (ICAPS). *Int J Intercult Relat.* 2001;25:483–510
65. Bochner S. Culture shock due to contact with unfamiliar cultures. In: Lonner WJ, Dinnel DL, Hayes SA, Sattler DN, eds. *Online Readings in Psychology and Culture.* Volume 8, chapter 7. Bellingham, WA: Center for Cross-Cultural Research, Western Washington University; 2003
66. Brehm SS. *Intimate Relationships.* New York, NY: Random House; 1985
67. Betancourt JR, Green AR, Carillo JE, Ananeh-Firempong O. Defining cultural competence: a practical framework for addressing racial/ethnic disparities in health and health care. *Public Health Rep.* 2003;118:293–302
68. Purnell L. The Purnell model for cultural competence. *J Transcult Nurs.* 2002;13(3): 193–196
69. Arends-Tóth J, van de Vijver FJR. Assessment of psychological acculturation. In: Sam DL, Berry JW, eds. *The Cambridge Handbook of Acculturation Psychology.* Cambridge, MA: Cambridge University Press; 2006:142–160
70. National Center for Children in Poverty. 2008
71. Lam TK, McPhee SJ, Mock J, et al. Encouraging Vietnamese-American women to obtain pap tests through lay health worker outreach and media education. *J Gen Intern Med.* 2003;18(7):516–524
72. Lewin SA, Dick J, Pond P, et al. Lay health workers in primary and community health care. *Cochrane Database Syst Rev.* 2005;CD004015
73. Oandasan IF, Barker KK. Educating for advocacy: exploring the source and substance of community-responsive physicians. *Acad Med.* 2003;78:S16–S19
74. Kumagai AK, Lypson ML. Beyond cultural competence: critical consciousness, social justice, and multicultural education. *Acad Med.* 2009;84:782–787
75. Vaughn LM. *Psychology and Culture: Thinking, Feeling and Behaving in Global Contexts.* New York, NY: Psychology Press; 2010
76. McPhatter AR. Cultural competence in child welfare: what is it? How do we achieve it? What happens without it? *Child Welfare.* 1997;76:255–278

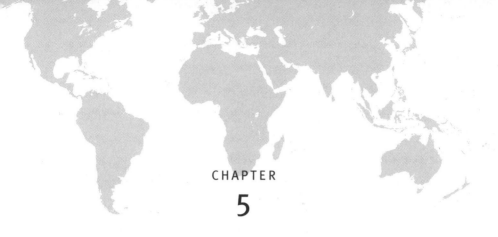

CHAPTER

5

International Law and Health

Peter J. Hammer, JD, PhD

■ DIAGNOSING THE PROBLEM OF CHILDREN'S HEALTH: THE ROLE OF LAW AND GOVERNANCE

From a medical perspective, we already know the leading causes of child mortality—acute respiratory infections, diarrheal diseases, and neonatal infections.[1] For the vast majority of cases, we also know the appropriate medical treatments. The difficult challenge and tragedy of global children's health lies in applying proven solutions to known problems. In *The State of the World's Children 2008: Child Survival*, the United Nations Children's Fund (UNICEF) identifies the "[u]nderlying and structural causes of maternal and child mortality."[1] Among other factors, the report lists "[p]oorly resourced...health and nutrition services," "[l]ack of hygiene and access to safe water or adequate sanitation," and exclusion from essential health services "due to poverty and geographic or political marginalization."[1]

This list hints at structural concerns that raise basic issues of governance, not medicine. The report also acknowledges that these are complex and multidimensional problems in need of multidimensional solutions: "Their wide-ranging nature and interrelatedness require them to be addressed at different levels—community, household, service provider, government and international—in an integrated manner to maximize effectiveness and reach."[1] This is a daunting challenge, but it is ultimately a challenge of effective governance, calling for frameworks that can facilitate exactly these forms of effective cooperation.

Problems of water and sanitation help show the often hidden link between governance and health. The medical implications of unclean water and poor sanitation are clear.

> *In developing countries, 1 in 5 people do not use safe water, and roughly half are without adequate sanitation. The repercussions are often deadly. The number of children under five worldwide dying from diarrhoea is estimated at almost 2 million per year; in many countries the proportion of child deaths due primarily to diarrhoea is around 20 percent. An estimated 88 percent of diarrhoeal deaths are attributed to poor hygiene practices, unsafe drinking-water supplies and inadequate access to sanitation.[1]*

Popular understandings of the link between health and sanitation, characteristic of the "great sanitary awakening," are old and predate scientific understandings of the causes of disease.[2] Furthermore, the basic solutions to these problems are also well understood. The issue is not what to do but how to do it. There can be no clean water or proper sanitation without effective forms of local cooperation, typically facilitated by local governments. As such, the presence of clean water and proper sanitation can be used as a proxy for the existence of effective governance. Conversely, poor sanitation is an indication, among other things, of the absence of effective forms of local cooperation.

Making the diagnosis is easier than remedying its causes. Providing clean water and proper sanitation requires surmounting all the difficult historical challenges involved in establishing effective forms of local governance in the first place. This is not an easy task. Indeed, the baseline expectation should be that structures enabling effective cooperation are the exception and not the rule, as they are difficult to establish and maintain. Moreover, areas where effective structures of local governance have not historically taken root (as witnessed by the absence of clean water and sanitation) are likely to be among the most difficult settings in which to build cooperative frameworks. Sustainable public health progress, however, is not possible if one focuses on clean water without also focusing on governance. Developing countries are full of wells donated by well-intentioned organizations that quickly fall into disrepair because technology was inserted in the absence of a supportive social infrastructure.

The underlying lessons are even broader. Improved governance is critical for improving water and sanitation, but it is also critical for almost every other aspect of policy implementation addressing maternal and child health. This reality is again recognized in the UNICEF report, which stresses the need to establish a "continuum of care" linking households, communities, and health facilities.[1] There are important, although often not stated, dimensions of governance behind every aspect of this continuum of care. But to classify the problem of children's health in terms of governance is also to open a Pandora's box of problems. Specific interfaces of the continuum of care are multiple and varied, calling not only for various effective local actions but complicated inter-linkages from the local through the national and ultimately to the international community. These are complicated and difficult challenges. Any notion of law and governance being up to the challenge must itself be open, flexible, and multidimensional.

■ APPRECIATING THE MULTIDIMENSIONAL NATURE OF LAW AND GOVERNANCE

There is no single or simple answer to the question, "What is law?" Popular conceptions often view law as a series of commands or directives—a list of things citizens must do or must refrain from doing. Other popular conceptions view law as creating a series of entitlements— enforceable demands that citizens can make against the state. Common to both of these understandings is the implicit assumption that whatever law is, it can be enforced and its violations punished. There are certainly social domains in which these views ring true and provide workable frameworks to understand what law is and what it can do.

In the domain of global health governance, however, neither of these understandings is very useful. To begin with, whatever law and governance means for global children's health, its meaning must exist in a world where there is no effective enforcement of its mandates. International law exists without international police or effective international enforcement. With the notable exceptions of the World Trade Organization (WTO) mandatory dispute resolution process and certain matters under the purview of the UN Security Council, there are few established enforcement mechanisms for the breach of international law. International law may declare that there is a right to health, but this right must mean something substantially different in the international realm than a comparable declaration would mean in a domestic setting where legal mandates can be backed by a state's police powers. The perennial challenge of law and governance in the international setting is to establish goals, set objectives, and enable effective forms of cooperation in the absence of traditional state enforcement mechanisms.

Defining the issue in this manner rightly suggests that the problem of global health governance has more in common with private law than public law. Private actors (individuals, businesses, and nonprofit and nongovernmental organizations [NGOs]) often face the challenge of forging effective voluntary agreements in which the prospect of state enforcement is remote. How private actors do this, what models and techniques they use, and how these methods map on to a wide range of varied local conditions are potentially fruitful avenues of investigation. Ironically, business schools, rather then law schools, might be a better source of inspiration for physicians and public health advocates concerned with global health governance.

This is not to say that law and institutional structures do not matter—they do. What is important about law in this setting is not its ability to command, which it cannot, but its ability to help establish frameworks that can facilitate more effective forms of voluntary cooperation. Again, the sources of inspiration may be surprising.

The best primer for those concerned about global health governance may be a course in institutional economics, which covers focused training in the role of incentives, transaction costs, information failures, coordination, collective action, and agency problems.[3,4] Institutional economics teaches an important set of tools, but it also counsels a different temperament in approaching policy making.

One hallmark of institutional economics is the value of institutional agnosticism. The focus is on function, not form. The same public health function can be provided through a wide range of different institutional forms—public-regulatory, private-market, or hybrid public-private partnerships. No one form is appropriate in all settings. Moreover, the desired form will often be influenced, in a path-dependent manner, by a country's historical mix of institutional structures. In this setting, policy making should consist of a rigorous exercise in comparative institutional analysis—objectively comparing the plausible range of institutional solutions and selecting the least worse. This is an intensely empirical investigation of alternatives in which evidence should matter. Prior ideologic beliefs about the competing virtues of the state and market are best left aside.

While no unitary model of governance emerges from this analysis, it is possible to produce fairly systemized processes of decision-making as to how governance problems can be approached. Consistent with mainstream economics and international relations theory, the basic behavioral assumption adopted here is that actors, state and non-state, act in what they believe to be their own best interest, although the values underlying each actor's perceived self-interest may vary widely. A flow-chart for addressing public health issues can take the following form:

Problem → Bases of Cooperation → Tools → Strategy

1. Clearly understand the nature of the public health problem.
2. Identify the range of potential bases of cooperation that can build self-interested coalitions for action around the problem.
3. Examine the range of possible tools and models available through which to act.

These 3 steps can lead to the construction of appropriate public health strategies or policies.

This is a problem-driven approach. Everything depends on an honest and thorough understanding of the public health problem. Appropriate strategies will change, sometimes radically, as the nature of the public health problem changes. An authentic understanding of the problem will suggest which bases of cooperation are possible. While neither exhaustive nor mutually exclusive, the following list includes potential useful bases of cooperation for global public health problems. Different coalitions and different actors will have different motivations. Bases of cooperation include

• Health as security
• Health as a global public good
• Health as development
• Health as a human right
• Health as a humanitarian concern

The list suggests a hierarchy in terms of each mandate's strength, at least from a traditional nation-state perspective. States are most likely to act when there is a security threat and are least likely to act when the concern is predominately humanitarian or a matter of human rights. Different international organizations and international NGOs often define their missions in a manner more consistent with one basis of cooperation than another. The World Bank, for example, is chiefly motivated by health as development, while the World Health Organization (WHO) functions more comfortably within the model of health as a human right or humanitarian concern.

Each basis for cooperation, in combination with each particular problem, creates its own mandate for action. The strength of these mandates will vary widely, with some being more effective than others. Bioterrorism and highly contagious infectious diseases such as pandemic influenza have clear national security implications, while childhood diarrhea clearly does not. Correspondingly, the security mandate for action in the former case will be stronger than the latter.

Whether and how HIV/AIDS fits into the security paradigm raises interesting questions and has its own revealing history.[5] The international surveillance function necessary to detect infectious diseases and emerging public health threats is one of the best examples available of a genuine global public good. As such, the mandate for action underlying the WHO Revised International Health Regulations,[6] a combination of security threats and a global public good, was particularly strong.

At the same time, each basis for cooperation has its own boundaries and limits. There is a tendency in the literature to overstate the reach of the public-good mandate, but not every public health concern is a genuine global public good. Moreover, the nature of public good can change at different units of analysis. What may be a public good at the local or national level may not be a public good at the international level. Caution is appropriate. When the mandate for action is misidentified or overstated, the very foundation for building an effective framework for cooperation can be undermined from the beginning. If effective coalitions are to be built, it is important to be brutally honest about which bases of cooperation are implicated, as well as the strength of their various warrants. To do otherwise is akin to building a house on sand. The sad reality is that global children's health implicates a range of some of the weaker warrants for international cooperation—health as development, health as a human right, and health as a humanitarian concern. It is wiser to be creative and effective within these realms than to attempt to overstretch the potential bases of cooperation.

Once the problem and bases of cooperation are understood, policy makers need to examine the range of available tools and models for action. The choice of tools will clearly depend on the nature of the problem and whether action is intended at the international, national, or local level. Staying at the international level for the time being, the range of available tools and models might consist of

- Hard-law legal instruments, such as traditional treaties (Convention on the Rights of the Child [1989])[7] or the treaty-based convention-protocol framework (WHO Framework Convention on Tobacco Control [2003])[8]
- Soft-law recommendations, statements, declarations, or goals (Declaration of Alma-Ata [1978],[9] Millennium Development Goals [MDGs],[10] WHO International Code of Marketing of Breast-milk Substitutes[11)]

- Creation of a new international organization (The Global Fund to Fight AIDS, Tuberculosis and Malaria)[12] or a looser network-based coalition of existing international organizations and national governmental and NGOs (Global Alliance for Vaccines and Immunisation [GAVI])[13]
- A range of possible public-private partnerships (Malaria Vaccine Initiative)

The process of understanding the problem and selecting the appropriate bases of cooperation and proper set of tools ultimately produces a strategy or policy for taking action on the issue. While this discussion focuses primarily on the international level, the same heuristic approach can also be applied at the national and local levels.

■ INTERNATIONAL LAW AND GOVERNANCE IN THE SERVICE OF CHILDREN'S HEALTH

Every global effort to assist children's health has some aspect of governance. What is lacking is a systematic appreciation of the importance of governance and the need for structures that can better coordinate disparate and often uncoordinated initiatives. This section examines a broad range of undertakings—the historic role of treaty making to improve children's health, different forms of network-based actions to improve public health, and efforts to facilitate more effective local governance and grassroots participation.

What is obviously missing from this list is the role of national health system development. Without doubt, national health systems are a critical part of the governance equation and substantial international aid and attention has been directed at improving national structures. This is an important topic deserving separate treatment. International law and governance often act as surrogates for national governance in those states with the weakest or most corrupt national structures. In these states, international and NGOs frequently serve functions that the state would otherwise serve. Unfortunately, these functions are often performed without sufficient appreciation of the quasi-public nature of the role. This makes a more express appreciation of the role of governance even more important.

The Role and Limits of Classic International Law in Children's Health

It is common for international lawyers to distinguish between *hard law* and *soft law*. Hard law consists of formal treaty obligations negotiated and assented to by individual sovereign states. Hard law (a treaty) is what most people think of when they think of international law. Soft law consists of a range of nonbinding resolutions, recommendations, and policy statements issued by various international organizations and institutions.

There is no shortage of hard law concerning children's health. Standard references include the WHO Constitution,[14] the International Covenant on Economic, Social and Cultural Rights (1966),[15] and the Convention on the Rights of the Child (1989).[7] These instruments can collectively be interpreted as creating a right to health.[16]

The WHO Constitution is a treaty instrument that speaks of a fundamental right to health, which is defined as "a state of complete physical, mental, and social well-being and not merely the absence of disease or infirmity."[14] The WHO Constitution makes only 2 express references to children. The first is in the preamble: "Healthy development of the child is of basic importance; the ability to live harmoniously in a changing total environment is essential to such development."[14] The second reference is in article 2, stating that one of the basic functions of the WHO is "to promote maternal and child health and welfare and to foster the ability to live harmoniously in a changing total environment."[14]

The right to health is further articulated by the International Covenant on Economic, Social and Cultural Rights.[15] Article 12 of the covenant broadly defines a right to health: "The States Parties to the present Covenant recognize the right of everyone to the enjoyment of the highest attainable standard of physical and mental health."[15] Among other measures, the treaty obligates signatories to take all steps necessary for the "reduction of the stillbirth rate and of infant mortality and for the healthy development of the child."[15]

In terms of children's health, the most important treaty is the Convention on the Rights of the Child.[7] Article 24 of the convention, dealing with the health of children, provides in full

1. States Parties recognize the right of the child to the enjoyment of the highest attainable standard of health and to facilities for the treatment of illness and rehabilitation of health. States Parties shall strive to ensure that no child is deprived of his or her right of access to such health care services.
2. States Parties shall pursue full implementation of this right and, in particular, shall take appropriate measures:
   a. To diminish infant and child mortality;
   b. To ensure the provision of necessary medical assistance and health care to all children with emphasis on the development of primary health care;

    c. To combat disease and malnutrition, including within the frame-work of primary health care, through, inter alia, the application of readily available technology and through the provision of adequate nutritious foods and clean drinking water, taking into consideration the dangers and risks of environmental pollution;

    d. To ensure appropriate pre-natal and post-natal health care for mothers;

    e. To ensure that all segments of society, in particular parents and children, are informed, have access to education and are sup-ported in the use of basic knowledge of child health and nutri-tion, the advantages of breastfeeding, hygiene and environmental sanitation and the prevention of accidents;

    f. To develop preventive health care, guidance for parents and family planning education and services.

3. States Parties shall take all effective and appropriate measures with a view to abolishing traditional practices prejudicial to the health of children.

4. States Parties undertake to promote and encourage international co-operation with a view to achieving progressively the full realiza-tion of the right recognized in the present article. In this regard, par-ticular account shall be taken of the needs of developing countries.[7]

In addition to hard law, there are countless soft-law declarations and resolutions addressing children's health. The most important are probably the Declaration of Alma-Ata[9] and the MDGs.[10] In 1978, the Declaration of Alma-Ata reaffirmed health as a fundamental human right and called for "the attainment by all peoples of the world by the year 2000 of a level of health that will permit them to lead a socially and economically productive life."[9] The declaration advocated a focus on primary health care that included, among other things, particular attention to "an adequate supply of safe water and basic sanitation," "maternal and child health care, including family planning," and "immunization against the major infectious diseases."[9]

The MDGs are a set of 8 quantifiable targets that members of the international community committed themselves to obtain by 2015.[10] While each target has implications for children's health, MDG 1 (pov-erty/nutrition), MDG 4 (child mortality), MDG 5 (maternal health), MDG 6 (combating HIV/malaria), MDG 7 (clean water and sanitation), and MDG 8 (global partnerships) are particularly salient.[10] To their credit, the MDGs provide an effective framework to help coordinate activities by the international community in pursuit of these objectives. Indeed, this soft-law instrument, through its efforts to create more effective frameworks for cooperation, has probably done more to advance children's health than any hard-law instrument.

When reading the various hard- and soft-law instruments, 2 equally strong reactions are common. The first is a genuine respect for the scope, depth, and intensity of the formal international commitment to children's health as a basic human right. The second is a sense of a large gap existing between the aspirational goals established by these international instruments and the actual facts. These dual impressions help delineate the strengths and limitations of international law as a tool for improving children's health.

The shortcomings of traditional international law are well known. First, it is very difficult to speak of meaningful rights in the absence of enforcement mechanisms, yet the absence of effective means of enforcement is a defining hallmark of international law. Human rights are typically enforced through a process of naming and shaming—report writing and commission findings. In the end, however, if a country fails to comply with its obligations, such as those in the Convention on the Rights of the Child, there is very little the international community can do about it (although extreme cases of human rights abuses can generate ad hoc regimes of economic and political sanctions). A second limitation is the substantive construction of the right itself. Positive rights, like the right to health, are self-constrained by the principle of *progressive realization*. At most, countries commit themselves to do the best they can, given the resources they have.

While not being overly critical of the human rights paradigm, it is necessary to understand what it can and cannot accomplish. Human rights have a role to play. Human rights are particularly important in the hands of individuals and advocacy groups because these rights are the principal means that individuals have to make claims on the international community. Traditionally, international law was the exclusive domain of the nation-state. Not only was there no participatory role for the individual in this game, but international law imposed no obligations on the state's conduct toward its own people. The treatment of citizens was a concern beyond the reach of traditional international law. The development of human rights marked a radical change in this orientation. The international community now recognizes that nations have obligations to their citizens and that, in limited ways, individuals can press their claims against states in an international setting.

Indeed, these tools can and should be more aggressively pursued. To do this more effectively, human rights lawyers must join ranks with epidemiologists and other public health experts. New and creative ways need to be developed to demonstrate that insufficient resources are being devoted to children's health, even under the constraints of the doctrine of progressive realization. Cross-sector analyses can be conducted under defensible measures of social welfare to show that money could be more efficiently reallocated to public health. Analogies could be drawn to emerging trade law, such as under the WTO Agreement on the Application of Sanitary and Phytosanitary Measures (1995),[17] where article 5(5) permits the disparate treatment of "like risks" to be used as a basis for inferring discriminatory treatment.[17,18] Similar arguments could be marshaled in public health matters. Disparate treatment by governments of comparable sectors of public spending could be used to demonstrate a failure of the state to progressively realize its commitment to children's health and other economic, social, and cultural rights.

In the end, however, even this use of human rights law is really a tactic to establish political pressure. This suggests the real power of the human rights paradigm. Human rights are powerful not because they are an effective source of legal entitlement but because they can be effective levers for social change. This change happens not only at the policy level but also at the level of redefining social norms and values.

The human rights paradigm can help change the way people think. The human rights framework can build bridges of empathy to socially and geographically distant, disadvantaged communities that can be the basis for reordering international priorities. As such, the human right paradigm is most useful in combination with other bases of cooperation, such as health as development or as a humanitarian concern in the formation of workable frameworks for cooperation. Human rights can be a catalyzing force and glue that helps hold these coalitions together. On its own, however, its force is fairly limited. Human rights are just one of many necessary building blocks for effective action.

From Nations to Networks: The Role of Cooperative Frameworks

Law is much more than a source of mandates or entitlements and the international community is more than a collection of independent nation-states. One of the most important functions of law is its ability to establish cooperative frameworks. This approach to law provides a more useful template for addressing issues of global governance, particularly when confronting complicated social problems such as public health or the environment. But this vision of law must be combined with a more pragmatic understanding of the international community that reaches beyond the nation-state as the only relevant building block for action. International organizations and other non-state actors must also be part of the solution. We need to move from nations to *networks* as the primary unit for addressing public health problems such as children's health.[19]

Dodgson and Lee provide a useful mapping of the actors involved in global health governance.[20] In the tightest circle, there is the WHO, the World Bank, and the US government—3 actors that approach public health from very different perspectives and have very different understandings of their own missions and self-interests. For purposes of children's health, UNICEF would have to be added to the inner circle as well. One circle removed, Dodgson and Lee list developed countries (along with their bilateral aid agencies), developing countries as descriptive blocks, the WTO, and a range of UN agencies with health-related mandates, such as the International Labour Organization and the UN Population Fund. The next circle includes various groups of non-state actors comprising global civil society—religious groups, social movements, individuals, media, epistemic communities, and research institutions. As an illustration of how fast things are changing, the Bill & Melinda Gates Foundation and the Global Fund to Fight AIDS, Tuberculosis and Malaria would have to be added to the map and placed at or near the inner circle.

The mapping of actors is just the first step. For effective action to take place there must be mutual understanding of the nature of the problem to be addressed, an agreed-to strategy that is consistent with the missions and perceived self-interest of the leading actors (a basis for cooperation), and an organizational structure through which the strategy can be implemented. As suggested earlier, there are no one-size-fits-all solutions to these problems. The relevant actors must sit around the proverbial negotiating table and hammer out a solution that best fits whatever problem is being addressed. This is an exercise in which creativity and problem solving are essential skills.

While there are no one-size-fits-all solutions, there are a number of different models that can serve as sources of inspiration. Each of these illustrates a different type of network-based cooperation. Three examples will be considered here: the Global Fund to Fight AIDS, Tuberculosis and Malaria[12]; the WHO Framework Convention on Tobacco Control[8]; and Global Alliance for Vaccines and Immunisation (GAVI).[13]

The Global Fund represents an innovative effort to combat 3 diseases plaguing the international community. Legally, the Global Fund is a private foundation registered under Swiss law. However, the government of Switzerland entered into a headquarters agreement with the Global Fund that recognizes it as an international legal personality and grants it certain legal privileges and immunities similar to those granted to intergovernmental organizations.[12] Voting members of the board consist of representatives from developed (8 members) and developing (7 members) countries, as well as representatives of civil society and the private sector (5 members). Representatives from the WHO, Joint UN Programme on HIV/AIDS, and World Bank and a Swiss citizen serve as ex officio board members. Funding proposals are generated by and implemented through a newly created, nation-based infrastructure of country coordinating mechanisms, which themselves comprise new forms of public-private partnerships. While certainly not the only way to imagine mounting a global fight against AIDS, tuberculosis, and malaria, the Global Fund stands as an ambitious example of a new type of network-based cooperation in the service of global health governance.

The WHO Framework Convention on Tobacco Control serves as a different model.[8] Formally, the convention is a treaty and, therefore, an instrument of hard international law. There are 2 things that distinguish this exercise from traditional treaty-making processes. First, the convention-protocol framework is dynamic in nature and initiates an ongoing governance process. Effectively used in the field of international environmental law, the convention establishes a general commitment by all members to broad goals and establishes a governance structure that enables the international community to continue to work the issue. Series of specific protocols can then be negotiated and adopted (each also a treaty) to address particular aspects of the larger social problem. The second distinguishing factor is how, through the auspices of the WHO, the broader epistemic community of public health professionals played a substantial role in pushing forward the tobacco control agenda and shaping the treaty's contents.[21,22] This process was substantially different from the exclusive nation-state orientation of traditional treaty making. Both aspects of the WHO Framework Convention on Tobacco Control make it an interesting model for future cooperative action in public health. Larry Gostin, for example, has advocated the use of the convention-protocol framework as the basis for addressing a wide range of global public health problems.[23,24]

GAVI, the final model, is a looser network-based form of action. In the face of stalled international progress, the Gates Foundation spearheaded efforts to renew international action concerning childhood immunizations.[13] Rather than start a brand new international organization like the Global Fund, and rather than work exclusively through an existing international organization, GAVI was formed. GAVI is best understood in terms of a structure that enables more effective cooperation and action among existing stakeholders in the campaign for childhood vaccinations. GAVI has a lean secretariat housed in UNICEF offices in Geneva. It has a 12-member board consisting of representatives from developing world governments, WHO, UNICEF, World Bank, pharmaceutical companies, NGOs, research institutes, and the Gates Foundation. As the Gates Foundation explained, "The strategy was to create an inclusive decision-making body to bring new coordination to a disjointed, inefficient marketplace."[13]

Costello and Osrin have argued for new network-based action with respect to maternal and child health.[25] They advocate for the creation of a new global fund dedicated to meeting the needs of maternal, neo-natal, and child health. Their proposal is consistent with the views pro-posed here—the need to develop frameworks that enable more effective forms of cooperation. There are many challenges to making sustained improvements in children's health. Many developing countries have limited public health infrastructures and limited capacity at the national level to oversee or coordinate the multiplicity of international, bilateral, and nongovernmental actors working in the field. What could a new global fund do to help? In addition to potentially attracting additional resources, a new global fund could play important administrative and governance functions. The authors observed that "donor countries want assurances that their investments are managed well, transparently accounted for, and achieve results."[25] Costello and Osrin outline how these functions might be structured and performed. The governance functions need not take the exact form these authors advocate, but their proposal highlights the need to pay more attention to the role of governance, as well as the need for new frameworks to facilitate more effective forms of cooperation among existing actors in the name of public health.

Asking the question, "What bases of cooperation might support an initiative such as a new global fund for maternal and child health?" suggests the many challenges that any such effort would face. To begin, the problems of children in developing countries do not constitute a direct security threat to those countries. There is no strong security mandate. While aspects of the public health infrastructure necessary to address children's health (clean water and sanitation) might constitute a public good from a local and perhaps even national perspective, it is difficult to characterize them as a global public good. There is no strong global public good mandate. Health as development raises more dif-ficult questions. There are undoubtedly some economic benefits from investing in basic children's health. The value of such an investment, however, is immediately discounted from an economic perspective by the young age of the child and the potentially high background rate of child mortality. This obviously sounds harsh, but most developing societies implicitly recognize this same harsh reality by having compensatory high numbers of children. Similarly, in some cultures with high rates of child mortality, families postpone naming children and forming other types of bonds until the child reaches an age at which survival is more likely. From a short or intermediate time frame, the health as development mandate is relatively weaker for children's health than other public health investments. In contrast, AIDS was considered a particularly strong threat to the economies of developing countries because it hit people in the most productive years of their economic lives. Significantly, the development case for children's health is stronger when one examines basic infrastructure investments (ie, water, sanitation, and education) that have potential crossover benefits, as well as public health investments that protect the health of the mother and hence the entire family. There is a development case to be made, but it is of a more targeted and selective nature.

The ultimate cooperative bases for children's health must be found in the relatively weaker warrants of health as a human right and health as a humanitarian concern, with health as development playing a supporting role. As sketched previously, the human rights case for children's health is well established. Similarly, children's health rates particularly high on the humanitarian scale. The challenge is to creatively leverage these bases of cooperation into a more effective framework for network-based action. Many dimensions of improved governance in this regard are fairly self-evident and would be commonly acknowledged. More effective donor coordination (a governance function) is clearly needed. Efforts to think holistically in terms of integrated packages of services, continuums of care, and more cost-effective forms of intervention need to be extended. In addition, better planning that makes more seamless the connection between global and local dimensions of governance is certainly in order.

Linking Global and Local: Building Governance at the Grassroots Level

In the developing world, most children die outside the reach of health facilities. Children's health cannot be sustainably improved until a global public health infrastructure is established that can effectively reach into individual homes in the world's most remote rural communities. This requires creative thinking about governance at the most grassroots levels. There is good news and bad news in this regard. The bad news is that in many countries, like Cambodia, the notion of the village is completely unrelated to any notion of established administrative structures providing public services.[26] All too often, the notion of the village is also unrelated to notions of strong communal bonds or ties. The good news is that the potential bases of cooperation on behalf of children's health at the local level are much stronger than at the international level. The challenge at the global level is that the health of children in third-world countries does not affect the direct self-interests of developed countries. At the household and village level, where these children live and die, the story is very different.

The health of the mother (wife/daughter/sister) and child directly affects the well-being of the family and, by extension, the community and village. The strongest self-interest and, therefore, the strongest allies are potentially at the local level. To be sure, there are substantial obstacles to effective local cooperation as well. Health status typically tracks socioeconomic status. As a result, the sickest members of society are often the most politically marginalized and disenfranchised. Gender and the status of women add additional complications. Effective action will require surmounting numerous social, economic, cultural, and political barriers. Nevertheless, empowering stakeholders at the local level and encouraging various forms of participation and cooperation are potentially fruitful strategies.

Again, these views reflect an emerging consensus. Most people working in the field understand the importance of greater grassroots participation. The challenge is how to best accomplish this objective and how to conceptualize the role of local participation within a larger integrated framework of global network-based governance. There are no one-size-fits-all solutions. Chapter 3 of the UNICEF report, *The State of the World's Children 2008: Child Survival*, describes many innovative efforts to improve children's health.[1] Some of these initiatives include integrated management of neonatal and childhood illness in India,[1] Arranque Parejo en la Vida (Equal Start in Life) program in Mexico, safe water systems in Afghanistan, school sanitation and hygiene education in Bangladesh, and community-based HIV prevention and treatment in Botswana.[1] In addition, UNICEF supports the innovative Seth Koma program in Cambodia, in partnership with parallel processes fostering deconcentration and decentralization of state functions, to empower women in participation with village development councils in a process to improve public health.[27] Similar ambitious undertakings can be found in the UN Millennium Villages Project.[28] Building on these and other successes, the Global Fund to Fight AIDS, Tuberculosis and Malaria is

now targeting community systems strengthening as a central component of its future action.[29] Building frameworks of cooperation from
the grassroots level up is one of the most important frontiers in global
public health. But local participation is not a panacea for public health
problems and establishing effective local cooperation will not be easy.
Building frameworks for effective network-based participation at the
international level requires identifying bases of cooperation that could
lead to a convergence of the perceived self-interest of disparate actors.
The same is true at the local level. Too often, participation becomes a
tactic used by international organizations to implement preestablished
agendas. Such efforts can not establish real or effective grassroots participation. The participation of local stakeholders must be authentic and
self-sustaining. Local actors must be provided real opportunities to give
input and their views must help shape the agenda of any cooperative
undertaking. The same governance heuristic employed at the international level must be employed at the local level.

Problem → Bases of Cooperation → Tools → Strategy

What is the nature of the local public health problem? What are the
potential bases of cooperation between local actors and between local
and international actors? What are the available tools and models? If
international objectives do not correspond to the perceived needs and
self-interest of local actors, and if local actors are not given proper incentives to participate, effective local cooperation and governance cannot
be maintained.

Governance is critical to global children's health and a more considered understanding of governance is essential for the construction of
more effective public health programming. Nation-states, particularly
in developing countries, are often constrained by the limited reach of
their administrative structures and the underdeveloped and ineffective
status of their bureaucratic institutions. Health ministries often have
difficulties projecting power much beyond the nation's capital and the
largest provincial towns. International organizations are constrained
in different ways but face their own challenges in extending programming to remote areas. This is a serious problem because the basic needs
of children require effective and ongoing forms of public health services
that can only be provided at the most local of local levels. Without
more effective forms of public health governance, substantial progress cannot be made in improving children's health and meeting the
MDGs. National and international actors have had only sporadic success in effectively connecting the international and national apparatus
to the local level. This remains the most important challenge to law,

governance, and public health. More creative understandings of law and an express appreciation of the need to create frameworks that enable more effective forms of cooperation offer partial insights into ways to move forward.

■ KEY POINTS

- Some of the most important obstacles to improving children's health concern issues of law and governance, not medicine.
- The presence of clean water and proper sanitation can be used as a proxy for the existence of effective governance. Conversely, poor water and sanitation is an indication, among other things, of the absence of effective forms of local cooperation.
- International law can be interpreted as creating a fundamental right to children's health, but a large gap exists between the aspirational goals set by this right and the reality the world confronts.
- International law is best approached not as a set of mandates but as a set of tools and tactics that can help establish frameworks that can facilitate more effective forms of cooperation.
- A flowchart for addressing public health issues can take the following form:

  Problem → Bases of Cooperation → Tools → Strategy
- Bases of cooperation for international law include
  — Health as security
  — Health as a global public good
  — Health as development
  — Health as a human right
  — Health as a humanitarian concern
- Progress on children's health will require building multidimensional networks of cooperation effectively linking global, national, and grassroots efforts.

REFERENCES

1. United Nations Children's Fund. *The State of the World's Children 2008: Child Survival.* http://www.unicef.org/sowc08/docs/sowc08.pdf
2. Institute of Medicine. A history of the public health system. In: *The Future of Public Health.* Washington, DC: National Academy Press; 1988:56–72
3. Eggertsson T. *Economic Behavior and Institutions.* Cambridge, MA: Cambridge University Press; 1990
4. Kasper W, Streit ME. *Institutional Economics: Social Order and Public Policy.* Northampton, MA. Edward Elgar Pub; 1999
5. Singer PW. AIDS and international security. *Survival.* 2002;44(1):145–158

6. World Health Organization. *International Health Regulations*. 2nd ed. Geneva, Switzerland, World Health Organization; 2005. http://www.who.int/csr/ihr/ IHR_2005_en.pdf

7. International Conventions on the Rights of the Child. 1989. http://untreaty.un.org/ English/TreatyEvent2001/pdf/03e.pdf

8. World Health Organization. *WHO Framework Convention on Tobacco Control*. 2003. http://www.who.int/tobacco/framework/WHO_FCTC_english.pdf

9. Declaration of Alma Ata. 1978. http://www.who.int/hpr/NPH/docs/declaration_ almaata.pdf

10. United Nations. General Assembly. 55th Sess. Resolution 55/2. United Nations' Millennium Declaration. 2000. http://www.un.org/millennium/declaration/ ares552e.pdf

11. World Health Organization. *International Code of Marketing of Breast-Milk Substitutes*. 1981. http://www.who.int/nutrition/publications/code_english.pdf

12. Global Fund to Fight AIDS, Tuberculosis and Malaria. Framework document of the Global Fund to Fight AIDS, Tuberculosis and Malaria. 2002. http://www.theglobalfund. org/documents/TGF_Framework.pdf

13. Bill and Melinda Gates Foundation. Ensuring the world's poorest children benefit from lifesaving vaccines. 2008:1–5. http://www.gatesfoundation.org/learning/Documents/ GAVI.pdf

14. World Health Organization. Constitution. 2006. http://www.who.int/governance/eb/ who_constitution_en.pdf

15. Covenant on Economic, Social and Cultural Rights. 1966. http://www2.ohchr.org/ english/law/pdf/cescr.pdf

16. United Nations High Commissioner for Human Rights and World Health Organization. *The Right to Health*. Fact Sheet No. 31. 2008. http://www.ohchr.org/Documents/ Publications/Factsheet31.pdf

17. World Trade Organization. *Agreement on the Application of Sanitary and Phytosanitary Measures*. 1995. http://trade.wtosh.com/english/tratop_e/sps_e/spsagr_e.htm

18. World Trade Organization. Report of the Appellate Body. Ab–1997–4. EC Measures Concerning Meat and Meat Products (Hormones). 1998. http://www.wto.org/english/ tratop_e/dispu_e/cases_e/ds26_e.htm

19. Kickbush I. The development of international health policies B: accountability intact? *Soc Sci Med*. 2000;51:979–989

20. Dodgson R, Lee K. Global health governance: a conceptual review. In: Wilkinson R, Hughes S, eds. *Global Governance: Critical Perspectives*. London, England: Routledge; 2002:92–110

21. Wipfli H, Bettcher DW, Subramaniam C, et al. Confronting the tobacco epidemic: emerging mechanisms of global governance. In: McKee M, Garner P, Scott R, eds. *International Co-operation in Health*. Oxford, UK: Oxford University Press; 2001:127–149

22. Jacob GF. Without reservation. *Chic J Int Law*. 2004;5(1):287–302

23. Gostin LO. Why rich countries should care about the world's least healthy people. *JAMA*. 2007;298(1):89–92

24. Gostin LO. Meeting the survival needs of the world's least healthy people: a proposed model for global health governance. *JAMA*. 2007;298(2):225–228

25. Costello A, Osrin D. The case for a new global fund for maternal, neonatal and child survival. *Lancet*. 2005;366:603–605

26. Ovesen J, Trankell IB, Ojendal J. When every household is an island: social organisation and power structures in rural Cambodia. *Uppsala Research Reports in Cultural Anthropology*. No. 15. Stockholm, Sweden; 1996

27. United Nation Children's Fund. Report on the Qualitative Assessment of Community Action for Child Rights (Seth Koma) Programme (Part I) and An Assessment of the Collaboration of Seth Koma and Selia for UNICIEF Cambodia (Part II). 2002

28. Millennium Villages. http://millenniumvillages.org. Accessed August 1, 2011

29. Global Fund to Fight AIDS, Tuberculosis and Malaria. *Community Systems Strengthening Framework May 2010.* http://www.theglobalfund.org/documents/rounds/10/R10_InfoCSS_Note_en. Accessed August 1, 2011

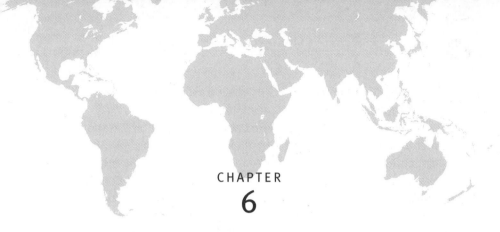

CHAPTER

6

Maltreatment and Advocacy

Vincent J. Palusci, MD, MS, FAAP
Dena Nazer, MD, FAAP

■ INTRODUCTION

Not only are large numbers of the world's children adversely affected by economics, politics, and war, but they are also harmed by immediate and long-term effects of child abuse and neglect.[1] Studies in countries throughout the world have documented the growing recognition of harmful parental and societal practices. There is a growing body of knowledge supporting intervention to prevent physical and emotional injuries and illnesses during childhood, which will affect victims throughout their life.[2-5] Pediatricians and other professionals caring for children, in addition to their training and experience in recognizing and responding to child abuse and neglect, will have to incorporate into their practices the many international variations in cultures, parenting, and reporting laws and practices, and a growing international movement supporting children.

The United Nations Convention on the Rights of the Child (UNCRC) was enforced in 1990 (General Assembly Resolution 44/25) subsequent to being ratified by all countries except the United States and Somalia.[6] Specific provisions deal with a child's right to protection from all forms of violence, abuse, and exploitation; this applies to all children with their families, refugees, and those in armed conflict. It also contains provisions addressing economic, sexual, and other forms of exploitation and torture. In addition, the UNCRC contains specific references to the plight of indigenous children that are not contained in other human rights treaties; there are also provisions about parents' rights and responsibilities.

The UNCRC brought fundamental change to the international community despite ongoing discussion about its limitations.[7,8] Violence against children is not only morally and socially unacceptable but it now violates a fundamental right to respect for and protection of inherent human dignity, physical and mental integrity, and equal protection under the law. By ratification, 193 countries committed themselves and are legally bound to respect, protect, and fulfill the rights of children. These countries also took many legislative, social, and other measures to bring their laws and practices into compliance with the UNCRC. In addition, nongovernmental organizations (NGOs), United Nations Children's Fund (UNICEF), and other UN agencies with growing involvement of professional groups, such as pediatricians and the corporate sector, support the UNCRC implementation.

It is in the context of varying levels of national commitment to and implementation of the UNCRC that the pediatrician will face varying definitions, legal procedures, and societal responses to child maltreatment and exploitation. Professionals caring for children outside the United States should acquaint themselves with local cultural and legal practices and community resources to best provide for the health, safety, and protection of children. While injury pathophysiology, biomechanics, and stress mechanisms do not change from continent to continent or country to country, the pediatrician should not expect the same level of systematic societal response to child maltreatment in developing countries as it might receive in the United States. Depending on cultural background and exposure, the pediatrician will also face a variety of parenting practices, poverty, socially accepted norms, and physical discipline that will test sensitivity to and understanding of complementary and alternative medicine practices that will refocus the pediatrician's energies on truly promoting child health in the international setting.

■ DEFINITIONS

While a variety of definitions have been used, *child maltreatment* generally falls into 5 types: physical abuse, sexual abuse, neglect, psychological maltreatment, and other exploitation. The World Health Organization (WHO) broadly defined these types of maltreatment for data collection and intervention (Box 6-1). The UNCRC states that a child is "[e]very human being below the age of eighteen years unless, under the law applicable to the child, majority is attained earlier" and that child maltreatment consists of "all forms of physical or mental violence, injury and abuse, neglect or negligent treatment, maltreatment or exploitation, including sexual abuse." It also includes "intentional use of physical force or power, threatened or actual, against a child, by an individual or group that either results in or has a high likelihood of resulting in actual or potential harm to the child's health, survival, development or dignity."

Child maltreatment occurs primarily in the family but also in schools, alternative care institutions and detention facilities, places where children work, and communities. The definition was extended to include exploitation of children in inappropriate work settings that are likely to be hazardous or interfere with the child's education, or are harmful to the child's health or physical, mental, spiritual, moral, or social development. Children who are exploited in armed conflict generally fall outside these child maltreatment regulations but are covered under

---

Box 6-1. World Health Organization Conceptual Definitions of Child Maltreatment

PHYSICAL ABUSE
Intentional use of force against a child that results in, or has a high likelihood of resulting in, harm to the child's health, survival, development, or dignity, which includes hitting, beating, kicking, shaking, biting, strangling, scalding, burning, poisoning, and suffocating. This may or may not be with the objective of punishment.

SEXUAL ABUSE
Involvement of a child in sexual activity that he or she does not fully comprehend, to which he or she is unable to give informed consent or for which the child is not developmentally prepared, or that violates the laws or social taboos of society. This can be by adults or other children who, by virtue of their age or development, are in a position of responsibility, trust, or power over the child.

PSYCHOLOGICAL MALTREATMENT
A pattern of failure over time on the part of the parent or caregiver to provide bonding and a developmentally appropriate and emotionally supportive environment; other acts include restricting movement, belittling, blaming, threatening, frightening, discriminating against, ridiculing, and other nonphysical hostile treatment.

NEGLECT
Isolated incidents and patterns of failure over time on the part of the parent or caregiver, when in a position to provide food, clothing, shelter, health, education, nutrition, and safety for the child.

EXPLOITATION
Commercial or other exploitation of a child refers to use of the child in work or other activities for the benefit of others. This includes, but is not limited to, child labor and child prostitution. These activities are to the detriment of the child's physical or mental health, education, or spiritual, moral, or social-emotional development.

From World Health Organization. *Preventing Child Maltreatment: A Guide to Taking Action and Generating Evidence.* Geneva, Switzerland: WHO Press; 2006; and World Health Organization. *Report of the Consultation on Child Abuse Prevention, WHO, Geneva,* 29-31 March 1999. Document WHO/HSC/PVI/99.1. http://whqlibdoc.who.int/hq/1999/WHO_HSC_PVI_99.1.pdf. Accessed March 15, 2011

other local and international statutes and the mandate of the Office of the Special Representative of the UN Secretary-General for Children and Armed Conflict. Therefore, the professional caring for children during war will have to rely on international regulations concerning the rights of combatants (such as the Geneva convention) outside the realm of child abuse and neglect.

An additional form of child maltreatment, *medical neglect* or medical care neglect, was defined separately from neglect in some jurisdictions. For example, 7 US states specifically define medical neglect as failing to provide any special medical treatment or mental health care that a child needs.[9] In addition, 4 US states define medical neglect as withholding medical treatment or nutrition from disabled infants with life-threatening conditions. The American Academy of Pediatrics (AAP) notes that medical neglect usually takes 1 of 2 forms: failure to heed obvious signs of serious illness or failure to follow a physician's instructions once medical advice is sought. Either of these situations can be fatal or lead to chronic disability.[10] Several factors are considered necessary for diagnosing medical neglect.

1. A child is harmed or is at risk of harm from lack of health care.
2. The recommended health care offers significant net benefit to the child.
3. The anticipated benefit of the treatment is significantly greater than its morbidity so that reasonable caregivers would choose treatment over nontreatment.
4. It can be demonstrated that access to health care is available and not used.
5. The caregiver understands the medical advice given.

A caveat applies when medical resources are limited or nonexistent. Medical care neglect usually identifies that the family failed to provide needed care when otherwise able to do so. Thus, the pediatrician will have to consider the resources available in addition to parental factors when considering this form of child maltreatment.

■ EPIDEMIOLOGY OF CHILD MALTREATMENT ACROSS THE WORLD

As the United Nations reports, child maltreatment is "a global problem" with "reports of cruel and humiliating punishment, genital mutilation of girls, neglect, sexual abuse, homicide, and other forms of violence against children...long recorded, but the grave and urgent nature of this global problem has only recently been revealed."[11]

It is difficult to precisely determine the incidence and prevalence of child maltreatment across the world due to variations in the application of definitions in law and in practice, different numbers of cases generated with voluntary versus mandated reports, parenting and cultural practices, acceptability of corporal punishment and other family violence, and resources available for systematic epidemiologic case ascertainment. Some jurisdictions have little or no information about child maltreatment, while data systems have been in place in many countries for more than 20 years.[12]

Currently, published international child maltreatment information usually comes from governmental administrative data systems, large-scale international surveys, or multi-country samples using specific survey tools that often assess specific types of child maltreatment. Several models were developed in various countries to capture the number of children coming to the attention of social services or legal authorities or the prevalence of behaviors that place children at risk for child maltreatment.[13]

Population-based surveys using the parent-child Conflict Tactics Scale, the Adverse Childhood Experiences questionnaire, the Lifetime Victimization Screening Questionnaire, and International Society for Prevention of Child Abuse and Neglect (ISPCAN) screening tools have all been variably used to assess child maltreatment worldwide.[4] The reader is referred to several organizations, such as ISPCAN, and available child maltreatment textbooks and journals, such as *Child Abuse & Neglect: The International Journal, Child Maltreatment,* and *Child Abuse Review,* as well as numerous publications addressing child maltreatment types, human development, and child psychology. The ISPCAN Working Group on Child Maltreatment Data is working to make strategies available for more standardized data, greater data collection, and greater availability of existing data for policy development.[12]

There are a variety of country reports concerning the incidence or prevalence of child maltreatment. The United States, Canada, England, and Australia often report all types of child maltreatment rates at 3% to 5% with fewer than half receiving investigation and fewer than a quarter being legally substantiated. Increasingly, non–English-speaking countries, such as the Netherlands, Greece, and Croatia, are reporting population-based rates that are not substantially different.[12] When individual countries such as the United States possess the resources to accurately count child maltreatment cases, additional obstacles often prevent an accurate comparison. Organizations such as the WHO have decried poor public health surveillance of child maltreatment across the world, and there is active discussion on the world stage about measuring and reporting strategies. Each country (and sometimes provinces or states) has its own policy and practice around child maltreatment definitions and reporting and whether a report is substantiated. Such difficulties occur within countries over time as well. Even with similar standards, the social acceptability and professional stance on reporting can make similar case scenarios result in different reporting and governmental responses.

Fatality and hospital discharge data have been compared across continents, but research comparisons are limited by the application of commonly used *International Classification of Diseases* coding and underutilization of external cause-of-injury codes (E codes).[14] The homicide rate of children in 2002 was twice as high in lower-income countries compared with higher-income countries (2.58 versus 1.21 per 100,000 population). The highest child homicide rates occur in adolescents, especially boys between the ages of 15 and 17 years (3.28 for girls; 9.06 for boys) and among newborns to children 4 years of age (1.99 for girls; 2.09 for boys). The following was determined using limited country-level data:

- An estimated 53,000 children died worldwide in 2002 as a result of homicide.
- Eighty percent to 98% of children suffered physical punishment in their homes.
- One third or more of children experienced severe physical punishment from the use of implements.
- Twenty percent to 65% of school-aged children were verbally or physically bullied in the past 30 days.
- One hundred and fifty million girls and 73 million boys younger than 18 years experienced forced sexual intercourse or other forms of sexual violence in 2002.
- One-hundred million to 140 million girls and women worldwide underwent some form of female genital mutilation (FGM) or cutting.
- One-point-eight million children were sexually exploited in prostitution and pornography in 2000 according to estimates by the International Labour Organization (ILO).[11]

Variations in the use of corporal punishment were identified. Multiple Indicator Cluster Surveys were used in one study of 124,916 children in 28 developing and transitional countries to determine the prevalence of psychological and moderate to severe physical abuse during the previous month.[15] The survey found that a majority (83%) of African children experienced psychological abuse, with moderate and severe physical abuse affecting 64% and 43%, respectively. Comparable rates were lower in transitional countries in central Europe. At one end of the spectrum, the use of any violent punishment by parents is noted in even greater numbers (greater than 75%) in countries such as Guyana, Iraq, Gambia, Jamaica, Ghana, Togo, Cameroon, Vietnam, and Yemen.[12] Corporal punishment was noted to be highly accepted in some countries—92% in Syria and 56% in Sierra Leone.[15] At the other end of the spectrum, the secretive nature of human trafficking makes information about these children even more difficult to ascertain; their plight is thought to be more perilous.[16]

While studies of risk and protective factors among countries are problematic due to methodologic and definitional differences, studies clearly confirm child maltreatment to be an international problem with common themes among countries. Surveys of child maltreatment in large nonclinical adult populations have been conducted in many countries, including the United States and Canada; early studies found low rates due to under-recognition and underreporting. More recent studies found rates in line with comparable North American research; for example, rates for sexual abuse ranged from 7% to 36% for women and 3% to 29% for men.[3,17] Most studies find females to be sexually abused 1 to 3 times more than males. Economic development, status, age, sex, and gender are among the many factors associated with the risk of lethal violence. Studies suggest that young children are at greatest risk of physical violence, while sexual violence predominantly affects those who reached puberty or adolescence. Boys are at greater risk of physical violence than girls, while girls face greater risk of sexual violence, neglect, and forced prostitution.

Social and cultural patterns of conduct, stereotyped roles, and socioeconomic factors such as income and education also play an important role. Small-scale studies reveal that some groups of children are especially vulnerable to violence.[11] These groups include children with disabilities, ethnic minorities and other marginalized groups, street children, children in conflict with the law, and refugees and other displaced children.

Stable family units can be a powerful source of protection from violence for children in all settings. Factors that are likely to be protective in the home and other settings include good parenting, strong bonds between parents and children, and positive nonviolent discipline. Factors that are likely to protect against violence at school include school-wide policies and effective curricula that support the development of nonviolent and nondiscriminatory attitudes and behaviors.

High levels of social cohesion are shown to have a protective effect against violence in the community, even when other risk factors are present.

International initiatives are underway to expand knowledge about the epidemiology of child maltreatment beyond currently available statistics. The ISPCAN Child Abuse Screening Tool (ICAST) children's instrument is 1 of 3 tools designed by a panel of child maltreatment experts from 40 countries to study the prevalence of childhood victimization. Other tools have been designed to study child victimization from parents' perspectives on their child rearing and from the young adult on childhood experiences.[18] Using the parent version, approximately 15% of children were shaken, 24% were hit on the buttocks with an object, and 37% were spanked. Two percent of parents reported choking and smothering their child.[19] A retrospective version was also tested.[20] Further assessment and wider implementation of the surveys are planned.

■ VARIATIONS IN PARENTING METHODS AND PRACTICES

While many cultural practices exist, pediatricians will encounter complementary and alternative medicines and variations in parenting across the world that potentially cross over into child abuse and neglect, including the use of physical discipline and corporal punishment, FGM, cupping, moxibustion, therapeutic burning, and coining.

Physical Discipline and Corporal Punishment

Effective discipline requires 3 essential components: a positive, supportive, loving relationship between the parent(s) and child; positive reinforcement strategies to increase desired behaviors; and removing reinforcement or punishment to reduce or eliminate undesired behaviors. All components must function well for discipline to be successful.[21] Punishment can be verbal or corporal and can range from restraining or slapping the hand of a child about to touch a hot stove to identifiable child abuse, such as beatings, scaldings, and burnings.

Spanking and other forms of corporal punishment are widely accepted and used throughout the world. Using a modified parent-child Conflict Tactics Scale to address parental discipline of children in Brazil, Chile, Egypt, India, Philippines, and the United States, nearly all 14,239 mothers surveyed used nonviolent discipline and verbal or psychological punishment.[22] Physical punishment was used in at least 55% of the families. Spanking rates (open hand on buttocks) ranged from a low of 15% in an educated community in India to a high of 76% in a Philippine community. Similarly, there was a wide range in the rates of children who were hit with objects (9% to 74% [median: 39%]) or beaten by their parents (0.1% to 28.5%).

Spanking and less traumatic forms of physical discipline were found to increase the chance of physical injury, and the child may not understand the connection between the behavior and the punishment.[21] Although the child may react with shock from being spanked and stop the undesired behavior, repeated spanking may cause agitated, aggressive behavior in the child that may lead to physical altercations between the child and parent. Spanking and threats of spanking lead to strained parent-child relationships, making discipline substantially more difficult when physical punishment is no longer an option, such as with adolescents. Spanking is no more effective as a long-term strategy than other methods of discipline, and relying on spanking makes other discipline strategies less effective.[23] Time-out and positive reinforcement of other behaviors are more difficult to implement and take longer to become effective when spanking was previously a primary discipline method. The more children are spanked, the more anger they report as adults, the more likely they are to spank their own children and approve of hitting a spouse, and the more marital conflict they experience. Spanking is associated with higher rates of physical aggression, more substance abuse, and increased risk of crime and violence when used with older children and adolescents.[23]

There is consensus against using extremely harsh methods of physical punishment, such as burning or smothering, which are rare in all countries. Shaking continues to be used; 20% of parents in 9 communities admitted shaking children younger than 2 years.[22] In a larger survey of discipline practices by Gray,[12] 33% to 94% of children reported receiving violent punishment in countries ranging from Bosnia and Herzegovina (33%) to Yemen (94%); 1% to 44% experienced severe physical discipline. Similar parental acceptance of physical punishment was reported in children as young as 2 years. More violent discipline is used in countries where more domestic violence, polygamy, and child labor is reported. More education and more books in the home were associated with a greater use of nonviolent discipline strategies.

Corporal punishment in schools was prohibited in at least 108 countries worldwide. However, at least 78 of these did not prohibit corporal punishment as a disciplinary measure in penal institutions for children in conflict with the law, and 43 did not prohibit it as a judicial sentence of the courts for young people convicted of an offense.[24] Box 6-2 shows the 29 nations that have specific laws protecting children from all corporal punishment and the year the law was instituted.

Box 6-2. Nations With Specific Laws Protecting Children From All Corporal Punishment	
Kenya (2010)	Romania (2004)
Tunisia (2010)	Ukraine (2004)
Poland (2010)	Iceland (2003)
Liechtenstein (2008)	Germany (2000)
Luxembourg (2008)	Israel (2000)
Republic of Moldova (2008)	Bulgaria (2000)
Costa Rica (2008)	Croatia (1999)
Spain (2007)	Latvia (1998)
Venezuela (2007)	Denmark (1997)
Uruguay (2007)	Cyprus (1994)
Portugal (2007)	Austria (1989)
New Zealand (2007)	Norway (1987)
Netherlands (2007)	Finland (1983)
Greece (2006)	Sweden (1979)
Hungary (2005)	

From Global Initiative to End All Corporal Punishment of Children. End all corporal punishment of children. http://www.endcorporalpunishment.org/pages/progress/prohib_states.html. Accessed June 14, 2011

In addition, in 1996, the supreme court in Rome declared all corporal punishment to be unlawful. In Nepal in 2005, the supreme court declared null and void the legal defense that allowed parents, guardians, and teachers to administer a "minor beating."[24] In some nations, corporal punishment of children now falls under assault laws, but in most cases the ban is educational and there are no provisions for criminal penalties but rather for public education, help, and support for parents. Social change resulted in significantly reduced acceptance and use of corporal punishment on children decades after the enactment of a ban in Sweden.

Female Genital Mutilation

Female genital mutilation, also referred to as female genital cutting and female circumcision, includes procedures that physically or symbolically alter or injure female genitalia for nonmedical reasons. It is considered a form of child abuse in the United States and a violation of human rights by the WHO and UNICEF. The practice is most common in the western, eastern, and northeastern regions of Africa; in some countries in Asia and the Middle East; and among certain immigrant communities in North America and Europe. In Africa, about 92 million girls 10 years and older are estimated to have undergone FGM, with the most severe types performed among Somalian and Sudanese populations.

Female genital mutilation is mostly carried out on young girls sometime between infancy and 15 years of age, although it is performed on newborns in certain countries. According to the WHO, FGM is classified into the following 4 major types (Figure 6-1 shows normal female genitalia):

- *Type 1—clitoridectomy.* Partially or totally removing the clitoris and, in very rare cases, only the prepuce (Figure 6-2).
- *Type 2—excision.* Partially or totally removing the clitoris and the labia minora with or without excising the labia majora (Figure 6-3).
- *Type 3—infibulation (most severe).* Narrowing the vaginal opening by creating a covering seal that is formed by cutting and repositioning the inner or outer labia with or without removing the clitoris (Figure 6-4).

Figure 6-1. Normal Female Genital Anatomy

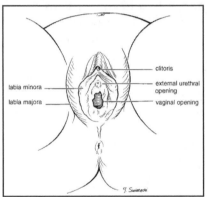

From American Academy of Pediatrics Committee on Bioethics. Ritual genital cutting of female minors. *Pediatrics.* 2010;125(5):1088–1093

Figure 6-2. Type 1 Female Genital Mutilation—Clitoridectomy

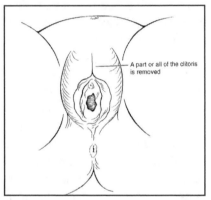

From American Academy of Pediatrics Committee on Bioethics. Ritual genital cutting of female minors. *Pediatrics.* 2010;125(5):1088–1093

Figure 6-3. Type 2 Female Genital Mutilation—Excision

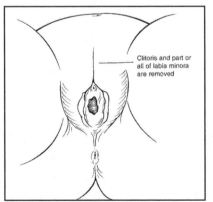

From American Academy of Pediatrics Committee on Bioethics. Ritual genital cutting of female minors. *Pediatrics.* 2010;125(5):1088–1093

Figure 6-4. Type 3 Female Genital Mutilation—Infibulation

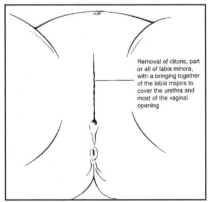

From American Academy of Pediatrics Committee on Bioethics. Ritual genital cutting of female minors. *Pediatrics.* 2010;125(5):1088–1093

- *Type 4.* All other harmful procedures to the female genitalia for non-medical purposes (eg, pricking, piercing, incising, scraping, cauterizing the genital area).[25]

Female genital mutilation has no health benefits but does have adverse effects. Complications depend on the degree of FGM and how it is performed. The practice is often carried out by non-medically trained operators with rare administration of antibiotics and anesthesia. Equipment includes old, rusty scissors, knives, or pebbles that are not usually washed. A girl's legs are subsequently bound around the ankles and thighs and she is kept in bed for a week. Immediate complications include severe pain, shock, bleeding (hemorrhage, anemia, and death), tetanus or sepsis, urine retention, open sores in the genital region, and injury to nearby genital tissue. Long-term complications are more common in types 2 and 3, including urinary complications (urethral strictures, meatal obstruction, chronic urinary tract infection, meatitis, and urinary crystals), scarring (fibrosis, keloids, partial fusion, complete fusion, hematocolpos, inclusion/sebaceous cyst, and vulvar abscess), pain (neuromas, chronic vaginal infections, dyspareunia, vaginismus, dysmenorrheal, and menorrhagia), and infertility (vaginal stenosis, infibulated scar, dyspareunia, and apareunia).

Female genital mutilation has been performed due to a mix of cultural, religious, and social factors within families and communities. Where FGM is a social convention, the social pressure to conform to what others do and have been doing is a strong motivation to perpetuate the practice. Parents initiate the practice for their daughters and, as most females in those regions underwent the procedure, many females do not feel they themselves are mutilated. Female genital mutilation is often considered a necessary part of raising a girl properly and a way to prepare her for adulthood and marriage. Female genital mutilation is often motivated by beliefs about what is considered proper sexual behavior, linking the procedure to premarital virginity and marital fidelity. Although no religious scripts require the practice, practitioners often believe it has religious support. Local structures of power and authority, such as community leaders, religious leaders, circumcisers, and even some medical personnel, support the practice.

The WHO and UNICEF recognize FGM as a violation of human rights of girls and women. Female genital mutilation is illegal and subject to criminal prosecution in several countries, including Sweden, Norway, Australia, and the United Kingdom. In 1997, the WHO issued a joint statement with UNICEF and the United Nations Population Fund against the practice of FGM. A new statement, with wider UN support, was then issued in February 2008 to support increased advocacy for FGM abandonment.[26] In 2008, the World Health Assembly passed a resolution (WHA61.16) on FGM elimination, emphasizing the need for concerted action in all sectors—health, education, finance, justice, and women's affairs.

The WHO strongly urges health professionals to not perform such procedures. However, because of immigration, pediatricians, obstetricians, and gynecologists increasingly encounter girls and women who are victims of this practice; parents may even request that a physician perform the procedure on their daughter. Over the last decade, there has been a dramatic increase in the proportion of FGM operations carried out by trained health care personnel (94% of women in Egypt, 76% in Yemen, 65% in Mauritania, 48% in Côte d'Ivoire, and 46% in Kenya), which may reduce immediate side effects. In the United States, the AAP[27] reaffirmed its position opposing all types of FGM that pose risks of physical or psychological harm, including the clitoral nick, which is forbidden under US federal law. The AAP counsels its members not to perform such procedures, recommends that they actively seek to dissuade families from carrying out harmful forms of FGM, and urges them to provide patients and their parents with compassionate education about the harms while remaining sensitive to the cultural and religious reasons that motivate parents to seek this procedure for their daughters.

Therapeutic Cultural Practices

Various cultural practices are used to treat diseases around the world. Parents may seek these forms of therapy because of cultural beliefs in their benefit or limited access to medical care. Although not intentionally abusive, these practices can have many adverse effects and may result in findings that mimic child abuse. Furthermore, they may result in the delay or refusal of standard medical practices. Pediatricians need to be aware of such practices so they can educate parents on their adverse side effects and about other forms of medical therapy. It is important to be sensitive to other cultures yet help parents understand the importance of not taking health risks that can affect their children. Recognition and education is essential for pediatricians who may see children with skin burns and bruises as a result of these practices that mimic physical abuse. Frequently, patients and families do not offer this information when they see their physician out of embarrassment and fear of judgment.

Cupping

Cupping is one of the oldest methods of traditional Chinese medicine. The earliest recorded use of cupping dates back to the early fourth century, and books written during the Tang and Qing dynasties describe cupping in great detail to treat a variety of health conditions in all age groups. In China, cupping is used primarily to treat respiratory conditions such as bronchitis, asthma, and congestion; arthritis; gastrointestinal disorders; and certain types of pain. Some practitioners also use cupping to treat depression and reduce swelling. Fleshy parts on the body, such as the back and abdomen (and to a lesser extent, the arms and legs), are the preferred sites for treatment. A cup is placed over the skin and the skin is then drawn up into the cup; this is believed to open the skin's pores, stimulate blood flow, break up obstructions, and create an avenue to draw out toxins in the body. Practitioners originally used hollowed-out animal horns for cups.

Today, most practitioners use cups made of thick glass or plastic, although bamboo, iron, and pottery cups are still used in some countries. Glass cups are preferred because they do not break or deteriorate and they allow the practitioner to see the skin and evaluate the treatment. In a typical session, glass cups are warmed using a cotton ball or other flammable substance which is soaked in alcohol, ignited, and then placed inside the cup. This burning removes the oxygen and warms the air to create a vacuum. As the substance burns, the cup is turned upside down so the practitioner can place it over a specific area of the body. The vacuum that is created anchors the cup to the skin and pulls it upward as the air inside cools. Depending on the condition being treated, the cup will be left in place for 5 to 10 minutes; several cups may be placed on a patient's body at the same time.

Some practitioners will also apply small amounts of lubricants or medicated or herbal oils to the skin before the cupping procedure. Lubricants are used to move the cup around once it is placed on the skin to cover a wider area, which results in linear purpuric streaks rather than circular (Figure 6-5). Other variations to the technique include wet cupping, which involves incising the skin before the cup is placed or during the process of suctioning, with needles placed at the base of the cup being

Figure 6-5. Cupping—Circular Areas of Erythema Over the Back

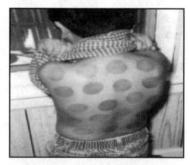

From American Academy of Pediatrics. *Visual Diagnosis of Child Abuse on CD ROM.* 3rd ed. Elk Grove Village, IL: American Academy of Pediatrics; 2008

used. Modern appliances that use a manual hand pump to create the suction are also currently available and used.

In a systematic literature review of 550 clinical studies published between 1959 and 2008, it was noted that the quality and quantity of randomized, controlled trials on cupping therapy appears to have improved during the past 50 years in China, and the majority of studies show potential benefit for pain conditions, herpes zoster, and other diseases. However, further rigorous designed trials in relevant conditions are warranted to support its use in practice.[28]

While cupping is considered relatively safe, it can cause some swelling and bruising on the skin. As the skin is drawn up under the cup, superficial blood vessels in the papillary dermis are broken, thereby creating distinctive circular cutaneous lesions and bruises on the areas where the cups were applied. Because the procedure is slow and controlled, the application of the cup and subsequent bruises are usually painless, and any marks disappear within a few days of treatment; however, these marks can be confused with physical abuse.[29]

Patients with inflamed skin, high fever, or convulsions, and patients who bleed easily, are not suitable candidates for cupping. Pregnant women should not have cupping on their abdomen or lower back. Cupping should not cross bony areas, such as spine ridges or shoulder blades. Lubricants can cause contact dermatitis with erythema, edema, blisters, and scaling in areas of direct contact. Cutaneous burns may result when proper attention is not exhibited during the procedure, resulting in heating the cup too much as well as the air inside it. Children with significant pain from cupping, long-lasting marks, or inappropriate use of the procedure can be considered abused or neglected.

Moxibustion

Moxibustion is a traditional Chinese medicine technique for all ages that involves burning the herb mugwort (*Artemisia vulgaris,* also known as moxa and traveler's herb) to facilitate healing. Moxibustion has been used throughout Asia for thousands of years. Its purpose is to strengthen the blood, stimulate the flow of body energy (referred to as chi), and maintain general health. In direct moxibustion, a small, cone-shaped amount of moxa is placed on top of an acupuncture point and burned. This type of moxibustion is categorized into 2 types, scarring and non-scarring. With scarring moxibustion, the moxa is placed on a point, ignited, and allowed to remain on the point until it burns out completely. This may lead to localized blisters and scarring after healing (Figure 6-6). With non-scarring moxibustion, the moxa is placed

Figure 6-6. Moxibustion—Scars Resulting From Burns Surrounding the Umbilicus

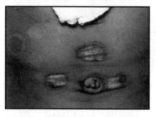

From Feldman KW. Pseudoabusive burns in Asian refugees. *Am J Dis Child.* 1984;138(8):768–769, with permission from American Medical Association.

on the point and lit but is extinguished or removed before it burns the skin. The patient will experience a sensation of heat that penetrates deep into the skin but should not experience any pain, blistering, or scarring unless the moxa is left in place for too long. In indirect moxibustion, a practitioner lights one end of a moxa stick and holds it close to the area being treated until the area turns red. Another form uses acupuncture needles and moxa. A needle is inserted into an acupoint and retained. The tip of the needle is then wrapped in moxa and ignited, generating heat to the point and the surrounding area. After the desired effect is achieved, the moxa is extinguished and the needle(s) removed.

Moxibustion is usually taught as part of a qualified acupuncture or traditional Chinese medicine degree program. Although there are no licensing or accreditation requirements, a practitioner in the United States must have an acupuncture license to perform moxibustion. In Western medicine, moxibustion has successfully been used to turn breech babies into a normal head-down position prior to childbirth; one study published in 1998 found that up to 75% of women with breech presentations had fetuses rotated to the normal position after receiving moxibustion.[30] Other studies show that moxibustion increases the fetus' movement in pregnant women and may reduce the symptoms of menstrual cramps when used in conjunction with traditional acupuncture.[30,31]

Although moxibustion has been safely used in traditional Chinese medicine for centuries, it is not for everyone. Children with direct moxibustion can have significant pain and scarring after the procedure. It can result in circular or target-like burns and sometimes scarring, which may be confused with intentional child abuse, particularly cigarette burns. Burning moxa also produces a great deal of smoke and a pungent odor and can cause respiratory problems in susceptible individuals. Children with significant pain, scarring, or respiratory effects can be considered abused or neglected.

Maqua (Therapeutic Burning)

Maqua is a form of therapeutic burning used by healers in some parts of the Middle East and Africa. This therapy uses a red-hot iron, a burning coal, or a pinch of hot cinder to cauterize and burn the skin, resulting in full-thickness burns that are usually limited to small circular areas (Figure 6-7). Therapeutic burning can result in many complications, including infections, septicemia, contractures, and even death.[32] Furthermore, it has no medical benefit and may delay seeking appropriate medical care.

Coining

One of the most common folk remedies practiced among Southeast Asians is coining. Also called coin rubbing or cao gio, coining is a dermabrasive therapy used to relieve a variety of illnesses, such as aches, pains, fever, seizures, chills, headaches, cough, vomiting, colds, nausea, abdominal pain, and symptoms related to changes in the weather. These illnesses are caused by an excess of "wind" in the body, which can be treated by "releasing" it from the body. Coining pulls the wind to the surface of the body and creates a pathway for its release. The amount of wind is measured by the degree of redness that appears on the body after coining. Balms or oils, such as Tiger Balm or liquid herbal medicines containing camphor, methanol, wintergreen oil, eucalyptus oil, peppermint oil, and cinnamon oil, are most commonly used. The skin is first lubricated with a balm or oil and the coin rubbed firmly and repeatedly in a linear pattern until blood appears under the skin, usually along the spine and ribs (Figure 6-8).[29] The technique is considered effective when it produces prominent marks that usually last only a few days.

There are complications associated with coining and misunderstanding the red marks found on patients. Children usually describe the procedure as soothing, but pain and bruising can result when the procedure is misapplied. Hyperpigmentation may also persist after the marks resolve. The

Figure 6-7. Maqua (Therapeutic Burns) in a Child With Abdominal Pain
Notice the circular scars on her chest and abdomen.

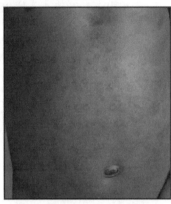

Reprinted with permission from Nazer D, Smyth M. Cutaneous conditions mimicking child abuse. In: Palusci VJ, Fischer H, eds. *Child Abuse and Neglect: A Diagnostic Guide for Physicians, Surgeons, Pathologists, Dentists, Nurses, and Social Workers.* London, UK: Manson Publishing; 2010: 69–90

Figure 6-8. Coining—Linear Lines of Petechiae and Ecchymoses on a Child's Back

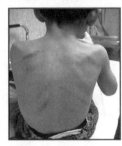

From American Academy of Pediatrics. *Visual Diagnosis of Child Abuse on CD ROM.* 3rd ed. Elk Grove Village, IL: American Academy of Pediatrics; 2008

lubricants used may cause burns, contact dermatitis, and toxicity. Tiger Balm or other oils contain camphor, which is absorbed transdermally when applied or rubbed on the skin. Camphor intoxication exhibits neurologic manifestations such as irritability, hyperreflexia, myoclonic jerks, confusion, coma, and apnea. Seizures are common and may be the first manifestation, with death sometimes resulting from respiratory failure or status epilepticus. The effectiveness of coining to treat ailments such as aches and pains can be attributed to these balms and oils, but their therapeutic use in children is limited and toxicities have been described.[33] Children with significant pain, bruising, scarring, or toxicity can be considered abused or neglected.

Other Cultural Practices

Other folk remedies have caused confusion with child abuse or have resulted in adverse health effects and even death. The therapeutic use of garlic has been reported to cause chemical burns after prolonged application.[29] Rue is a material sometimes used to treat the Hispanic folk illnesses mal ojo (evil eye) and empacho (presumed intestinal blockage). Rue may cause phytophotodermatitis, which may be mistaken for abusive burns. Herbal teas, folk remedies containing lead, and compounds containing theophylline, opium, caffeine, aspirin, or acetaminophen can poison children. In addition to the danger imposed, their use may be confused with intentional poisoning. Salting newborns by applying salt to the skin is an Asian custom that is still practiced in some areas of Turkey. It is thought to keep the skin healthy. However, this practice may lead to hypernatremia if the skin is damaged and the salt is absorbed.

Some cultures believe that scarification can serve as a preventive measure in infancy to ensure lifelong health. Scarification is also called cicatrization and is a form of body modification in which a design or pattern is cut, etched, or scratched into human skin to make a permanent scar. Like most body modifications, there are many reasons why people choose to be scarified. Sometimes it is for cultural identity; sometimes, for health treatment. Scarification is frequent in Africa and may be as significant an issue as cupping and coining.

The calves and intrascapular region are common sites for preventive scarification in Greece. The act of scarifying has been compared to tattooing because it permanently changes the skin. It has also been identified with self-harm because people have used it to cover self-inflicted wounds. Scarification began as cultural identification, especially in Maori and African societies. Other cultures may use it for religious reasons, and nearly all cultures use it for aesthetics. Facial scarification, as done in Africa and New Guinea, may be mistaken for abuse if the proper cultural context is not considered. It has been argued that although there is a reasonable case for permitting competent adults to use scarification, the practice should not be made available to minors.[34]

■ INTERNATIONAL ISSUES IN CHILD MALTREATMENT REPORTING

When practicing in a new country, pediatricians should acquaint themselves with local practices and standards applied to child maltreatment identification and reporting. While reporting is required in all US states and territories, there are variable mandated and voluntary reporting requirements in several countries depending on laws and resources (Box 6-3). Reporting can be mandated by law, allowed by law (voluntary reporting), or not specifically enumerated in a country's laws or regulations. Sexual abuse and sexual assault are often covered more specifically by criminal statutes than by child protection regulations. It is important to realize that these can result in severe criminal penalties in certain jurisdictions and a report can result in the death penalty on conviction or severe ostracism for the child and family. Some countries have a child protective orientation that emphasizes legalistic interventions; others have a family service orientation that emphasizes therapeutic interventions.[35] Information about these practices can be determined using information from ISPCAN as well as from pediatricians who are internationally based.[36,37]

Countries with mandated reporting usually have laws that apply to licensed professionals, such as medical practitioners and pediatricians. The pediatrician should ascertain whether the regulations in these countries apply to them in their visiting capacity and what exactly is required. A full listing of specific country and regional laws is beyond the scope of this chapter, but the pediatrician needs to realize that while many countries do have legally required reporting, they may only require that the most serious forms of physical and sexual abuse be reported (neglect and psychological abuse not being reportable); the basis for such reports may differ from the US "reasonable cause to suspect" standard; there are varying legal protections for making reports; and reports may go to police, governmental child protective services or community-based NGOs, social workers, or other special centers. The outcome for the child and family may rely significantly on the organization that investigates and provides services in a particular locality. For example, confidential doctors have been used in the Netherlands to investigate possible child maltreatment and to direct services without resorting to public reporting systems.[38]

Box 6-3. Child Maltreatment Reporting Requirements by Country

PROFESSIONAL REPORTING REQUIRED BY LAW

Argentina
Armenia
Australia
Bangladesh
Belarus
Benin
Bolivia
Bosnia and Herzegovina
Brazil
Bulgaria
Canada
Chile
Colombia
Denmark
Democratic Republic of Congo
Egypt
England
Estonia
Ethiopia
Finland
France
Greece
Guatemala
Honduras
Hungary
Iceland
India
Israel
Italy
Japan
Korea
Kyrgyzstan
Lebanon
Malaysia
Mauritius
Mexico
Mongolia
Montenegro
Morocco
Nepal
Peru
Philippines
Portugal
Romania
Russia
Rwanda
Serbia
Sierra Leone
South Africa
Spain
Sweden
Taiwan
Tajikistan
Thailand
Togo
Turkey
Turkmenistan
Ukraine
United States
Yemen
Zambia

PROFESSIONAL REPORTING ALLOWED BY LAW

Afghanistan
Bahrain
Cameroon
China
Fiji
Germany
Hong Kong, SARC
Netherlands
New Zealand
Nigeria
Pakistan
Poland
Portugal
Saint Lucia
Scotland
Singapore
Sri Lanka
Switzerland
Uganda

NO COUNTRYWIDE REPORTING SYSTEM

Albania
Georgia
Iraq
Ivory Coast
Saudi Arabia
Somalia
Syria

Adapted from Daro D, ed. *World Perspectives on Child Abuse.* 7th ed. Aurora, CO: International Society for Prevention of Child Abuse and Neglect; 2006; and Daro D, ed. *World Perspectives on Child Abuse.* 8th ed. Aurora, CO: International Society for Prevention of Child Abuse and Neglect; 2009

Several countries have voluntary professional reporting or general-ized reporting requirements that are not specific for pediatricians. As with mandated reporting, the pediatrician should ascertain what is to be reported and to whom, the process for investigation, and what resources are available for the reporter and family after a report is made. A vol-untary reporting system offers the pediatrician the flexibility to better understand child maltreatment issues in a family, assist with services, and preserve the family unit's integrity and child's safety. Historically, jurisdictions with voluntary reporting noted fewer child maltreatment cases, and many children and families received services without ever being officially reported. However, the pediatrician must also realize that poverty, a lack of follow-up, and the potential for future harm may mitigate the ability to effectively intervene. This is heightened in coun-tries with no specific reporting requirements where the pediatrician's only choice may be to call law enforcement authorities. Pragmatically, a police report may result in services and protection for the child, but it may also result in punishment of the child or family or no response at all when little or no resources are available or corruption has made the police response ineffective. The pediatrician should consult other practitioners and NGOs when practicing outside the United States to determine child maltreatment reporting requirements and best practices for services for families and children affected by child maltreatment.

■ STEPS FOR THE VISITING PEDIATRICIAN

The visiting pediatrician will be faced with varying cultures, parenting practices, child maltreatment definitions, laws, and reporting require-ments when practicing outside the United States. The pediatrician will have to understand these psychosocial and societal challenges to success-fully diagnose and treat disease among international child populations. In addition, child maltreatment is an important cause of physical and emotional harm in and of itself, and the pediatrician seeking to improve child health and advocate for the needs of the child and family will have to proactively prepare for specific cultural and legal practices that apply to the jurisdiction where that pediatrician will practice.

International practice requires pediatricians to become knowledgeable about specific types of child maltreatment identified in local law and custom as well as specific requirements and processes for reporting child maltreatment. They should learn specific steps to take when they suspect abuse so as to comply with local law and custom, to assist in governmen-tal intervention, and to best treat the child and family without creating inappropriate family ridicule or endangerment. Pediatricians also need to learn about services and agencies available to provide ongoing social and psychological support to prevent child maltreatment in high-risk families after it occurs.

Pediatricians should talk with culturally knowledgeable leaders and practitioners to understand the use of alternative and complementary medical practices in the community and local opinion about their proper use and abuse. When certain practices are known to be harmful or injurious, a health care professional may have little recourse other than working with the family to mitigate harm or working within local systems to provide services and assistance for children and families. Steps available to protect the child and reduce harm need to be thought out *before* the maltreated child is brought for medical care.

Beyond practice, several recommendations were made by international child maltreatment professionals.[39] To improve social context, pediatricians can participate in movements to create, implement, or monitor a national plan to prevent violence. They can increase multidisciplinary collaboration and assist with child maltreatment data collection and research on the incidence, outcomes, and costs associated with child maltreatment. They can also work to strengthen and expand child maltreatment primary prevention activities as well as treatment options for child maltreatment victims, including international models for medical team responses to child maltreatment.[40] This includes evaluating whether successful prevention programs, such as home visiting, can be adapted for local use.[41] Perhaps most importantly, a pediatrician practicing outside the United States should be nonjudgmental and should assume that parents, if they were provided with adequate personal, social, and financial resources, would optimally care for their children and protect them from abuse and neglect. It is in the best tradition of pediatrics and the special physician-family relationship for the pediatrician to recognize and respond to the psychosocial needs of families, to protect their health and safety, and to advocate for their needs in the medical system and within society.

■ KEY POINTS

- Child maltreatment consists of all forms of physical or mental violence, injury and abuse, neglect or negligent treatment, and maltreatment or exploitation, including sexual abuse, and includes intentional use of physical force or power, threatened or actual, against a child, by an individual or group that results in or has a high likelihood of resulting in actual or potential harm to the child's health, survival, development, or dignity.

- Although difficult to precisely determine its incidence, child maltreatment is a global problem. Professionals caring for children, in addition to their training and experience in recognizing and responding to child maltreatment, will have to incorporate into their practices the many international variations in cultures, parenting, and reporting laws and practices. They will also have to acquaint themselves with community resources to best provide for the health, safety, and protection of children.

- Corporal punishment is one of the parenting practices a pediatrician will encounter that may cross over into child abuse. Some nations classify corporal punishment of children under assault laws, but in most cases the ban is educational. Some forms like spanking are widely accepted and used throughout the world. Pediatricians should educate parents against the use of corporal punishment against children. In addition to the physical injuries that may result, corporal punishment is an ineffective mode of discipline and associated with higher rates of physical aggression, more substance abuse, and increased risk of crime and violence when used with older children and adolescents.

- Many cultural practices may have potential harmful side effects or may mimic findings after abuse. Pediatricians, while sensitive to parents' cultural and religious reasons, need to dissuade parents from practices that are harmful to children.
  - Female genital mutilation is one of the practices that is considered a form of child abuse and a violation of human rights. Pediatricians are urged not to perform such procedures and to educate their parents about the harms of such procedures.
  - Other alternative medical practices may result in bruises (eg, coining, cupping) or burns (eg, moxibustion, maqua). In addition to their harmful side effects, they may be confused with injuries from child abuse. Pediatricians need to be aware of such practices and educate parents about their use in a culturally sensitive way.

- Pediatricians visiting other countries should become more knowledgeable about varying definitions of child maltreatment and reporting laws and resources available for families. They need to be nonjudgmental and culturally sensitive to different practices. They need to be first and foremost advocates for children and educators for families in an effort to prevent child maltreatment globally and to improve child health.

■ REFERENCES

1. Kaljee LM, Stanton B. The foundation of global child health. In this text
2. Gelles RJ, Cornell CP. International perspectives on child abuse. *Child Abuse Negl.* 1983;7:375–386
3. Finkelhor D. The international epidemiology of child sexual abuse. *Child Abuse Negl.* 1994;18:409–417
4. World Health Organization, International Society for Prevention of Child Abuse and Neglect. *Preventing Child Maltreatment: A Guide to Taking Action and Generating Evidence.* Geneva, Switzerland: World Health Organization, International Society for Prevention of Child Abuse and Neglect; 2006. http://whqlibdoc.who.int/publications/2006/9241594365_eng.pdf. Accessed June 17, 2011
5. World Health Organization. *Report of the Consultation on Child Abuse Prevention, 29–31 March 1999.* Geneva, Switzerland: World Health Organization; 1999. http://whqlibdoc.who.int/hq/1999/WHO_HSC_PVI_99.1.pdf. Accessed February 21, 2011
6. Doek JE. The CRC 20 years: an overview of some of the major achievements and remaining challenges. *Child Abuse Negl.* 2009;33(11):771–782
7. Svevo-Cianci K, Lee Y. Twenty years of the Convention on the Rights of the Child: achievements in and challenges for child protection implementation, measurement and evaluation around the world. *Child Abuse Negl.* 2010;34(1):1–4
8. Mulinge MM. Persistent socioeconomic and political dilemmas to the implementation of the 1989 United Nations' Convention on the Rights of the Child in sub-Saharan Africa. *Child Abuse Negl.* 2010;34(1):10–17
9. US Department of Health and Human Services, Administration for Children and Families. Definitions of child abuse and neglect: summary of state laws. 2010. http://www.childwelfare.gov/systemwide/laws_policies/statutes/define.cfm. Accessed November 20, 2010
10. Jenny C, American Academy of Pediatrics Section on Child Abuse and Neglect. Recognizing and responding to medical neglect. *Pediatrics.* 2007;120:1385–1389
11. Pinheiro PS. *World Report on Violence Against Children: Report of the Independent Expert for the United Nations Study on Violence Against Children.* New York, NY: United Nations General Assembly; 2006
12. Gray J, ed. *World Perspectives on Child Abuse.* 9th ed. Aurora, CO: International Society for Prevention of Child Abuse and Neglect; 2010
13. AlEissa MA, Fluke JD, Gerbaka B, et al. A commentary on national child maltreatment surveillance systems: examples of progress. *Child Abuse Negl.* 2009;33:800–814
14. Scott D, Tonmyr L, Fraser J, Walker S, McKenzie K. The utility and challenges of using ICD codes in child maltreatment research: a review of existing literature. *Child Abuse Negl.* 2010;33:791–808
15. Akmatov KS. Child abuse in 28 developing and transitional countries—results from the multiple indicator cluster surveys. *Int J Epidemiol.* 2010:1–9
16. Gjermenia E, Van Hook MP, Gjipali S, Xhillari L, Lungue F, Hazizi A. Trafficking of children in Albania: patterns of recruitment and reintegration. *Child Abuse Negl.* 2008; 32:941–948
17. Pereda N, Guilera G, Forns M, Gómez-Benito J. The international epidemiology of child sexual abuse: a continuation of Finkelhor (1994). *Child Abuse Negl.* 2009;33(6):331–342
18. Zolotor AJ, Runyan DK, Dunne MP, et al. ISPCAN Child Abuse Screening Tool Children's Version (ICAST-C): instrument development and multi-national pilot testing. *Child Abuse Negl.* 2009;33(11):833–841

19. Runyan DK, Dunne MP, Zolotor AJ, et al. The development and piloting of the ISPCAN Child Abuse Screening Tool-Parent version (ICAST-P). *Child Abuse Negl.* 2009;33(11):826–832

20. Dunne MP, Zolotor AJ, Runyan DK, et al. ISPCAN Child Abuse Screening Tools Retrospective version (ICAST-R): Delphi study and field testing in seven countries. *Child Abuse Negl.* 2009;33(11):815–825

21. Runyan DK, Shankar V, Hassan F, et al. International variations in harsh child discipline. *Pediatrics.* 2010;126(3):e701–e711

22. American Academy of Pediatrics Committee on Psychosocial Aspects of Child and Family Health. Guidance for effective discipline. *Pediatrics.* 1998;101:723–728

23. Straus MA, Donnelly DA. *Beating the Devil Out of Them: Corporal Punishment in American Families.* New York, NY: Lexington Books; 1994

24. Global Initiative to End Corporal Punishment. End all corporal punishment of children. http://www.endcorporalpunishment.org. Accessed November 21, 2010

25. World Health Organization. Female genital mutilation. 2010. http://www.who.int/mediacentre/factsheets/fs241/en. Accessed November 16, 2010

26. World Health Organization. *Eliminating Female Genital Mutilation: An Interagency Statement.* Geneva, Switzerland: World Health Organization; 2008. http://whqlibdoc.who.int/publications/2008/9789241596442_eng.pdf. Accessed on June 17, 2011

27. American Academy of Pediatrics. Policy statement: ritual genital cutting of female minors. *Pediatrics.* 2010;126:191

28. Cao H, Han M, et al. Clinical research evidence of cupping therapy in China: a systematic literature review. *BMC Complement Altern Med.* 2010;10(1):70

29. Nazer D. Cutaneous conditions mimicking child abuse. In: Palusci VJ, Fischer H, eds. *Child Abuse and Neglect: A Diagnostic Guide.* London, England: Manson Publishing; 2011:69–90

30. Cardini F, Weixin H. Moxibustion for correction of breech presentation: a randomized controlled trial. *JAMA.* 1998;280:1580–1584

31. Wang XM. Observations of the therapeutic effects of acupuncture and moxibustion in 100 cases of dysmenorrhea. *J Tradit Chin Med.* 1987;7(1):15–17

32. Raza S, Mahmood K, et al. Adverse clinical sequelae after skin branding: a case series. *J Med Case Rep.* 2009;3:25

33. Rampini SK, Schneemann M, Rentsch K, Bachli EB. Camphor intoxication after cao gio (coin rubbing). *JAMA.* 2002;288(1):45

34. Oultram S. All hail the new flesh: some thoughts on scarification, children and adults. *J Med Ethics.* 2009;35:607–610

35. Gilbert N. Introduction. In: Gilbert N, ed. *Combatting Child Abuse: International Perspectives and Trends.* New York, NY: Oxford University Press; 1997:3–6

36. International Society for Prevention of Child Abuse and Neglect. *World Perspectives on Child Abuse.* 7th ed. Chicago, IL: International Society for Prevention of Child Abuse and Neglect; 2006

37. Daro D, ed. *World Perspectives on Child Abuse.* 8th edition. Aurora, CO: International Society for Prevention of Child Abuse and Neglect; 2009

38. Roelofs MAS, Baartman HEM. The Netherlands: responding to abuse—compassion or control? In: Gilbert N, ed. *Combatting Child Abuse: International Perspectives and Trends.* New York, NY: Oxford University Press; 1997:192–211

39. Mian M. World report on violence and health: what it means for children and pediatricians. *J Pediatr.* 2004;145(1):14–19

40. Harr C, Souza L, Fairchild S. International models of hospital interdisciplinary teams for the identification, assessment, and treatment of child abuse. *Soc Work Health Care.* 2008;46(4):1–16

41. Palusci VJ, Haney ML. Strategies to prevent child maltreatment and integration into practice. *APSAC Advisor.* 2010;22:8–17

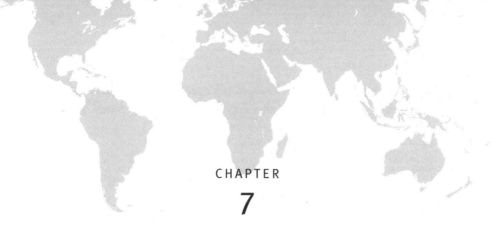

7

Environmental Hazards

Ruth A. Etzel, MD, PhD, FAAP

■ INTRODUCTION

Children's exposure to pollutants in the air, water, soil, and food—whether in the form of short-term, high-level, or long-term, low-level exposure—is a major contributor to increased morbidity and mortality, especially in developing countries. The World Health Organization (WHO) estimates that approximately one third of the disease burden in developing countries is attributed to modifiable environmental factors, including indoor and outdoor air pollution, unsafe water, inadequate sanitation, and hygiene. This is 2 to 3 times higher than the attributable portion in the most developed countries. Box 7-1 shows the WHO definition of the modifiable environment.[1] Figure 7-1 shows the higher burden of disease in African and Asian countries due to air, water, soil, and food contamination compared with the countries of North America and Europe.[2,3]

■ INDOOR AIR POLLUTION

Smoke From Biomass Fuel Combustion

About 2.5 billion people use solid fuels (biomass or coal) for cooking and breathe the air that is heavily polluted from burning these fuels. Ninety percent of rural households in low-income countries and a total of two thirds of the households in developing countries use biomass fuels for cooking or heating. The smoke contains particulates, carbon monoxide (CO), nitrogen oxides, sulfur oxides, benzene, formaldehyde, and polyaromatic hydrocarbons. Indoor sources of air pollution can produce

Box 7-1. Definition of the Modifiable Environment

- Air, soil, and water pollution with chemicals or biological agents
- Ultraviolet and ionizing radiation
- Built environment
- Noise, electromagnetic fields
- Occupational risks
- Agricultural methods, irrigation schemes
- Anthropogenic climate changes, ecosystem degradation
- Individual behaviors related to the environment, such as hand washing, food contamination with unsafe water or dirty hands

Excluded from the definition: Individual choices, such as alcohol and tobacco consumption, drug abuse, and diet; natural environments that cannot reasonably be modified (rivers, etc); unemployment (provided that it is not linked to the degradation of the environment); natural biological agents (eg, pollen); and person-to-person transmission that cannot reasonably be prevented by environmental interventions.

From World Health Organization. *Preventing Disease Through Healthy Environments: Towards an Estimate of the Environmental Burden of Disease.* http://www.who.int/quantifying_ehimpacts/publications/preventingdisease.pdf. Accessed June 15, 2011

Figure 7-1. Environmental Burden of Disease Globally

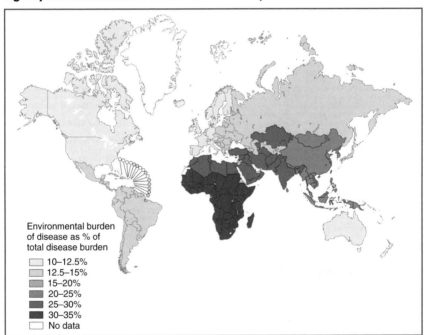

Environmental burden of disease as % of total disease burden

- 10–12.5%
- 12.5–15%
- 15–20%
- 20–25%
- 25–30%
- 30–35%
- No data

From World Health Organization. Health and Environmental Linkages Initiative. Priority environmental and health risks. http://www.who.int/heli/risks/en. Accessed August 1, 2011

very high exposure levels; concentrations of particulate matter less than 10 μm in aerodynamic diameter (PM_{10}) up to 2,000 μg/m³ are produced by burning biomass fuel (much higher than the WHO air quality guidelines [Table 7-1]).[4]

Most of the particulate matter from burning solid fuels is fine particles smaller than 2.5 μm in aerodynamic diameter. Infants and young children spend many hours very close to fires while their mothers cook.[5] High concentrations of indoor air pollution and long periods of exposure increase the risk of lower respiratory illness and tuberculosis among children.[6-8] In an analysis by the WHO in 2002, the indoor smoke from solid fuels accounted for the third highest disability-adjusted life years for children 0 to 4 years of age[9] (Figure 7-2).

In addition to cleaner burning stoves and fuels, behavioral interventions, such as keeping children away from the stove while their mother is cooking, using dry wood, and cooking outdoors whenever possible, can help reduce children's exposure to smoke from biomass fuel combustion.

Table 7-1. World Health Organization Air Quality Guidelines		
POLLUTANT	AIR QUALITY GUIDELINE VALUE	AVERAGING TIME
Carbon monoxide	100 mg/m³ 60 mg/m³ 30 mg/m³ 10 mg/m³	15 min 30 min 1 h 8 h
Nitrogen dioxide	200 μg/m³ 40 μg/m³	1 h annual
Ozone	100 μg/m³	8 h, daily maximum
Particulate matter		
$PM_{2.5}$	10 μg/m³ 25 μg/m³	1 y 24 h
PM_{10}	20 μg/m³ 50 μg/m³	1 y 24 h
Sulfur dioxide	500 μg/m³ 20 μg/m³	10 min 24 h

From World Health Organization. Air Quality Guidelines Global Update 2005. http://www.euro.who.int/__data/assets/pdf_file/0005/78638/E90038.pdf. Accessed July 6, 2011

Figure 7-2. Attributable Burden of Disease for Children 0 to 4 Years of Age

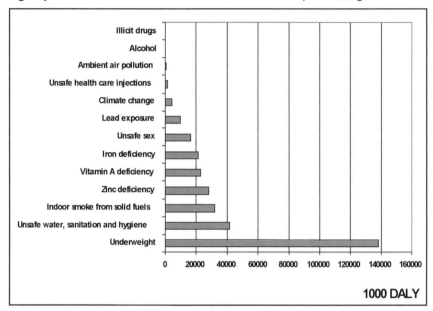

From Etzel RA. Indoor and outdoor air pollution: tobacco smoke, moulds and diseases in infants and children. *Int J Hyg Environ Health.* 2007;201:611–616, with permission from Elsevier.

Tobacco Smoke

More than 1 billion adults smoke worldwide. Tobacco, more than any other agent, kills approximately 5 million people a year—almost 14,000 every day. Tobacco will kill 8 million people a year by 2030; 70% of these deaths will be in developing countries. Around 700 million, almost half of the world's children, breathe air that is polluted by secondhand smoke. Secondhand smoke contains particulate matter and more than 4,000 different chemical compounds, many of which are poisons. Exposure to high levels of secondhand smoke causes mucous membrane irritation and respiratory effects that result in rhinitis, cough, exacerbation of asthma, headache, nausea, eye irritation, sudden infant death syndrome, and some cancers.[10,11] Exposure to secondhand smoke may also increase tuberculosis risk.[12] Using data from 192 countries, the WHO estimated the burden of disease worldwide from exposure to secondhand smoke to be approximately 1% of total mortality and 0.7% of total worldwide burden of disease in disability-adjusted life years (DALYs).[13] There is no safe level of exposure to secondhand smoke. The WHO urged all countries to pass laws requiring that all indoor public places be 100% smoke free.[14] Pediatricians can take an active role in educating parents and supporting smoke-free public policies. Blending smoking cessation counseling with secondhand smoke exposure reduction counseling can increase the attempts to quit made by lower-income mothers with young children.[15]

Carbon Monoxide

Carbon monoxide is produced by incomplete fuel combustion. Sources of CO include heating and cooking fuels, automobile exhaust, propane-fueled ice resurfacers (in ice arenas),[16] and cigarettes. Carbon monoxide poisonings increase after disasters such as hurricanes with the use of gasoline-powered generators to run refrigerators, air conditioners, and entertainment devices, including televisions and video games.[17] The symptoms and signs of mild CO poisoning (headache, nausea, vomiting, light-headedness, general malaise, dyspnea, confusion, and syncope) are nonspecific and may resemble influenza, tension or migraine headache, gastroenteritis, food poisoning, or depression. Children with higher exposures to CO may have seizures, coma, or dysrhythmias. A high index of suspicion is needed to identify CO poisoning.

Biological Particles

Exposures to airborne biological matter, including pollen and fungi, are associated with increased respiratory illness in children. Exposure to high levels of airborne fungi in damp and water-damaged indoor environments is linked to asthma exacerbations in children[18] and acute pulmonary hemorrhage in infants.[19]

■ OUTDOOR AIR POLLUTION

Children may be exposed outdoors to various mixtures of air contaminants (PM, nitrogen dioxide, sulfur dioxide, ozone, and other photo-chemical oxidants) depending on where they live and attend school, as well as other factors, such as how near their homes and schools are to polluting industries, power plants, areas of high traffic, and outdoor waste burning. Rapid industrialization has resulted in very high levels of particulate matter in some Asian cities.[20] Children exposed to outdoor air pollution and very high concentrations of particulate matter have an increased risk of acute and chronic respiratory diseases and decrements in lung function. The smallest particles result in the greatest lung damage. The WHO published a global update on air quality guidelines in 2005.[18] The air quality guidelines in Table 7-1 are recommended everywhere (indoors and outdoors) to significantly reduce the adverse health effects of pollution.

■ WATER POLLUTION

Unsafe Water, Poor Sanitation, and Hygiene

Nearly 1.1 billion people throughout the world are still without access to safe drinking water. Nearly 2.6 billion people, including half of all Asians, lack access to sanitary means to dispose excreta.[21] Proper sanitation and hygiene and safe drinking water can decrease diarrhea by 22% and decrease deaths resulting from diarrhea by 65%. Diarrhea accounts for 12% of deaths of children younger than 5 years.

Contaminated water causes a range of water-related diseases. A variety of viruses, bacteria, and parasites can contaminate drinking water and cause gastrointestinal diseases in infants and young children. Mortality and morbidity due to waterborne gastrointestinal diseases, mainly diarrheal, are still high in countries and communities where a substantial proportion of the population does not have access to proper water and sanitation. Effects from a lack of safe water and sanitation may also be indirect and long term; eg, repeated gastrointestinal infections represent a secondary cause of impaired growth, cognitive development, and school performance.[22,23]

Hygiene and household water treatment interventions have the greatest effect on diarrheal illness.[24] Eliminating open defecation should be a priority along with promoting the construction of basic sanitation facilities in households and providing safe water facilities close to people's homes that the community can operate and maintain.

Arsenic

Children are exposed to arsenic mainly through drinking water. Arsenic is naturally high in water in some areas of the world, including West Bengal, India; Bangladesh; Mongolia; China; Chile; and some parts of Africa. Arsenic is deposited in river systems over thousands of years from arsenic-rich material. Approximately 40 years ago, local authorities installed tube wells in Bangladesh and other areas to provide a clean source of drinking water uncontaminated by biological agents. In 1993, however, high levels of arsenic were discovered in the ground water in Bangladesh. A testing program revealed that about 1 in 5 tube wells were using water with high arsenic levels (greater than 50 parts per billion). A massive information campaign is under way to teach people in Bangladesh about the danger of drinking water with high arsenic levels.[25]

In addition to its natural presence in water, arsenic is also produced by a variety of activities, such as smelting and coal burning. Food crops, such as cassava, cocoyam, and other tuber crops grown in communities with mining and smelting activities, can take up arsenic from the soil.[26] Arsenic can also be found in herbal remedies.[27–29]

Arsenic is linked to neurodevelopmental problems in children. Overt symptoms of arsenic poisoning are rare in children but are seen in children as young as 3 years in Inner Mongolia.[30] After 20 or more years of exposure to high arsenic levels in drinking water, arsenic causes bladder, kidney, lung, and skin cancers. Neurologic effects, cardiovascular and pulmonary disease, skin lesions, and diabetes are also associated with arsenic exposure from drinking water.[31–33]

Fluoride

Drinking water in some parts of the world is contaminated with high levels of fluoride. Fluorosis is a potentially crippling disease caused by ingesting too much fluoride. Fluorosis is widespread in some parts of the world including the eastern part of Africa and some parts of China. High concentrations of fluoride in water can affect children's growth and intelligence.[34] Endemic goiter in children living in 6 villages in South Africa was associated with an excess of fluoride in the drinking water, presumably due to its influence on thyroid hormones.[35] Although drinking water is traditionally considered the main source of fluoride, food items may be a contributing factor in areas with high concentrations of fluoride in the soil.[36]

Other Chemicals

Chemical contamination of natural aquatic ecosystems by hospital wastewater is another, although less urgent, concern. Disinfectants, pharmaceuticals, radionuclides, and solvents are widely used in hospitals for medical purposes and research. In some low- and middle-income countries, hospital discharge of chemical compounds into the natural environment can lead to the pollution of water resources and risks for human health.[37]

■ FOOD-BORNE HAZARDS

Contamination of food with viruses and bacteria is a major cause of food-borne illnesses. Children are also at risk from a variety of chemical food-borne hazards in the environment, which include natural hazards such as mycotoxins and persistent organic pollutants.

Mycotoxins

Mycotoxins are toxic chemicals produced by certain fungi that can grow on crops in the field or during storage. Growth of fungi on grains, nuts, and other crops is influenced by temperature, humidity, and rainfall.

Mycotoxins can harm children's immune systems and lead to acute respiratory illness, gastrointestinal illness, tremors, and cancer.

Aflatoxins

Aflatoxins are poisonous substances that occur in food as a result of mold growth in peanuts and corn. High levels of aflatoxin cause acute aflatoxicosis.[38] Aflatoxin exposure during pregnancy (30% or more in tropical Africa) results in poor growth in the child's first year of life.[39] Aflatoxins are associated with jaundice in newborns and may be a cause of kwashiorkor.[40] In some parts of West Africa, about one third of children are exposed to food contaminated with more than 100 ppb aflatoxins[41]; these high levels of aflatoxin exposure may reduce secretory IgA in saliva.[42] In parts of East Africa, 49% of milk samples have high levels of aflatoxin M_1.[43]

Ochratoxin A

Ochratoxin A, produced by some molds, is toxic to the kidneys. Ochratoxin A contaminates many foods, including cereals, cereal-derived foods, dry fruits, beans, cocoa, coffee, beer, wine, poultry, eggs, pork, and milk.[44] Ochratoxin A is teratogenic, immunotoxic, genotoxic, mutagenic, and carcinogenic. In some parts of West Africa, approximately 35% of healthy people show ochratoxin A.

Fumonisins

Fumonisins are contaminants of cornmeal and cereals. Eating foods contaminated with fumonisins increases the risk of having a child with a neural tube defect and the risk of developing esophageal cancer during adulthood.

In developing countries, there is a need to ensure that children's foods do not contain excessive amounts of aflatoxins, ochratoxin A, or fumonisins.[45]

Other Chemicals

Persistent Organic Pollutants

Persistent organic pollutants include compounds such as polychlorinated biphenyls and dioxins, which are very resistant to biological degradation and remain in the environment for decades. The major source of children's exposure to persistent organic pollutants is through food.[46] The effects of these chemicals, which have been extensively investigated, include neurotoxicity and carcinogenesis.

Mercury

Mercury comes from combustion sources such as municipal waste incinerators and coal-burning power plants because coal contains mercury. The mercury is deposited into lakes and rivers and converted into methylmercury by bacteria, which then accumulates in fish that mothers and children eat. Methylmercury is toxic to the nervous system and can produce adverse neurodevelopmental effects on the fetus through the maternal diet.[10]

■ OTHER CONTAMINANTS

Lead

Children can be exposed to lead from a wide variety of sources. Leaded gasoline (petrol) was previously a major source of lead exposure. Currently, all but 9 countries have phased out leaded gasoline. Children may also be exposed from living or playing near areas where mining occurs, from lead in paint or ceramic dishes, from the use of lead ore in eye cosmetics, and from backyard cottage industries (eg, battery recycling). A mass lead intoxication occurred in Dakar, Senegal, during 2007 and 2008, which resulted in the deaths of 18 children. Their parents were engaged in recycling used lead-acid batteries and sieving and storing lead-contaminated soil in their residences.[47] In 2010, a lead poisoning epidemic in northern Nigeria resulted in the deaths of more than 200 children in communities where ore was mechanically ground as part of informal gold-mining activities. Children may also be exposed to lead in waste sites through ground, surface, and drinking water, as well as surface soil, sediments, consumable plants, or animals.

Lead is toxic to the nervous system; effects are particularly severe during the early development of the central nervous system, causing attention disorder and other developmental disabilities.[48–49] Children with elevated lead levels have lower intelligence scores, more language difficulties, attention problems, and behavior disorders.[48] These adverse effects on intellectual development of children are seen at blood-level concentrations below 10 µg/dL.[48] Blood-lead concentrations well above this level are frequently reported in children from many countries.[50,51]

Mercury

Children in low- and middle-income countries may be exposed to mercury from many sources.[52] For example, mercury is released from small-scale gold-mining sectors. Gold is extracted using mercury amalgamation, which poses a threat to human health.[53] Unmonitored releases of mercury from gold amalgamation has caused considerable environmental contamination and human health complications in the Amazon basin in South America and in rural sub-Saharan Africa.[54,55]

Skin lightening (bleaching) cosmetics and toiletries are widely used in some African countries. The active ingredients in these cosmetic products are mercury, hydroquinone, and corticosteroids. Skin absorption of mercury is enhanced because these products are used for a long duration on a large body surface area and under hot and humid conditions; fatalities have occurred.[56]

Cadmium

Children are primarily exposed to cadmium through food, secondhand smoke, and house dust. Recently, shiny children's jewelry manufactured in China was also documented to contain cadmium. Cadmium is toxic to kidney, liver, bone, and gonads and causes cancer. A study in the United States documented that behavioral problem scores at 5 and 7 years of age tended to increase with increasing blood cadmium; however, the trend was not significant. The study did not document significant effects of cadmium on children's neurodevelopment or blood pressure.[57]

Waste Sites

Uncontrolled hazardous waste sites may pose a hazard to children; these sites include waste storage and treatment facilities, landfills, former industrial sites, military facilities, waste recycling facilities, and unsanctioned wastewater discharge. Some of the substances found in uncontrolled waste sites include heavy metals such as lead, chromium, and arsenic, and organic solvents such as trichloroethylene and benzene.

Chemicals From Electronic Waste

Poor countries have become a destination for electronic waste (e-waste), including many tons of used desktop computers, fax machines, cell phones, and other electronic equipment. Although many of these machines can be repaired and resold, up to 75% of the electronics shipped to Africa is junk.[58] When dumped, this equipment may leach lead, mercury, and cadmium into the environment; when burned, it may release carcinogenic dioxins and polyaromatic hydrocarbons into the air. Children living in towns where primitive e-waste recycling occurs may have high blood levels of lead and cadmium.[59]

Pesticides

Pesticides (especially anticholinesterase-type) are some of the most common causes of acute poisonings among children in the developing world.[60] Even at low levels, these pesticides adversely affect children, including neurotoxicity and possibly endocrine disruption. Children heavily exposed to pesticides performed significantly worse on developmental tests than those less heavily exposed.[61]

Some of the older pesticides were designed to persist and can still be found in water and soil worldwide. Newer pesticides degrade more quickly but still contaminate water and soil and, consequently, food.

Nanoparticles

Nanoparticles, also called ultrafine particles, are particles with one dimension less than 100 nm and are in a wide variety of consumer products, including clothes, cosmetics, electronics, food, medicines, sunscreens, and sporting equipment. Children also breathe in nanoparticles because all gas combustion appliances, such as natural gas or propane cooking stoves, produce multiwall carbon nanotube aggregates—their concentrations are 10 times higher indoors than outdoors.[62] For low-solubility, low-toxicity materials, ultrafine particles are more toxic and cause more inflammation than fine particles.[63] Studies of children's exposure are needed but are hindered by a lack of information on the concentration of nanoparticles in many consumer products. Exposure estimates indicate that the application of sunscreen containing 2% nanoparticles results in an exposure of 56.7 mg/kg of body weight per day for a 2-year-old child.[64] The potential health effects are unknown.

■ RADIATION

Ionizing Radiation

Children can be significantly exposed to ionizing radiation from radioactive fallout (ie, after disasters such as those at the Fukushima and Chernobyl nuclear power plants)[65] and medical diagnostic equipment (ie, x-ray and radioisotopes). Abandoned medical scanners, food processing devices, and mining equipment that contains radioactive metals such as Cs-137 and Co-60 are often picked up by scrap collectors and sold to recyclers. Such items may be hidden inside beer kegs and lead pipes to prevent detection. Smelting these items contaminates recycled metal used to make new products (including consumer goods) and the furnaces that process the material. Many atomic devices were not licensed when they were first widely used by industry in the 1970s.

While most countries tightened regulations, it is difficult to track first-generation equipment that is now coming to the end of its useful life.

Acute effects of overexposure to ionizing radiation include acute radiation sickness (nausea, vomiting, diarrhea, declining white blood cell count, and thrombocytopenia), epilation (loss of hair), and death. Delayed effects are largely caused by mutagenesis, teratogenesis, and carcinogenesis. Ionizing radiation causes chromosome breaks in somatic cells (eg, lymphocytes, skin fibroblasts) that presumably account for the increased rates of cancer observed after exposure in childhood or adulthood.[66]

An excess of thyroid cancer occurred in Japanese children who were exposed to the atomic bomb beginning at 11 years of age. Thyroid cancer developed in hundreds of children in Ukraine and Belarus after a latent period of only 3 years following the partial meltdown of the nuclear reactor in Chernobyl in 1986.[67] Intrauterine exposure to ionizing radiation may cause small head size alone or severe mental retardation. Children are more sensitive to radiation than middle-aged adults by a factor of 10.[68] The health effects are greater if children are iodine deficient.

Radon

Children are constantly exposed to radon, which accounts for a large proportion of background radiation. Radon gas comes from radioactive decay of radium, a product of uranium deposits in rocks and soil. Radon enters homes through cracks in the foundation, porous cinderblocks, and granite walls. Most of the dose of radon and radon decay products is delivered to the lungs, resulting in an increased risk of lung cancer during adulthood; some of the dose goes to the bone marrow. An ecologic study in France showed an association between indoor radon concentration and acute myeloid leukemia in children younger than 10 years. Pediatricians should advise families about the hazards of radon exposure and point out that cigarette smoking adds to the radon-induced risk of lung cancer.

Solar Radiation (Ultraviolet Light)

Exposure to ultraviolet light induces skin cancer. Skin cancers rarely occur in childhood because of the long latent period except when there is markedly heightened sensitivity, as in xeroderma pigmentosum or albinism. The incidence of melanoma is increasing more rapidly than most cancers and children who experience repeated sunburns are at increased risk.

■ GLOBAL CLIMATE CHANGE

Climate change could affect child health in a number of different ways. Ecologic changes triggered by climate change could increase malnutrition, allergies, and exposure to mycotoxins, vector-borne diseases, and emerging infectious diseases. Also, environmental changes associated with greenhouse gases could lead to respiratory diseases, sunburn, melanoma, and immunosuppression.[69]

Exposure of children to the environmental hazards mentioned in this chapter is preventable. Pediatricians need to be aware of the adverse health effects from these hazards and work toward their control and eventual elimination.

■ KEY POINTS

With indoor air pollution, the main risks for child health include
- Increased incidence and severity of respiratory disorders such as acute lower respiratory tract illness, bronchitis, and asthma
- Mucous membrane irritation, headache, and discomfort

With outdoor air pollution, the main effects on child health include
- Increased incidence and severity of respiratory disorders such as acute lower respiratory tract infections, bronchitis, and asthma
- Long-term effects: chronic respiratory effects and cancer

With poor water supply, inadequate sanitation, and food contamination, the main effects on child health include
- Increased incidence and severity of diarrheal disease
- Indirect effects: impaired growth due to repeated infections

With poisoning, the main risks for child health include
- Acute toxicity (lead, mercury, or organophosphate poisoning)
- Chronic neurotoxicity: lower IQ, neurodevelopmental disorders

With radiation, the main risk for child health is childhood malignancy.

■ REFERENCES

1. World Health Organization. Preventing disease through healthy environments—towards an estimate of the environmental burden of disease. Geneva, Switzerland: World Health Organization; 2006. http://www.who.int/quantifying_ehimpacts/publications/preventingdisease.pdf
2. World Health Organization. Health and Environmental Linkages Initiative. Priority environmental and health risks. http://www.who.int/heli/risks/en
3. Smith KR, Corvalan CF, Kjellstrom T. How much global ill health is attributable to environmental factors? *Epidemiology.* 1999;10(5):573–584

4. World Health Organization. *WHO Air Quality Guidelines. Global Update 2005*. Geneva, Switzerland: World Health Organization; 2005. http://www.euro.who.int_data/assets/pdf_file/0005/78638/E90038.pdf

5. Barnes B, Mathee A, Moiloa K. Assessing child time-activity patterns in relation to indoor cooking fires in developing countries: a methodological comparison. *Int J Hyg Environ Health*. 2005;208(3):219–225

6. Bruce N, Perez-Padilla R, Albalak R. Indoor air pollution in developing countries: a major environmental and public health challenge. *Bulletin of the World Health Organization*. 2000;78(9):1078–1092

7. Ezzati M, Kammen D. Indoor air pollution from biomass combustion and acute respiratory infections in Kenya: an exposure-response study. *Lancet*. 2001;358(9282):619–624

8. Tipayamongkholgul M, Podhipak A, Chearskul S, Sunakorn P. Factors associated with the development of tuberculosis in BCG immunized children. *Southeast Asian J Trop Med Public Health*. 2005;36(1):145–150

9. World Health Organization. *World Health Report 2002. Reducing Risks, Promoting Healthy Life*. Geneva, Switzerland: World Health Organization; 2002. http://www.who.int/whr/2002/en

10. Etzel RA, Balk SJ, eds. *Pediatric Environmental Health*. 3rd ed. Elk Grove Village, IL: American Academy of Pediatrics; 2003

11. Best D, American Academy of Pediatrics Committee on Environmental Health, Committee on Native American Child Health, Committee on Adolescence. Secondhand and prenatal tobacco smoke exposure. *Pediatrics*. 2009;124:e1017–e1044

12. Lin HH, Ezzati M, Murray M. Tobacco smoke, indoor air pollution and tuberculosis: a systematic review and meta-analysis. *PLoS Med*. 2007;4(1):173–189

13. Oberg M, Jaakola MS, Woodward A, et al. Worldwide burden of disease from exposure to second-hand smoke: a retrospective analysis of data frm 192 countries. *Lancet*. 2011;377(9760):139–146

14. World Health Organization. *WHO Framework Convention on Tobacco Control*. Geneva, Switzerland; World Health Organization; 2005. http://www.who.int/tobacco/framework/en

15. Liles S, Melbourne FH, Matt GE, et al. Parent quit attempts after counseling to reduce children's secondhand smoke exposure and promote cessation: main and moderating relationships. *Nicotine Tob Res*. 2009;11(12):1395–1406

16. Salonen RO, Pennanen AS, Vahteristo M, Korkeila P, Alm S, Randell JT. Health risk assessment of indoor air pollution in Finnish ice arenas. *Environ Int*. 2008;34(1):51–57

17. Fife CE, Smith LA, Maus EA, et al. Dying to play video games: carbon monoxide poisoning from electrical generators used after hurricane Ike. *Pediatrics*. 2009;123(6): e1035–e1038

18. World Health Organization. *WHO Guidelines for Indoor Air Quality: Dampness and Mold*. Copenhagen, Denmark; 2009

19. Etzel RA, Montana E, Sorenson WG, Kullman GJ, Allan TM, Dearborn DG. Acute pulmonary hemorrhage in infants associated with exposure to *Stachybotrys atra* and other fungi. *Arch Pediatr Adolesc Med*. 1998;152:757–762

20. Jahn HJ, Schneier A, Breitner S, et al. Particulate matter pollution in the megacities of the Peal River Delta, China—a systematic literature review and health risk assessment. *Int J Hyg Environ Health*. 2011

21. Bartram J, Lewis K, Lenton R, et al. Focusing on improved water and sanitation for health. *Lancet*. 2005;365(9461):810–812

22. Neihaus MD, Moore SR, Patrick PD, et al. Early childhood diarrhea is associated with diminished cognitive function 4 to 7 years later in children in a northeast Brazilian shantytown. *Am J Trop Med Hyg.* 2002;66:590–593
23. Lorntz B, Soares AM, Moore SR, et al. Early childhood diarrhea predicts impaired school performance. *Pediatr Infect Dis J.* 2006;25:513–528
24. Fewtrell L, Colford JM Jr. Water, sanitation and hygiene in developing countries: interventions and diarrhoea—a review. *Water Sci Technol.* 2005;52(8):133–142
25. Smith AH, Lingas EO, Rahman M. Contamination of drinking water by arsenic in Bangladesh: a public health emergency. *Bulletin of the World Health Organization.* 2000;78(9):1093–1103
26. Zheng N, Wang Q, Zheng D. Health risk of Hg, Pb, CD, Zn, and Cu to the inhabitants around Huludao Zinc Plant in china via consumption of vegetables. *Sci Total Environ.* 2007;383:81–89
27. Street RA, Kulkarni MG, Stirk WA, Southway C, Van Staden J. Variation in heavy metals and microelements in South African medicinal plants obtained from street markets. *Food Addit Contam Part A Chem Anal Control Expo Risk Assess.* 2008;25(8):953–960
28. Steenkamp V, Stewart MJ, Curowska E, Zuckerman M. A severe case of multiple metal poisoning in a child treated with a traditional medicine. *Forensic Sci Int.* 2002;128(3):123–126
29. Obi E, Akunyili DN, Ekpo B, Orisakwe OE. Heavy metal hazards of Nigerian herbal remedies. *Sci Total Environ.* 2006;369(1-3):35–41
30. Xia Y, Liu J. An overview on chronic arsenism via drinking water in PR China. *Toxicology.* 2004;198(1-3):25–29
31. Khan MM, Sakauchi F, Sonoda T, Washio M, Mori M. Magnitude of arsenic toxicity in tube-well drinking water in Bangladesh and its adverse effects on human health including cancer: evidence from a review of the literature. *Asian Pac J Cancer Prev.* 2003;4(1):7–14
32. Liaw J, Marshall G, Yuan Y, Ferreccio C, Steinmaus C, Smith AH. Increased childhood liver cancer mortality and arsenic in drinking water in northern Chile. *Cancer Epidemiol Biomarkers Prev.* 2008;17(8):1982–1987
33. von Ehrenstein OS, Poddar S, Yuan Y, et al. Children's intellectual function in relation to arsenic exposure. *Epidemiology.* 2007;18(1):44–51
34. Wang SX, Wang ZH, Cheng XT, et al. Arsenic and fluoride exposure in drinking water: children's IQ and growth in Shanyin county, Shanxi province, China. *Environ Health Perspect.* 2007;115(4):643–647
35. Jooste PL, Weight MJ, Kriek JA, Louw AJ. Endemic goitre in the absence of iodine deficiency in schoolchildren of the Northern Cape Province of South Africa. *Eur J Clin Nutr.* 1999;53(1):8–12
36. Kjellevold Malde M, Maage A, Macha E, Julshamn K, Bjorvatn K. Fluoride content in selected food items from five areas in East Africa. *J Food Compost Anal.* 1997;10:233–245
37. Emmanuel E, Pierre MG, Perrodin Y. Groundwater contamination by microbiological and chemical substances released from hospital wastewater: health risk assessment for drinking water consumers. *Environ Int.* 2009;35(4):718–726
38. Centers for Disease Control and Prevention. Outbreak of aflatoxin poisoning—Eastern and Central Provinces, Kenya, January–July 2004. *MMWR Morb Mortal Wkly Rep.* 2004;53:790–793
39. Turner PC, Collinson AC, Cheung YB, et al. Aflatoxin exposure in utero causes growth faltering in Gambian infants. *Int J Epidemiol.* 2007;36(5):1119–1125

40. Hendrickse RG. Of sick turkeys, kwashiorkor, malaria perinatal mortality, heroin addicts and food poisoning: research on the influence of aflatoxins on child health in the tropics. *Ann Trop Med Parasitol.* 1997;91(7):787–793

41. Turner PC, Mendy M, Whittle H, Fortuin M, Hall AJ, Wild CP. Hepatitis B infection and aflatoxin biomarker levels in Gambian children. *Trop Med Int Health.* 2000;5:837–841

42. Turner PC, Sophie E, Moore SE, Hall AJ, Prentice AM, Wild CP. Modification of immune function through exposure to dietary aflatoxin in Gambian children. *Environ Health Perspect.* 2003;111:217–220

43. Kang'ethe EK, M'Ibui GM, Randolph TF, Lang'at AK. Prevalence of aflatoxin M1 and B1 in milk and animal feeds from urban smallholder dairy production in Dagoretti Division, Nairobi, Kenya. *East Afr Med J.* 2007;84(11 Suppl):S83–S86

44. Sangare-Tigori B, Moukha S, Kouadio JH, et al. Ochratoxin A in human blood in Abidjan, Côte d'Ivoire. *Toxicon.* 2006;47(8):894–900

45. Food and Drug Administration Compliance Program Guidance Manual. http://www.cfsan.fda.gov/~acrobat/cp07001.pdf

46. World Health Organization. *Persistent Organic Pollutants: Impact on Child Health.* Geneva, Switzerland: World Health Organization; 2010. http://www.who.int/ceh/publications/persistent_organic_pollutant/en/index/html

47. Haefliger P, Mathieu-Nolf M, Lociciro S, et al. Mass lead intoxication from informal used lead-acid battery recycling in Dakar, Senegal. *Environ Health Perspect.* 2009;117:1535–1540

48. World Health Organization. *Childhood Lead Poisoning.* Geneva, Switzerland: World Health Organization; 2010. http://www.who.int/ceh/publicatons/childhoodpoisoning/en/index.html

49. Needleman HL, et al. The long-term effects of exposure to low doses of lead in childhood. An 11-year follow-up report. *N Engl J Med.* 1990;322(2):83–88

50. Njoroge GK, Njagi EN, Orinda GO, Sekadde-Kigondu CB, Kayima JK. Environmental and occupational exposure to lead. *East Afr Med J.* 2008;85(6):284–291

51. He K, Wang S, Zhang J. Blood lead levels of children and its trend in China. *Sci Total Environ.* 2009;407(13):3986–3993

52. World Health Organization. *Children's Exposure to Mercury Compounds.* Geneva, Switzerland: World Health Organization; 2010. http://www.who.int/ceh/publicatons/children_exposure/en/index.html

53. Hilson G, Hilson CJ, Pardie S. Improving awareness of mercury pollution in small-scale gold mining communities: challenges and ways forward in rural Ghana. *Environ Res.* 2007;103(2):275–287

54. Hilson G. Abatement of mercury pollution in the small-scale gold mining industry: restructuring the policy and research agendas. *Sci Total Environ.* 2006;362(1-3):1–14

55. Spiegel SJ, Savornin O, Shoko D, Veiga MM. Mercury reduction in Munhena, Mozambique: homemade solutions and the social context for change. *Int J Occup Environ Health.* 2006;12(3):215–221

56. Olumide YM, Akinkugbe AO, Altraide D, et al. Complications of chronic use of skin lightening cosmetics. *Int J Dermatol.* 2008;47(4):344–353

57. Cao Y, Chen A, Radcliffe J, et al. Postnatal cadmium exposure, neurodevelopment, and blood pressure in children at 2, 5, and 7 years of age. *Environ Health Perspect.* 2009;117(10):1580–1586

58. Schmidt CW. Unfair trade: e-waste in Africa. *Environ Health Perspect.* 2006;114(4):a232–a235

59. Zheng L, Wu K, Li Y, et al. Blood lead and cadmium levels and relevant factors among children from an e-waste recycling town in China. *Environ Res.* 2008;108(1):15–20

60. Tagwireyi D, Ball DE, Nhachi CF. Toxicoepidemiology in Zimbabwe: pesticide poisoning admissions to major hospitals. *Clin Toxicol (Phila).* 2006;44(1):59–66

61. Kuruganti K. Effects of pesticide exposure on developmental task performance in Indian Children. *Child Youth Environ.* 2005;15(1):83–114

62. Murr LE, Garza KM, Soto KF, et al. Cytotoxicity assessment of some carbon nanotubes and related carbon nanoparticle aggregates and the implications for anthropogenic carbon nanotube aggregates in the environment. *Int J Environ Res Public Health.* 2005;2(1):31–42

63. Stone V, Johnston H, Clift MJ. Air pollution, ultrafine and nanoparticle toxicology: cellular and molecular interactions. *IEEE Trans Nanobioscience.* 2007;6(4):331–340

64. Hansen SF, Michelson ES, Kamper A, Borling P, Stuer-Lauridsen F, Baun A. Categorization framework to aid exposure assessment of nanomaterials in consumer products. *Ecotoxicology.* 2008;17(5):438–447

65. Christodouleas JP, Forrest RD, Ainsley CG, et al. Short-term and long-term health risks of nuclear-power-plant accidents. *N Engl J Med.* 2011

66. Bithell JF, Stewart AM. Prenatal irradiation and childhood malignancy: a review of British data from the Oxford survey. *Br J Cancer.* 1975;31:271–287

67. Tronko MD, Bogdanova TI, Komissarenko IV, et al. Thyroid carcinoma in children and adolescents in Ukraine after the Chernobyl nuclear accident: statistical data and clinicomorphologic characteristics. *Cancer.* 1999;86:149–156

68. Slovis TL, et al. Executive summary: conference on the ALARA concept in pediatric CT intelligent dose reduction (18–19 Aug 2001). *Pediatr Radiol.* 2002;32:221

69. Bunyavanich S, Landrigan CP, McMichael AJ, Epstein PR. The impact of climate change on child health. *Ambul Pediatr.* 2003;3(1):44–52

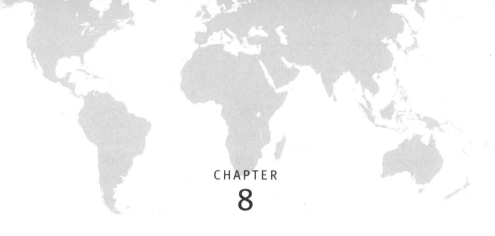

CHAPTER

8

Medical Work in Resource-Limited Countries

Cliff O'Callahan, MD, PhD, FAAP

■ THE YEARNING TO HELP

It is without a doubt that truly incredible needs exist for children around the world—in the more affluent higher-income countries and in economically and developmentally emerging nations. In fact, the majority of the globe's children and their families live in challenging situations where food, shelter, security, and access to medical and educational services are scant.[1]

It is also true that more people of all backgrounds in developed nations are aware of these disparities and wish to help rectify the situation. There is a growing tangible yearning to reach out and help, to respond to the images bombarding us, and to participate in some meaningful way. Unfortunately, it can become difficult, even for those in the medical profession, to determine the best way to do that.

The Reality That Drives the Yearning to Respond

Every few seconds a child younger than 5 years dies despite the fact that most of these deaths could reasonably be averted through evidence-based interventions at the family, community, and regional level. Every day 1,500 women die in pregnancy or childbirth, leaving their families worse off than before. The disparity in wealth, life expectancy, and access to services such as health, education, and water is growing ever wider among and within countries.[2] The burden of living in miserable conditions and suffering inordinate childhood mortality is increasingly concentrated in fewer regions, all of which are far from our higher-income realities and attention. This is powerfully demonstrated in Figure 8-1, in which each dot represents the death of 5,000 children younger than 5 years.

A hypothetical random sampling of the general US population will reveal that there is an awareness that horrible situations exist "over there" and organizations and individuals are responding. Many are at least vaguely aware of some of the efforts to improve the health and well-being of our global neighbors—Bono's concerts and his (RED) program, the US President's Emergency Plan for AIDS Relief, the Clinton Global Initiative, the Bill & Melinda Gates Foundation, Dr Paul Farmer's work in Haiti because of Tracy Kidder's book *Mountain Beyond Mountains,* and the United Nations Children's Fund (UNICEF). A very few may have heard of the Millennium Development Goals (MDGs).

On further questioning our respondents would be able to list some of the situations that pose dire threats to children—hunger, HIV/AIDS, malaria, and cleft palates. These answers reflect the images portrayed in advertisements from organizations looking for donations and from episodic reports in the news. It is rare that internal military conflicts, child trafficking, access to services, corruption, family and national debt burden, neglected diseases, and even tuberculosis are mentioned.

Figure 8-1. Worldwide Distribution of Child Deaths

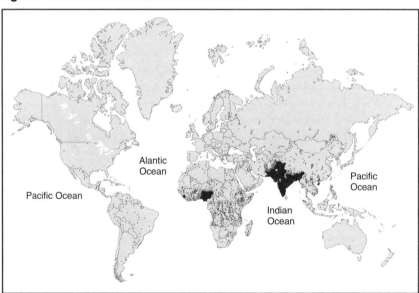

From Black RE, Morris SS, Bryce J. Where and why are 10 million children dying every year? *Lancet.* 2003;361(9376):2226–2234, with permission from Elsevier.

Many in the health field would respond similarly to those in the general population, but over the last decade there has been a remarkable increase in a deeper awareness of the realities—and the desire to respond—led in no small part by our younger colleagues. A defining moment in the accessibility of lucid information was the *Lancet* child survival series in the summer of 2003,[3] which crystallized the state of the globe's neediest in terms of mortality, etiologies, evidence-based health interventions, and economic and political responses. This was followed by similar series on maternal[4] and neonatal[5] situations and needs.

Clarifying the crushing needs in such a pithy manner has paralleled the frequency of presentations at conferences and discussions in academic centers, leading to increased interest among health professionals to respond. Furthermore, the recognition that health as a component of general well-being is a fundamental human right, based in the UN Convention on the Rights of the Child,[6] means that participation in global health efforts becomes a logical means to aid the global family in attaining the realization of this philosophy.

Yearning to Help: The Response

Historically, the response to medical needs around the world originated through a combination of religious, political, and military influences. The Order of Malta formed around 1048 during the crusades when the first knights built a hospital in Jerusalem. Over the centuries a variety of Catholic orders dedicated themselves to service of the sick; after the reformation other Christian religions began ministries to the sick at home and abroad, often following in the footsteps of explorers and colonization.

Presently, a considerable proportion of the medical aid provided, especially in Africa and the Americas, is through faith-based organizations. Jewish and Islamic medical aid organizations are also becoming increasingly active throughout the world. It is only relatively recently that medical aid organizations have been created without a religious underpinning. Henry Dunant's efforts in response to the atrocities of war led to the adoption of the Geneva Convention as well as the formation of the International Committee of the Red Cross in 1863, and Doctors Without Borders came into being in 1971, ostensibly as an areligious and apolitical entity; these are 2 of the most recognizable organizations. However, until recently, relatively few people undertook these efforts. Albert Schweitzer's 1931 book, *On the Edge of the Primeval Forest*, was perhaps the first book to popularize the work of those rare health care workers in developing regions.

Presently, there appear to be 3 populations in health fields with a burgeoning interest to respond to the needs of families in challenging situations. The first and fastest growing population is the learners—undergraduates, health science students, and residents. The second population is those in the workforce, and the third population is the retired.

Surveys conducted over the last quarter century reflect this growing interest. Very few physicians, a paltry 0.32%, were involved with global health activities in 1984.[7] Assuming that offering residency training and electives reflects expressed interest, one can see the remarkable increase in programs offering international health courses or special programs; the proportion of US medical students who took international electives rose from 6% in 1984 to 26% in 2007.[8]

Pediatric residencies offering global health electives mirrored that trend by increasing from 25% of surveyed US and Canadian programs in 1996[9] to 52% in the most recent survey of residencies in the United States, Puerto Rico, and the Caribbean in 2007.[10] The 2008 American Academy of Pediatrics (AAP) survey of graduating residents contained illuminating responses; training in global health topics was available to 59% of respondents, and 21% participated in such training. Moreover, the opportunity to participate in global health training was an essential or very important factor in selecting a residency program for 22% of respondents. Remarkably, about one third of respondents were definitely or very likely planning to work or volunteer in a developing country after residency.[11]

The only time that international health interest and activities were assessed in practicing pediatricians occurred with the ninth AAP Periodic Survey of Fellows in late 1989. With a response rate of 71% from 1,000 surveys, 38% of respondents said they would serve or may be interested in serving in some capacity in a developing country within the next 3 years. Even then, 20 years ago,

> *Sixteen pediatricians (about 2% of all respondents) said they participate in overseas health programs, and have devoted an average of 122.3 hours in those activities during the past year. Among these pediatricians, 69% volunteered their time, 19% participated for a reduced fee, and 12% participated for a full fee. The pediatricians were equally divided on how they participated in the overseas health programs: 33% each said they did direct patient care, participated as an advocate/consultant, and did both direct patient care and advocacy/consultation.[12]*

Medical academies and societies are also responding to the interests and needs of their membership by dedicating staff and programs to support global health activities. Examples include the American Academy of Family Physicians (AAFP) Center for International Health Initiatives, created in 2000; the American Congress of Obstetricians and Gynecologists Department of International Activities; and the American College of Physicians International Activities Coordinating Committee. The Canadian Paediatric Society and Royal College of Paediatrics and Child Health in Britain have international health sections, while the AAP has a dedicated Office of International Affairs as well as the member-driven Section on International Child Health.

The number of organizations dedicated to working on issues in developing regions has increased dramatically over recent years. Of the 5,400 larger nongovernmental organizations (NGOs) that Charity Navigator[13] tracks, 500 are involved in international activities. GuideStar[14] currently tracks 9,505 nonprofits under the category of international health. Even this does not reflect the multitude of small grassroots groups that exist within developing countries or the small 501(c)(3) nonprofits that community groups or individuals create for their specific projects. Furthermore, it is difficult to estimate the total number and types of health-related organizations because one might argue that groups involved in agriculture, land rights, microenterprise, and human rights can improve general health and should be included.

Pediatric-related NGOs within the NGO Committee on UNICEF increased from 13 in 1949 (when it first began) to 80 presently, with 191 NGOs having consultative status with UNICEF in 2006. Nongovernmental organizations having a relationship with the World Health Organization (WHO) increased from around 10 in 1948 to 185 in official consultative status as of January 2009.[15]

Governments and intergovernmental organizations increasingly involve themselves in responding to needs in poorer regions. Younger-than-5 mortality trends are good proxy measures of national health status and intervention efforts; the rate decreased substantially from 1960 to 1990 because of enormous efforts after the Declaration of Alma-Ata. However, since then the rate of decline in childhood mortality has slowed from 2.5% to 1.1% per year. This reality led to a renewed and coordinated response through the September 2000 UN MDGs,[16] whose signatories represent all 189 UN member states. Tracking from 1990 through 2008 produced a worldwide average reduction rate of 1.8%, which translates into 3.7 million fewer children dying each year, a commendable achievement.[17] However, for the 8.8 million children who do die yearly (as of 2008), there remains an urgent call to more intense action.

The governments of the 20-some wealthy nations that comprise the Development Assistance Committee of the Organisation for Economic Co-operation and Development recently reaffirmed their promise to increase economic aid to 0.7% of gross national income (GNI) (formally GNP or GDP). Unfortunately, they have a dismal record of complying with the agreement, which was first made in 1970 with the goal of reaching that level by the mid-1970s.[18] Currently, they voice intent to reach the goal in the MDG 2015 time frame—45 years late. The United States is well below its commitment at 0.2% GNI (Figure 8-2). At this time, only 5 countries meet the goal.[19]

How to Operationalize the Yearning to Help

The previous section's brief overview of the magnitude and generalized responses to global need is a necessary prelude to this next section. How might any one individual who is responding to the yearning to help consider proceeding? The following is based on my experience advising a variety of students, physicians, and other health professionals during

Figure 8-2. Net Official Development Assistance in 2008 as Percent of Gross National Income

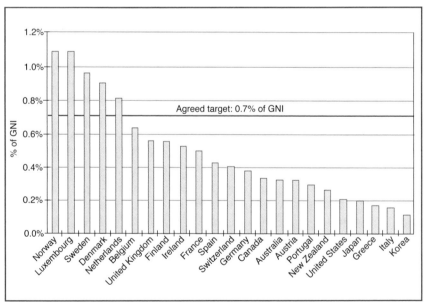

From Shah A. Causes of poverty. Global Issues Web site. http://www.globalissues.org/issue/2/causes-of-poverty. Updated June 5, 2011. Accessed June 15, 2011

the working part of their lives, as well as retirees, over the past 15 years. It is wonderful to see such enthusiasm and altruism in those who are gifted with intelligence and skills. It is sad to see the idealism fade as the pressures of study, family, and work pry many of them away from their dreams as they failed to find a way to channel their energies during the period in their lives when they were open to making the difficult decisions that might set them on a road less traveled.

The desire to respond to the yearning is powerful. To actualize that dream, it is imperative to go through a process of self-discernment to determine a realistic path. One must be open to a variety of options and truthful about the limitations that exist. It can be helpful to lead people through a simple discernment process.

Figure 8-3 presents a generalized decision tree for those early in their career decision-making process, often at the undergraduate level, when determining an area of concentration. It is fairly self-explanatory, but

Figure 8-3. Generalized Logic Decision Tree

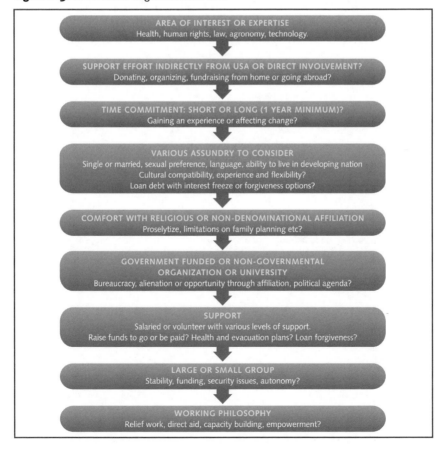

volumes could be written about each step. Despite the fact that the second level asks whether one will actually go abroad to be involved in global issues or do so from their developed nation, most learners do not understand how critical that step is until the other parameters are considered, and they often end up back at that point. The sequence of decision steps is not necessarily fixed and must sometimes be rearranged based on the unique priorities of the individual.

Following the same logic, Figure 8-4 illustrates a more specific pathway for those in the medical field. It is not exhaustive and there are most likely unique life choices not covered. Its aim is to paint broad swaths of choices to help learners determine what they are certain of and what they are equivocal about and, therefore, what they still need to research.

For the purposes of this chapter, it will be assumed that the reader is following the path in Figure 8-4 down to working abroad for a long-term block of time with an organization. However, someone who only gets partway down the decision tree should not be dissuaded from becoming involved in work abroad. There are innumerable examples of physicians from private, health maintenance organization, community clinic, and Indian Health Service settings who travel abroad episodically and

Figure 8-4. Medical Jobs Off the Beaten Path

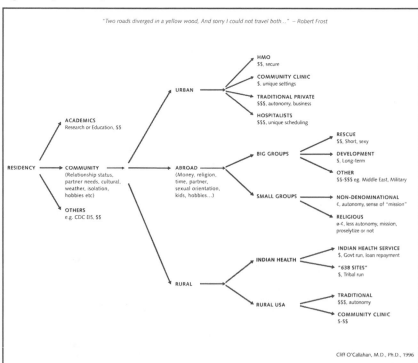

support efforts from home. There is a growing body of pediatricians, especially hospitalists and emergency physicians, who are becoming adept at negotiating unique job schedules. Many pediatricians contract to work in blocks or job share to amass time for work abroad.

Alternatively, another route to involvement with global health improvement is through academic institutions. Collaborative partnerships created between academic centers and communities or institutions in other countries can be extremely powerful catalysts for change for the learners and academicians of both parties. Table 8-1 lists a few examples of such partnerships.

For those pediatricians, regardless of their primary work environment, who truly feel they can go abroad for episodic short-term or longer tours, ongoing discussions are warranted with mentors who can help them filter the choices found in the many aid agency listings.

Perhaps the most critical step in the self-discernment process is to determine the capacity in which one wishes to work. Is one drawn to disaster relief, refugee aid, education, direct patient care in hospitals or clinics, community organizing, public health, or research on a particular disease entity? Once this becomes clear it is easier to negotiate the daunting lists.

Obvious next issues to address and research are whether one is comfortable working within an organization with religious overtones or a mission to proselytize; it becomes immediately clear that the vast majority of organizations listed are, to some degree, religiously affiliated. However, affiliation with a denomination does not automatically indicate religious overtones in the provision of care and demonstrates the need to research each option carefully.

The ability to search for opportunities is much easier in the digital age, but there are also some superb printed resources. The AAP Section on International Child Health maintains an up-to-date catalog of groups who use pediatricians in its book *Working in International Child Health*[23]

Table 8-1. Academic Centers and Community Partnerships		
NAME	ACADEMIC PARTNER	HOST PARTNER
Shoulder to Shoulder[20]	10 US academic medical centers	Honduras
The Canadian Neonatal Network[21]	11 Canadian universities	China
Welbodi Partnership[22]	Welsh ABM University Health Board	Sierra Leone

Abbreviation: ABM, Abertawe Bro Morgannwg.

and on its Web site.[24] Other texts are useful from a general medicine perspective, such as the accessible *Finding Work in Global Health*[25] and the quite extensive *Awakening Hippocrates: A Primer on Health, Poverty, and Global Service.*[26] The latter's companion volume, *A Practical Guide to Global Health Service,* contains an extensive list titled, "The Omni Med database of international health service opportunities."[27] Particular positions of a wider spectrum that would include public health, consulting, administrative, and managerial work with agencies and universities can be found in other sources such as the Global Health Council Global Health Career Network.[28]

Evaluating an organization for which one might consider working or donating is also more easily accomplished now. A variety of resources are available and can be found in Box 8-1. However, it can still be difficult to research background on small nonprofit organizations with budgets below $1 million per year.

Box 8-1. Resources for Evaluating Organizations

American Institute of Philanthropy at www.charitywatch.org critically evaluates more than 500 groups.

Charity Navigator at www.charitynavigator.org rates more than 5,000 groups using Form 990.

Ministry Watch at www.ministrywatch.com rates more than 500 evangelical groups.

Evangelical Council for Financial Accountability at www.ecfa.org rates 1,400 groups.

GuideStar at www.guidestar.org facilitates access to the Form 990 that nongovernmental organizations submit to the Internal Revenue Service for 700,000 charities.

Great Nonprofits at www.greatnonprofits.org is a blog-like review site.

Transparency International at www.transparency.org tracks corruption.

■ BARRIERS TO BECOMING INVOLVED

The algorithms for self-discernment allude to barriers that might preclude working in certain categories. It is important to take time and examine these honestly with one's self, family, and mentors.

Burden of Debt

One of the most common and insurmountable barriers is the burden of debt when finishing residency. The Association of American Medical Colleges estimates that more than 86% of graduating medical students have educational debt. In 2008, the average US medical school graduate carried a debt burden of more than $145,000 from public medical schools and $180,000 from private medical schools. European medical students incur less debt burden because very few pay tuition. Their situation may be slowly changing. Britain is now charging students from more affluent families. However, on the positive side, some British physicians in training can take up to 3 years and work abroad in an out-of-program experience with the ability to return to the program and stage they left.

Very few loans offer the option to freeze interest accruement and defer principle payments while working in volunteer positions. Sporadic groups on an individual basis have covered the interest accruement as part of their support package for volunteers during their service. The Baylor International Pediatric AIDS Initiative (BIPAI), for example, offers a competitive salary and significant loan repayment. The MedSend model of covering a volunteer's monthly loan payment is a powerful example of what is possible but is limited to those who are comfortable with an overtly Christian agenda. As an alternative to working abroad, many choose to work in Indian Health Service sites where loan repayment can be up to $24,000 per year. Others pursue the Centers for Disease Control and Prevention Epidemic Intelligence Service, in which they earn a domestic salary and are often able to work abroad.

There is a glimmer of hope for the future in the form of legislative changes, such as the Global Health Expansion, Access to Labor, Transparency, and Harmonization Act of 2010 (HR 4933), which might make moneys available for professionals expanding the health workforce abroad. Significant changes to loan repayment programs recently became effective through the College Cost Reduction and Access Act of 2007; section 203 creates a new income-based repayment program that can result in substantially lower monthly payments for those with a high-debt/low-income ratio, even if not involved in public service activities. In this program, remaining debt is forgiven after 25 years. For those who seriously consider full-time work in a public service setting or for a nonprofit 501(c)(3) and have a similar high-debt/low-income ratio, section 401 provides forgiveness of remaining debt after just 10 years (which does not have to be continuous). While this legislation was written and designed to aid law graduates working in public service settings, the law is broadly applicable. A superb description of the background to and explanation of this legislation can be found at www.law.georgetown.edu/news/releases/documents/Forgiveness_000.pdf.

Time

The ability to affect change and improve the lives of children and their families depends on many factors; the time we can dedicate to the task is certainly one of the most important. However, the reality for many in the health field is that there are forces pulling us to remain on more typical paths—the weight of building a career in academics or practice, finding a life partner, raising a family, paying off loans, fearing the unknown. The great majority of health professionals who involve themselves with global volunteerism or work do so in short stints of a week to a month at a time. Some find ways to make their short interventions productive and nondisruptive. However, if the MDGs are to be met, it will require more health professionals dedicating longer periods working in nontraditional settings.

The NGOs engaged in long-term work generally recognize that one must commit to at least 1 to 2 years of service to realistically contribute to the program. This time frame likely reflects summiting the steep learning curve that leads to a better understanding of the particular program philosophy, the local security and social norms, the different clinical environment and treatment stratagems, and the comfort of living in another milieu that can be potentially challenging, such as rural or urban poverty, linguistic and sociocultural isolation, physical separation from friends and family, weather patterns, work ethics, availability of social outlets, and others. It is quite similar to the well-recognized temporal improvement in physician efficacy and comfort when transitioning from residency to work life in a new area but compounded by a multitude of more unique variables.

The length of this transitional phase that brings one from novice to contributing participant is realistically affected by the number and length of prior experiences and the quality and depth of prior training and orientation—both of which are consciously modifiable. On the other hand, the unique combination of resiliency, flexibility, fortitude, and gumption that any individual possesses, and which allows that person to not only survive in challenging environments but thrive, is less modifiable. It must be determined through experiences and followed by reflection and truthful introspection before embarking on further or more extensive endeavors.

Calculating one's unique comfort level in a lower-income country setting is a critical part of the discernment process to know whether one should follow the short-term or long-term experience pathway. For this reason, educational institutions sending learners abroad must provide good preparatory education, as well as create excellent opportunities where a learner can be challenged and supported, and have sensitive mentors or faculty on site to facilitate the reflection process.

Family and Relationships

One very real barrier for many idealistic learners finishing residency and wishing to pursue their dream of working in global health is relationships. For some, the barrier to going abroad is concern for the safety of their spouse, parents, or other family members. For others it is the time pressure to encounter a compatible life partner. This is potentially more complicated depending on one's gender, race, religion, and sexual orientation in relation to the contemplated region or culture. Furthermore, a greater proportion of women are entering the health profession and expressing an interest in global and community health activities. The pressure to start a family, the safety concerns about where to be pregnant and deliver children, and the issues surrounding raising and schooling dependents abroad are all valid preoccupations and potential barriers to short- and long-term involvement abroad.

Fear

Fear of working in the developing world is a very real barrier that must be honestly recognized. There is a substantial increase in risk to self, depending on the length of time abroad, that includes illnesses, stress resulting in mental health issues, and work-related hazards such as blood-borne pathogens.[29] The rates of road and travel injuries are rising exponentially in lower-income countries even as they decrease in the industrialized world.[30] Fortunately, there remain many opportunities for those who discern that they are not suited to living in an emerging nation, or even visiting for short-term collaborations. All organizations and institutions can benefit from volunteers who work on the home front teaching, mentoring, organizing, and fund raising.

■ ETHICAL CONSIDERATIONS WHEN INTERVENING IN OTHER'S LIVES

Health professionals channel their efforts to address the needs of those less fortunate in a variety of ways; many choose a long-term commitment of more than a year to work and live in developing nations providing direct care, public health assistance, community development, teaching, or conducting research. Many more professionals and almost all learners choose a shorter time frame because of time restraints, loans, family commitments, fear of the unknown, and the inability to break away from a comfortable existence.

These shorter experiences may be offered through government or university affiliations, NGOs with a religious or secular bent, and small private groups that are often church based. Many argue that these short visits are helpful[31] while others contend that they offer little beyond immediate respite, provide substandard care, and squander millions of dollars.[32–36] Regardless, short visits will continue. Those visiting from the educational realm can be a valuable means of raising consciousness and skills in our future medical professionals.[37,38]

The fact that we have the wealth and political advantage to travel abroad and visit a developing country where the vast majority of our hosts will never have such an opportunity creates an immediate and inevitable power imbalance that gives us pause and could prompt reflective discussion among participants before embarking on a journey.

From the collective experience of many colleagues, Sue Hammerton, with whom I worked in Guatemala for many years, and I developed a set of ethical principles that I now offer as a discussion piece and framework for visiting medical groups so they might effectively and ethically work with local health structures in the communities they visit, with the hope that the intervention will affect recipients and visitors in a positive manner.

The principles that guide medical education in our developed country's institutions, such as the Accreditation Council for Graduate Medical Education (ACGME) competencies in the United States, need not be different than the principles that guide medical work in developing country settings. Professionalism, medical knowledge pertinent to the area, appropriate system-based practice and care, particular emphasis on cultural and linguistic sensitivity in patient care and interpersonal skills, and the goal of continuous learning and improvement from the experience are necessary components for planning a medical visit or long-term stay—as necessary as a passport and plane ticket. Various countries, such as India, Nepal, El Salvador, and Jamaica, place restrictions and oversight on visiting groups.[39] It is reasonable to suggest that it is even more important that a group aims for the highest standards when a guest in regions where there is no explicit oversight or accountability, realizing the challenges of monitoring outcomes and providing follow-up in a vulnerable population.[40]

The overarching goal of these recommendations is that the host community and visiting group have a *mutually beneficial ethical relationship*. Professionals come with good will and energetic plans for intervention, but oftentimes these visitors may be misguided or influenced by a naive personal agenda. Therefore, it is not surprising that the resulting effort does not affect the community in positive health improvements and programs.

Guidelines for how a traveler might optimally behave while abroad have been developed. The International Society of Travel Medicine created a guide for "the responsible traveler" that is applicable to anyone going abroad.[41]

A 1997 editorial in *BMJ* led to a conference in Cambridge, MA, in 2000 with the theme "Shared Statement of Ethical Principles for Everyone in Health Care." The published report[42] nicely summarizes the discussions around the 6 major principles proposed.

1. Health care is a human right.
2. The care of the individual is at the center of health care, but the whole system needs to work to improve the health of populations.
3. The health care system must treat illness, alleviate suffering and disability, and promote health.
4. Cooperation with each other, those served, and those in other sectors is essential for all who work in health care.
5. All who provide health care must work to improve it.
6. Do no harm.

These principles, though quite broad, can certainly be used when designing or examining a global health program.

Guidelines that are more directed at medical professionals interested in short-term medical work abroad have been postulated.[40] The most recent and excellent is the product of the Working Group on Ethics Guidelines for Global Health Training and elucidates a broad array of guidelines broken down into categories under "Sending and host institutions," "Trainees," and "Sponsors" that are particularly pertinent to global health training programs.[43]

The framework that Sue Hammerton and I first created in 2004 (Box 8-2) proposes 7 principles that we felt were imperative to incorporate into a visit conducted by *any* medical group who claims they are there to contribute to the improvement of global health at the community level.

Box 8-2. Framework for a Mutually Beneficial Ethical Relationship

Discernment of self and visiting group
Expressed felt need of host community
Cultural and linguistic competency
Benefit to host community
Benefit to visiting group
Ethically acceptable material benefits
Ethical relationship

Discernment of Self and Visiting Group

One of the most important but often overlooked steps in the process of arranging for a medical visit abroad is *intention*—the process of discernment and planning whereby the individual and group reflect on the impetus to make such a visit and explicitly clarify their goals. Many of us would, on serious reflection, acknowledge the wish to journey abroad for reasons that might include altruism, adventure, compassion, proselytizing, guilt, learning, escape, and personal gain. The last might include admiration from others, professional advancement, and research and project completion. All may be valid if realized in a thoughtful way.

The importance of this first principle is that the discerning process can determine every aspect of the visit, ultimately determining whether the great effort in getting to a community resulted in a mutually positive experience or, alternatively, a few stories in the local paper about the visitors and plastic bags of out-of-date sample medicine for nebulous ills in the hands of confused locals.

Expressed Felt Need of Host Community

For the relationship to be mutually beneficial, the visiting group must determine the expressed felt needs of the host community.[44] This implies creating a space of time, commitment, and effort whereby the visiting institution, because of its discernment process and resultant goal setting, meets with a community to learn with them and provide services perceived to be vital by the host community. This is in contrast to medical visits that seldom have an effect beyond the immediate distribution of services and medicine. The glaring need that initially inspired the effort to visit rarely results in a change in the overall state of well-being for the hosts. However, incorporating the most basic rural public health initial assessment tools[45] into a first step, the visiting group could meet with established leaders, elders, and elected and medical representatives. Additionally, it should also make it a point to meet with local women's groups to get an accurate reflection of maternal and child needs. This process takes time and may seem to delay the intentions of the visitors. We trust that embracing this kind of relationship will eventually result in a richer experience. Demonstrating thoughtful planning and implementation is especially important for our learners and colleagues.

The importance of this principle is the acknowledgment that local people know their own needs and visiting medical guests can respect their host's dignity and intelligence by helping them to address necessary issues. There are a growing number of examples of such collaboration.[46-48]

Cultural and Linguistic Competency

This principle reflects how we act and interact with the host community. For a visiting group to accurately assess and clarify a mutually expressed felt need with a host community, it must proceed with cultural and linguistic competence. Medical institutions in the United States are expected to provide patients with access to translation services. We hold our medical learners and providers to a high standard of cultural integrity through regulations, despite the challenge of actually meeting those expectations.[49] For example, in the United States these regulations originate with the ACGME and the Joint Commission, while in Britain it is with the General Medical Council. It is equally vital to strive toward those expectations of language and cultural competency while working as guests among vulnerable populations. Visiting preceptors of medical learners bear an even greater responsibility to acquire linguistic skills or quality translators, and model cultural awareness and sensitivity. In many cases it is possible to find local organizations and individuals who can help with this process of acculturation.

Benefit to Host Community

Most visiting medical professionals would claim that sharing the wealth of knowledge and skills they possess, with the goal of improving health for the chosen host community, is one of the most important motivating factors for traveling on a medical delegation or living and working abroad. Providing ambulatory care to long lines of villagers might give the perception that needs are being addressed. However, most resulting interventions have exceedingly short-term results because of a lack of continuing care and medicine. Moreover, the presence of foreign doctors can often undermine the confidence that hosts have with their local providers. Conversely, by working in conjunction with local physicians, rural nurses, health promoters, and midwives, visitors create the opportunity to play a critical role in improving health system capacity and quality.[50] It is necessary that a visiting group acts in ways that reflect a conscious choice to put the good of their hosts above their own needs.

One of the most simple yet profound benefits that host communities express is the joy they feel in knowing that others from more powerful nations know and care about them as they work together in solidarity.

Benefit to Visiting Group

The purpose of this principle is to optimize the benefit to visitor and host while minimizing harm to the host community. One of the most powerful transformative aspects of working in economically, environmentally, or politically challenged resource-poor areas is to be exposed to the reality of life beyond a developed country. Physicians attracted to this work know that they will gain much more than they could ever hope to give and will benefit tremendously from the experience.[51] Being forced to diagnose using clinical skills and bearing witness to advanced stages of disease with little recourse for cure crystallizes the effect of public and interventional health, economics, policy, and geography on the well-being of our neighbors in lower-income settings. Coupled with built-in time for reflection and directed instruction, the lessons learned in such settings can improve our provision of care to large immigrant and indigent populations in developed regions and can be the catalyst for novel and ongoing collaborations.[52,53] Such partnerships between higher-income and lower-income areas are critical if there is to be an improvement in global health to meet the MDGs.[54–56]

There are unique situations that bear continued scrutiny and reflection, such as the experiences surgical trainees gain from performing surgeries abroad that are rarely if ever performed in their home institutions.

Ethically Acceptable Material Benefits

Health systems in the developed world generate an enormous amount of medical waste, and some of it can certainly be used in less well-supplied regions. Many examples exist at the local and regional level for collecting medicines, supplies, and equipment for donation.[57] The challenge behind this sixth principle is that the recipient must be provided some choice in what is brought, often at great expense, and that the material is appropriate. Durable medical equipment should be in good working order and accompanied by spare parts and instructions in the recipient's language. Reference material and journals are best in the local language, although English is moderately universal as a medical language, and should be less than 5 to 10 years old, depending on the type, as stated by AAP and AAFP book repositories. Patient-directed educational material should be language and culture appropriate. Medicines should be appropriate in type, quantity, and expiration date.[58]

It is worth considering whether collecting monetary donations and buying materials and medicines in country might benefit the community on a larger scale.

The Shelf-Life Extension Program that the Food and Drug Administration administers for the US military demonstrates that many drugs can be used beyond their expiration date,[59] but donating expired medicines can be offensive to our hosts and illegal for many countries' ministry of health to accept. If a decision is made to use expired medicines, the visiting group must take responsibility to communicate this decision with the host, repackage, and explain the change of expiration dates. Samples of medicines rarely used and of amplified spectrum should be avoided. A guiding principle could be to bring only high-quality generics from the WHO lists, general and pediatric, of essential medicines[60] that have a remaining 12-month shelf life.

Ethical Relationship

Both words in this principle are important—everything that a visiting or collaborating group does should be based on ethical standards of practice and conducted within a relationship *with* the host community. Mutual respect and shared goals achieved over an extended period have much more likelihood of fostering good will and positive outcomes for all involved. Eliciting the perceptions of the host community can be extremely valuable and remarkably revealing.[61]

Group leaders, those involved in research projects, and all precepting health professionals bear an enormous responsibility. They are the ambassadors of the institution they represent and the country from which they originate. These health ambassadors have a tremendous effect on their learners and colleagues as well as on host participants and patients. Their attention to details such as providing quality orientation and daily feedback, ensuring good patient documentation and follow-up, and maintaining communication with host representatives can ensure a positive ongoing relationship. The lack of such detail can be devastating.[62]

All short- and long-term visitors, and the institutions, NGOs, and churches they represent, need to take responsibility in maintaining the highest standards of medical care. Significant insightful work published on ethical principles for students needs to be adopted and incorporated.[63]

The guiding principles outlined here are merely a framework, leaving more to be discussed and built. Based on discussions during various international health conferences, it is probable that many would support proposing the development of a similar set of expanded principles to evaluate the work of NGOs because they work with the most marginalized and expend enormous amounts of resources in the name of improving global health.

■ GLOBAL WORK FROM HOME

If the process of engaging in quality experiences and reflection with trusted and thoughtful mentors results in a discernment that precludes living or working abroad, that is a positive outcome. It prevents disappointment and stress in the individuals trying to force themselves to live a dream in a manner to which they are not suited, and saves time and resources for the organization.

It is true that some barriers, such as debt or raising young children, are temporary and that when life circumstances change, other paths may open up. For example, a significant number of senior and retired physicians are exploring opportunities to work or teach in underserved settings.

For many, the simplest route to getting involved is through charitable giving. If one feels he or she does not have the skills, time, or interest in actually working abroad at the global level, that person can certainly donate monetarily. Investing wisely by researching a recipient organization is now much easier by using the tools in Box 8-1. Consciously choosing to donate the equivalent of one's most common visit level or procedure, or a block of time, on a regular basis (eg, deciding to donate the equivalent of what one earns from the most common US clinic visit billed, such as **99213,** or a 30-minute salary equivalent for someone in the National Health Service Corps, every 2-week pay period) is a concrete way of donating skills and energy toward meeting the MDGs, albeit through another.

Some professionals might consciously choose not to go abroad on a short-term intervention so that they might divert the money otherwise used in lost productivity at home, travel, and lodging toward engaging and paying for more local involvement in the host community. For example, the money that a plastic surgeon loses by taking a week of vacation, flying to South America, and staying in a hotel to perform a couple dozen operations could otherwise employ a local physician for months. That locally trained equivalent would perform many times that number of operations and would be there to provide follow-up and respond to complications.

■ GOING MEANS RETURNING: REENTRY PHENOMENON

Returning to a home country after a short stay away can be jolting, but there is often profound and ongoing psychological anguish after an extended period abroad. This is certainly recognized and described among returning missionaries, diplomatic corps members, military, students, and even businesspeople. Various religious groups have programs to address this, as does the US Department of State and military. The business community recognizes it as a potential threat to employee satisfaction and longevity among its most experienced managers.

The literature is sparse on this subject, but some commonalities emerge—individuals who indicate a change toward a more global identity experience high satisfaction with life. However, it is also found that those who embrace a more global cultural identity tend to feel more estranged from their original identity and exhibit much higher distress during repatriation.[64]

There is a brief practical learning module on medical worker reverse culture shock available on the Web[65]; each institution and organization should consciously develop and incorporate such a program into its structure. The existence of proactive reentry training can be an important method of evaluating groups and academic institutions on comprehensive support.

■ KEY POINTS

People tend to be happier when they are involved in activities beyond their usual work life that are for the benefit of others. *Global* implies more than simply "abroad or international" and may mean becoming involved in our own communities. Further richness can be attained by learning how our neighbors in more challenging settings live and work by spending time with them and determining, together, how to affect lasting change. However, the further one's dream takes him or her from the typical medical trajectory, the deeper one needs to contemplate the journey and its perils and rewards.

- Interest in global health activities is increasing among learners, those in practice, and retirees.
- Governmental and nongovernmental involvement in global health issues has proliferated over the past century.
- A process of discernment can be critical for the individual or organization contemplating involvement in global health activities.
- Significant barriers exist that must be considered and surmounted before embarking on any long-term global health activities.
- A set of ethical principles or guidelines is presented to stimulate discussion and reflection in those contemplating spending time in developing regions and those already engaged in activities.
- Anyone can be actively involved in global health improvements without even leaving home.

■ REFERENCES

1. United Nations Children's Fund. *The Annual Report 2008*. July 2009. http://www.unicef.org/publications/index_49924.html
2. Gapminder. http://www.gapminder.org
3. Black RE, Morris SS, Bryce J. Where and why are 10 million children dying every year? *Lancet*. 2003;361(9376):2226–2234

4. Filippi V, Ronsmans C, Campbell O, Graham W, Mills A, Borghi J. Maternal health in poor countries: the broader context and a call for action. *Lancet*. 2006;368(9546): 1535–1541. http://www.who.int/pmnch/media/pmnch.in.the.press/lancetseries/en/ index.html

5. Darmstadt D, Bhutta Z, Cousens S, Adam T, Walker N, de Bernis L. Evidence-based, cost-effective interventions: how many newborn babies can we save? *Lancet*. 2005;365(9463):977–988

6. Convention on the Rights of the Child. http://www.unicef.org/crc

7. Baker T, Weisman C, Ellen Piwoz E. US physicians in international health: report of a current survey. *JAMA*.1984;251(4):502–504

8. Bazemore A, Henein M, Goldenhar L, Szaflarski M, Lindsell C, Diller P. The effect of offering international health training opportunities on family medicine residency recruiting. *Fam Med*. 2007;39(4):255–260. Updated data from http://www.aamc.org/ data/gq/allschoolsreports/2007.pdf

9. Torjesen K, Mandalakas A, Kahn R, Duncan B. International child health electives for pediatric residents. *Arch Pediatr Adolesc Med*. 1999;153(12):1297–1302

10. Nelson B, Lee A, Newby P, Chamberlin R, Huang C. Global health training in pediatric residency programs. *Pediatrics*. 2008;122:28–33

11. Anspacher M, Denno D, Pak-Gorstein S, et al. Pediatric resident training in global health. *PAS Abstract*. In press

12. American Academy of Pediatrics Division of Child Health Research. Periodic Survey of Fellows #9. 1989. http://www.aap.org/research/periodicsurvey/surv2arc.htm

13. Charity Navigator. http://www.charitynavigator.org. Accessed October 2, 2009

14. GuideStar. http://www2.guidestar.org. Accessed October 3, 2009

15. World Health Organization. http://www.who.int/civilsociety/relations/en. Accessed September 27, 2009

16. United Nations Non-Governmental Liaison Service. Millennium Development Goals. http://www.un-ngls.org/orf/mdg.htm. Accessed October 3, 2009

17. You D, Wardlaw T, Salama P, Jones G. *Lancet*. 2009. DOI:10:1016/ S0140-6736(09)61609-9

18. UN General Assembly. Resolution 2626 (XXV), October 24, 1970, paragraph 43. http://daccessdds.un.org/doc/RESOLUTION/GEN/NR0/348/91/IMG/NR034891. pdf?OpenElement

19. Shah A. US and foreign aid assistance. *Global Issues*. http://www.globalissues.org/ article/35/us-and-foreign-aid-assistance based on data from http://www.oecd.org/ dataoecd/50/17/5037721.htm. Accessed September 27, 2009

20. Shoulder to Shoulder. http://www.shouldertoshoulder.org. Accessed October 3, 2009

21. The Canadian Neonatal Network. http://www.canadianneonatalnetwork.org/shanghai/ announcement.shtml. Accessed October 3, 2009

22. The Welbodi Partnership. http://www.welbodipartnership.org/index.html. Accessed October 3, 2009

23. Dueger C, O'Callahan C, eds. *Working in International Child Health*. 2nd ed. Elk Grove Village, IL: American Academy of Pediatrics; 2008

24. American Academy of Pediatrics Section on International Child Health. http://www. aap.org/cgi-bin/overseas/aapartcl.cfm. Accessed October 3, 2009

25. Osborn G, Ohmans P, eds. *Finding Work in Global Health: A Practical Guide for Jobseekers or Anyone Who Wants to Make the World a Healthier Place*. 2nd ed. Saint Paul, MN: Health Advocates Press; 2005

26. O'Neil E. *Awakening Hippocrates: A Primer on Health, Poverty, and Global Service*. Chicago, IL: American Medical Association; 2006
27. O'Neil E. *A Practical Guide to Global Health Service*. Chicago, IL: American Medical Association; 2006
28. Global Health Council. Global Health Career Network. http://careers.globalhealth.org. Accessed October 5, 2009
29. Wilkinson D, Symon B. Medical students, their electives, and HIV. *BMJ*. 1999;318: 139–140
30. World Health Organization, United Nations Children's Fund. World report on child injury prevention. 2009. http://www.who.int/violence_injury_prevention/child/injury/world_report/en/index.html. Accessed October 5, 2009
31. VanTilburg C. Attitudes towards medical aid to developing countries. *Wilderness Environ Med*. 1995;6(3):264–268
32. Bezruchka S. Medical tourism as medical harm to the Third World: why? For whom? *Wilderness Environ Med*. 2000;11(2):77–78
33. Rees T, Lluberas G, Bezruchka S. Letters and author response. *Wilderness Environ Med*. 2001;12:63–65
34. Fenton P. Health hijack. *Lancet*. 1999;353:1887–1888
35. Garrett L. The challenge of global health. *Foreign Affairs*. 2007 Jan/Feb
36. DeCamp M. Scrutinizing global short-term medical outreach. *Hastings Center Report*. 2007;37(6):21–23
37. Panosian C, Coates TJ. The new medical "missionary"—grooming the next generation of health care workers. *N Engl J Med*. 2006;354:1771–1773
38. Kamat D, Armstrong R. Global child health: an essential component of residency training. *J Pediatr*. 2006;149:735–736
39. Bishop R, Litch JA. Medical tourism can do harm. *BMJ*. 2000;320(7240):1017
40. Walsh D. A framework for short-term humanitarian health care. *Int Nurs Rev*. 2004; 51(1):23–26
41. International Society of Travel Medicine. 7 tips for the responsible traveler. http://www.istm.org/WebForms/Members/MemberResources/publications/handouts/responsible.aspx. Accessed February 28, 2011
42. Hanlon CR. Ethical principles for everyone in health care. *J Am Coll Surg*. 2001;192(1): 72–78
43. Crump JA, Sugarman J, the Working Group on Ethics Guidelines for Global Health Training (WEIGHT). Ethics and Best Practice Guidelines for Training Experiences in Global Health. *Am J Trop Med Hyg*. 2010;83(6):1178–1182
44. Schaffer G. Personal communication. San Lucas Toliman, Guatemala
45. Werner D, Bower B. *Helping Health Workers Learn: A Book of Methods, Aids, and Ideas for Instructors at the Village Level*. Palo Alto, CA: Hesperian Press; 1982
46. Suchdev P, Ahrens K, Click E, et al. A model for sustainable short-term international medical trips. *Ambul Pediatr*. 2007;7:317–320
47. Clutter P. Project Helping Hands: medical mission organization increases educational focus with village health care provider seminar in Caranavi, Bolivia. *J Emerg Nurs*. 2004;30(5):A27–A28
48. Heck J, Bazemore A, Diller P. The shoulder to shoulder model—channeling medical volunteerism toward sustainable health change. *Fam Med*. 2007;39(9):644–650
49. Flores G. Lost in translation? Pediatric preventive care and language barriers. *J Pediatr*. 2006;148(2):154–157

50. Rowe A, de Savigny D, Lanata C, Victora CG. How can we achieve and maintain high-quality performance of health workers in low resource settings? *Lancet.* 2005;366:1026–1035

51. Cardiello PU. Tremendous benefits. *J Med Assoc Ga.* 1999;88(1):23–25

52. Gupta AR, Wells CK, Horwitz RI, Bia FJ, Barry M. The International Health Program: the fifteen-year experience with Yale University's Internal Medicine Residency Program. *Am J Trop Med Hyg.* 1999;61:1019–1023

53. Miller WC, Corey GR, Lallinger GT, Durack DT. International health and internal medicine residency training: the Duke University experience. *Am J Med.* 1995;99(3):291–297

54. Murray CJL, Laakso T, Shibuyak K, Hill K, Lopez AD. Can we achieve Millenium Development Goal 4? New analysis of country trends and forecasts of under-5 mortality to 2015. *Lancet.* 2007;370:1040–1054

55. Evans DB, Lim S, Adam T, Tan-Torres Edejer T. Evaluation of current strategies and future priorities for improving health in developing countries. *BMJ.* 2005;331:1457–1461

56. Byass P, Ghebreyesus TA. Making the world's children count. *Lancet.* 2005;365(9465):1114–1116

57. Remedy. http://www.remedy.org

58. World Health Organization Department of Essential Drugs and Other Medicines. Guidelines for drug donations. 1999. http://whqlibdoc.who.int/hq/1999/who_edm_par_99.4.pdf. Accessed September 29, 2009

59. Abramowicz M. Drugs past their expiration date. *Med Letter.* 2002;44:1–2. http://www.medletter.com/freedocs/expdrugs.pdf

60. World Health Organization. http://www.who.int/medicines/publications/essentialmedicines/en. Accessed September 28, 2009

61. Green T, Green H, Scandlyn J, Kestler A. Perceptions of short-term medical volunteer work: a qualitative study in Guatemala. *Global Health.* 2009;5:4

62. Wolfburg A. Volunteering overseas—lessons from surgical brigades. *N Engl J Med.* 2006;354:443–445

63. Pinto A, Upshur R. Global health ethics for students. *Dev World Bioeth.* 2009;9(1):1–10

64. Sussman N. Testing the cultural identity model of the cultural transition cycle: sojourners return home. *Int J Intercult Relat.* 2002;26:391–408

65. http://www.uniteforsight.org/cultural-competency/module13. Accessed October 25, 2009

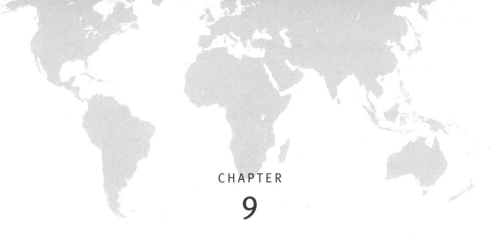

9

Disaster Relief

Sachin N. Desai, MD (corresponding author)
Michael U. Callaghan, MD
Bonita Stanton, MD, FAAP

■ INTRODUCTION

The first exposure to global health for many pediatric health care workers may be during a disaster relief trip. Disaster situations present unique challenges, particularly in settings with poor infrastructure and poverty. Natural disasters, defined by the World Health Organization (WHO) as any sudden ecologic phenomenon of sufficient magnitude requiring external assistance, have been responsible for a large amount of death, injuries, and homelessness. In the past decades, new strategies in disaster assessment, evaluation, and management have unfolded. In the past, aid volunteers would arrive and assist with basic relief, focusing on immediate medical care, shelter, and food.

Recent disasters, such as the earthquake in Haiti and the tsunami in Asia, demonstrate that disaster relief is increasingly being provided by small groups, including pediatric professionals, in addition to the traditional large-scale disaster relief organizations. The health cluster approach has served to bring together agencies working on similar mandates, such as health, sanitation, nutrition, and protection. For emergency operations, the WHO serves as the lead agency for the health cluster and is responsible for coordinating activities between international and local agencies.

Unfortunately, improvements in disaster response have resulted in minimal success with little change in mortality figures and human suffering despite increased scrutiny by the international scientific community.[1,2] All too often, the tragedy is all but forgotten in the ensuing weeks as the rest of the world returns to its daily lives.[3] Largely, it is the destruction of infrastructure (eg, roads, communication, transportation) that increases the challenge of providing immediate disaster relief. An effective response relies on a proper needs assessment to ensure relief supplies and personnel are delivered when and where they are needed most.[4]

With a rapid growth of urban centers, the developing world is projected to be home for 80% of the world's population by 2025,[5] with much of this growth in areas of high population density,[6] poverty, and limited infrastructure support. Taken together, these factors place the developing world at high risk for enduring mass casualties.

Care of minor injuries comprise the majority of medical care provided following most natural disasters. Clean water, food, clothing, shelter, and sanitation are the primary needs of acute disaster relief. Climate change has heightened the concern for severe weather events and a subsequent increase in vector-borne diseases.[6] The large-scale displacement of people, most of whom are women and children, is common in the aftermath of natural disasters. Programs focusing on maternal and child healthcare (Box 9-1) are essential when addressing the substantial morbidity and mortality often associated with these highly vulnerable groups.

Box 9-1. Essential Components of Maternal, Child, and Reproductive Health Programs

Health education and outreach

Prenatal delivery/postnatal care

Nutritional supplementation

Immunization/weight monitoring for infants

Encouragement and education for breastfeeding

Family planning

Education of sexual transmitted infection and HIV prevention

From Noji EK. Public health in the aftermath of disasters. *BMJ*. 2005;330(7504):1379–1381

■ SPECIAL NEEDS OF CHILDREN

Children are often disproportionately affected by natural disasters. The risk is usually compounded because they are often raised in poverty, resulting in lower baseline nutritional status, decreased immunization rates, higher load of intestinal parasites, and limited access to health care.[7] Splitting up of families and death of caregivers can occur as a result of severe disasters. Unaccompanied orphans can be found roaming the streets in the initial weeks after the destruction. Disasters often create an even greater socioeconomic burden on countries already struggling with poor governance and impoverished residents. The economic effect can be devastating—an initial rise in food prices can lead to increased malnutrition rates and overcrowding of urban centers, further exacerbating the effect of poverty in severe emergencies. Delayed recovery can worsen acute and chronic adverse psychological sequelae of the disaster.[8]

To survive, families often must sell household possessions in addition to sacrificing expenditures on basic necessities, such as education and clothes, to obtain food. Vulnerable child populations are of great concern when considering the lack of resources available for protecting them in many developing countries. Damage to schools and health clinics contributes to disruption in child welfare. Depending on the amount of destruction, schools are commonly used as shelters. Communities are faced with the decision of when to evacuate those driven from their homes so that classes may resume and some semblance of normalcy can return for affected children.[9] Children are already at a greater risk of abuse, abandonment, and even trafficking in many of these poverty-stricken areas. As populations cluster to accommodate temporary makeshift settlements, the population density and scarcity of resources amplify the risks for violence and crime.

Increased attention is being focused on the significant psychological trauma children experience in these settings, as evidenced by physical violence, exposure to drugs, and forced separation from their families. Poverty and political instability coexist in many instances. The tragedy of natural disasters is further complicated by human-driven conflict. As many as 300,000 children younger than 18 years were involved in some combat role in more than 50 countries in 2001.[7] Management strategies of childhood psychological emergencies include active intervention versus removing children from these harmful exposures and restoring normalcy as quickly as possible through family reunification.[10,11] A high proportion of children exposed to disasters experience some degree of post-traumatic stress disorder, depression, or anxiety.[8]

Children, particularly infants, differ anatomically and physiologically from adults, which markedly affects how they should be medically managed in disasters. They have much higher surface area-to-volume ratios than adults, which increases their risk of dehydration, hypothermia, and exposure-related toxicities. Increased respiratory rates place children at elevated risk from aerosol exposures. Children may not be able to sense and avoid dangers associated with the disaster. Age and developmental stages markedly influence how children will respond psychologically to disasters and the events surrounding them. For all of these reasons, pediatric health professionals are essential to disaster response efforts.

■ SPECIAL NEEDS OF WOMEN

Women play a central role in the recovery of an area affected by disaster. Women heading households are often given responsibility for distributing food and relief supplies because of a greater assurance that the supplies will be equitably allocated among family members. To survive the direst circumstances, women employ many strategies and often deny themselves basic provisions in favor of their children or male partners. Severe desperation can force mothers into compromising situations involving transactional sex, which also increases the risk of HIV transmission and other sexually transmitted infections (STIs) in what may be an already higher-risk community. Organizations such as the Red Cross, International Rescue Committee, and United Nations High Commissioner for Refugees are fundamental in working with local organizations to track down and reunite women with their children and families. Many of these international and local partnerships have been essential in helping displaced women form small businesses, enabling them with money, food, and the confidence to cope in a crisis.

Special subpopulations of particular vulnerability are newborn babies and women who are pregnant, in labor, or postpartum. In 2005 Hurricane Katrina affected approximately 56,000 such women and 75,000 infants.[12] Box 9-2 lists important considerations for these populations.

Box 9-2. Planning for the Care of Pregnant Women and Newborns During a Disaster

Triaging of women in labor

Identifying location of where women will give birth

Availability of birth kits

Ability to care for newborns

Appropriate shelter facilities for those in labor and for immediate postpartum care

---

Adapted from Pfeiffer J, Avery MD, Benbenek M, et al. Maternal and newborn care during disasters: thinking outside the hospital paradigm. *Nurs Clin North Am.* 2008;43(3):449–467

■ NEEDS ASSESSMENTS OF HUMANITARIAN CRISES

Disasters can involve large numbers of displaced populations, disruption of normal services, a high risk of epidemics, or the threat of conflict. These commonly encountered scenarios require additional preparation and training by aid workers who plan to assist in these crises. Although the public outcry for immediate action can be vocal, for effective aid relief to reach the greatest in number of people and be effective in need, it must be appropriately targeted.[13]

Rapid needs assessments best assist in using the limited resources that are available. Small teams can be sufficient to address food, water, supplies, communication, and transport. Teaming with local agencies and sharing information assists in more efficient and clear reporting and minimizes duplication of efforts. Well-coordinated and cooperative efforts are essential to optimize international effort. Many factors, including the nature and effect of the disaster, play an important role in defining consequences and relief planning.

Organizational efforts such as the Sphere Project and People in Aid offer strategies to help maximize the potential for optimizing humanitarian assistance. The Red Cross and other international nongovernmental organizations introduced the Sphere Project in 1997 as a means to improve assistance quality by developing universal standards in 5 core areas (Box 9-3). The project aims to identify populations affected by disasters and define their rights to organize effective planning and implementation of humanitarian relief. Similarly, People in Aid was founded to improve human resources management focusing on organizational decisions that affect aid workers.

Box 9-3. Organizations Working to Improve Humanitarian Assistance Standards

The Sphere Project (www.sphereproject.org)
  Water supply, sanitation, and hygiene promotion
  Food security and nutrition
  Food aid
  Shelter, settlement, and nonfood items
  Health services

People in Aid (www.peopleinaid.org)
  Learning, training, and development
  Briefing and debriefing
  Performance management and support
  Motivation and reward

From the Sphere Project (www.sphereproject.org) and People in Aid (www.peopleinaid.org).

Major life-threatening issues involve the lack of nonmedical necessities, including access to drinking water, sanitation, food, and shelter. Provision of an emergency water supply for hydration and hygiene is of greatest importance. After water, sanitation is the greatest need. Planning must ensure that there is no less than 1 latrine per 20 persons and that these facilities are no more than a minute's walk from living quarters. Increased mortality is noted when food energy intake falls below 1,500 kcal per adult per day. The WHO recommends nutritional intake of 2,100 kcal per person per day. Temporary shelters should be avoided if at all possible because these are rarely replaced. However, there may be no other options when such vast destruction occurs. Medical issues primarily revolve around the transmission of infectious diseases secondary to crowded and unsanitary conditions.

The immediate urge to send rescue teams and supplies must be balanced by their tendency to divert valuable resources. Typically, survivors provide most rescue efforts and survival from entrapment decreases rapidly after 24 to 36 hours.[14] Emergency health kits from the WHO can be distributed quickly and matched to population size and needs.

■ CRITICAL PUBLIC HEALTH INTERVENTIONS

Prioritizing public health interventions is critical in minimizing respiratory infections, diarrhea, and other communicable diseases. Well-known risk factors include overcrowding, inadequate hygiene and sanitation, and contaminated water supplies. Quick implementation of a good water and waste disposal system is instrumental in reducing further spread of disease. Well-planned emergency settlements with special attention to shelter location, layout, spacing, and type are vital post-disaster measures. Other factors influencing disease transmission include preexisting disease incidence, immunization rates, utility damage, and the presence of disease vectors that facilitate spread of disease.

Water Supply and Waste Disposal

The United Nations High Commissioner for Refugees recommends a minimum of 15 to 20 L of clean water for drinking, washing, and bathing. Adequate amounts of clean and safe water are favored over smaller amounts of high-quality water. Water distribution points that provide lidded buckets of chlorinated water and solid waste pickup locations, although labor intensive, have proven to be highly effective preventive measures when instituted early in the post-emergency phase. Together with health education, availability of bathing and washing facilities with soap are other important components of the post-emergency phase.

Vector control relies on disrupting the source of disease transmission, such as control of mosquitoes, flies, fleas, and rats. Insecticide-treated bed nets are shown to reduce the mosquito burden, which is the disease vector of malaria.[15,16] Interventions should be culturally appropriate for sanitation measures to be deemed effective. In the early phase while latrine construction is underway, initial sanitation action may focus on separating areas of defecation from sources of potable water.

Repercussions of poor sanitation, water, and hygiene extend beyond childhood morbidity and mortality. Children, especially girls, are denied the right to education because of lack of acceptable sanitation facilities.

Shelter

Alternate forms of shelter, such as resettlement camps, are instituted when housing losses exceed 25%. In poor communities, this decision can lead to the unintentional evolution of permanent slums, which can attract additional homeless and destitute populations. The WHO recommends 30 m^2 of personal living space with a minimum of 3.5 m^2 floor space per person in these emergency shelters.

Information Technology in Disaster Response

Surveillance must be ongoing to optimize the relief effort management response. Early field surveys may be simple, providing immediate answers to assist in basic needs, while later surveys can help with assessing long-term efforts and the rebuilding process. Crude mortality rates serve as the most critical indicator of current health status, as well as a baseline for the affected population.

Information technology (IT) can be used to reconnect families whose members become lost during a natural disaster. For example, the Google Person Finder (http://haiticrisis.appspot.com) was reported to have tracked more than 50,000 displaced individuals.

Principles of medical care in emergency situations must be altered to achieve the best overall result. Care should be based on simple field-tested protocols, such as those provided by Doctors Without Borders (www.doctorswithoutborders.org) and the WHO (www.who.int/hac/techguidance/en). These protocols and the use of items on the essential drug lists maximize the efficient use of limited resources and help all available health care workers to provide appropriate care. Innovations in field-appropriate technology also assist in delivering care to those in need. For example, evaluation of ultrasonography in mass casualty and extreme environments demonstrated that it was an ideal triage tool that provided rapid, portable, and effective means in identifying intra-abdominal and intrathoracic injuries.[17] Likewise, wireless transmission is applicable to redirect trauma triage in extreme environments.[17-20] Although there are many reports that cite the use of IT in disaster planning, preparation, and warning, few reports exist on these applications during the emergency relief phase.[21-23] The Pan American Health Organization developed a free inventory software program, SUMA Humanitarian Supply Management System (www.disaster-info. net/SUMA/english/index.htm), as well as a government warehouse to assist in standardized procurement and distribution of essential medical supplies, Programme de Médicaments Essentiels (PROMESS) (http://new. paho.org/hai/index.php?option=com_content&task=view&id=7006&I temid=230&lang=en). Both have been integral in the emergency relief response in recent disasters, such as the 2010 Haitian earthquake and ensuing cholera outbreak.

The Internet is also a valuable resource for sharing information during a crisis. The Cambodian government used the Internet following the 1997 flood to obtain snake antivenom to treat 100 victims.[24] The emergence of powerful and durable personal digital assistants and wireless technology will support the trend to further advance the use of IT applications for out-of-hospital disaster response. These technologies have been used for employing database systems, needs assessment applications, messaging systems, geographic information systems, and even transferring clinical or radiographic images in resource-limited areas.[25-27]

■ UNIQUE CIRCUMSTANCES ASSOCIATED WITH SPECIFIC NATURAL DISASTERS

With weak infrastructure and the inability to move to safer places, poverty is the most important factor in determining vulnerability. Trauma secondary to these disasters affect children disproportionally, with child mortality generally higher than that of adults. However, with respect to earthquakes, newborns and young infants were often protected because they often slept with their mothers. In the case of floods, tropical storms, and tornadoes, children younger than 10 years accounted for the largest proportion of deaths because members of this age group were not able to hold onto stationary objects, such as trees, to avoid being swept away.

Earthquakes

Earthquakes are one of the deadliest and most destructive natural events, responsible for greater than 1 million deaths and injuries in the past 2 decades.[28] Building collapse and entrapment pose the greatest risks. Loss of power and water can cripple an affected community. In a time when they are needed most, hospital equipment and facilities are unable to function properly. The most successful rescues take place within the first 24 hours and most lives are saved by immediate actions of survivors.[29] Health concerns following an earthquake are related to entrapment, including hypoxia, inhalation injury, hypothermia, dehydration, drowning, crush syndrome, and infected wounds.[30]

Although trauma is the primary cause of death and injury, many victims require care for acute exacerbations of chronic disease, such as diabetes, cardiac problems, asthma and other respiratory diseases, sickle cell disease, or mental health problems. Numerous studies suggest that the ability to reduce earthquake mortality relies on search-and-rescue action within the first 2 days following the disaster.[31-34]

A tsunami is a very large wave or series of waves resulting from an underwater earthquake or volcano. This can result in immediate building destruction and deaths secondary to drowning and crushing. Infectious sequelae following seawater aspiration lead to pneumonias and soft tissue infections, as was observed in the South Asian tsunami in December 2004.[35]

Floods

Floods are the most common natural disaster worldwide, affecting and killing the most people.[36] Seventy percent of all deaths from floods occur in India or Bangladesh, although they exist in almost every country.[37] Injury occurs due to fast-flowing debris and boulders as well as fallen trees. While the main cause of death is drowning, damage to community agriculture and housing can result in food shortages and homelessness. Contaminated water supply can lead to infections, especially cholera. The 2010 Pakistan floods affected more than 20 million people, caused approximately 2,000 deaths,[38] and were responsible for more than US \$9.7 billion in damage.[39] A rise in snakebites was documented from forced migration to higher ground after rising water levels.[40] Increased numbers of fires were also noted due to breaks in oil and gasoline tanks.[36]

Tropical Storms

Tropical rotating storm systems are called *cyclones, hurricanes,* or *typhoons,* depending on which region of the globe they occur. These events primarily affect coastal areas with a recent increase in injuries and deaths as a result of population growth in these locales.[41] Together with strong damaging winds, secondary effects can include tornadoes and flooding. Drowning is the leading cause of death, although other etiologies include trauma from flying or fast-flowing objects as well as entrapment.

Tornadoes

Tornadoes consist of violently strong winds with a vacuum vortex that is often responsible for extensive damage to non-reinforced buildings in their path. High-velocity winds can throw debris causing fatal injuries and high rates of secondary infected lacerations.

Volcanic Eruptions

Areas surrounding volcanoes are often well populated because volcanic ash provides highly fertile soil. The greatest immediate risks of a volcanic eruption include suffocation and respiratory ailments from ash inhalation, superheated stream, and even lethal gas.[42,43] Imminent concerns following an eruption include potential complications of flowing volcanic debris. Although slow and predictable, lava flows destroy everything in their path. Pyroclastic flows are fast currents of extremely hot gases (greater than 1,000°C) that can move at several hundred kilometers per hour, posing a considerable risk to life because they are hard to escape. Scalding hot mudflows occur when heavy rains mix with volcanic ash and debris, which also can advance downhill speeds up to 100 km per hour. Long-standing respiratory conditions can develop, such as excessive mucous production and asthma exacerbations, dehydration, burns, and eye infections.

■ COMMUNICABLE DISEASE CONTROL OF EPIDEMIC MANAGEMENT

Malnutrition, diarrheal diseases, measles, acute respiratory infections, and malaria account for the majority of deaths among those who are displaced. With the possibility of disrupted water supplies and sewage treatment facilities, concern for disease outbreaks commonly surface, especially in areas of high population density and displacement. Adequate provision of water, basic sanitation, community outreach, and effective case management based on international protocols using essential drugs and supply lists have been instrumental in saving countless numbers of lives. Ensuring ongoing primary care health interventions, such as coverage with measles vaccine, vitamin A, and deworming medication, in addition to providing insecticide-treated bed nets (in malaria endemic areas), are vital in reducing mortality in humanitarian crises.

The spread of STIs such as HIV and syphilis are exacerbated by disaster situations. The Joint United Nations Programme on HIV/AIDS has issued guidelines for emergency situations (Box 9-4).[44]

Heavy rains and flooding can lead to the migration of animal populations and washing away of insecticide spray, which can disrupt vector-control efforts, also resulting in increased disease transmission.

Box 9-4. Guidelines for HIV/AIDS Prevention in Emergency Situations

Minimum response to be conducted even in the midst of emergency
1.1 Establish coordination mechanism.
2.1 Assess baseline data.
2.2 Set up and manage a shared database.
2.3 Monitor activities.
3.1 Prevent and respond to sexual violence and exploitation.
3.2 Protect orphans and separated children.
3.3 Ensure access to condoms for peacekeepers, military, and humanitarian staff.
4.1 Include HIV considerations in water/sanitation planning.
5.1 Target food aid to affected and at-risk households and communities.
5.2 Plan nutrition and food needs for population with high HIV prevalence.
5.3 Promote appropriate care and feeding practices for people living with HIV/AIDS.
5.4 Support and protect food security of HIV/AIDS-affected and at-risk households and communities.
5.5 Distribute food aid to affected households and communities.
6.1 Establish safely designed sites.

Adapted from Inter-Agency Standing Committee. *Guidelines for HIV/AIDS Interventions in Emergency Settings.* http://www.unaids.org/en/resources/unaidspublications/2005. Accessed August 7, 2011

Unburied dead bodies pose minimal risks of health hazards; these risks can be limited through measures directed toward those assisting with handling dead bodies, such as appropriate training and vaccination against hepatitis B and tuberculosis, using disposable gloves and body bags, washing hands, and disinfecting transport materials. There are also national networks of morticians who can be called on in natural disasters to help properly handle decaying bodies.

Respect for local customs and practices should be instituted when possible; however, when there are large numbers of victims, mass burial is most often the appropriate method of disposal. Proper body burial has not been shown to pose significant contamination risk to groundwater used for drinking.

Immunization

Mass vaccination is employed only when an increased number of cases are noted despite recommended sanitary measures. There are several vaccines with certain characteristics that would be deemed useful in this setting (Box 9-5). Measles vaccination is shown to save many children's lives throughout the developing world in emergency settings. All children 6 months to 5 years of age are recommended to receive measles immunization. Several recent large-scale cholera outbreaks led to the recommendation of using cholera vaccines in conjunction with other prevention and control strategies in areas where the disease is endemic and in areas at risk for outbreaks.[45] Although it is a challenge to implement

Box 9-5. Characteristics That Make a Vaccine Useful in Post-disaster Settings

Proven efficacy with high safety and low adverse effects

Easy to administer (single dose)

Confers rapid and long-lasting protection for people of all ages

Available in sufficient quantities to guarantee vaccine supply for the entire population at risk

Low-cost vaccines

From Noji EK, Lee CY. Natural disaster medicine. In: Auerbach PS, ed. *Wilderness Medicine*. 5th ed. Philadelphia, PA: Mosby; 2007: 1854

vaccination in settings with an overburdened health system, a new inexpensive oral cholera vaccine may be a feasible option to save thousands of lives thanks to a large observed herd immunity effect.[46]

Nutrition

Shortages in food are present following an absolute reduction in food and often a problem with distribution systems. Vulnerable groups such as pregnant or lactating women, children younger than 5 years, and the elderly should be targeted when instituting emergency feeding programs. More than one third of all deaths in children younger than 5 years are attributable to undernutrition as a direct cause or through the weakening of the body's resistance to illness. The risk is substantially elevated following a disaster. Provision of fortified foods and micronutrient supplements is an integral component of response. Promotion of breastfeeding is fundamental to prevent undernutrition and mortality among newborns and infants in emergencies. Use of infant and young child feeding counselors are instrumental in offering support and training for these issues, in addition to other needs, such as feeding of young children separated from their families in the acute period following a disaster.

Mental Health and Psychosocial Development Needs

Natural disasters disrupt all aspects of life for children; their immediate nutritional and physical needs may not be met; their families may be lost or killed; their community links, including their schooling, religion, and other daily life aspects, may be destroyed; and the safety provided by law and order may be nonfunctional. Despite widespread recognition of the need for disaster relief efforts to address the mental health and psychosocial developmental needs of children,[47] the evidence base to direct such efforts remains weak.[48] An expert panel recommended that in addition to traditional emergency approaches based on protection (and therefore focusing on vulnerabilities of children and their communities) and reconnecting family members, relief workers should also focus on children's strengths and reestablish some familiar routines for children as quickly as possible. For example, while it may not be possible to reopen schools, ad hoc schooling should be initiated. This approach is based on social ecology models of child development, notably that of Bronfenbrenner,[49] which underscore the importance of social environment to children in crisis. It is believed that a rapid return to tasks and activities with which children are familiar and which may represent normal life will mitigate the adverse effect of disasters.[48,50]

Psychological Aspects of Providing Medical Humanitarian Aid

Catastrophe relief aid is an experience that will change the lives of all involved in the effort. Misery and grief are unavoidable consequences when encountering the multitudes of homeless and traumatized children. It is essential to realize that relief teams are guests in the country and should not impose their beliefs on others. As is often the case, prevention is better than cure and efforts to return communities to normalcy should be the underlying focus. Reuniting families, returning children to school, and providing work for adults all provide psychological benefits to survivors. Mental illness is rarely a priority in resource-limited areas, but specific psychosocial issues that surface involve caring for interpersonal violence victims (ie, abuse, rape, and torture), disabled people, and soldiers. Those suffering sequelae associated with mental illness have the same basic needs as everyone else, including clean water, food, and shelter.

■ KEY POINTS

- All disasters have unique aspects, but recognition of common features permits rapid and orderly facilitation of much-needed healthcare services.
- Critical services requiring immediate reestablishment include adequate clean water, sanitation, nutrition, shelter, immunizations, and vector-control measures.
- Lack of access to medical reports from agencies out in the field can hamper and obstruct the quality and rapidity of provided aid. When possible, access sites such as ReliefWeb (www.reliefweb.int) and the Cochrane Collaboration Evidence Aid project (www2.cochrane.org/evidenceaid/project.htm).
- Women and children represent vulnerable populations throughout the world, even in non-disaster settings.

■ REFERENCES

1. Noji EK, Lee CY. Natural disaster management. In: Auerbach PS, ed. *Wilderness Medicine*. 5th ed. Philadelphia, PA: Mosby Elsevier; 2009:1843–1856

2. Secretariat I. *International Decade for Natural Disaster Reduction: Action Plan for 1998–1999*. United Nations Office for the Coordination of Humanitarian Affairs; 1998:1–2

3. Noji E. Disasters: introduction and state of the art. *Epidemiol Rev*. 2005;27:3

4. Sunders KO, Birnbaum ML, eds. *Health Disaster Management Guidelines for Evaluation and Research in the Utstein Style*. World Association for Disaster and Emergency Medicine, Nordic Society for Disaster Medicine; 2003. http://www.wadem.org/guidelines.html. Accessed June 17, 2011

5. Ahern M, Kovats RS, Wilkinson P, Few R, Matthies F. Global health impacts of floods: epidemiologic evidence. *Epidemiol Rev*. 2005;27:36–46

6. Senior C, Jones R, Lowe J, Durman C, Hudson D. Predictions of extreme precipitation and sea-level rise under climate change. *Philos Transact A Math Phys Eng Sci*. 2002;360:1301

7. Seaman J, Maguire S. ABC of conflict and disaster: the special needs of children and women. *BMJ*. 2005;331:34

8. Kronenberg ME, Hansel TC, Brennan AM, Osofsky HJ, Osofsky JD, Lawrason B. Children of Katrina: lessons learned about postdisaster symptoms and recovery patterns. *Child Dev*. 2010;81:1241–1259

9. Balsari S, Lemery J, Williams TP, Nelson BD. Protecting the children of Haiti. *N Engl J Med*. 2010;362:e25

10. Bracken PJ, Petty C. *Rethinking the Trauma of War*. London, England: Free Association Books; 1998

11. Sphere Project. *Humanitarian Charter and Minimum Standards in Disaster Response*. Oxford, UK: Oxfam Publishing; 2004

12. Pfeiffer J, Avery M, Benbenek M, et al. Maternal and newborn care during disasters: thinking outside the hospital paradigm. *Nurs Clin North Am*. 2008;43:449–467

13. Krin C, Giannou C, Seppelt I, et al. Appropriate response to humanitarian crises. *BMJ*. 2010;340:c562

14. Redmond A. ABC of conflict and disaster: natural disasters. *BMJ*. 2005;330:1259

15. Eisele TP, Larsen D, Steketee RW. Protective efficacy of interventions for preventing malaria mortality in children in Plasmodium falciparum endemic areas. *Int J Epidemiol*. 2010;39(Suppl 1):i88–i101

16. Lengeler C. Insecticide-treated bed nets and curtains for preventing malaria. *Cochrane Database Syst Rev*. 2004:CD000363

17. Ma O, Norvell J, Subramanian S. Ultrasound applications in mass casualties and extreme environments. *Crit Care Med*. 2007;35:S275

18. Sarkisian A, Khondkarian R, Amirbekian N, Bagdasarian N, Khojayan R, Oganesian Y. Sonographic screening of mass casualties for abdominal and renal injuries following the 1988 Armenian earthquake. *J Trauma*. 1991;31:247

19. Keven K, Ates K, Yagmurlu B, et al. Renal Doppler ultrasonographic findings in earthquake victims with crush injury. *J Ultrasound Med*. 2001;20:675

20. Strode C, Rubal B, Gerhardt R, et al. Satellite and mobile wireless transmission of focused assessment with sonography in trauma. *Acad Emerg Med*. 2003;10:1411–1414

21. Arnold J, Levine B, Manmatha R, et al. Information-sharing in out-of-hospital disaster response: the future role of information technology. *Prehosp Disaster Med*. 2004;19:201–207

22. Noji E. The nature of disaster: general characteristics and public health effects. The public health consequences of disasters. 1997:3–20

23. Stephenson R, Anderson P. Disasters and the information technology revolution. *Disasters*. 2002;21:305–334

24. Information transmission through the Internet for the preparedness against venomous snakes as the aftermath of Cambodian Flood in 1997. The 4th Asia-Pacific Conference on Disaster Medicine; 1998; 81

25. Chandrasekhar C, Ghosh J. Information and communication technologies and health in low income countries: the potential and the constraints. *Bull WHO*. 2001;79:850–855

26. Cabrera M, Arredondo M, Rodriguez A, Quiroga J. Mobile technologies in the management of disasters: the results of a telemedicine solution. American Medical Informatics Association; 2001:86

27. The use of a personal digital assistant and network geographic information systems for a first aid drill for a greatly number of injured people at a regional toxic disaster. International Symposium on Recent Advances in Disaster Prevention; Taipei, Taiwan; National Institute of Injury Prevention; 2002

28. The potential impacts of climate variability and change on health impacts on extreme weather events in US. *Environ Health Perspect*. 2001;109:191–198

29. Hamilton R. *International Decade for Natural Disaster Reduction (IDNDR) Early Warning Programme: Report on Early Warning Capabilities for Geological Hazards: IDNDR Secretariat.* Geneva, Switzerland; 1999:A1–A36

30. Schultz C, Koenig K, Noji E. A medical disaster response to reduce immediate mortality after an earthquake. *N Engl J Med*. 1996;334:438

31. Arnold C, Durkin M. *Hospitals and the San Fernando Earthquake of February 1971: The Operational Experience.* San Mateo, CA: Building Systems Development Inc; 1983

32. De Bruycker M, Greco D, Annino I, et al. The 1980 earthquake in southern Italy: rescue of trapped victims and mortality. *Bull WHO*. 1983;61:1021

33. Noji E. Medical consequences of earthquakes: coordinating medical and rescue response. *Disaster Manag Response*. 1991;4:32–40

34. Zhi-Yong S. Medical support in the Tangshan earthquake: a review of the management of mass casualties and certain major injuries. *J Trauma*. 1987;27:1130

35. Kongsaengdao S, Bunnag S, Siriwiwattnakul N. Treatment of survivors after the tsunami. *N Engl J Med*. 2005;352:2654

36. Floods, hurricanes and tsunamis. In: Baskett P, Weller R, eds. *Medicine for Disasters*. 1988:291–307

37. National Resource Council. *Confronting Natural Disasters: An International Decade for Natural Disaster Reduction.* Washington DC: National Academy Press; 1987

38. United Nations Office for the Coordination of Humanitarian Affairs. *Pakistan Floods Emergency Response Plan, Revision.* http://www.reliefweb.int/rw/rwb.nsf/db900SID/VDUX-89DTJ3?OpenDocument

39. Asian Development Bank Assess Pakistan Flood Damage at $9.7 Billion. ADB News Release. Brussels, Belgium: World Bank; 2010

40. Ussher JH. Philippine flood disaster. *J R Nav Med Serv*. 1973;59:81

41. Sheets R. *The US Hurricaine Problem: An Assessment for the 1990s.* Miami National Hurricaine Center; 1994

42. Baxter P, Bernstein R, Falk H, French J, Ing R. Medical aspects of volcanic disasters: an outline of the hazards and emergency response measures. *Disasters*. 1982;6:268–276

43. Bernstein R, Baxter P, Falk H. Immediate public health concerns and actions in volcanic eruptions: lessons from the Mount St. Helens eruptions, May 18–October 18, 1980. *Am J Public Health.* 1986;76:25

44. Joint United Nations Programme on HIV/AIDS. *Guidelines for HIV/AIDS Interventions in Emergency Settings.* 2008. http://data.unaids.org/Publications/External-Documents/iasc_guidelines-emergency-settings_en.pdf

45. World Health Organization. Cholera vaccines: WHO position paper. *Wkly Epidemiol Rec.* 2010;85(13):117–128

46. Clemens J, Holmgren J. Urgent need of cholera vaccines in public health-control programs. *Future Microbiol.* 2009;4(4):381–385

47. United Nations Children's Fund. Humanitarian action report 2008. http://www.unicef.org/har08/index_index.html

48. Ager A, Stark L, Akesson B, Boothby N. Defining best practice in care and protection of children in crisis-affected settings: a Delphi study. *Child Dev.* 2010;81:1271–1286

49. Bronfenbrenner U. *The Ecology of Human Development: Experiments by Nature and Design.* Cambridge, MA: Harvard University Press; 1979

50. Kostelny K. A culture-based, integrative approach. In: Boothby N, Strang A, Wessells M, eds. *A World Turned Upside Down: Social Ecological Approaches to Children in War Zones.* Bloomfield, CT: Kumarian Press, Inc; 2006:19–37

Caring for Pediatric Travelers and Immigrants

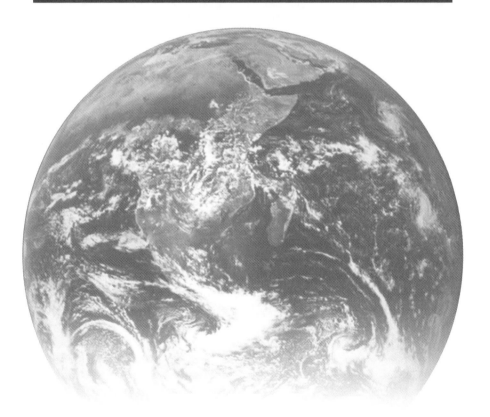

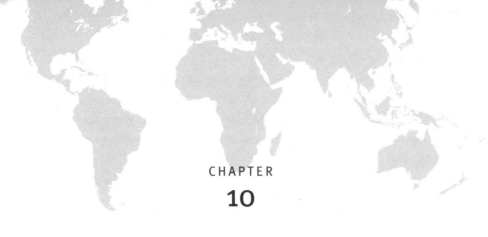

CHAPTER

10

Travel Clinics

John C. Christenson, MD, FAAP

■ INTRODUCTION

Every year, close to 1 billion people travel across international boundaries. More than 50 million people travel to a developing country. Countries within sub-Saharan Africa, Asia, and Latin America are frequently visited by children. Many of these countries are endemic for malaria, dengue fever, and yellow fever. In addition, traveler's diarrhea is one of the most common diseases acquired while traveling in the developing world. These diseases are preventable. All individuals traveling to a developing country should seek pretravel medical advice with the goal of preventing travel-related illnesses. In addition, administering specific vaccinations and prescribing prophylactic medications against malaria are important means of preventing disease. While some clinicians are comfortable providing this type of medical care to their patients, many seek the assistance of experts in travel medicine. Vaccines specific to international travel, such as those for yellow fever and typhoid fever, are not available in most primary care practices. Web sites and printed materials can help clinicians prepare their patients for travel. Travelers can also easily access these sources. However, these sources may be too basic or too difficult for some to assess the precise risk in a given region, thus necessitating an expert in travel medicine to provide needed advice. Travel clinics are the most reliable assets in these circumstances. Education, risk assessment, medical advice, vaccinations and prescriptions for chemoprophylaxis can all be obtained in a single place.[1]

Pediatric travelers pose a great challenge because they require different considerations for recommended antimalarial chemoprophylaxis agents with dosing according to body weight and possible contraindications for certain vaccines in younger children. Vaccines protective against typhoid fever and yellow fever cannot be administered to those younger than 2 years and 4 months, respectively. Infants whose families want to take them to areas of the world at risk for high-altitude illness require specialized attention, family education, and chemoprophylaxis. At times, travel advice is insufficient for the type of region and anticipated activities.[2] Unfortunately, many travelers, especially those visiting friends and relatives, do not visit travel clinics or receive preventive medical advice.[3] It is imperative that clinicians become more knowledgeable in most aspects of travel medicine and learn how to access pertinent sources of information.[4] In some primary care settings, clinicians with travel medicine expertise successfully integrate travel medicine consultation into their practice.[5,6]

This chapter specifically discusses the multiple aspects needing consideration when developing a travel clinic, whether as a freestanding practice or an integrated component of a large medical practice. Emphasis is given to pediatric travelers and their families.

■ A POPULATION AT RISK: THE PEDIATRIC TRAVELER

Infants and children travel to most regions of the developing world. They visit endemic areas with malaria and yellow fever, such as sub-Saharan Africa and South America.[7] Travelers visit friends and family, vacation, study abroad, participate in humanitarian missions, or move because of parental work assignments. Common complaints, such as diarrhea, abdominal pain, and fevers, were reported among children in 16.9 (14.3–19.7) episodes per 100 person weeks.[8] Nonspecific fevers, malaria, bacillary dysentery, diarrhea, and dengue fever are frequent causes of fevers in children returning from the tropics.[9,10] Travel to South Asia to visit family is a risk factor for typhoid fever acquisition. Diarrhea is a frequent medical problem of the traveling pediatric population. Forty percent of small children between the ages of 3 and 6 years were affected by diarrhea.[11] In younger children, the clinical course is more severe and the illness lasts longer. Some of these children required hospitalization. In another study, an attack rate of 47.1% was reported among pediatric travelers who visited Angola.[12] While medical problems are common during long stays, unfortunately, immigrants visiting friends and relatives are at higher risk because many do not receive appropriate chemoprophylaxis, vaccines, and medical advice.[3]

■ SOURCES FOR TRAVEL ADVICE, VACCINES, AND CHEMOPROPHYLAXIS

Parents of traveling children need accessible sources of reliable information to educate themselves and their children on the most appropriate means of disease prevention. Travel magazine articles and books are reasonable initial sources, but some do not contain the most up-to-date information. Frequently accessed Internet sites are the Centers for Disease Control and Prevention (CDC) Travelers' Health (www.cdc.gov/travel) and World Health Organization International Travel and Health (www.who.int/ith/en/index.html). While these sites contain useful information, navigating through them may be cumbersome for many non–medically trained individuals.

Pediatric travelers visiting a developing country may be referred to a travel clinic by their primary care professional; others are self-referred. Unfortunately, travel clinics may not be available locally for some. In these cases, the primary care professional will be asked to provide the necessary advice. Multiple review articles on travel medicine have been published,[4,13] which clinicians may find useful.

Travel clinics are frequently affiliated with large medical centers. Some are contained within clinical infectious disease programs. Many clinics are self-sustaining private clinics or part of a primary care medical practice. Travel vaccines are now available through many local pharmacies and nurse-based immunization services. In addition, city- or county-based health departments may provide vaccination services for travelers. There are few travel clinics that exclusively cater to the pediatric age group and their families. Within travel clinics, the level of comfort in providing services to infants and children varies.

■ WHERE CAN ONE FIND A TRAVEL CLINIC?

Two easily accessible Internet sites provide a list of clinics: the American Society of Tropical Medicine and Hygiene (www.astmh.org/source/ClinicalDirectory) and the International Society of Travel Medicine (www.istm.org). These Web sites contain a list of travel clinics within the United States and other countries and provide information on travel medicine providers with special certifications in travel health. Church groups with prior travel experiences usually know where to obtain vaccines, prescriptions, and advice, and frequently refer friends, relatives, and members to these sources. Community centers of various ethnic groups will refer members to specific clinics for vaccinations. In some communities, travelers planning to visit friends and family will only visit a travel clinic or immunization center because a yellow fever vaccine is required to enter a country.

■ VISITING A TRAVEL CLINIC

Patients' medical history, past travel experience, and immunization history influence their needs. For a travel medicine provider to be able to offer the best advice, various components of a travel clinic consultation need to be assessed. In most cases, travelers or their parents or guardians will complete a clinic visit questionnaire in which this information will be recorded. The form allows space for the travel clinic provider to record useful information about the visit.

Travel Destinations

Travel advice, vaccines, and need for antimalarial chemoprophylaxis are based on a traveler's expected risk. Travelers must identify countries or regions they plan to visit. Detailed maps should be available for research. A comprehensive, detailed world atlas is an essential tool for all travel clinics. Risks may vary within a country. For example, travelers visiting Costa Rica and spending time exclusively in the capital of San José will not be exposed to malaria. However, if visiting jungle areas, they may need antimalarial chemoprophylaxis. Most of South Africa is malaria-free and travelers will not require antimalarial prophylaxis; however, visits to Kruger National Park in the northeastern region will require it.

Travel Activities

The type of activities planned may affect risk. The risk of acquiring certain infections such as hepatitis A and diarrhea vary greatly. A careful businessperson staying with family in a 5-star hotel will have a lower risk than a student backpacking in rural areas of the same country. Knowing these plans beforehand allows the provider an opportunity to give specific recommendations. For example, travelers wanting to participate in white-water rafting may place themselves at risk for leptospirosis, necessitating a discussion about doxycycline chemoprophylaxis, while travel with infants may trigger discussions about safe travel practices during flight and on land.

Building an Educational Handout

Starting with this information, an individualized educational handout for travelers can be built. The handout will include general recommendations addressing travel, required and recommended vaccines, and need for antimalarial chemoprophylaxis. Information about the country (eg, culture, crime, embassy contact information) and regions can be included. Web sites such as www.cdc.gov and www.who.int/en can be used. In addition, commercial sites such as Travax (www.travax.com) and tropimed (www.tropimed.com) can be used to obtain up-to-date information including maps. These latter sites require an annual subscription fee. Advice on food and beverage precautions, swimming, sexual activity, animal bites, altitude illness, and safety can be provided. The information provided to the traveler should be documented on clinic visit forms. During the visit, the travel medicine provider can decide which items should be discussed in person. Depending on the number of travelers, the complexity of the trip, and past travel experiences, a clinic visit may take 1 to 2 hours. Because it would be impossible to cover all aspects of travel and provide vaccines, most of the needed information can be provided through the printed handout, allowing travelers to review and read it at home before their trip.

Topics that may require discussion during a clinic visit include
- Immunizations (benefits and potential side effects)
- Antimalarial chemoprophylaxis
- Insect bite prevention
- Jet lag
- Motion sickness
- Travel-related thrombosis
- Altitude illness
- Accident and injury prevention
- Traveling with young children
- Animal bites
- Crime
- Travel and medical evacuation insurance
- Swimming
- Treatment of traveler's diarrhea (eg, rehydration, antibiotics)
- Food and beverage precautions
- Food preparation
- Country-specific access to health care

Travel Dates and Duration

Departure dates and travel duration also influence risk. In some countries, certain periods are associated with a higher risk of disease, such as the rainy season (malaria) and the dry season (meningococcal disease). Prolonged stays increase the risk of acquiring most travel-related illnesses, such as traveler's diarrhea, malaria, typhoid fever, and Japanese encephalitis virus infection.

Medical History

Most travelers are healthy, but many have chronic medical problems. A current list of medications and past illnesses is important. A list of allergies, especially severe allergies to egg products, vaccines, and medications, should be obtained and the following questions asked:

* Is the traveler currently immunosuppressed?
* Does the traveler suffer from gastrointestinal disorders such as inflammatory bowel disease?

Many disorders may increase the risk of illness while traveling, increase the risk of adverse reactions from medications or vaccines, or pose contraindications for receiving a given vaccine or medication. Examples include a history of depression, which would contraindicate the use of mefloquine as antimalarial chemoprophylaxis, and immunosuppressed individuals, who should not receive live vaccines such as yellow fever, oral typhoid Ty21a, or measles, mumps, and rubella.

Immunization Record

Past immunizations must be recorded. Travelers are encouraged to bring their vaccine records to the travel clinic visit. Vaccines should not be repeated unnecessarily. While hepatitis A vaccine is frequently recommended for travel to developing countries, in the United States most children will routinely receive it at 1 year of age. Eleven- to 12-year-olds and adolescents routinely receive the quadrivalent meningococcal conjugate vaccine, which is recommended for travel to countries in the sub-Saharan Africa meningitis belt during the dry season and when planning pilgrimage (Hajj) trips to Saudi Arabia. For each vaccine administered in the clinic, a CDC Vaccine Information Statement (VIS) should be provided; they can be obtained from the CDC Web site (www.cdc.gov/vaccines/pubs/vis). Administered vaccines must be recorded in the traveler's clinic visit form, including injection site, dose, log numbers, and expiration dates. It should also be documented that potential vaccine side effects were discussed and VISs provided.

Prescribed Medications

Medications prescribed for antimalarial chemoprophylaxis, self-treatment of traveler's diarrhea, and prevention of altitude illness should be recorded. It should be documented that their potential side effects were discussed. The dosage and number of doses prescribed should also be recorded. Preprinted prescription pads may be useful for some practitioners.

Patient/Parent Acknowledgment

The clinic visit form should include a general acknowledgment or disclosure paragraph stating that potential benefits, side effects, and costs of vaccines and chemoprophylactic medicines were discussed with travelers and their families. The traveler or parent should sign a statement affirming this. The form should state which information was provided, including antimalarial agent adverse reactions, insect bite prevention, safety, sexual activity, altitude illness, animal bites, and jet lag. The educational handout will usually contain much of this information.

Costs and Billing

Because of the potential costs of vaccines and medications, a visit to a travel clinic can be concerning. To avoid unnecessary expenses and potential side effects, the travel medicine provider should have a good understanding of the traveler's needs. Most private and public insurers will not offer coverage for travel-related clinic visits, vaccines, or medications. To avoid collection delays or lack of compensation, most travel clinics require payment at the time of service. Forms and receipts can be provided to travelers so they can bill insurers if they would like.

Billing forms containing appropriate coding information may facilitate payment to the traveler (if available). In the United States, *Current Procedural Terminology 2011* codes are available for travel-related counseling and vaccines (Box 10-1).

Vaccines

Travel clinics stock a variety of vaccines. Vaccines against typhoid fever, Japanese encephalitis virus, and yellow fever require special purchasing and are not routinely available in the offices of primary care physicians. Clinicians are required to have prior authorization from the state health department to administer yellow fever vaccine—an official stamp is needed. If a practitioner is expecting a large volume of travelers in the practice, the clinic could purchase and stock necessary vaccines. For most vaccines, storage requirements are similar to those of other vaccines. Like other vaccines, practitioners must be familiar with administration routes and potential side effects. Clinics belonging to local health departments or larger medical centers (who can negotiate better contracts based on volumes) can offer many travel vaccines at a lower cost to the traveler. The primary care practitioner could administer some recommended vaccines; good examples are tetanus-diphtheria boosters (including tetanus, diphtheria, and acellular pertussis vaccine),

Box 10-1. *Current Procedural Terminology* **Codes for Travel-Related Counseling and Vaccines**

PREVENTIVE MEDICINE, INDIVIDUAL COUNSELING

99401	15 minutes
99402	30 minutes
99403	45 minutes
99404	60 minutes

PREVENTIVE MEDICINE, GROUP COUNSELING

99411	30 minutes
99412	60 minutes

IMMUNIZATION ADMINISTRATION, FOR VACCINES

90460	18 years or younger; first injection
90461	each subsequent injection
90471	Older than 18 years and adults; first injection
90472	each subsequent injection

COMMONLY USED VACCINE CODES

90632	Hepatitis A, adult
90633	Hepatitis A, pediatric
90636	Hepatitis A and B (Twinrix)
90675	Rabies
90690	Typhoid Ty21a, oral
90691	Typhoid polysaccharide Vi, injectable
90707	Measles, mumps, and rubella
90713	Poliovirus, inactivated
90715	Tetanus, diphtheria, and acellular pertussis
90717	Yellow fever
90734	Meningococcal, quadrivalent conjugate
90735	Japanese encephalitis virus

meningococcal vaccines for an adolescent, and hepatitis A for a 1-year-old. These are frequently covered by the traveler's primary insurance and would not require out-of-pocket payment (other than a co-payment).

■ TIMING OF VISIT TO TRAVEL CLINIC

Depending on the type of travel, duration, destination, and prior vaccination experiences, travelers should plan for sufficient time to complete all necessary vaccinations and to initiate antimalarial chemoprophylaxis if necessary. Two to 4 weeks is usually sufficient for most pediatric travelers whose routine immunizations are up-to-date. Adults with limited travel experience may require multiple visits and months to complete a vaccine series, such as parents traveling to adopt a child and who require hepatitis B vaccination (which may require 6 months to complete).

Depending on the antimalarial agent selected, initiation may be required up to 2 weeks prior to travel. For some vaccines, accelerated schedules may be available (eg, hepatitis B, hepatitis A and B, Japanese encephalitis virus), but they still require at least 2 to 3 weeks to complete. Travel medicine providers should be familiar with these schedules. Primary care physicians must educate patients and parents to plan ahead and seek travel advice with sufficient time to complete needed vaccinations and other preventive measures.

■ MEDICAL CARE DURING AND AFTER TRAVEL

A clinician knowledgeable in travel-related illnesses should be available for the returning traveler, if needed. Fevers, skin ailments, and diarrhea are frequent problems. If the individual providing pretravel advice is uncomfortable providing this care, a referral to an infectious disease specialist or an expert in travel medicine (www.istm.org or www.astmh. org) is pertinent. Travelers benefit from having information on how to access health care abroad. Medical insurance plans are not accepted in many lower-income countries; the traveler will be expected to pay for services at the time of the visit. However, the traveler may enroll beforehand in an international medical and evacuation insurance program that provides coverage for himself and his family while traveling. Many of these may even help coordinate medical care, if needed (eg, International SOS). Individuals with chronic medical problems should have specific information on specialists or hospital centers in areas being traveled. When traveling, travelers should have a list of all medications, by generic name, and doses in case medical care is needed.

Preparation and provision of appropriate pretravel education and needed vaccines and prescriptions are useful tools in the prevention of travel-related illnesses. Where travel clinics are unavailable, a well-prepared and knowledgeable primary care practitioner can be just as efficient as a travel medicine provider. The pediatric traveler requires special attention and consideration. The traveler must enjoy the activities surrounding a visit to relatives and friends, humanitarian work, or studying abroad. Staying healthy will help ensure this. Most travel-related illnesses are preventable.

■ KEY POINTS

- Travel clinics provide necessary medical preventive advice, required and recommended vaccinations, and antimalarial chemoprophylaxis for at-risk travelers.

- Destinations, travel duration, planned activities, and medical and immunization history help determine the degree of risk travelers will experience during a trip.
- A comprehensive educational handout is an integral part of travel clinic visits.
- Most public and private insurers do not pay for pretravel consultations and vaccinations.

■ REFERENCES

1. Blair DC. A week in the life of a travel clinic. *Clin Microbiol Rev.* 1997;10:650–673
2. Dwelle TL. Inadequate basic preventive health measures: survey of missionary children in Sub-Saharan Africa. *Pediatrics.* 1995;95:733–737
3. Bacaner N, Stauffer B, Boulwire DR, Walker PF, Keystone JS. Travel medicine considerations for North American immigrants visiting friends and relatives. *JAMA.* 2004;291:2856–2864
4. Stauffer W, Christenson JC, Fischer PR. Preparing children for international travel. *Travel Med Infect Dis.* 2008;6:101–113
5. Backer H, Mackell S. Potential cost-savings and quality improvement in travel advice for children and families from a centralized travel medicine clinic in a large group-model health maintenance organization. *J Travel Med.* 2001;8:247–253
6. Walter EB, Clements DA. Travel consultation for children in a university-affiliated primary care setting. *Pediatr Infect Dis J.* 1998;17:841–843
7. Christenson JC, Fischer PR, Hale DC, Derrick D. Pediatric travel consultation in an integrated clinic. *J Travel Med.* 2001;8:1–5
8. Newman-Klee C, D'Acremont V, Newman CJ, Gehri M, Genton B. Incidence and types of illness when traveling to the tropics: a prospective controlled study of children and their parents. *Am J Trop Med Hyg.* 2007;77:764–769
9. Klein JL, Millman GC. Prospective, hospital based study of fever in children in the United Kingdom who had recently spent time in the tropics. *BMJ.* 1998;316:1425–1426
10. Riordan FAI, Tarlow MJ. Imported infections in East Birmingham children. *Postgrad Med J.* 1998;74:36–37
11. Pitzinger B, Steffen R, Tschopp A. Incidence and clinical features of traveler's diarrhea in infants and children. *Pediatr Infect Dis J.* 1991;10:719–723
12. Silva FG, Figueiredo A, Varandas L. Traveler's diarrhea in children visiting tropical countries. *J Travel Med.* 2009;16:53–54
13. Hill DR, Ericsson CD, Pearson RD, et al. The practice of travel medicine: guidelines by the Infectious Diseases Society of America. *Clin Infect Dis.* 2006;43:1499–1539

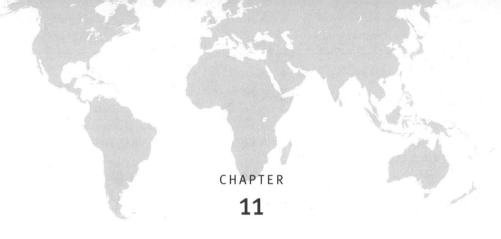

CHAPTER

11

Pretravel Care

Jocelyn Y. Ang, MD, FAAP
Ambika Mathur, PhD

■ INTRODUCTION

International travel continues to increase. According to the United Nations World Tourism Organization, there were 924 million international tourist border crossings in 2008, which is an increase of 16 million (2%) from 2007.[1] The purpose for international travel can include pleasure, visiting friends and relatives, or business. Children often accompany adults during travel. Traveling with family can be an educational and entertaining experience for children. Unfortunately, information about the incidence of pediatric illnesses associated with international travel is limited because the numbers of children traveling are fewer than adults. Health issues related to pediatric international travel are complex because of variable immunity, different age-related behaviors reflecting varied activities, exposure, and age-specific health risks. The most common reported health problems related to travel include diarrheal illnesses, malaria, and motor vehicle- and water-related injuries. Children traveling to developing countries are at higher risk for a variety of travel-related infectious health problems, including malaria, intestinal parasite infestations, and tuberculosis. Risk of acquiring illness during travel depends on the geographic area visited and individual factors such as age, baseline health conditions, length of stay, and activities planned.

The consulting pediatric health professional has a key role in preparing the family for prevention of travel-related illnesses and helping reduce health risks so the entire family can enjoy their travel.

■ PLANNING FOR HEALTHY TRAVEL

Precaution and Prevention

Prior to travel, practitioners should provide the following key advice to traveling families:

- *Child identification documentation.* The child should carry identification and travel destination(s). Long travel times, layovers, and non-familiarity with new areas and locations can result in the separation of children and parents.

- *Travel insurance coverage.* Families should purchase health insurance coverage for travel because accidents are the leading cause of mortality in young travelers.[2] If the families' regular health plan does not have coverage for international travel, they should purchase travel and evacuation insurance, as the cost of an evacuation could range from $25,000 to $100,000 per person.

- *Documentation for child traveling with one parent.* Because of increasing incidents of child abduction in disputed custody cases, a letter of authorization giving permission for the travel from the non-accompanying parent should be obtained. It is advisable to have the letter notarized so its validity will not be questioned. In addition, a notarized copy of the custodial document or death certificate is required if the accompanying parent is divorced or widowed.

■ MINIMIZING TRAVEL ANXIETY

Stress management techniques should be discussed with families to minimize children's anxiety about traveling to new areas.

- *Planning process.* Parents should include the child in the planning process of the anticipated trip by creating excitement with videos, books, pictures, food, and the Internet. Children can help plan for sites and people they will visit and foods they would like to eat. These activities give children a sense of control and ownership of the travel process.

- *Items of security/familiarity.* Allowing the child to carry a special toy, blanket, or picture helps establish a sense of security and familiarity during travel.

- *Disruption of normal routines.* Children should be made aware that they might encounter situations that could disrupt their normal routines, such as long delays, irregularly scheduled meals, and unusual schedules and nap times.

■ PRETRAVEL INTERVENTION

Chemoprophylaxis

Malaria

Malaria is endemic throughout the tropical areas of the world. It is caused by 1 of 5 *Plasmodium* species, which are intraerythrocytic protozoa: *P falciparum, P vivax, P ovale, P malariae,* or *P knowlesi. P knowlesi* is a parasite of the Old World monkeys but has been increasingly reported to cause human disease in Southeast Asia. Malaria is usually acquired from the bite of a nocturnal-feeding female *Anopheles* mosquito. Symptoms of malaria include high-grade fever with chills, rigors, and headache and can be paroxysmal. Anemia and thrombocytopenia are commonly seen. Jaundice can occur because of hemolysis. Infection with *P falciparum* is potentially fatal and can manifest as cerebral edema with varying neurologic manifestations including seizures, mental confusion, coma, and death.

According to the 2008 World Health Organization malaria report,[3] an estimated 247 million malaria cases occurred among 3.3 billion at-risk people in 2006 with an estimated 881,000 deaths. The majority (more than 75%) of deaths occurred in Africa and in children younger than 5 years.

In the United States and other higher-income countries, the majority of malaria infections occur among persons who traveled to areas with ongoing malaria transmission. Children account for a considerable proportion of total malaria cases imported into non-endemic countries.[4] From 1992 through 2002, more than 17,000 cases of imported malaria in children 18 years and younger were reported in 11 non-endemic countries, including the United States, United Kingdom, and France; most cases (more than 70%) were acquired in Africa.[4] The largest overall percentage of cases occurred among children 15 to 17 years of age.[4] Visiting friends and relatives in the country of origin was a risk factor for acquiring malaria.

All travelers should be counseled about taking appropriate antimalarial chemoprophylaxis, as well as various preventive measures to avoid mosquito bites. It is important to emphasize that no antimalarial agent is 100% effective in protecting against the risk of contracting malaria. The appropriate antimalarial agent must be combined with personal protective measures, such as insect repellent, long sleeves and pants. An insecticide-treated bed net is essential to protect against mosquito bites when accommodations are not adequately screened or air-conditioned.

A recommendation for appropriate antimalarial chemoprophylaxis is determined by the risk of acquiring malaria and the prevalence of antimalarial drug resistance in the destination. The possibility of drug interaction and drug allergies should also be considered.

In many areas of the world, resistance to antimalarial agents has developed. Currently, *P falciparum* resistance to chloroquine was confirmed in all areas with *P falciparum* malaria except in the Dominican Republic, Haiti, Central America west of the Panama Canal, Egypt, and some countries in the Middle East.[5] Resistance to mefloquine was reported on the borders of Thailand along Burma (Myanmar) and Cambodia, on the border between Burma and China, in Laos along the borders of Laos and Burma, and the adjacent parts of the Thailand-Cambodia border, as well as in southern Vietnam.[5] For up-to-date information on antimalarial-resistant patterns, health care professionals should consult the Centers for Disease Control and Prevention (CDC) Travelers' Health Web site at www.cdc.gov/travel.

Indications for prophylaxis in children are the same as those in adults except for doxycycline, which should not be given to children younger than 8 years because of the risk of dental staining. In addition, the use of atovaquone and proguanil (Malarone) is not established in children weighing less than 5 kg. Drug dosages in children should be calculated based on their current weight and should not exceed adult dosages. Drug doses for malaria chemoprophylaxis are provided in Table 11-1. In the United States, mefloquine and chloroquine phosphate are available only in adult tablet forms, while atovaquone and proguanil is available in pediatric tablet form. These drugs have bitter tastes. Pharmacists can pulverize the tablets and prepare gelatin capsules according to calculated pediatric doses. Gelatin capsules can then be opened and mixed in a small amount of food or drink to administer to children.

Because antimalarial chemoprophylaxis is not completely effective and some may elect not to take prophylaxis, travelers should be aware of the signs and symptoms of malaria (eg, fever, chills, flu-like symptoms) and seek medical attention immediately if these signs and symptoms develop. If prompt medical attention is not available, self-treatment with atovaquone and proguanil (Malarone), if not already taking for prophylaxis, should be initiated immediately because malaria can be fatal if treatment is delayed. For patients already taking atovaquone and proguanil (Malarone) for prophylaxis, the use of the same drug at therapeutic doses is not recommended; artemether-lumefantrine (Coartem) can be an option for presumptive self-treatment for malaria. Despite self-treatment for possible malaria, travelers still need to seek urgent medical

Table 11-1. Drugs Used in the Prophylaxis of Malaria

DRUG	USAGE	ADULT DOSE	PEDIATRIC DOSE	COMMENTS
Atovaquone and proguanil (Malarone)	Prophylaxis in all areas	Adult tablets contain 250 mg atovaquone and 100 mg proguanil hydrochloride. One adult tablet orally, daily.	Pediatric tablets contain 62.5 mg atovaquone and 25 mg proguanil hydrochloride. 5–8 kg: ½ pediatric tablet daily > 8–10 kg: ¾ pediatric tablet daily > 10–20 kg: 1 pediatric tablet daily > 20–30 kg: 2 pediatric tablets daily > 30–40 kg: 3 pediatric tablets daily > 40 kg: 1 adult tablet daily	Begin 1 to 2 days before travel to malarious areas. Take daily at the same time each day while in the malarious area and for 7 days after leaving such areas. Contraindicated in persons with severe renal impairment (creatinine clearance <30 mL/min). Atovaquone and proguanil should be taken with food or a milky drink. Not recommended for prophylaxis for children weighing < 5 kg, pregnant women, and women breastfeeding infants weighing < 5 kg. Partial tablet dosages may need to be prepared by a pharmacist and dispensed in individual capsules.
Chloroquine phosphate (Aralen and generic)	Prophylaxis only in areas with chloroquine-sensitive malaria	300 mg base (500 mg salt) orally, once per week	5 mg/kg base (8.3 mg/kg salt) orally, once per week, up to maximum adult dose of 300 mg base	Begin 1 to 2 weeks before travel to malarious areas. Take weekly on the same day of the week while in the malarious area and for 4 weeks after leaving such areas. May exacerbate psoriasis.
Doxycycline (Many brand names and generic)	Prophylaxis in all areas	100 mg orally, daily	8 years and older: 2 mg/kg up to adult dose of 100 mg/day	Begin 1 to 2 days before travel to malarious areas. Take daily at the same time each day while in the malarious area and for 4 weeks after leaving such areas. Contraindicated in children younger than 8 years and in pregnant women.

Table 11-1. Drugs Used in the Prophylaxis of Malaria, continued

DRUG	USAGE	ADULT DOSE	PEDIATRIC DOSE	COMMENTS
Hydroxy-chloroquine sulfate (Plaquenil)	An alternative to chloroquine for prophylaxis only in areas with chloroquine-sensitive *P falciparum*	310 mg base (400 mg salt) orally, once per week	5 mg/kg base (6.5 mg/kg salt) orally, once per week, up to maximum adult dose of 310 mg base	Begin 1 to 2 weeks before travel to malarious areas. Take weekly on the same day of the week while in the malarious area and for 4 weeks after leaving such areas.
Mefloquine (Lariam and generic)	Prophylaxis in areas with chloroquine-sensitive malaria	228 mg base (250 mg salt) orally, once per week	≤9 kg: 4.6 mg/kg base (5 mg/kg salt) orally, once per week 10–19 kg: ¼ tablet once per week 20–30 kg: ½ tablet once per week 31–45 kg: ¾ tablet once per week >46 kg: 1 tablet once per week	Begin at least 2 weeks before travel to malarious areas. Take weekly on the same day of the week while in the malarious area and for 4 weeks after leaving such areas. Contraindicated in persons allergic to mefloquine or related compounds (eg, quinine, quinidine) and in persons with active depression, a recent history of depression, generalized anxiety disorder, psychosis, schizophrenia, other major psychiatric disorders, or seizures. Use with caution in persons with psychiatric disturbances or a previous history of depression. Not recommended for persons with cardiac conduction abnormalities.

Table 11-1. Drugs Used in the Prophylaxis of Malaria, continued

DRUG	USAGE	ADULT DOSE	PEDIATRIC DOSE	COMMENTS
Primaquine[a]	Prophylaxis for short-duration travel to areas with principally *P vivax*	30 mg base (52.6 mg salt) orally, daily	0.5 mg/kg base (0.8 mg/kg salt) up to adult dose orally, daily	Begin 1 to 2 days before travel to malarious areas. Take daily at the same time each day while in the malarious area and for 7 days after leaving such areas. Contraindicated in persons with G6PD deficiency. Also contraindicated during pregnancy and lactation unless the infant being breast-fed has a documented normal G6PD level.
	Used for presumptive anti-relapse therapy (terminal prophylaxis) to decrease the risk of relapses of *P vivax* and *P ovale*	30 mg base (52.6 mg salt) orally, once per day for 14 days after departure from the malarious area	0.5 mg/kg base (0.8 mg/kg salt) up to adult dose orally, once per day for 14 days after departure from the malarious area	Indicated for persons who have had prolonged exposure to *P vivax*, *P ovale*, or both. Contraindicated in persons with G6PD deficiency. Also contraindicated during pregnancy and lactation unless the infant being breast-fed has a documented normal G6PD level.

Abbreviation: G6PD, glucose-6-phosphate dehydrogenase.

[a]All persons who take primaquine should have a documented normal G6PD level prior to starting the medication.

Adapted from Centers for Disease Control and Prevention. *CDC Health Information for International Travel 2010*. Atlanta, GA: US Department of Health and Human Services, Public Health Service; 2010

attention—this is only a temporary measure. Doses of atovaquone and proguanil (Malarone) and artemether-lumenfantrine (Coartem) for self-treatment are provided in Table 11-2.

Traveler's Diarrhea

Traveler's diarrhea (TD) is common among infants and children, and signs and symptoms tend to be more prolonged and more severe.[6] Leading etiologies[7] of TD in children are the same as adults, including bacterial causes: *Escherichia coli* (enterotoxigenic, enteroaggregative), *Campylobacter, Salmonella,* and *Shigella.* Other causes of TD

Table 11-2. Presumptive Self-treatment of Malaria

DRUG	ADULT DOSE	PEDIATRIC DOSE	COMMENTS
Atovaquone and proguanil[a] (Malarone). Self-treatment drug to be used if professional medical care is not available within 24 hours. Medical care should be sought immediately after treatment.	4 tablets (each dose contains 1,000 mg atovaquone and 400 mg proguanil) orally as a single daily dose for 3 consecutive days	Daily dose to be taken for 3 consecutive days. 5–8 kg: 2 pediatric tablets 9–10 kg: 3 pediatric tablets 11–20 kg: 1 adult tablet 21–30 kg: 2 adult tablets 31–40 kg: 3 adult tablets >41 kg: 4 adult tablets	Contraindicated in persons with severe renal impairment (creatinine clearance <30 mL/min). Not recommended for self-treatment in persons on atovaquone and proguanil prophylaxis. Not currently recommended for children weighing <5 kg, pregnant women, and women breastfeeding infants weighing <5 kg.
Artemether-lumefantrine (Coartem)	1 tablet = 20-mg artemether and 120-mg lumefantrine	A 3-day treatment schedule with a total of 6 oral doses is recommended for adult and pediatric patients based on weight. The patient should receive the initial dose, followed by the second dose 8 hours later, then 1 dose orally twice a day for the following 2 days.	5–<15 kg: 1 tablet per dose 15–<25 kg: 2 tablets per dose 25–<35 kg: 3 tablets per dose ≥35 kg: 4 tablets per dose

Adapted from Centers for Disease Control and Prevention. *CDC Health Information for International Travel 2010.* Atlanta, GA: US Department of Health and Human Services, Public Health Service; 2010 and Centers for Disease Control and Prevention. Malaria. http://www.cdc.gov/malaria/diagnosis_treatment/treatment.html. Accessed July 6, 2011

include viruses (ie, rotavirus, norovirus) and protozoa (eg, *Giardia, Cryptosporidium, Cyclospora*).

To prevent TD, families should be counseled not to consume unsafe foods; the "cook it, boil it, peel it, or forget it" rule should be followed; families should practice water and food safety measures; and anticipatory guidance on diarrhea treatment should be given. Use of an oral rehydration solution to prevent dehydration should diarrhea develop should be emphasized. While prophylaxis with nonantibiotic agents, such as bismuth subsalicylate (BSS), as well as antibiotics is used in adults to prevent TD, it is not recommended in children because of the lack of data on its efficacy. Furthermore, the BSS dose for prevention of TD in children is currently unknown. Frequent and prolonged use of BSS can potentially cause salicylate intoxication from salicylate absorption[8] as well as increase the risk of developing Reye syndrome in patients with influenza or chickenpox.

Antimicrobial prophylaxis for TD can lead to the development of resistant enteric pathogens, allergic reactions, and antibiotic-associated enterocolitis. Antimicrobial prophylaxis for TD is not recommended in children because the potential risks outweigh the benefits. Similarly, antibiotic prophylaxis is generally not recommended in adults.[9] However, fluoroquinolones are usually the antibiotics of choice when considering chemoprophylaxis for TD.[9] Recently, fluoroquinolone use has been associated with predisposition to infection with hypervirulent strains of *Clostridium difficile* associated with increased morbidity and mortality.[10] Fluoroquinolones use in children is limited because of the concern of cartilage damage in weight-bearing joints among beagle pups seen in animal toxicology studies.[11] Reported fluoroquinolone-associated musculoskeletal events in children were none[12] or transient and reversible.[13]

Presently, ciprofloxacin is the only Food and Drug Administration–approved fluoroquinolone for use in children and it is only approved for inhalational anthrax and complicated urinary tract infections and pyelonephritis.[14] Although some probiotics appear to prevent TD in adults,[15] data showing effectiveness in children are still limited.

■ AIR TRAVEL

Air travel has become a convenient and accessible form of transportation; more families, including children, travel by air. Illness associated with air travel is usually related to changes in air pressure and oxygen concentration, immobility during flights, or transmission of communicable diseases caused by close proximity to other passenger with infectious diseases.

Age

For healthy children, including newborns and infants, air travel is generally safe.[16] However; it is advisable to delay travel 1 to 2 weeks after birth to ensure that the newborn is indeed healthy and free of congenital defects or cardiovascular and pulmonary disease. Most commercial airlines reach cruising altitudes of 11,000 to 13,000 m (36,000 to 40,000 feet) and this would lead to hypoxia if uncompensated. The aircraft cabin is therefore pressurized to atmospheric pressure of 1,500 to 2,400 m (5,000 to 8,000 feet). At this altitude, the barometric pressure (P_B) in the aircraft cabin is around 560 mm Hg, which is equivalent to 15% oxygen and is lower compared with the normal value of 760 mm Hg and oxygen pressure of 21% at sea level.

While healthy children may be asymptomatic from lower oxygen concentrations, children with preexisting medical conditions, such as cardiopulmonary diseases, anemia, and sickle cell, as well as upper or lower respiratory symptoms at the time of travel, may be at risk for hypoxia and increased risk of exacerbation of their disease during the flight. Consultation with a physician should be done before the scheduled flight so arrangements can be made with the airline to provide oxygen and monitoring equipment if needed.

Otolaryngologic Conditions

Barotitis Media

To equalize cabin air pressure, air in the middle ear and sinuses expands during ascent and contracts during descent. Middle ear barotrauma is characterized by otalgia and is secondary to the inability to equilibrate tympanic cavity and atmospheric pressures because of eustachian tube obstruction.[17] Barotitis media is an acute or chronic inflammation of the middle ear caused by barotrauma[17] and characterized by an acute onset of ear pain, hearing loss, or vertigo. The prevalence of barotitis in young children is 25% compared with 5% in adults[18]; ear pain is reported in 55% of children and 20% of adults during descent.[18] Equalization of pressure in the middle ear can be facilitated by swallowing motions, such as breastfeeding or bottle-feeding babies. Older children can chew gum, blow up a balloon, or close their nose with their thumb and index finger and exhale gently with the mouth closed (Valsalva maneuver).[19]

Otitis Media

Otitis media is not thought to preclude flight if appropriate antibiotics are administered for at least 48 hours and the eustachian tube is patent. While limited to expert opinion, it has been recommended that children wait 2 weeks after treatment for acute otitis media before flying.[15] Recent surgical procedures involving structures of the inner or middle ear may be affected by pressure changes and are a contraindication to flight. Children who underwent recent procedures, such as tympanomastoidectomy, stapedectomy, labyrinthectomy or acoustic neurectomy, mastoidectomy, or other otologic surgeries, should not fly until cleared by their otolaryngologist.[16] Myringotomy or ear tube placement is not a contraindication to flying because they actually protect against middle ear barotraumas by minimizing pressure changes.[16] Children with chronic otitis media rarely suffer from barotraumas; it is not a contraindication to air travel.[20]

Thromboembolic Disease

Healthy children are not known to be at risk for developing deep vein thrombosis during a prolonged flight.[17] However, children with hypercoagulable states as well as those with a history of thromboembolic events, major surgery within 6 weeks, or a malignancy may be at increased risk of developing deep venous thrombosis as a result of immobility. They should consult their own physicians who may advise prophylaxis with low molecular weight heparin or acetylsalicylic acid.

In-flight Transmission of Communicable Diseases

The enclosed environment of the aircraft cabin, including limited ventilation, recirculated air, and close proximity to fellow passengers, has the potential for disease transmission.[21] Within this confined environment, the risk of disease transmission is not well known. The most studied in-flight transmission of an airborne pathogen is *Mycobacterium tuberculosis* (TB).

The risk of TB transmission aboard commercial aircraft remains low. Several studies of potential transmission of TB infection during air travel were reported in the mid-1990s. Subsequently, contact investigations revealed a probable link of transmission of infection in 2 investigations by conversion to a positive tuberculin skin test, but active TB disease was not found in any of the infected individuals. Limited data suggest the risk of disease transmission to other passengers is associated with sitting within 2 rows of a contagious passenger for more than 8 hours.[22] Other airborne diseases, including measles, meningococcal disease, severe acute respiratory syndrome, and influenza, are rarely implicated in aircraft transmission. Transmission of norovirus gastroenteritis on airplanes has also been reported rarely. Mode of transmission of norovirus gastroenteritis is generally by person-to-person spread via the fecal-oral route or through contaminated food or water. However, on an aircraft with high incidence of vomiting among infected individuals, airborne transmission may occur with subsequent ingestion of viral particles.[23]

Despite these cases, the chance of contracting a respiratory infection during air travel is quite small; the quality of aircraft cabin air is well controlled.[24] Most commercial aircraft recirculate 50% of the air in the cabin in an effort to conserve fuel. The recirculated air in the cabin passes through a series of high-efficiency particulate air (HEPA) filters; the same type of HEPA filters are also used in hospitals and can remove 99.97% of dusts, bacteria viruses, and fungi at a size of 0.3 μm. In addition, the air exchanges in the aircraft cabin range from 20 to 30 times per hour compared with 12 air exchanges per hour in most office buildings. To minimize the risk of transmission of communicable diseases, passengers who are unwell should postpone travel until they are recovered. Furthermore, passengers who appear to have a communicable disease may be denied boarding by the airline.

Use of Restraining Devices

According to the Federal Aviation Administration (FAA), the safest place for a child on an airplane during turbulence or an emergency is in an approved child restraint system (CRS) or a child safety device—not on a parent's lap.[25] The FAA strongly encourages the use of a CRS or an FAA-approved child safety device. However, the FAA does not mandate CRS use, as it requires families to purchase an extra airline ticket. Some families may even decide to drive, which is statistically more dangerous than flying.[26]

A CRS is a hard-backed safety seat approved by the government for use in aircraft and motor vehicles. Each CRS contains the wording, "This restraint is certified for use in motor vehicles and aircraft." The FAA recommends that children weighing less than 20 pounds use a rear-facing CRS. Children weighing 20 to 40 pounds should use a forward-facing CRS. Children weighing more than 40 pounds can be secured with an airplane seat belt.[25]

An alternative to using a CRS is a child safety device, which is a harness-type restraint appropriate for children between 22 and 44 pounds. The FAA approved the child safety device for use on aircraft only; it contains the wording, "FAA Approved in Accordance with 14CFR 21.305(d), Approved for Aircraft Use Only."[25]

While other vehicular restraint systems (eg, booster seats, harness vests) enhance safety in vehicles, the FAA prohibits their use on airplanes during takeoff, taxiing, and landing. These restraints should not be brought into the cabin but rather checked as baggage. In addition, "belly belts" or supplemental lap restraints are not approved for use in airplanes or vehicles in the United States.

Jet Lag

Jet lag is a group of symptoms associated with rapid, long-haul flights across different time zones. It is characterized by sleeping disturbances, daytime fatigue, irritability, and generalized malaise.[27] It is still not known to what extent children experience jet lag. Travel to different time zones, jet lag, and schedule disruptions can disturb sleep patterns in infants, children, and adults. Parents should help children adapt to new time zones as quickly as possible by encouraging them to stay active and exposing them to natural light during the day. Melatonin has been used to reduce the symptoms of jet lag and improve sleep after travel to multiple time zones.[27] However, it is not recommended because of insufficient evidence to conclude its effectiveness in children with jet lag. Diphenhydramine can be useful for some children but may cause oversedation or paradoxical agitation; a test dose should be administered before travel to determine the effect on the individual child.

Motion Sickness

Motion sickness is the discomfort experienced when perceived motion disturbs the organs of balance. Nausea, vertigo, pallor, and cold sweats are common manifestations of motion sickness in children.[28] Ataxia and nausea are the most frequent symptoms in children younger than 5 years and in children older than 12 years, respectively. The most common medications used to control motion sickness in children are dimenhydrinate and diphenhydramine. For symptomatic treatment, dimenhydrinate, 1 to 1.5 mg/kg per dose, or diphenhydramine, 0.5 to 1 mg/kg per dose up to 25 mg, can be given 1 hour before travel and every 6 hours thereafter during the trip. A test dose should be given before departure because some children can have paradoxical reaction to these drugs. Parents should also be advised of sedative side effects.

Safety data on other antiemetic compounds in children are limited. Antidopaminergic agents, such as metoclopramide and prochlorperazine, are not recommended because of their ineffectiveness to control motion sickness and their association with extrapyramidal symptoms in children.[29] Scopolamine is also not recommended due to its known side effects and lack of clinical use in children.[30] Alternatives to medical treatment include directing fresh, cool, ventilated air on the face; avoiding seats toward the rear of the aircraft; focusing on the horizon or a stable object; not reading books or playing video games; limiting head movement; and reclining whenever possible.[28]

■ OTHER TRAVEL-RELATED HEALTH RECOMMENDATIONS

Food-Borne and Waterborne Illness

Using common sense when handling and preparing food is the best way to reduce the risk of food-borne and waterborne illnesses in infants and children. Parents should use purified bottled water for drinking, brushing teeth, preparing food, and mixing infant food. It should be stressed that washing hands with soap and water is the best way to reduce the number of germs prior to touching, preparing, or eating food. If soap and water are not available, an alcohol-based hand sanitizer containing at least 60% alcohol should be used. The family should carry finger foods or snacks when traveling due to the irregularity of mealtimes. Food sold by street vendors should be strictly avoided.

Accidents

Vehicle-related accidents are the leading cause of death among travelers.[2] Children weighing less than 40 pounds should be restrained in age-appropriate car seats or booster seats while traveling.[25] Car seats should be brought from home, as well-maintained and approved seats may not be available at the travel destination.

Drowning is the second-leading cause of death among travelers.[2] Children must be well supervised around water. In addition, parents should closely monitor tides, currents, and warnings.

Sun Exposure

Approximately 23% of a person's lifetime sun exposure reportedly occurs before 18 years of age.[31] Strong evidence exists of a relationship between cumulative sun exposure and skin cancer. Therefore, infants and children should be kept away from direct sunlight. If in sunlight, appropriate protective clothing, such as hats and long-sleeved, loose-fitting shirts, should be worn to decrease sun exposure. Waterproof sunscreen with a sun protection factor of 15 or higher, which is known to reduce the lifetime incidence of skin cancer, should be used.[32]

Protection Against Insects and Other Arthropods

Several infections (eg, malaria, yellow fever, dengue fever) can be transmitted via insect bites; it is important that travelers avoid these insects. Children should wear light-colored, protective clothing (eg, long-sleeved shirts, long trousers, socks).

Insect repellents can help reduce exposure to mosquito bites that may carry viruses. Based on research reviewed by the CDC, repellents containing DEET or picaridin (KBR 3023) typically provide longer lasting protection than other products, and oil of lemon eucalyptus (p-men-thane-3,8-diol) provides longer lasting protection than other plant-based repellents such as soy or citronella. However, there is limited information on the effectiveness of plant-based repellents.

DEET is safe and effective. A concentration of 30% or less is considered safe and can be used on children 2 months and older.[33] Products with a concentration of 20% to 33% provide protection lasting for 6 to 12 hours.[34] Specifically, a product containing 23.8% DEET provided an average of 5 hours of protection from mosquito bites; 20% DEET provided almost 4 hours of protection; 6.65% DEET provided almost 2 hours of protection; and 4.75% DEET provided approximately 1 hour and 30 minutes of protection. DEET should only be applied to exposed skin. Avoid areas around the eyes and mouth and over cuts, wounds, or irritated skin.

The American Academy of Pediatrics has not yet issued specific recommendations or opinions concerning the use of picaridin or oil of lemon eucalyptus for children.

Permethrin is a highly effective insecticide and repellent derived from the chrysanthemum flower.[34] It can be used on clothing, shoes, and bed nets. Refer to the product's label for instructions on reapplying the insecticide repellent. Permethrin should not be sprayed onto skin.

Altitude Illness

Like adults, infants and children can suffer from altitude illness, including acute mountain sickness (AMS), high-altitude cerebral edema (HACE), and high-altitude pulmonary edema (HAPE).[36] Young children may present with nonspecific symptoms of fussiness and alterations in appetite, activity, or sleep patterns during or following recent exposure to altitude.[35] Acute mountain sickness is usually a benign disorder but may progress to HACE or HAPE if not promptly treated. Treatment for AMS depends on the severity of symptoms.[36] For mild AMS, treatment includes halting ascent, hydrating, resting, and taking analgesics.[36] For more severe symptoms, treatment includes descent, steroids, and oxygen. For prevention of AMS, a slow-graded ascent is recommended to achieve acclimatization.[36] *Acclimatization* refers to physiologic changes that allow the body to function at relative hypoxia. When a slow-graded ascent is not possible, the use of acetazolamide to aid in acclimatization may be needed.[36] Acetazolamide extended-release capsules have been used for prophylaxis or amelioration of symptoms of AMS in patients 12 years and older—500 to 1,000 mg orally extended-release capsule once a day; during rapid ascent, 1,000 mg per day is recommended;

initiate 24 to 48 hours before ascent and continue for 48 hours or longer while at high altitude. Acetazolamide is contraindicated in children with a known sulfa allergy.[37]

Parasitic Infestations

Children are more likely than adults to become exposed to various parasites (eg, ascaris, trichuris, hookworm, strongyloides, cutaneous larva migrans) because they are more likely to come in contact with soil or sand. Children should wear protective footwear and parents should lay down a sheet or towel before placing the child on the ground. In addition, parents should not dry clothes or diapers on the ground. Cutaneous infestations with fly larvae (myiasis) can be prevented by ironing clothes that are dried in open air.

■ COUNSELING FOR CHILDREN WITH CHRONIC MEDICAL CONDITIONS

Children with preexisting medical conditions pose a different set of challenges. It is important for the parents of such children to consult with a travel medicine specialist prior to traveling. It is essential for parents to carry an adequate supply of medications (eg, seasonal allergy medication) in their carry-on luggage. All medications should be transported in their original containers. An adequate supply of syringes and needles should be provided, along with a letter justifying their need, for children with insulin-dependent diabetes. An oral or topical steroid burst can be carried for eczema or asthma, while a preloaded epinephrine syringe (EpiPen) should be carried for children with a history of allergic and anaphylactic reactions (eg, bee stings, shellfish or peanut allergies). Pediatric-dose EpiPens are available for children weighing less than 30 kg. Children with more complicated conditions such as cystic fibrosis, HIV/AIDS, congenital heart disease, and renal disease should be managed in consultation with their respective specialists.

Parents should be advised to carry a medical kit containing prescription medications and other items (Table 11-3). Parents should also be instructed to seek medical attention at early signs and symptoms of disease. Such symptoms might include high fever, lethargy, unexplained fussiness, crying without tears, dry mouth, high respiratory rate, labored breathing, or a toxic appearance (the child "looks sick").

■ KEY POINTS

The travel experience is important for families. Health care professionals can help minimize stress related to travel by counseling families and providing medical and commonsense advice. Practitioners can also refer

Box 11-1. Suggested Items to Carry in a Medical Kit

- Adequate supply of prescription medications in original containers
- Analgesics/antipyretics (eg, ibuprofen, acetaminophen)
- Antihistamine/antipruritic (eg, diphenhydramine)
- Epinephrine auto-injector (especially if there is history of severe allergic reaction)
- Bandages and wound dressings
- DEET-based repellent and permethrin (when appropriate)
- Diaper rash ointment (eg, A+D, zinc oxide, Aquaphor)
- Disinfectant solutions (eg, 10% povidone-iodine, chlorhexidine)
- Oral rehydration solutions or packets
- Sunscreen of greater than 15 SPF and active against UVA and UVB
- Thermometer
- Tweezers
- Scissors
- Antibacterial ointment
- Antimalarial drugs (if applicable)

Abbreviation: SPF, sun protection factor.

to several electronic resources related to travel listed in Table 11-3 for more information.

Summary of pretravel physician visit

- Assess routine childhood immunization.
- Assess the need for any travel-specific vaccines and malaria chemoprophylaxis.
- Provide anticipatory guidance about monitoring children carefully for signs and symptoms of illness.
- Explain that children with fever, unexplained irritability, or signs of dehydration should be evaluated urgently.
- Ensure families know when and where to seek medical attention.
- Provide the family with a list of resources on traveling with infants and children.

Summary of physician advice to traveling family

- Carry documentation.
- Involve children in the planning process.
- Bring medications to combat jet lag and motion sickness.
- Secure children in appropriate seating device while traveling.
- Wash hands with soap and water before touching, preparing, or eating food.
- Alcohol-based hand sanitizer (at least 60% alcohol) may be used if soap and water are not available.
- Use bottled water for drinking, brushing teeth, and preparing food.
- Avoid disease-causing insects and animals.
- Avoid sun exposure.

Table 11-3. Selected Travel Medicine-Related Web Sites for Practitioners

AUTHORITATIVE TRAVEL MEDICINE RECOMMENDATIONS	
CDC Travelers' Health	www.cdc.gov/travel
CDC Travelers' Health—Yellow Book	www.cdc.gov/yellowbook
US Department of State Country Specific Consular Information	http://travel.state.gov/travel/cis_pa_tw/cis/cis_4965.html
WHO International Travel and Health	www.who.int/ith/en
The Practice of Travel Medicine: Guidelines by the Infectious Diseases Society of America	www.journals.uchicago.edu/doi/pdf/10.1086/508782
EMERGING DISEASES AND OUTBREAKS	
WHO Global Alert and Response (GAR)	www.who.int/csr/en
WHO Global Alert and Response (GAR) Disease Outbreak News	www.who.int/csr/don/en
WHO Global Alert and Response (GAR) Diseases Covered by GAR	www.who.int/csr/disease/en
CDC Health Alert Network Archive	www2a.cdc.gov/HAN/ArchiveSys
GeoSentinel: The Global Surveillance Network of the International Society of Travel Medicine and CDC	www.geosentinel.org
ProMED-mail, the Program for Monitoring Emerging Diseases	www.promedmail.org
HealthMap—Global Health, Local Information	www.healthmap.org/en
SURVEILLANCE AND EPIDEMIOLOGIC BULLETINS	
CDC *Morbidity and Mortality Weekly Report*	www.cdc.gov/mmwr
WHO *Weekly Epidemiological Record*	www.who.int/wer
Eurosurveillance	www.eurosurveillance.org
PAHO/WHO National Epidemiological Surveillance Information	www.paho.org/English/DD/AIS/vigilancia-en.htm
Armed Forces Health Surveillance Center Global Emerging Infections Surveillance and Response Systems Operations Division	www.afhsc.mil/geis

Table 11-3. Selected Travel Medicine-Related Web Sites for Practitioners, continued

VACCINE RESOURCES

CDC US Advisory Committee for Immunization Practices Recommendations	www.cdc.gov/vaccines/pubs/ACIP-list.htm
CDC Vaccine Information Statements	www.cdc.gov/vaccines/pubs/vis/default. htm
CDC Current Vaccine Shortages & Delays	www.cdc.gov/vaccines/vac-gen/shortages/ default.htm
American Academy of Pediatrics *Red Book Online* Vaccine Status Table	http://aapredbook.aappublications.org/ news/vaccstatus.shtml
CDC *Epidemiology and Prevention of Vaccine-Preventable Diseases: The Pink Book*	www.cdc.gov/vaccines/pubs/pinkbook/ default.htm
CDC *The Pink Book:* Appendices	www.cdc.gov/vaccines/pubs/pinkbook/ pink-appendx.htm
Quick Chart of Vaccine-Preventable Disease Terms in Multiple Languages	www.immunize.org/izpractices/p5122.pdf
Institute for Vaccine Safety Package Inserts and Manufacturers for some US Licensed Vaccines and Immunoglobins	www.vaccinesafety.edu/package_inserts. htm
PATH Vaccine Resource Library	www.path.org/vaccineresources

CONSUMER-ORIENTED TRAVEL HEALTH INFORMATION AND PRODUCTS

High Altitude Medicine Guide	www.high-altitude-medicine.com
Travel Health Online	www.tripprep.com
MDtravelhealth.com	www.mdtravelhealth.com
Chinook Medical Gear, Inc.	www.chinookmed.com
Magellan's	www.magellans.com
Travel Medicine	www.travmed.com

OVERSEAS MEDICAL AND SAFETY ASSISTANCE

US Department of State Tips for Traveling Abroad	http://travel.state.gov/travel/tips/ tips_1232.html
US Department of States Overseas Security Advisory Council Bureau of Diplomatic Security	www.osac.gov

Table 11-3. Selected Travel Medicine-Related Web Sites for Practitioners, continued

FAA International Aviation Safety Assessments Program	www.faa.gov/about/initiatives/iasa/more
International Association for Medical Assistance to Travelers	www.iamat.org
International SOS	www.internationalsos.com/en
MedEx Global Solutions Worldwide Travel Assistance & International Medical Insurance	www.medexassist.com
DISABILITY RESOURCES	
MossRehab ResourceNet	www.mossresourcenet.org/travel.htm
US Department of Transportation Aviation Consumer Protection and Enforcement	http://airconsumer.ost.dot.gov
Society for Accessible Travel & Hospitality	www.sath.org
Mobility International USA	www.miusa.org
MAPS AND COUNTRY INFORMATION	
University of Texas at Austin Perry-Castañeda Library Map Collection	www.lib.utexas.edu/Libs/PCL/Map_collection/map_sites/map_sites.html
CIA: The World Factbook	https://www.cia.gov/library/publications/the-world-factbook
US Department of State Background Notes	www.state.gov/r/pa/ei/bgn
United Nations Cartographic Section Department of Field Support	www.un.org/Depts/Cartographic/english/htmain.htm
Global Gazetteer Version 2.2	www.fallingrain.com/world
PROFESSIONAL MEDICAL SOCIETIES WITH A MAJOR FOCUS ON TRAVELERS' HEALTH	
International Society of Travel Medicine	www.istm.org
American Society of Tropical Medicine and Hygiene	www.astmh.org
Divers Alert Network	www.diversalertnetwork.org
Wilderness Medical Society	www.wms.org
Undersea & Hyperbaric Medical Society	www.uhms.org
American Travel Health Nurses Association	www.athna.org
Christian Medical & Dental Associations	www.cmdahome.org

Table 11-3. Selected Travel Medicine-Related Web Sites for Practitioners, continued

DISEASE PAGES

WHO Global Health Atlas	www.who.int/GlobalAtlas
CDC Diseases & Conditions A-Z Index	www.cdc.gov/DiseasesConditions
Malaria Atlas Project	www.map.ox.ac.uk
CDC Seasonal Influenza (Flu)	www.cdc.gov/flu
Global Polio Eradication Initiative	www.polioeradication.org
PAHO/WHO Malaria	www.paho.org/english/ad/dpc/cd/malaria.htm
PAHO/WHO Featured Surveillance Items	www.paho.org/english/ad/dpc/cd/dengue.htm

GENERAL TRAVEL AIDS

US Department of State Foreign Embassy Information & Publications	www.state.gov/s/cpr/rls
Electronic Embassy	www.embassy.org/embassies/index.html
The World Clock—Time Zones	www.timeanddate.com/worldclock
Tourism Offices Worldwide Directory	www.towd.com
Visa ATM Locator	http://visa.via.infonow.net/locator/global/jsp/SearchPage.jsp
Mastercard ATM Locator	www.mastercard.com/cardholderservices/atm

US ORGANIZATIONS OFFERING TRAINING IN TRAVEL MEDICINE

Gorgas Courses in Clinical Tropical Medicine	www.gorgas.org
Tulane University School of Public Health and Tropical Medicine	www.sph.tulane.edu/tropmed
University of Washington School of Medicine Continuing Medical Education	http://depts.washington.edu/cme/home

Abbreviations: CDC, Centers for Disease Control and Prevention; CIA, Central Intelligence Agency; FAA, Federal Aviation Administration; PAHO, Pan American Health Organization; PATH, Program for Appropriate Technology in Health; WHO, World Health Organization.

Adapted from Centers for Disease Control and Prevention. *CDC Health Information for International Travel 2010*. Atlanta, GA: US Department of Health and Human Services, Public Health Service; 2010

■ REFERENCES

1. United Nations World Tourism Organization. UNWTO World Tourism Barometer. 2009. http://www.worldtourism.org/facts/eng/pdf/barometer/UNWTO_Barom09_2_en_excerpt.pdf. Accessed July 15, 2009

2. Guse CE, Cortes LM, Hargarten SW, Hennes HM. Fatal injuries of US citizens abroad. *J Travel Med.* 2007;14(5):279–287

3. World Health Organization. *World Health Organization Malaria Report 2008.* http://apps.who.int/malaria/wmr2008/malaria2008.pdf. Accessed July 15, 2009

4. Stager K, Legros F, Krause G, et al. Imported malaria in children in industrialized countries, 1992–2002. *Emerg Infect Dis.* 2009;15(2):185–191

5. Centers for Disease Control and Prevention. *The Yellow Book.* 2008. http://wwwn.cdc.gov/travel/yellowbook/2008/ch4/malaria.aspx

6. Pitzinger B, Steffen R, Tschopp A. Incidence and clinical features of traveler's diarrhea in infants and children. *Pediatr Infect Dis J.* 1991;10(10):719–723

7. Mackell S. Traveler's diarrhea in the pediatric population: etiology and impact. *Clin Infect Dis.* 2005;41(Suppl 8):S547–S552

8. Pickering LK, Feldman S, Ericsson CD, Cleary TG. Absorption of salicylate and bismuth from a bismuth subsalicylate–containing compound (Pepto-Bismol). *J Pediatr.* 1981;99(4):654–656

9. Drugs for traveler's diarrhea. *Med Lett Drugs Ther.* 2008;50(1291):58–59

10. Razavi B, Apisarnthanarak A, Mundy LM. Clostridium difficile: emergence of hypervirulence and fluoroquinolone resistance. *Infection.* 2007;35(5):300–307

11. Stahlmann R, Kuhner S, Shakibaei M, et al. Chondrotoxicity of ciprofloxacin in immature beagle dogs: immunohistochemistry, electron microscopy and drug plasma concentrations. *Arch Toxicol.* 2000;73(10–11):564–572

12. Yee CL, Duffy C, Gerbino PG, et al. Tendon or joint disorders in children after treatment with fluoroquinolones or azithromycin. *Pediatri Infect Dis J.* 2002;21(6):525–529

13. Grady R. Safety profile of quinolone antibiotics in the pediatric population. *Pediatr Infect Dis J.* 2003;22(12):1128–1132

14. American Academy of Pediatrics Committee on Infectious Diseases. The use of systemic fluoroquinolones. *Pediatrics.* 2006;118(3):1287–1292

15. McFarland LV. Meta-analysis of probiotics for the prevention of traveler's diarrhea. *Travel Med Infect Dis.* 2007;5(2):97–105

16. Aerospace Medical Association Medical Guidelines Task F. Medical Guidelines for Airline Travel, 2nd ed. *Aviat Space Environ Med.* 2003;74(5 Suppl):A1–A19

17. Air travel and children's health issues. *Paediatr Child Health.* 2007;12(1):45–59

18. Stangerup SE, Tjernstrom O, Harcourt J, Klokker M, Stokholm J. Barotitis in children after aviation; prevalence and treatment with Otovent. *J Laryngol Otol.* 1996;110(7):625–628

19. Tompkins O. Ears and air travel. *AAOHN J.* 2007;55(8):336

20. Sade J, Ar A, Fuchs C. Barotrauma vis-a-vis the "chronic otitis media syndrome": two conditions with middle ear gas deficiency. Is secretory otitis media a contraindication to air travel? *Ann Otol Rhinol Laryngol.* 2003;112(3):230–235

21. Zitter JN, Mazonson PD, Miller DP, Hulley SB, Balmes JR. Aircraft cabin air recirculation and symptoms of the common cold. *JAMA.* 2002;288(4):483–486

22. Kenyon TA, Valway SE, Ihle WW, Onorato IM, Castro KG. Transmission of multidrug-resistant Mycobacterium tuberculosis during a long airplane flight. *N Engl J Med.* 1996;334(15):933–938

23. Kirking HL, Cortes J, Burrer S, et al. Likely transmission of norovirus on an airplane, October 2008. *Clin Infect Dis*. 2010;50(9):1216–1221

24. Bull K. Cabin air filtration: helping to protect occupants from infectious diseases. *Travel Med Infect Dis*. 2008;6(3):142–144

25. Federal Aviation Administration. *Child Safety on Airplanes 2008*. http://www.faa.gov/passengers/fly_children/crs. Accessed July 16, 2009

26. Federal Aviation Administration. *Flying with Children 2008*. http://www.faa.gov/passengers/fly%5Fchildren. Accessed July 16, 2009

27. Morgenthaler TI, Lee-Chiong T, Alessi C, et al. Practice parameters for the clinical evaluation and treatment of circadian rhythm sleep disorders. An American Academy of Sleep Medicine report. *Sleep*. 2007;30(11):1445–1459

28. Stauffer W, Konop R, Plotnikoff G, Deepak K. "Stop the car, Mom, I'm going to be sick!" *Contemp Pediatr*. 2002;19(7):43–56

29. Manteuffel J. Use of antiemetics in children with acute gastroenteritis: are they safe and effective? *J Emerg Trauma Shock*. 2009;2(1):3–5

30. Spinks AB, Wasiak J, Villanueva EV, Bernath V. Scopolamine (hyoscine) for preventing and treating motion sickness. *Cochrane Database Syst Rev*. 2007(3):CD002851

31. Godar DE, Urbach F, Gasparro FP, van der Leun JC. UV doses of young adults. *Photochem Photobiol*. 2003;77(4):453–457

32. Stern RS, Weinstein MC, Baker SG. Risk reduction for nonmelanoma skin cancer with childhood sunscreen use. *Arch Dermatol*. 1986;122(5):537–545

33. Pickering LK, Long SS, McMillan JA, eds. Prevention of mosquitoborne infections. In: *Red Book: 2006 Report of the Committee on Infectious Diseases*. 27th ed. Elk Grove Village, IL: American Academy of Pediatrics; 2006:197–199

34. Katz TM, Miller JH, Hebert AA. Insect repellents: historical perspectives and new developments. *J Am Acad Dermatol*. 2008;58(5):865–871

35. Duster MC, Derlet MN. High-altitude illness in children. *Pediatr Ann*. 2009;38(4):218–223

36. Pollard AJ, Niermeyer S, Barry P, et al. Children at high altitude: an international consensus statement by an ad hoc committee of the International Society for Mountain Medicine, March 12, 2001. *High Alt Med Biol*. 2001;2(3):389–403

37. Micromedex 1.0 Healthcare Series Drug Point Summary on Acetazolamide. http://dmc-micromedex/hcs/librarian/ND_T/HCS/ND_PR/Main/CS/285940/DUPLICATIONSHIELDSYNC/A12095/ND_PG/PRIH/ND_B/HCS/SBK/1/ND_P/MainPFActionId/hcs.common.RetrieveDocumentCommon/DocId/004140/ContentSetId/100/SearchTerm/acetazolamide/SearchOption/BeginWith

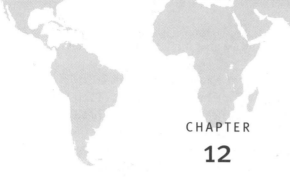

CHAPTER

12

Adolescent Travelers Without Parents

Linda S. Nield, MD, FAAP
Deepak M. Kamat, MD, PhD, FAAP

■ INTRODUCTION

Adolescence is a time for significantly remodeling the brain's gray and white matter.[1] Risk taking may ensue as adolescents strive to be more independent. As part of the journey to independence, the opportunity for international travel without parental supervision may arise. The adolescent's decision-making skills will be tested as total freedom from parental authority may be experienced for the first time.

Parents may seek the counsel of the pediatrician to determine if the adolescent is mature enough to travel without them. To assess if a child could travel alone responsibly, the parents should consider circumstances from the recent past in which the child displayed decision-making skills. The adolescent's reasonable management of past and present difficulties, especially emergency situations, provides some reassurance that he is capable of coping with unpredictable events that may arise while traveling abroad. A pattern of reckless sexual behavior and substance abuse is worrisome because these unhealthy activities may increase while the adolescent is away from parental authority.[2,3] It is mandatory that before an adolescent is allowed to travel independently, he is already considered dependable and trustworthy by parents, teachers, and other adults who supervise the adolescent in various capacities. Consistent contact between parents and the adolescent via telephone or the Internet should be guaranteed before solo travel is even allowed.

Once the decision for adolescent travel is made, the pediatrician may be consulted about potential medical implications of international travel. Therefore, the pediatrician must be well versed in health-related issues associated with adolescent travel. The travel's health implications will vary depending on the destination, reason, and length of stay. This chapter addresses those implications to which adolescents are particularly susceptible so the pediatrician is able to provide effective pretravel advice.

■ EPIDEMIOLOGY

The travel industry touts youth tourism—travel among individuals 16 to 24 years of age—as the most rapidly growing age group in the 21st century.[4] Approximately one tenth or 3 million of the total travelers from the United States were students visiting overseas destinations in 2007.[5] Results of a study from 2005 and 2007 revealed that more than 70% of surveyed households included a 12-year-old to 18-year-old member who traveled on a group trip without the family, and approximately 8% of trips were taken to international locations.[6] Along with recreation and study, adolescents will travel for several purposes (Box 12-1). Some teenagers may participate in international youth exchange programs or travel overseas after high school or college graduation. European countries in particular are popular international destinations for study,[7] but adolescents may travel to various areas all over the world. Many adolescents and young adults are drawn to adventure travel or travel that involves aggressive physical activity on potentially dangerous terrain, such as mountain climbing and other strenuous sports. Participation in ecotourism may provide the adolescent with the opportunity to visit remote

---

Box 12-1. Reasons for Adolescent Travel

- Adventure travel
- Cultural exploration
- Club activity
- Ecotourism
- Missionary projects
- Performing arts
- Recreation
- Religious pilgrimages
- Sporting events
- Study
- Visitation of friends and relatives
- Volunteerism
- Work

areas of the world and obtain an appreciation for other ways of life that may not include modern conveniences found in the United States.

Spring break is typically a 1-week pleasure vacation for American high school and college students occurring in the months of February through April. This annual jaunt has become synonymous with binge drinking, taking drugs, and being promiscuous.[8] It is estimated that approximately a half-million students (spring breakers) will visit national or international destinations every year.[8] Some students will admit to choosing a vacation spot that has lenient alcohol laws and caters to entertaining young adults. In recent decades, Mexican resorts have become popular spring break destinations. Whether the travel is brief and solely for recreation or lengthier and for more altruistic purposes, health-related issues (Box 12-2) may arise and will vary depending on the details of the travel agenda.

Infectious Diseases

Parental worry about an adolescent acquiring an infection while on vacation is the likely reason for a pretravel health care visit. Although there are no studies that address the acquisition of infections in adolescent travelers specifically, there are some studies available that include young adults in the surveyed populations.[9–12] The most common health complaints during travel include upper respiratory and gastrointestinal symptoms. Common viral illnesses such as influenza, rather than exotic local pathogens, are more likely to be the cause of respiratory symptoms emerging during travel. An outbreak of *Histoplasma capsulatum,* a febrile respiratory tract disease, is an example of a travel-acquired illness in adolescents vacationing in Acapulco, Mexico, in 2001.[13] Reports such as this are rare. Steffen et al reported that teenagers and young adults are at particular risk of acquiring traveler's diarrhea; the risk-taking behavior of this age group and perhaps the tendency to not comply with safe eating practices may explain the increased risk.[14]

In general, longer travel duration is associated with a higher risk of infection acquisition in developing countries.[10] Malaria and dengue fever are often listed in the top 5 infections encountered from travel to

---

Box 12-2. Health Issues of Adolescent Travel

- Infectious diseases
- Sexual hazards
- Noninfectious diseases
- Trauma
- Substance use
- Crime

developing or tropical destinations.[9–12] Measles outbreaks occur around the world, even in Europe. The vast majority of measles in the United States are secondary to importations from other countries.[15] Other infections that can spread in travelers include typhoid and hepatitis B. Risk factors for hepatitis B acquisition are more common among younger travelers on longer trips.[16] Hospitalization, sexual activity, or body piercings or tattoos while traveling are some of the reported risk factors for acquiring hepatitis B.[16,17]

Obtaining a tattoo or body piercing may go hand in hand with risk-taking behaviors like alcohol and marijuana use.[18] Along with the acquisition of hepatitis B, some potential infectious complications of body modification include acquisition of other viral hepatitides and other blood-borne viral and bacterial pathogens, skin abscesses, and endocarditis. Adolescents and young adults vary in their appreciation of the importance of proper hygienic practices required for body modification and in their awareness of the possible health implications associated with obtaining a tattoo or piercing.[19]

Sexual Hazards

There is no doubt that adolescents are at risk for sexually transmitted infections (STIs) while traveling. *Chlamydia,* gonorrhea, human papillomavirus (HPV), syphilis, hepatitis, and HIV are some of the infections spread during travel. Shah and colleagues tracked STIs in US citizens post-travel and found a significant peak in March and May, perhaps coinciding to spring break return.[20] During travel, adolescents may be more uninhibited because of freedom from adult supervision. The adolescent's first sexual encounter may occur while vacationing and is often viewed as a negative experience; girls may have persistent feelings of worthlessness, depression, and worry about pregnancy.[3] Being male and younger than 20 years is associated with a high frequency of casual sexual encounters during travel.[21] However, adolescent girls are also very sexually active during travel, and some may use alcohol to justify risky behavior.[22] Casual sex while traveling abroad correlates to casual sex in the home country.[23]

Experiencing multiple sex partners, unprotected sex, and sex while intoxicated are high-risk behaviors for contracting an STI.[24] Common reasons for not using condoms include poor judgment due to alcohol use, lack of condom availability, and lack of consideration of long-term consequences of unsafe sex.[23] One third of spring break travelers admitted to having sex with a new partner they met at the vacation location. Many of the travelers reported that they rarely or never worried about contracting an STI.[24]

HIV is particularly worrisome because young adults bear the major burden of this infection worldwide. The immaturity of the adolescent cervix makes girls more vulnerable to STIs like herpes simplex, which increases the susceptibility to HIV.[25] Certain areas of the world have very high infection rates and the adolescent's destination is a factor in the degree of likely exposure. The risk of acquiring HIV is highest for travel to Africa, followed by South Asia.[26]

A potential noninfectious health consequence of increased and unprotected sexual activity is pregnancy. The risk of an adolescent conceiving while traveling is unknown.[27] Researchers of a survey of adolescent girls reported that 15% of respondents were concerned about the possibility of being pregnant after vacationing for a week with other adolescents and without parental authority.[3]

Noninfectious Diseases

Because younger and fitter travelers are more likely to engage in strenuous outdoor activities, especially if participating in adventure travel, they will be exposed to the natural elements of the surroundings. Heat or cold injuries, animal bites, insect and marine creature stings, and acute mountain or altitude illness are some of the potential consequences of exposure to environmental dangers (Box 12-3). Acute altitude illness is characterized by headache, dizziness, nausea or vomiting, insomnia, and fatigue, which results from hypobaric hypoxia at altitudes higher than 2,500 m above sea level.[28] Being more physically fit does not prevent one from suffering from altitude illness.[28] Triggers of acute altitude illness include overexertion within 24 hours of ascent, dehydration, hypothermia, smoking, and alcohol or sedative consumption.[28] Bite wounds and the need for rabies prophylaxis are more likely experienced in travelers in the third decade of life.[29]

Box 12-3. Potential Health Hazards During Adventure Travel	

• Altitude illness
• Bites
  —Animal
  —Arthropod
  —Marine life
• Cold injuries
• Dermatologic diseases
  —Contact dermatitis
  —Photodermatitis
  —Phytophotodermatitis
  —Sunburn
	• Dehydration
	• Drowning
	• Head injury
	• Heat illness
	• Lacerations
	• Musculoskeletal injuries
	  —Fractures
	  —Sprains

Trauma

Injuries are a major potential health concern for the adolescent traveler. Death is more likely to occur during travel due to an accident than secondary to an infectious disease or other physical illness.[30] Motor vehicle accidents (MVAs) and drowning are the main causes of injury while traveling abroad.[30,31] Travel to developing countries places the adolescent at a particularly high risk compared with developed countries. Characteristics of the young traveler and the host country place the young traveler at particular risk for MVAs. High-risk behaviors, such not using seat belts or driving under the influence of mind-altering substances, increase the odds that the adolescent will be an accident. Poor road conditions, poorly functioning vehicles, unfamiliar roads and road rules, and lack of law enforcement of road rules in the host country add to the danger.

Morbidity and mortality associated with bodies of water are mainly caused by drowning. Swimming alone in unfamiliar territory, inexperience with water sports such as diving or snorkeling, or being under the influence of mind-altering substances increase the chances of drowning or near-drowning experiences.

After a traumatic event occurs, there is no guarantee that effective health care is nearby, especially in developing countries. The parents and adolescent should keep in mind that emergency medical systems are not available everywhere in the world.

Substance Use

Substance use is more likely to occur in adolescents who vacation in popular locations known for a party atmosphere than those who travel to metropolitan areas, national parks, or small towns.[8] Binge drinking, cigarette and marijuana smoking, and other illicit drug use are common and can escalate during adolescent travel without parental guidance.[2,3] Spring break is a risk factor for heightened alcohol use,[8,32] along with traveling with friends.[2] College students vacationing with friends during spring break dramatically increased their alcohol use, as revealed in one study.[2] In a survey of spring break participants, the vast majority of men, some younger than 21 years, and more than three quarters of women admitted to drinking excessively in the past day.[8] Men are more likely to drink greater amounts, to the point of intoxication and sickness. However, female travelers also engage in more risky substance abuse. Fifteen percent of the respondents in a survey of adolescent female travelers sought medical care after sustaining injuries while under the influence of alcohol or another mind-altering substance.[3] The vast majority who engaged in sexual activity (86%) admitted to doing so while drunk.

The use of illegal drugs also may increase. Josiam and colleagues reported that approximately half of spring break vacationers were offered an illegal substance while traveling, but less than 5% admitted to trying the new drug.[33] Cigarette smoking doubled in a surveyed group of adolescent girls, and marijuana was smoked for the first time by some of the travelers.[3] Routine users of drugs admit to heightened drug use during spring break travel.[33]

Crime

The naive traveler who may be fatigued and overwhelmed in a new land is at risk for being a perpetrator and a victim of crime. Adolescent travelers may be more prone to frequent business establishments where crime is more likely to occur, such as nightclubs. If one ventures into unfamiliar and unsafe areas in the host country, the risk of becoming a victim of rape, thievery, assault and battery, or a terrorist attack is heightened.[30] Rape is not uncommon and 12% of polled female spring break travelers felt forced or pressured into engaging in sexual activity.[22] Popular spring break destinations such as Cancún, Mexico, and Daytona, FL, experience increased rates of crimes such as rape, assault, and arrests during the spring break time frame.[22]

Ignorance of the law is not a valid defense for committing a crime. More young men than women are arrested for crimes in other countries.[34] Narcotics and violence are often involved in the unlawful act. Possession of prescription medications, if not properly identified, may be a cause for legal woes in some foreign countries.

■ PRETRAVEL ADVICE

General

Providing pretravel advice (Box 12-4) reduces morbidity during travel in some instances.[29] Parents and the adolescent can be referred to helpful resources to ensure that all aspects of health care and travel preparations are considered before traveling from home.[27,35–38] Pretravel advice should focus on issues most likely to arise for the type of travel the adolescent will be taking. For instance, if adventure travel is planned, protection from environmental hazards should be emphasized. If study in Europe is planned, safety and responsible sexual and drinking habits should be emphasized. Student travelers are strongly urged to register their foreign travel with the US Department of State, which can contact the traveler or family if an emergency arises in the foreign land or at home.[39]

Box 12-4. Pretravel Advice

GENERAL
- Schedule pretravel appointment months in advance.
- Research the travel destination and proposed travel activities so specific potential health hazards are determined.
- Establish plans for potential health hazards that may arise.
- Invest in travel insurance, including evacuation insurance.
- Register travel plans with US Department of State.

ADOLESCENT WITH CHRONIC DISEASE
- Provide adolescent with strategies and information to control all aspects of daily living with chronic disease.
- Locate a physician in host country who may be called on if expertise is needed.
- Ensure adequate supply of maintenance and emergency medications.
- Provide brief review of pertinent medical records.

PREVENTION OF ACUTE INFECTIOUS DISEASE
- Ensure routine vaccinations required in United States are up-to-date.
- Receive location-specific vaccines.
- Determine need for malaria prophylaxis.
- Discuss proper hygiene practices for food consumption.

PREVENTION OF SEXUALLY TRANSMITTED INFECTIONS AND RELATED HEALTH HAZARDS
- Educate about acquisition and prevention of sexually transmitted infections.
- Encourage safe sex; provide condom samples.
- Provide adolescent with information about the link between alcohol and drug consumption, sexual activity, and date rape.

PREGNANCY PREVENTION
- Discuss proper use of emergency contraception and offer prescription.

PREVENTION OF TRAUMA/SUBSTANCE USE/CRIME-RELATED HEALTH HAZARDS
- Reinforce commonsense behavior and basic safety practices of routine seat belt and helmet use and obeying rules of the road.
- Discuss avoidance of driving, swimming alone, wild animals, excessive alcohol intake, illicit drug use, and potential crimes.
- Avoid walking or socializing alone or in areas with an unsafe reputation.
- Encourage discussion between adolescent and parent about emergency planning in the event of rape and other crimes.
- Remind patient that civil rights are not guaranteed outside the United States.
- Determine location of closest consulate (information available at US Department of State Bureau of Consular Affairs [www.travel.state.gov]).

The adolescent with a chronic illness, including psychiatric and physical disorders, is a special circumstance. Before independent travel can occur, the chronically ill adolescent must be in complete control of the disease (ie, knows the names and proper doses of all medications, is capable of administering medications, and has an emergency plan in place). The pediatrician can prescribe an adequate supply of emergency medications (eg, albuterol for asthma) and enough maintenance medications to last the entire trip. If several months of medication are required, perhaps a local physician should be found before travel in case a medical emergency arises or medical assistance is needed. The safest approach to traveling with medications is for the traveler to carry written information from her physician about the necessity of the prescription to avoid any legal consequences. A concise written review of the adolescent's chronic medical condition(s) should also be taken on the journey. Travel insurance, which covers evacuation, is strongly encouraged, as medical evacuation can cost tens of thousands of US dollars.[37]

Infectious Diseases

The need for vaccinations is the likely impetus for parents to seek pre-travel medical advice for their adolescent child. The ideal time for the pretravel clinic appointment is not known; if the clinic appointment is made too far in advance, pretravel counsel may be forgotten, but if made too late, there may not be enough time for adequate immunization and malaria prophylaxis. Two to 6 months in advance is a reasonable time frame so that some vaccine series will be complete before travel occurs and advice may be retained. For example, 2 hepatitis A vaccines administered 6 months apart is one particular dosing schedule. Even if a vaccine series cannot be completed before travel, some protection will be obtained from vaccine dosages already administered. As with any aged traveler, the destination will determine the need for certain vaccinations (eg, yellow fever vaccine for parts of Africa and South America), and the pediatrician should consult various resources, such as the Centers for Disease Control and Prevention, for the most up-to-date immunization recommendations. The adolescent should receive the full series of vaccines routinely recommended in the United States, including meningococcal, hepatitis A and B, human papillomavirus, and influenza. The meningococcal vaccine is particularly important for Hajj pilgrims or visitors to areas of outbreaks such as the sub-Saharan "meningitis belt"— a region stretching across mid-Africa from parts of Senegal to Ethiopia. Children with underlying immune deficiencies (terminal complement deficient or asplenic) are also at increased risk for meningococcal infection. Parents should ensure that their child receives 2 measles, mumps, and rubella vaccinations in their lifetime before travel because measles outbreaks occur worldwide.

A discussion about prevention of acute illness, infectious disease especially, and avoidance of environmental hazards should be part of pretravel advice. Hand washing is a major preventive measure for most respiratory and gastrointestinal disorders. Packing portable containers of liquid hand sanitizer is a practical tip. Hygienic eating practices are advocated for all travelers. Avoiding raw or undercooked food and drinking from local water supplies, especially in lower-income countries, is strongly recommended. The adolescent traveler should be warned that adherence to proper personal hygiene alone may not prevent traveler's diarrhea due to poor restaurant hygiene in most developing countries.[40]

If the adolescent develops diarrhea, maintaining proper hydration during acute illnesses should be encouraged. Supplying the adolescent with powdered electrolyte solution packets and the education to properly prepare the solutions with bottled water is advised. Empiric use of antibiotic prophylaxis for traveler's diarrhea is not routinely recommended in children, but adolescents may benefit from the administration of azithromycin or a fluoroquinolone if severe diarrhea develops.[41]

Malaria prevention will need to be addressed if the adolescent is traveling to tropical destinations or affected areas. Malaria prophylaxis recommendations will depend on the details of the travel agenda, especially the travel destinations. The specifics of the prescribed antimalarial chemoprophylaxis will depend on the presence of resistant strains along the journey's route. Compliance with chemoprophylaxis must be emphasized along with the implementation of steps to minimize mosquito contact and bites.[41] Mosquito avoidance is possible by wearing protective clothing, consistently applying insecticide, and using appropriate netting around bedding and windows.[41]

Sexual Hazards

Ideally parents should have already counseled their maturing child about sexual issues in everyday life[42]; if not, the potential consequences of reckless sexual behavior must be discussed openly and completely. Counseling should be individualized so that high-risk adolescents receive more warning about sexual hazards, but it should be kept in mind that traveling abroad can foster risky behavior in any adolescent who then engages in out-of-the ordinary activities.[23] Parents and children can be referred to sexual health resources[43] to become more knowledgeable about potentially life-altering and life-threatening STIs. Condoms and other birth control products should be made available to the traveling adolescent and consistent use of these products must be emphasized. In one report, taking condoms on the journey and reading information about STIs were predictors of practicing protected sex during travel.[44] Hepatitis B and HPV vaccination are especially important to the sexually active teen. Emergency contraception should be discussed with girls and perhaps a prescription provided so proper use can be discussed in the controlled setting of the familiar pediatrician's office.

Noninfectious Diseases

To avoid adverse environmental health effects, the adolescent should learn about the climate and potential hazards of the travel destination. Appropriate clothing and equipment should be brought on the journey. Avoiding wild animals and properly applying insect repellent will help deter bites. Soft-tissue injury is the main consequence of animal bites, but rabies may be a concern because it exists worldwide and is endemic to many areas, especially in South America. Aggressive application of sunscreen is a basic safety tenet to which an adolescent should adhere, especially if a tropical location is part of the journey. Adolescents should only participate in sporting events and adventure travel activities for which they are adequately trained. The importance of having experienced supervisors or guides present during adventure activities must be emphasized. Trying new hobbies, such as diving or snorkeling, may be very appealing to the young adult but should be discouraged if he received little or no training and consumed alcohol beforehand. The advantages of remaining well hydrated and well rested should be emphasized so the adolescent appreciates that staying healthy will improve the overall quality of his travel experience.

Trauma

Because death is more likely to occur secondary to an injury rather than an infectious disease or other illness, providing effective advice about accident prevention is especially important. Because MVAs occur frequently during travel, it is prudent to advise the adolescent against driving in the host country for legal and safety reasons. If available, the adolescent should use public transportation and avoid driving or being a passenger in a car with a driver who is unfamiliar with the roads. No one should swim or participate in water sports alone, and warning signs at beaches should be obeyed. The dangers of drinking alcohol or ingesting illicit drugs before driving or participating in sports cannot be overemphasized.

Substance Use

Because drug use can escalate while traveling, parents of a known drug user should strongly reconsider the decision to allow solo travel at all. Parents should also be aware of strong advertising campaigns that try to entice young travelers to venture to vacation spots with lenient alcohol laws. Alcohol and illicit substances may be readily available for consumption during a spring break vacation. Using educational brochures as the only tool to counsel about avoiding drug use is not effective in reducing this unwanted behavior; more aggressive counseling is needed for high-risk individuals.[45] References are available to help parents and pediatricians counsel adolescents about avoiding substance use[46] and other health-related issues.[47] Parents should seek educational programs that teach strategies to avoid consuming alcohol while on campus and traveling. Many college campuses are sponsoring student coalitions to promote healthier lifestyles in general and discourage excessive alcohol intake.[48]

Sharing practical information with the adolescent may deter drug use while she is traveling.[49] The adolescent should be warned that penalties for drug-related offenses in some areas of the world are much more severe than in the United States and may even include the death penalty. All young travelers should be encouraged to obey the laws of the host land, seek non–alcohol-focused activities, and use taxi or shuttle services from their lodging to establishments where alcohol may be consumed.[8]

Crime

Before traveling, the adolescent should know how to contact the closest US embassy or consulate if assistance in legal matters is needed. Basic safety practices, such as not walking alone at night or in unfamiliar or disreputable places, are an obvious part of crime deterrence. Public transportation and licensed taxi cabs should be the preferred mode of traveling around the host country, although adolescents should be warned that they may be targeted as crime victims at places of public transportation in foreign lands. Accepting food or drink from new acquaintances should be discouraged, especially because date rape drugs (eg, Rohypnol) can be unknowingly slipped into beverages.[27] Young women need to be warned that if rape occurs, authorities (ie, parents, local and US officials) must be informed and medical care sought. The possibility of contracting an STI and becoming pregnant must be addressed after a sexual assault. Self-administering emergency contraception does not address the legal, physical, and emotional consequences of rape.

The experience of being arrested while abroad can vary depending on the crime and country in which it was committed. Some crimes may involve very serious penalties compared with punishments administered in the United States. The right to legal counsel is not guaranteed in all lands. The young traveler should be reminded that participating in political demonstrations in foreign countries may have negative legal consequences, unlike in the United States. Using common sense and obeying local laws will protect the adolescent in most instances.

■ KEY POINTS

- Millions of American adolescents travel abroad every year, placing themselves at risk for travel-related morbidity.
- Travel-related issues that can adversely affect an adolescent's health include infectious and noninfectious diseases, sexual hazards, trauma, substance use, and crime.
- Pretravel advice should include information about each of the potential travel-related health issues, with emphasis on proper vaccination, sexual and substance use counseling, and safe and law-abiding behavior.
- Parents and adolescents should research travel destinations beforehand so hazards specific to the travel location and agenda can be anticipated.
- Emergency plans should be reviewed for potential crises that may arise during travel.
- Registering with the US Department of State and purchasing evacuation insurance should be strongly encouraged.

■ REFERENCES

1. Lenroot RK, Giedd JN. Brain development in children and adolescents: insights from anatomical magnetic resonance imaging. *Neurosci Biobehav Rev.* 2006;30(6):718–729
2. Grekin ER, Sher KJ, Krull JL. College spring break and alcohol use: effects of spring break activity. *J Stud Alcohol Drugs.* 2007;68(5):681–688
3. Schwartz RH, Milteer R, Sheridan MJ, et al. Beach week. A high school graduation rite of passage for sun, sand, suds, and sex. *Arch Pediatr Adolesc Med.* 1999;153:180–183
4. World Youth Student and Education Travel Confederation. Youth Tourism—The Travel Industry's Boom Sector. 2007. http://www.aboutwysetc.org/Docs/PR_UNWTOPartnership.pdf. Accessed January 22, 2009
5. US Department of Commerce, International Trade Administration, Manufacturing and Services, Office of Travel and Tourism Industries. *Profile of US Resident Travelers Visiting Overseas Destinations: 2007 Outbound.* Washington, DC
6. Holecek DF, Nicholls S, Collinson J. *Student and Youth Travel Research Institute. Characteristics, Scale and Economic Importance on Independent, Overnight Travel by 12 to 18-year-olds in the United States.* Lansing, MI: Michigan State University; 2008:1–19
7. Boffa E, Student Youth Travel Association. The Destination "Hot List" for Young Travelers. SYTA Announces Top 10 Most Popular Student Destinations. 2008. http://www.syta.org/uploads/StatResearch/Top%2010%20Destinations%20release%202008.pdf. Accessed December 16, 2008
8. Smeaton GL, Josiam BM, Dietrich UC. College students' binge drinking at a beachfront destination during spring break. *J Am Coll Health.* 1998;46(6):247–254
9. Klein JL, Millman GC. Prospective, hospital based study of fever in children in the United Kingdom who had recently spent time in the tropics. *BMJ.* 1998;316:1425–1426
10. Hill DR. Health problems in a large cohort of Americans traveling to developing countries. *J Travel Med.* 2000;7:259–266

11. Riordan FA, Tarlow MJ. Imported infections in East Birmingham children. *Postgrad Med J.* 1998;74:36–37

12. O'Brien D, Tobin S, Brown GV, et al. Fever in returned travelers: review of hospitalized admissions for a 3 year period. *Clin Infect Dis.* 2001;33:603–609

13. Centers for Disease Control and Prevention. Outbreak of acute respiratory febrile illness among college students—Acapulco, Mexico, March 2001. *MMWR.* 2001;50(14):261–262

14. Steffen R, Tornieporth N, Clemens SA, et al. Epidemiology of travelers' diarrhea: details of a global survey. *J Travel Med.* 2004;11: 231–237

15. Centers for Disease Control and Prevention. Update: Measles—United States, January–July 2008. *MMWR.* 2008;57(33):893–896

16. Connor BA, Jacobs RJ, Meyerhoff AS. Hepatitis B risks and immunization coverage among American Travelers. *J Travel Med.* 2006;13(5):273–280

17. Zuckerman JN, Hoet B. Hepatitis B immunization in travelers: poor risk perception and inadequate protection. *Travel Med Infect Dis.* 2008;6(5):315–320

18. Forbes GB. College students with tattoos and piercings: motives, family experiences, personality factors, and perception by others. *Psychol Rep.* 2001;89(3):774–786

19. Cegolon L, Miatto E, Bartolotto M, Benetton M, Mazzeoleni F, Mastrangelo G, VAHP Working Group. Body piercing and tattoo: awareness of health related risks among 4, 277 Italian secondary school adolescents. *BMC Public Health.* 2010;10:73

20. Shah AP, Smolensky M, Burau KD, et al. Recent change in the annual pattern of sexually transmitted diseases in the United States. *Chronobiology Internation.* 2007;24:947–960

21. Matteelli A, Carosi G. Sexually transmitted diseases in travelers. *Clin Infect Dis.* 2001;32:1063–1067

22. American Medical Association. Sex and intoxication among women more common on spring break according to AMA poll. http://www.ama-assn.org/ama/pub/category/print/16083.html. Accessed January 20, 2009

23. Gagneux OP, Blochliger CU, Tanner M, et al. Malaria and casual sex: what travelers know and how they behave. *J Travel Med.* 1996;3:14–21

24. Apostolopoulos Y, Sonmez S, Yu CH. HIV-risk behaviours of American spring break vaccinationers: a case of situational disinhibition. *Int J STD AIDS.* 2002;13:733–743

25. Futterman DC. HIV and AIDS in adolescents. *Adolesc Med Clin.* 2004;15:369–391

26. Richens J. Sexually transmitted infections and HIV among travelers: a review. *Travel Med Infect Dis.* 2006;4(3-4):184–195

27. Nield LS. Advising the adolescent traveler. *Clin Fam Pract.* 2005;7(4):761–772

28. Jafarian S, Gorouhi F, Ghergherechi M, Lotfi J. Respiratory rate within the first hour of ascent predicts subsequent acute mountain sickness severity. *Arch Iranian Med.* 2008;11(2):152–156

29. Boggild AK, Costiniuk C, Kain KC, et al. Environmental hazards in Nepal: altitude illness, environmental exposures, injuries, and bites in travelers and expatriates. *J Travel Med.* 2007;14:361–368

30. Spira AM. Preventive guidance for travel: trauma avoidance and medical evacuation. *Dis Mon.* 2006;52:261–288

31. Guse CE, Cortes LM, Hargarten SW, et al. Fatal injuries of US citizens abroad. *J Travel Med.* 2007;14(5):279–287

32. Lee CM, Maggs JL, Rankin LA. Spring break trips as a risk factor for heavy alcohol use among first-year college students. *J Stud Alcohol.* 2006;67(6):911–916

33. Josiam BM, Hobson JSP, Dietrick U, et al. An analysis of the sexual, alcohol and drug related behavioral patterns of students on spring break. *Tourism Manage.* 1998;19:501–513

34. MacPherson DW, Gushulak BD, Sandhu J. Arrest and detention in international travelers. *Travel Med Infect Dis.* 2007;5(4):217–222

35. Breuner CC. The adolescent traveler. *Prim Care.* 2002;29(4):983–1006

36. Centers for Disease Control and Prevention. Travelers' health. http://wwwn.cdc.gov/travel/default.aspx. Accessed January 12, 2009

37. US Department of State. Students abroad. http://studentsabroad.state.gov. Accessed January 12, 2009

38. American Medical Association. Discussing spring break. Top ten things to discuss with your college student before spring break. http://www. ama-assn.org/ama/pub/category/9914.html. Accessed January 20, 2009

39. US Department of State. https://travelregistration.state.gov

40. Shlim DR. Looking for evidence that personal hygiene precautions prevent traveler's diarrhea. *Clin Infect Dis.* 2005;41(Suppl 8):S531–S535

41. Immunization in special circumstances. In: Pickering LK, Baker CJ, Long SS, McMillan JA, eds. *Red Book: 2006 Report of the Committee on Infectious Diseases.* 27th ed. Elk Grove Village, IL: American Academy of Pediatrics; 2006:67–103

42. Thornton AC, Collins JD. Teaching parents to talk to their children about sexual topics. *Clin Fam Pract.* 2004;6:801–819

43. von Sadovszky V. Preventing women's sexual risk behaviors during travel. *JOGNN.* 2008;37:516–524

44. Croughs M, Van Gompel A, de Boer E, et al. Sexual risk behavior of travelers who consulted a pretravel clinic. *J Travel Med.* 2008;15(1):6–12

45. Paz A, Sadetzki S, Potasman I. High rates of substance abuse among long-term travelers to the tropics. *J Travel Med.* 2004;11:75–81

46. Kodjo CM, Klein JD. Prevention and risk of adolescent substance abuse: the role of the adolescent, families and communities. *Pediatr Clin North Am.* 2002;49:257–268

47. Cottrell LA, Nield LS, Perkins KC. Effective interviewing and counseling of the adolescent patient. *Pediatric Annals.* 2006;35(3):164–172

48. American Medical Association. A matter of degree. The national effort to reduce high-risk drinking among college students. http://www.ama-assn.org/ama/pub/category/3558.html. Accessed January 20, 2009

49. Sanford C. Urban medicine: threats to health travelers to developing world cities. *J Travel Med.* 2004;11:313–327

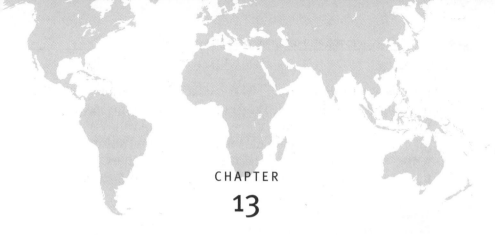

Immunization for Travelers

Chokechai Rongkavilit, MD

■ PRACTICAL GUIDE FOR IMMUNIZING TRAVELERS

Most international travelers need a combination of routine immunizations and special required travel immunizations. Certain population groups may be lacking routine immunizations (eg, hepatitis B, tetanus, varicella, influenza) while preparing for international travel. These groups should be updated with these immunizations. The completion of a full immunization schedule is important to protect against vaccine-preventable diseases and to avoid receiving medical care in a country in which the level of care may be insufficient. The following guidelines are designed to help health care professionals determine and provide appropriate immunizations for travelers:

1. *Review the traveler's itinerary.* The health care professional must be aware that the traveler's particular destination within a country and the nature and duration of the stay are important factors in determining immunization needs. For example, a volunteer planning to spend 3 months working in a rural village may need a different immunization than a businessman planning to spend 5 days in an urban area of the same country.

2. *Determine the traveler's medical status.* The health care professional should assess the medical history, physical examination, laboratory testing, and review of medical records as indicated to determine medical stability. At times it may be prudent to advise against international travel based on the traveler's medical condition.

3. *Determine immunizations that will be needed.* All routine immunizations should be reviewed and updated. The need for special international travel immunizations should be based on current information about international immunizations and disease patterns. One source of country-specific information is the Centers for Disease Control and Prevention (CDC) *Health Information for International Travel* (also known as the Yellow Book) and the CDC Travelers' Health Web site (www.cdc.gov/travel).

4. *Determine entry requirements.* When itineraries involve travel to Africa or South America, health care professionals should check up-to-date resources for yellow fever status and immunization entry requirements of these countries, as well as all countries that the traveler will subsequently visit. This is important because yellow fever vaccination is a regulated international immunization. When itineraries include travel to Saudi Arabia for purposes of participation in the annual Hajj, check up-to-date resources for special immunization requirements, as in recent years meningococcal immunization has been required.

5. *Complete the international immunization schedule.* Several factors complicate this evaluation.
   a. Number of required or recommended immunizations and their particular schedules
   b. Length of time until departure
   c. Compatibility of certain immunizations with other immunizations, antibiotics, and antimalarials
   d. Traveler's health status, including allergies
   e. Traveler's interest and personal or financial concerns

6. *Educate and inform the traveler about the immunization to be administered.*

7. *Immunize the traveler.*

8. *Record administered vaccines in the traveler's medical record.*

9. *Complete the International Certificate of Vaccination or Prophylaxis (ICVP).*

10. *Complete a letter if needed.* The letter, which may contain items such as exemption from yellow fever, justification of medications, and justification to carry sterile needles and syringes, may accompany travelers.

■ INTERNATIONAL CERTIFICATE OF VACCINATION OR PROPHYLAXIS

To prevent importation and indigenous transmission of yellow fever, the International Health Regulations allow a number of countries to require a certificate of vaccination or ICVP from travelers arriving from endemic areas, even if only in transit.[1] Travelers arriving without a completed ICVP may be quarantined or refused entry unless they submit to on-site vaccination. Such requirements may be strictly enforced, particularly for persons traveling from Africa or South America to Asia. Some countries in Africa require evidence of vaccination from all entering travelers; others may waive the requirements for travelers coming from non-endemic areas who are staying in the country fewer than 2 weeks.

For purposes of international travel, yellow fever vaccine produced by different manufacturers worldwide must be approved by the World Health Organization (WHO) and administered at a certified center in possession of an official Uniform Stamp that can be used to validate the ICVP. State health departments are responsible for designating non-federal yellow fever vaccination centers and issuing Uniform Stamps to health care professionals. The ICVP must be validated by the center that administers the vaccine.

Most city, county, and state health department immunization or travel clinics, as well as private travel clinics or individual health care professionals, are designated sites. Information about the location and hours of yellow fever vaccination centers may be obtained by contacting local or state health departments or visiting the CDC's Travelers' Health Web site (www.cdc.gov/travel). Vaccinees should receive a completed ICVP, signed and validated with the stamp of the center where the vaccine was administered. Only the most recent ICVP (form CDC 731) complies with 2005 International Health Regulations and should be used for any vaccine administered on or after December 15, 2007. Previously issued certificates remain acceptable proof of vaccination against yellow fever as long as the certificate is valid. This certificate is valid 10 days after vaccination and for a subsequent period of 10 years. The ICVP should be kept with the traveler's passport. Failure to secure validations can cause a traveler to be revaccinated, quarantined, or denied entry.

Some countries do not require an ICVP for infants younger than 6 or 9 months or 1 year. Travelers should be advised to check the individual country's requirements through the embassies or consulates or the CDC Travelers' Health Web site (www.cdc.gov/travel). If a physician concludes that a yellow fever vaccine should not be administered for medical reasons only, the traveler should be given a signed-and-dated exemption letter on the physician's letterhead stating that contraindication to vaccination is acceptable to certain governments outside the United States. Ideally, the letter should be written on letterhead and bear the stamp used by the health department and official vaccination centers to validate the ICVP.

When planning to use a waiver letter, the traveler should also obtain specific and authoritative advice from the embassy or consulate of the country or countries she plans to visit. Waivers of requirements obtained from embassies or consulates should be documented by appropriate letters and retained for presentation with the ICVP. Reasons other than medical contraindications are not acceptable for exemption from vaccination. The traveler should be advised that issuance of a waiver does not guarantee that the destination country will accept it; on arrival at the destination the traveler may be faced with quarantine, refusal of entry, or vaccination on site.

■ SPECIAL IMMUNIZATION

Hepatitis A Vaccines

General Information About Hepatitis A Infection

Hepatitis A virus is distributed worldwide, although the prevalence of infection varies considerably on the basis of hygiene and sanitation conditions. In areas with overcrowding, limited access to clean water, and inadequate sewage systems, hepatitis A infection occurs almost universally in people early in life. Because most young children who acquire hepatitis A are asymptomatic, disease rates in highly endemic areas of the world are low. Hepatitis A is rarely fatal in children and young adults; however, the case-fatality rate exceeds 2% among those older than 40 years and may be 4% for those aged 60 years or older. Although seronegative adults in such areas of the world are at high risk of infection and disease, outbreaks are unusual because of the high prevalence of antibody to hepatitis A virus in the population.[2]

The primary source for hepatitis A transmission is person to person through the fecal-oral route. On rare occasions, hepatitis A infection is transmitted by transfusion of blood or blood products collected from donors during the viremic phase of infection.[3] Since 2002, nucleic acid amplification tests, such as the polymerase chain reaction (PCR) assay, have been applied to the screening of source plasma used for the manufacture of plasma-derived products.[4]

Transmission is generally limited to close contacts, and hepatitis A is rarely spread by casual interactions. Transmission of hepatitis A within families is common. Hepatitis A can be acquired through exposure to contaminated water, ice, or shellfish harvested from sewage-contaminated water, or from fruits, vegetables, or other foods that are eaten raw and that were contaminated during harvesting or subsequent handling by an infected food handler. Stools from a hepatitis A virus–infected person are most infectious from approximately 14 to 21 days before to approximately 8 days after the onset of jaundice.[5] Hepatitis A RNA has been reported to be detectable in stool by PCR assay for up to 3 months after the acute illness[6]; children can shed hepatitis A for up to 10 weeks after the onset of clinical illness.[6]

The incubation period for hepatitis A averages 28 days (with a range of 15 to 50 days). Hepatitis A typically has an abrupt onset of symptoms that can include fever, malaise, anorexia, nausea, abdominal discomfort, dark urine, and jaundice. The likelihood of having symptoms with the hepatitis A virus is related to the infected person's age. In children younger than 6 years, most infections (70%) are asymptomatic; if illness does occur, its duration is usually less than 2 months. Although the hepatitis A virus is not excreted chronically, clinical relapses may occur in 10% to 15% of patients over a 6- to 9-month period and may be associated with recurring excretion of the virus in stool.[7]

Hepatitis A is the most important vaccine-preventable disease for travelers. The risk of hepatitis A is 4 to 30 cases per 100,000 months of stay in an area with endemic hepatitis A for travelers who are not immunized against hepatitis A.[8] In 2003, international travel was the source of hepatitis A for more than 25% of cases among children younger than 15 years. The vaccine should be considered for all travelers to areas with moderate to high risk of infection, and those at high risk of acquiring the disease should be strongly encouraged to be vaccinated regardless of where they travel. Spread of hepatitis A virus in child care settings has occurred from exposure to children who acquired the virus after visiting countries of their parent's birth.

Vaccine Information

The US Advisory Committee on Immunization Practices (ACIP) recommends routine hepatitis A immunization in all children between the ages of 12 and 23 months.[9] Two monovalent hepatitis A vaccines, Havrix and Vaqta, are currently licensed in the United States for persons at least 12 months of age. Both vaccines are safe and highly effective. Both are made of an inactivated hepatitis A virus adsorbed to aluminum hydroxide as an adjuvant. Havrix is prepared with 2-phenoxyethanol as a preservative, while Vaqta is formulated without a preservative. Both vaccines are available in 2 formulations based on the patient's age. Twinrix is a combined hepatitis A and hepatitis B vaccine licensed for persons older than 18 years, containing 720 enzyme-linked immunosorbent assay (ELISA) units of hepatitis A antigen (50% of the Havrix adult dose) and 20 μg of recombinant hepatitis B surface antigen protein (the same as the Engerix-B adult dose).

The different vaccine formulations are similarly immunogenic when given in their respective recommended schedules and doses. One dose of Havrix induced seroconversion by 15 days in 80% to 98% of children, adolescents, and adults and by 1 month in 96% to 100%. One month after a second dose, which was administered 6 months after the first dose, 100% of the children, adolescents, and adults had protective serum antibody concentrations with high geometric mean titers. One dose of Vaqta induced seroconversion in 69% of adults 2 weeks after the first dose. One month after the first dose of Vaqta, 94% to 97% of children, adolescents, and adults had seroconverted. One month after a second dose, which was administered 6 months after the first dose, 100% had seroconverted. The protective antibody response following primary vaccination in adults and children persists for more than 10 years.[10,11] Results from mathematic models indicate that after completion of the primary series, anti-hepatitis A antibodies probably persist for 25 years or more.[12] Booster doses are not recommended. Given the long incubation period of hepatitis A (average 2 to 4 weeks), the vaccine is recommended for healthy international travelers aged 40 years or younger regardless of their scheduled dates for departure.[13] The use of immunoglobulin is now virtually obsolete for the purposes of travel prophylaxis.

Indications for Vaccination

Besides routine immunization for all children 1 year of age (ie, 12 to 23 months), unvaccinated children between 2 and 18 years can be vaccinated at subsequent visits as part of catch-up vaccination. In addition, hepatitis A vaccination is recommended for adolescent and adult males who have sex with men, users of injection and non-injection illicit drugs, persons who work with hepatitis A–infected primates or with hepatitis A virus in a research laboratory, persons with clotting-factor disorders, and persons with chronic liver disease.[9]

Persons traveling to countries that have high or intermediate hepatitis A endemicity, including Central and South America, Africa, and most of Asia and Eastern Europe, should be vaccinated before departure. The risk of hepatitis A for persons traveling to certain areas of the Caribbean is unknown, although vaccination should be considered if travel is anticipated to areas with questionable sanitation.

Administration

All hepatitis A vaccines should be administered intramuscularly in the deltoid muscle.[9] The immunization schedule is shown in Table 13-1. Havrix and Vaqta are given in 2 doses. Twinrix requires 3 or 4 doses. The Food and Drug Administration (FDA) approved an accelerated schedule of Twinrix (ie, doses at days 0, 7, and 21) for travelers, with a booster dose to be given at 1 year. Given the long incubation period of hepatitis A (average 2 to 4 weeks), the vaccine can be administered up to the day of departure and still protect travelers.[13]

Side Effects

Adverse reactions are mild and include local pain and, less commonly, induration at the injection site. No serious adverse events attributed definitively to hepatitis A vaccine have been reported.

Table 13-1. Recommended Doses and Schedules for Inactivated Hepatitis A Vaccines[a]

AGE	VACCINE	HEPATITIS A ANTIGEN DOSE	VOLUME PER DOSE, ML	NO. OF DOSES	SCHEDULE
12 mo through 18 y	Havrix	720 ELISA units	0.5	2	Initial and 6 to 12 mo later
12 mo through 18 y	Vaqta	25 antigen units[b]	0.5	2	Initial and 6 to 18 mo later
19 y or older	Havrix	1,440 ELISA units	1.0	2	Initial and 6 to 12 mo later
19 y or older	Vaqta	50 antigen units[b]	1.0	2	Initial and 6 to 18 mo later
18 y or older	Twinrix[c]	720 ELISA units	1.0	3 or 4	Initial and 1 and 6 mo later **OR** Initial, 7, and 21 to 30 days, followed by a dose at 12 mo

Abbreviation: ELISA, enzyme-linked immunosorbent assay.

[a]Havrix and Twinrix are manufactured by GlaxoSmithKline Biologicals; Vaqta is manufactured and distributed by Merck & Co, Inc.
[b]Each unit is equivalent to approximately 1 μg of viral protein.
[c]A combination of hepatitis B (Engerix-B, 20 μg) and hepatitis A (Havrix, 720 ELISA units) vaccine (Twinrix) is licensed for use in people 18 years and older in 3- and 4-dose schedules.

Adapted from American Academy of Pediatrics. *Red Book: 2009 Report of the Committee on Infectious Diseases.* Pickering LK, Baker CJ, Kimberlin DW, Long SS, eds. 28th ed. Elk Grove Village, IL: American Academy of Pediatrics; 2009:332

Precautions and Contraindications

The vaccine should not be administered to people with hypersensitivity to any of the vaccine components. Safety data in pregnant women are not available, but the risk is considered to be low or nonexistent because the vaccine contains inactivated, purified, viral proteins. Limited data indicate that hepatitis A vaccine may be administered simultaneously with other vaccines. Vaccines should be given in a separate syringe and at a separate injection site. The immune response in immunocompromised people, including people with HIV infection, may be suboptimal.

Special Considerations

Vaqta and Havrix, when given as recommended, seem to be similarly effective. Studies among adults have found no difference in the immunogenicity of a vaccine series that mixed the 2 currently available vaccines, compared with using the same vaccine throughout the licensed schedule. Therefore, although completion of the immunization regimen with the same product is preferable, immunization with either product is acceptable.

Preimmunization testing for anti-hepatitis A antibodies generally is not recommended for children. Testing may be cost-effective for people who have a high likelihood of immunity from previous infection, including people whose childhood was spent in an area of high endemicity, people with a history of jaundice potentially caused by hepatitis A, and people older than 50 years. Post-immunization testing for anti-hepatitis A antibodies is not indicated because of the high seroconversion rates in adults and children. In addition, some commercially available anti-hepatitis A antibody tests may not detect low but protective concentrations of antibody induced by the first dose of vaccine.

For optimal protection, adults older than 40 years, immunocompromised persons, and persons with chronic liver disease or other chronic medical conditions planning to travel to an area in less than 2 weeks should receive the initial dose of vaccine along with immunoglobulin (0.02 mL/kg intramuscularly) at a separate anatomic injection site.[13] Travelers who are younger than 12 months, are allergic to a vaccine component, or otherwise elect not to receive vaccine should receive a single dose of immunoglobulin (0.02 mL/kg), which provides effective protection against hepatitis A for up to 3 months. Those who do not receive vaccination and plan to travel for longer than 3 months should receive an immunoglobulin dose of 0.06 mL/kg, which must be repeated if the duration of travel is longer than 5 months. Some experts recommend that hepatitis A vaccine be considered in children younger than

12 months when the benefits are deemed to be greater when the risk of exposure to the pathogen is high.[14]

Japanese Encephalitis Vaccine

General Information About the Disease

Japanese encephalitis (JE) is a considerable public health problem in most Asian regions but particularly in South Asia, Southeast Asia, East Asia, and the Pacific. The disease can cause irreversible neurologic damage. The JE virus is mainly transmitted by the mosquito *Culex tritaeniorhynchus,* which prefers to breed in irrigated rice paddies. This mosquito species and members of the *C gelidus* complex are zoophilic. Wading ardeid waterbirds (eg, herons, egrets) serve as virus reservoirs, but the virus regularly spills over into pigs, members of the *Equidae* family (eg, horses, donkeys), and humans. Japanese encephalitis is often confused with other forms of encephalitis. Differential diagnosis should therefore include other encephalitides (eg, conditions caused by other arboviruses and herpesviruses) and infections that involve the central nervous system (eg, bacterial meningitis, tuberculosis, cerebral malaria).

Because infected pigs act as amplifying hosts, domestic pig rearing is an important risk factor in the transmission to humans. Two distinct epidemiologic patterns of JE have been described. In temperate zones, such as the northern part of the Korean peninsula, Japan, China, Nepal, and northern India, large epidemics occur in the summer months; in tropical areas of southern Vietnam, southern Thailand, Indonesia, Malaysia, the Philippines, and Sri Lanka, cases occur more sporadically and peaks are usually observed during the rainy season.

Vaccine Information

An inactivated mouse brain (MB)-derived vaccine, JE-MB, the only vaccine licensed for use in children in the United States, is no longer available. Currently, the only vaccine available in the United States is the inactivated Vero cell culture–derived vaccine (Ixiaro [JE-VC]).[15] This vaccine is derived from the attenuated SA14-14-2 virus strain propagated in Vero cells. The vaccine is approved only for use in persons aged 17 years or older. It should be given as 2 doses (0.5 mL each) subcutaneously 28 days apart. The product does not include gelatin stabilizers, antibiotics, or thimerosal. Protective immune response was demonstrated in 97% of recipients after 2 doses, and the protective antibodies can be detected as early as 7 days after receiving the second dose of the vaccine. Up to 80% of recipients have the protective antibodies up to 12 months after vaccination.

Because JE-VC vaccine is not approved for children younger than 17 years, the options for vaccination against JE for pediatric travelers are limited. These options include (1) enroll in the ongoing JE-VC pediatric clinical trial at one of the US study sites; (2) administer JE-VC vaccine off-label using the study dosage (regular adult dose for children 3 years and older and half adult dose for children aged 2 months through 2 years); or (3) refer children to an international travelers' health clinic in Asia to receive the vaccine. Licensed JE vaccine available in Asia include a JE-MB vaccine manufactured in South Korea, an inactivated JE-VC vaccine manufactured in Japan, and a live-attenuated SA 14-14-2 vaccine manufactured in China. Each of these vaccines is licensed for routine pediatric use in several Asian countries.[16]

Considering the current existence of safe and effective JE vaccines at a relatively low cost for wide-scale use globally, the WHO continues to advise the integration of the JE vaccine (JE-MB or a live, attenuated vaccine) into the WHO immunization initiative in regions where this disease constitutes a public health risk.[17]

Indications for Vaccination

For most travelers to Asia, the risk for JE is very low; therefore, JE vaccine is not routinely recommended for all travelers to Asia.[18] In general, vaccine should be offered to persons spending a month or longer in endemic areas during the transmission season, especially if travel will include rural areas. Under specific circumstances, vaccine should be considered for persons spending less than 30 days in endemic areas (ie, areas experiencing epidemic transmission) and persons whose activities, such as extensive outdoor activities in rural areas, place them at high risk for exposure. In all instances, travelers should be advised to take personal precautions (eg, reduce exposure to mosquito bites). The decision to use JE vaccine should balance the risks for exposure to the virus and for developing illness, the availability and acceptability of repellents and other alternative protective measures, and the side effects of vaccination. Risk assessments should be interpreted cautiously because risk can vary within geographic areas and from year to year and because available data are incomplete. Estimates suggest that risk of JE in highly endemic areas during the transmission season can reach 1 per 5,000 per month of exposure; risk for most short-term travelers may be 1 per million.

Side Effects

Although JE-MB vaccine is reactogenic, rates of serious allergic reactions (generalized urticaria or angioedema) are low (1 to 104 per 10,000). The neural tissue substrate of the vaccine raised concerns about the possibility of vaccine-related neurologic side effects.[19] One case of Guillain-Barré Syndrome (GBS) temporally related to JE vaccination was reported; however, a causal relation between JE-MB vaccination and temporally related neurologic events has not been established. Local and systemic adverse events caused by JE-VC are similar to those reported for JE-MB or placebo adjuvant alone. No serious hypersensitivity reactions or neurologic adverse events were identified among JE-VC recipients in clinical trials. Additional post-licensure studies and monitoring of surveillance data are ongoing to evaluate the safety of JE-VC in a larger population.

Precautions and Contraindications

Vaccine recipients should be observed for a minimum of 30 minutes after immunization and warned about the possibility of delayed allergic reactions. The full course of immunization should be completed at least 10 days before departure. Vaccinees should be advised to remain in areas with access to medical care.

A history of allergy or hypersensitivity reaction to a previous dose of JE-MB vaccine is a contraindication to receiving additional doses. Persons with multiple allergies or a history of urticaria or angioedema for any reason may be at higher risk for allergic complications from this vaccine. This history should be considered when weighing the risks and benefits of the vaccine for an individual patient.

Special Considerations

No specific information is available on the safety of JE vaccine in pregnancy. Therefore, the vaccine should not be routinely administered during pregnancy. Japanese encephalitis acquired during pregnancy carries the potential for intrauterine infection and fetal death. Pregnant women who must travel to an area where risk of JE is high should be vaccinated when the theoretical risk of immunization is outweighed by the risk of infection.

Meningococcal Vaccines

General Information About Meningococcal Disease

Meningococcal disease is characterized by sudden onset of fever, intense headache, nausea, vomiting, stiff neck, and a rash with pink macules that develops petechiae. The case-fatality ratio may exceed 50%, but early diagnosis and treatment can lower the fatality rate to about 10%. Long-term sequelae among survivors include hearing loss, neurologic disability, or limb loss.[20] Up to 10% of populations in endemic countries carry *Neisseria meningitidis* asymptomatically in the nose and throat.[21]

Five major meningococcal serogroups associated with the disease are A, B, C, Y, and W-135.[22] Meningococci serogroups B and C are responsible for most disease in the Americas and Europe.[21,22] During the past years, serogroup Y emerged as a cause of disease in northern America. Serogroup A meningococci and, to a lesser extent, serogroup C account for most meningococcal disease cases in Africa and some areas in Asia. Serogroup W-135 has been associated with meningococcal disease epidemics in Saudi Arabia and Burkina Faso.[23,24]

Sporadic cases and outbreaks of meningococcal disease occur throughout the world. In the sub-Saharan African "meningitis belt," which stretches from Senegal in the west to Ethiopia in the east, peaks of serogroup A meningococcal disease occur regularly during the dry season (December through June).[25] In addition, major epidemics occur every 8 to 12 years. Travelers to sub-Saharan Africa may be at risk for meningococcal disease. Travelers to the meningitis belt during the dry season should be advised to receive meningococcal vaccine, especially if they will have prolonged contact with local populations. A serogroup W-135 epidemic occurred in Saudi Arabia in association with the Hajj pilgrimage.[23]

Vaccine Information

There are 2 meningococcal vaccines currently available, a tetravalent meningococcal polysaccharide vaccine (MPV4) and a tetravalent meningococcal polysaccharide-protein conjugate vaccine. Both protect against serogroups A, C, Y, and W-135. However, the conjugate vaccine is expected to be efficacious in young children, confer long-term protection, and provide herd immunity by reducing nasopharyngeal carriage and transmission.

Tetravalent Meningococcal Polysaccharide Vaccine

The antibody responses to each of the 4 polysaccharides in the tetravalent vaccine are serogroup specific and independent. The serogroup A polysaccharide induces antibody response among children as young as 3 months, although a response comparable to adults is not achieved until age 4 to 5 years; the serogroup C component is poorly immunogenic among young children.[26,27] The serogroups A and C vaccines show clinical efficacies of at least 85% among school-aged children and adults.[28-30] Serogroups Y and W-135 polysaccharides are safe and immunogenic among adults and children older than 2 years, although clinical protection has not been documented.[31] Measurable levels of antibodies against serogroup A and C polysaccharides decrease substantially during the first 3 years after a single dose of vaccine in children younger than 5 years. Among adults, antibody levels also decrease but are still detectable 10 years after vaccination.[32]

Tetravalent Meningococcal Conjugate Vaccine

There are currently 2 licensed tetravalent meningococcal conjugate vaccines, Menactra and Menveo. Menactra was found to not be inferior to MPV4 in terms of immunogenicity and safety. Two randomized, controlled trials conducted among persons 11 to 18 and 18 to 55 years of age compared immunogenicity of Menactra with MPV4. The percentages of subjects achieving at least a 4-fold rise in serum bactericidal antibody (SBA) titers were similar in Menactra and MPV4 groups. The percentage of subjects with at least a 4-fold rise in SBA was highest for serogroup W-135 and lowest for serogroup Y in both groups. The percentage of subjects achieving an SBA geometric mean titer of 128 or greater was high (greater than 97% for all serogroups) in both groups.[20,33]

The second tetravalent meningococcal conjugate vaccine (Menveo) was licensed in 2010. The capsular polysaccharide serogroups included in Menveo are the same as those contained in Menactra. The seroresponse to Menveo was found to be non-inferior to Menactra for all 4 serogroups.[34]

Indications for Vaccination

Tetravalent meningococcal polysaccharide-protein conjugate vaccine (Menactra and Menveo) is routinely recommended for all US children 11 to 18 years of age, including those at additional risk. Both are recommended for use in at-risk persons aged 11 to 55 years. Menactra can be used for at-risk children aged 2 to 10 years.[35] MPV4 can be used for at-risk persons older than 55 years. These at-risk groups include travelers to or residents of countries in which meningococcal disease is hyperendemic or epidemic, college freshmen living in dormitories, microbiologists who are routinely exposed to isolates of N meningitidis, military recruits, those with terminal complement component or properdin deficiencies, and those with anatomic or functional asplenia. Additionally, Menactra is preferred to MPV4 among children 2 to 10 years of age for control of meningococcal disease outbreaks. Providers may elect to vaccinate children aged 2 to 10 years who are infected with HIV. Persons aged 2 to 55 years who continue to be at risk for meningococcal infection, despite having been vaccinated with MPV4 three or more years earlier, are also candidates for revaccination with a meningococcal conjugate vaccine. The FDA has not approved the conjugate vaccines for use in children younger then 2 years or adults older then 55 years.

Vaccination is especially recommended for travelers visiting the parts of sub-Saharan Africa known as the meningitis belt during the dry season (December through June). Vaccination is required by the government of Saudi Arabia for all travelers to Mecca during the annual Hajj. Saudi Arabia requires that Hajj and Umrah visitors have a certificate of vaccination with a tetravalent (A, C, Y, W-135) meningococcal vaccine before entering the country. Advisories for travelers to other countries will be issued when epidemics of meningococcal disease caused by vaccine-preventable serogroups are detected; such information is available from international health clinics for travelers and state health departments or from the CDC Travelers' Health Web site, www.cdc.gov/travel.

Administration

A 0.5-mL dose of MPV4 contains 50 µg each of the 4 (A, C, Y, W-135) purified capsular polysaccharides. A 0.5-mL dose of Menactra contains 4 µg each of the 4 capsular polysaccharides conjugated to 48 µg of diphtheria toxoid. A 0.5-mL dose of Menveo contains 10 µg of serogroup A capular polysacharide and 5 µg each of the other 3 (C, Y, W-135) capsular polysaccharides conjugated to CRM197 diphtheria protein. Tetravalent meningococcal polysaccharide vaccine (MPV4) should be given subcutaneously. Tetravalent meningococcal polysaccharide-protein conjugate vaccine (Menactra and Menveo) should be given intramuscularly.[36]

Side Effects

Adverse reactions to meningococcal vaccines are usually mild; the most frequent reaction is pain and redness at the injection site, lasting for 1 to 2 days. Transient fever occurred among 5% or fewer of persons vaccinated, more commonly among infants. Allergic reactions (eg, urticaria, wheezing, rash) are rare. Anaphylaxis has been documented among fewer than 0.1 per 100,000 vaccine recipients. Neurologic reactions (eg, seizures, anesthesias, paresthesias) have also been reported infrequently.

Precautions and Contraindications

In 2005, reports suggested a possible association of GBS with Menactra, and ACIP recommended that persons with a past history of GBS not be vaccinated with Menactra unless they are at high risk for meningococcal disease.[37] Data are not available to evaluate the potential risk of

GBS following administration of Menveo. Tetravalent meningococcal polysaccharide vaccine is an acceptable short-term alternative for those with GBS.

Administration of Menactra, Menveo, or MPV4 is contraindicated among persons known to have a severe allergic reaction to any component of the vaccine, including diphtheria toxoid, or to natural latex rubber. Tetravalent meningococcal polysaccharide-protein conjugate vaccine and MPV4 are inactivated vaccines and may be given to immunosuppressed persons, but this may result in suboptimal immune response. No data are available about safety during pregnancy.

Rabies

General Information About the Disease

Rabies is still a serious public health threat in developing countries. More than 95% of human infections are of canine origin, mainly in Asia and Africa, in areas where dog rabies is endemic and inadequately controlled. Canine rabies virus infection remains 100% fatal among human beings. Given the increasing amount of international travel, the risk of rabies exposure remains an important public health issue worldwide. Furthermore, the potential for exposure to the virus in lower-income countries still exists via wild animals, including bats, foxes, raccoons, and skunks.[37]

Human rabies encephalitis can take 2 clinical forms: furious or agitated rabies and dumb or paralytic rabies. The latter is almost always seen in the victims of bat-transmitted rabies in the Americas, of vampire and insectivorous bat origin. Dog-transmitted virus may also cause paralytic rabies. The clinical manifestation may begin with nonspecific prodromal symptoms such as malaise, fever, and anorexia and specific local symptoms such as itchiness, pain, and paresthesia around the healed bite wound. This is followed by the acute neurologic phase with intense anxiety, agitation, confusion, high fever, convulsion, and pharyngeal or laryngeal muscle spasms (hydrophobia). Similar symptoms may also be induced when cool air blows on the face (aerophobia). Subsequently autonomic instability becomes extreme and hypotension, arrhythmia, hypoventilation, and coma will develop, resulting in death.

The diagnosis of rabies should be considered in any patient with unusual neurologic signs. In children especially, lack of a history of contact with a mammal should not deter the initiation of tests for rabies. It has long been known that children are more vulnerable to exposure to rabies infection, as they fail to recognize the danger or report animal contact. They are unable to run away and are more likely to have severe bites, especially on the head. The diagnosis of rabies could be made by viral isolation from saliva, brain tissues or cerebrospinal fluid, viral antigen detection from skin biopsy or corneal impression, rabies antibodies in cerebrospinal fluid, or viral gene detection by polymerase chain reaction.

Vaccine Information

The WHO recommends that the production and use of nerve tissue rabies vaccines in humans be discontinued and replaced by modern cell culture vaccines because nerve tissue vaccines have low potency and high incidence of serious, even fatal, neurologic complications, such as encephalomyelitis and GBS.[38] However, nerve tissue vaccines are still being used in some developing countries.

Modern cell culture vaccines are safe and immunogenic, with antibody response in more than 99% of vaccinees. Currently, human diploid cell vaccine (HDCV), purified chick embryo cell culture vaccine (PCECV), and purified Vero cell vaccine are available internationally. Human diploid cell vaccine and PCECV are licensed in the United States. Purified Vero cell vaccine is easier to produce and therefore cheaper to manufacture—an important factor for developing countries.[39] Rabies vaccination results in high titers of protective rabies virus–neutralizing antibodies as well as long-term immunologic memory. Originally, all vaccines were given intramuscularly; however, the reduced-dose intradermal vaccination was found efficacious and affordable especially for developing countries.[38]

Rabies immunoglobulin (RIg) is important in rabies prevention because it provides passive immunity when antibody response to the vaccine is mounting. Human RIg (HRIg) is the preferred product. However, if HRIg is in short supply or not available or affordable, purified equine immunoglobulin (ERIg) should be used. Most of the new ERIg preparations are potent, highly purified, safe, and less expensive. Rabies immunoglobulin can be administered at the same time as vaccination or up to day 7 of vaccination. It is not indicated beyond the seventh day of vaccination because antibody response to the vaccine has likely occurred.

Indications for Vaccination

Rabies Pre-exposure Prophylaxis

Pre-exposure prophylaxis is recommended for anyone at increased risk of exposure to the rabies virus. This includes laboratory staff, veterinarians, animal handlers, wildlife officers, and visitors to areas with a high risk of

Table 13-2. Rabies Pre-exposure Prophylaxis Schedule

VACCINATION	REGIMEN
Primary	HDCV or PCECV 1 mL intramuscularly on day 0, 7, and 28 (or 21 if time is limited) WHO also recommends HDCV, PCECV, or PVRV 0.1 mL intradermally on day 0, 7, and 28 (or 21 if time is limited).
Booster	HDCV or PCECV 1 mL intramuscularly on day 0

Abbreviations: HDCV, human diploid cell vaccine; PCECV, purified chick embryo cell culture vaccine; PVRV, purified Vero cell vaccine; WHO, World Health Organization.

Adapted from World Health Organization. Rabies vaccines. WHO position paper. *Wkly Epidemiol Rec.* 2007;82(49-50):425–435; and Manning SE, Rupprecht CE, Fishbein D, et al. Human rabies prevention—United States, 2008: recommendations of the Advisory Committee on Immunization Practices. *MMWR Recomm Rep.* 2008;57(RR-3):1–28

rabies (Table 13-2). Prophylaxis might offer partial immunity and protection if postexposure prophylaxis is delayed, and simplify postexposure management by eliminating the need for RIg and decreasing the number of vaccine doses.

Persons who receive pre-exposure prophylaxis should have a neutralization antibody test every 6 months or 2 years depending on the risk of exposure. For example, animal control workers who have a higher risk of rabies exposure may need more frequent antibody testing than those with less of an occupational risk. If the neutralizing antibody is less than 0.5 IU/mL or 1:5 serum dilution by the rapid fluorescent focus inhibition test, a single booster dose should be given (Table 13-2). If antibody testing is not available, booster vaccination every 5 years may be an acceptable alternative. If persons are exposed to rabies in the future, they are considered immunologically primed against rabies and simply require postexposure prophylaxis with days 0 and 3 vaccination.

Rabies Postexposure Prophylaxis

Prophylaxis after exposure to rabies virus should not await the results of laboratory diagnosis of the animal unless the species is unlikely to be infected with rabies and the test result can be obtained within 48 hours. Prophylaxis can also be postponed if the animal can be observed and rabies is not suspected. Prophylaxis should include prompt and thorough wound cleansing, passive immunization with RIg, and vaccination with cell culture rabies vaccines (tables 13-3 and 13-4). Prompt postexposure prophylaxis is nearly 100% effective in preventing rabies, even following high-risk exposure.[38] Recommendations addressing rabies postexposure prophylaxis depend on associated risks, including

Table 13-3. Rabies Postexposure Prophylaxis Schedule, United States	
TREATMENT	**REGIMEN**
Wound cleansing	Thorough cleansing with soap and water. If available, povidone-iodine solution should be used to irrigate the wound.
HRIg	20 IU/kg. If feasible, the full dose should be infiltrated around the wounds and any remaining volume should be given intramuscularly distant from vaccine administration.
Vaccine	HDCV or PCECV 1 mL intramuscularly (deltoid area if > 2 years of age, anterolateral thigh if < 2 years) on day 0, 3, 7, and 14
If a person previously completed pre-exposure or postexposure vaccination, HRIG is not needed and the vaccine can be given only on day 0 and 3.	

Abbreviations: HDCV, human diploid cell vaccine; HRIG, human rabies immunoglobulin; PCECV, purified chick embryo cell culture vaccine.

Adapted from Manning SE, Rupprecht CE, Fishbein D, et al. Human rabies prevention—United States, 2008: recommendations of the Advisory Committee on Immunization Practices. *MMWR Recomm Rep.* 2008;57(RR-3):1–28

1. *Type of exposure.* Bite exposure is more at risk for rabies than non-bite exposure. Prophylaxis is not indicated for non-bite exposure unless saliva or other potentially infected animal material is introduced into fresh, open cuts in skin or onto mucous membranes.

2. *Epidemiology of animal rabies and animal species in the area where the contact occurred.*

3. *Circumstance of the exposure incident.* An unprovoked attack might be more likely than a provoked attack to indicate that the animal is rabid. Bites as a result of feeding or handling an apparently healthy animal should generally be regarded as provoked.

4. *Availability of the animal for observation or rabies testing.*

The risk of rabies resulting from an encounter with a bat might be difficult to determine because of the minor injury usually inflicted and because some bat-related rabies viruses might likely result in infection after inoculation into a superficial epidermal layer. Although rare, human cases of rabies as a result of airborne transmission of the rabies virus have been reported[40]; this might be clinically important in view of bat cave exposures. If the person can be reasonably certain that a bite, scratch, or mucous membrane exposure did not occur, or if test results on the bat are negative for the virus, postexposure prophylaxis is not needed. Other situations that might qualify for prophylaxis include finding a bat in the same room with a person who might be unaware that

Table 13-4. Rabies Postexposure Prophylaxis Schedule, WHO

TREATMENT	REGIMEN
Wound cleansing	Thorough cleansing with soap and water for 15 minutes. If available, disinfect the wound with iodine solution or 70% alcohol.
RIG	Indicated for transdermal bites, scratches, or contamination of mucous membrane with saliva (ie, lick), exposure to bats. Not indicated for minor scratches or abrasions without bleeding or licks on broken/intact skin and nibbling of uncovered skin. 20 IU/kg for HRIG 40 IU/kg for ERIG If feasible, the full dose should be infiltrated around the wounds and any remaining volume should be given intramuscularly distant from vaccine administration.
Vaccine	HDCV, PCECV, and PVRV *Intramuscular route* 1 mL intramuscularly (deltoid area) on day 0, 3, 7, 14, and 28 or Two doses (1 mL each on left and right deltoid) on day 0, then 1 dose on day 7 and 21 *Intradermal route* 8-site regimen for HDCV and PCECV (8-0-4-0-1-1) Eight 0.1-mL injections on day 0, 4 injections on day 7, 1 on day 30 and 90 2-site regimen for PVRV and PCECV (2-2-2-0-1-1 or 2-2-2-0-2) Two 0.1-mL injections on day 0, 3, 7, and 1 injection on day 30 and 90 or Two 0.1-mL injections on day 0, 3, 7, and 28

If a person previously completed pre-exposure or postexposure vaccination, RIG is not needed and the vaccine can be given intramuscularly or intradermally only on day 0 and 3.

Abbreviations: ERIG, equine rabies immunoglobulin; HDCV, human diploid cell vaccine; HRIG, human rabies immunoglobulin; PCECV, purified chick embryo cell culture vaccine; PVRV, purified Vero cell vaccine; RIG, rabies immunoglobulin.

Adapted from World Health Organization. Rabies vaccines. WHO position paper. *Wkly Epidemiol Rec.* 2007;82(49–50):425–35; and World Health Organization. Current WHO guide for rabies pre and post-exposure prophylaxis in humans. http://www.who.int/rabies/PEProphylaxisguideline.pdf. Accessed June 16, 2011.

a contact occurred (eg, a sleeping person awakens to find a bat in the room; an adult witnesses a bat in the room with an unattended child, mentally disabled person, or intoxicated person). However, prophylaxis is not needed in those situations if test results on the bat are negative for rabies. Clinicians should seek assistance from public health officials for evaluating exposures or determining the need for postexposure management in situations that are not routine.

Side Effects

Cell Culture Vaccine

Local reactions, such as pain at the injection site, redness, and swelling, are common. Mild systemic reactions, such as fever, headache, and dizziness, have been reported. Systemic hypersensitivity reactions, including urticaria, pruritic rash, and angioedema, have been reported in up to 6% of persons receiving booster vaccination with HDCV.[41]

Rabies Immunoglobulin

Local reactions such as pain, redness, and induration are common. Headache is the most common systemic reaction. No serious adverse events, including hypersensitivity from HRIg, have been reported. There is a small risk of hypersensitivity reactions from ERIg. However, there are no scientific grounds for performing a skin test prior to administration of ERIg because the test is not predictive.

Precautions and Contraindications

Contraindications to postexposure prophylaxis following high-risk exposure do not exist because rabies is a lethal disease. This also pertains to postexposure prophylaxis in infants and pregnant women. For pre-exposure prophylaxis, previous severe reaction to any of the vaccine components is a contraindication for further use of the same vaccine.

Individuals with immune suppression, including HIV, should have neutralizing antibody testing 2 to 4 weeks after completing the pre-exposure series, and an additional dose of vaccination should be considered if the antibody response is not adequate. Immunosuppressive agents should not be given during postexposure prophylaxis unless essential. Neutralizing antibody testing 2 to 4 weeks after completing the postexposure series should be considered in immunosuppressed hosts. If the antibody response is not adequate, a specialist or public health official should be consulted. The intradermal route should be avoided and the intramuscular route should be used in immunocompromised individuals and in those who are taking corticosteroids or chloroquine.

Typhoid Fever

General Information About the Disease

Enteric (typhoid or paratyphoid) fever is a systemic illness caused by *Salmonella enterica* serotype *typhimurium* and *S enterica* serotype *paratyphi*. The organisms are highly adapted to humans and have no animal or environmental reservoirs. It is transmitted by the fecal-oral route. Excretion of the organisms by asymptomatic carriers or individuals who recently recovered from enteric fever is a major source of spread for an epidemic. Most cases are confined to lower-income countries with the greatest burden in the Indian subcontinent and Southeast Asia. Travelers visiting friends and relatives in endemic areas appear to be at increased risk for enteric fever compared with other travelers.[42] These travelers may have less control over their diet and be more likely to drink untreated water and eat uncooked foods while staying with friends or relatives.

Most people with enteric fever present with a nonspecific febrile illness, often with an insidious onset, after an incubation period of 1 to 2 weeks. Headache, malaise, myalgia, and dry cough are common. There are sudden episodes of shaking chills. Constipation and relative bradycardia are common but not necessary for the diagnosis. Rose spots (2 to 3 mm pink-red macules) on the chest and abdomen may appear. A variety of neuropsychiatric features may occur. Complications include gastrointestinal bleeding, intestinal perforation, and typhoidal encephalopathy. The case-fatality rate is highest among young children and elderly persons. Fewer than 5% will become long-term, asymptomatic carriers who may shed the organism in urine or stool for more than 1 year.[43]

Vaccine Information

All available vaccines are effective only against *S typhi*. None seem to provide any protection against *S paratyphi*, particularly *S paratyphi A*, which is increasing in the Indian subcontinent.[44]

Inactivated Whole-Cell Typhoid Vaccines

Although these early parenteral whole-cell vaccines are able to confer protection against typhoid fever, their global use as a public health tool for routine vaccination was undermined by their high reactogenicity, including fever, headache, and severe local pain. Consequently, the whole-cell vaccines were replaced by the well-tolerated virulence antigen (Vi)-based capsular polysaccharide vaccine and the oral live, attenuated Ty21a vaccine.

Vi-capsular Polysaccharide Typhoid Vaccines

This vaccine was developed by purifying Vi-capsular polysaccharide from wild type *S typhi* strain Ty2. The vaccine also contains phenol as a preservative. Previous exposure to *S typhi* does not seem to influence the immune response to vaccination. The protective efficacy of Vi polysaccharide vaccine in endemic areas was 72% over 17 months,[45] 64% over 21 months,[46] and 55% over 3 years.[47] A drawback of the parenteral Vi polysaccharide vaccine lies in its inability to stimulate mucosal immunity. In addition, revaccination does not elicit a booster effect because the immune response to the vaccine does not involve T cells; therefore, immunologic memory cannot be established. Covalent binding of Vi polysaccharide to recombinant *Pseudomonas aeruginosa* exotoxin A results in the induction of higher and more sustained antibody responses in comparison with pure Vi polysaccharide.[48] It also stimulates a booster response. A field trial in Vietnam showed a 2-dose immunization schedule resulted in 92% protection in children 2 to 5 years of age.[49]

Live, Attenuated Oral Typhoid Vaccine

The live oral vaccine is an attenuated *S typhi* strain, Ty21a, which is a mutant of the Ty2 strain. The strain lacks Vi antigen and is thus avirulent but contains immunogenic cell wall polysaccharides. The vaccine induces mucosal immunity (mucosal IgA) and serum antibodies, as well as cell-mediated immunity. An overall protective efficacy (as an enteric-coated capsule or a liquid formulation) of 67% to 80% was demonstrated for up to 7 years.[50-52] Herd immunity or indirect protection to non-immunized persons is also evidenced. Vaccinated individuals will be less likely to excrete virulent *S typhi* and there will be fewer temporary carriers in the community; these could result in reduction of infectious cases and transmission within a community.

Indications for Vaccination

Although the relevance to vaccine protection among travelers is unknown, the CDC and WHO recommend typhoid vaccination for persons traveling to countries where enteric fever is endemic, particularly the Indian subcontinent and Southeast Asia. These vaccines need to be given at least 2 weeks before departure. A unique phenomenon of typhoid vaccine immunity is that it can be overcome by a high inoculum dose (ie, ingestion of a large number of the organism). Thus, other protective measures, including drinking boiled or bottled water, eating thoroughly cooked food, and peeling fruits, must be followed despite vaccination. Persons with intimate exposure to a documented typhoid fever carrier, such as a household contact, a laboratory worker who has frequent contact with the organism, or those living in the endemic area of typhoid fever, should be vaccinated as well. Currently there are no commercially available vaccines for children younger than 2 years.

Administration

See Table 13-5 for administration of vaccines against typhoid fever.

Table 13-5. Administration of Vaccines Against Typhoid Fever

VACCINES	AGE OF RECIPIENTS, Y	REGIMEN	COMMENT
Oral live, attenuated Ty21a	> 6	Enteric coated capsule: 1 capsule by mouth every other day for 4 doses; booster given every 5 years. In Europe, it is available as a 3-dose vaccine.	Must be refrigerated before use. Taken with cool liquid 1 hour before meal. Concurrent use of antibiotics or antimalarials may interfere with antibody response.
Parenteral Vi-capsular polysaccharide	> 2	0.5 mL intramuscularly for 1 dose; booster given every 2 years	

Side Effects

Adverse systemic reactions from Vi-capsular polysaccharide vaccine are estimated to be about 2%. These include fever and headache. Adverse local reactions at the injection site are mostly mild and may occur in 10% to 40% of vaccines.[53] The adverse effects of oral live, attenuated vaccine are uncommon (less than 1%), including abdominal pain, nausea, and vomiting. Neither person-to-person transmission nor invasion of the bloodstream has been observed with the use of oral typhoid vaccine.

Precautions and Contraindications

A contraindication to vaccination includes a history of severe local or systemic reactions after a previous dose. No safety data are available for typhoid vaccines in pregnant women. Parenteral vaccine should not be given during an acute febrile illness. The oral live, attenuated vaccine should not be given to immunocompromised persons; the parenteral Vi polysaccharide vaccine may be an alternative. The oral vaccine requires replication in the gastrointestinal tract for effectiveness; it should not be given during gastrointestinal illness. The theoretical possibility for decreased immunogenicity when oral Ty21a vaccine is administered concurrently with antimicrobials has caused concern. Mefloquine can inhibit the growth of the live Ty21a strain in vitro; if this antimalarial is administered, vaccination with Ty21a should be delayed for 24 hours. The vaccine manufacturer advises that Ty21a vaccine should not be administered to persons receiving sulfonamides or other antimicrobial agents; Ty21a should be administered greater than or equal to 24 hours after an antimicrobial dose.[54]

Yellow Fever

General Information About the Disease

Yellow fever is a viral hemorrhagic fever caused by the yellow fever virus in the genus *Flavivirus*. Contrary to the misconception that yellow fever is an extinct disease, it remains endemic in many countries in tropical Africa and South America, principally in the Amazon region and contiguous grasslands. Several species of the *Aedes* and *Haemagogus* (South America only) mosquitoes transmit the virus. These mosquitoes are domestic (ie, they breed around houses), wild (ie, they breed in the jungle), or semi-domestic (ie, they display a mixture of habits). Yellow fever has a wide spectrum of illness, from mild nonspecific febrile symptoms to severe multiorgan failure and death.

The disease has 2 stages. The first stage, acute, is characterized by abrupt onset of fever, muscle pain, backache, headache, shivers, loss of appetite, nausea, and vomiting. The fever is paradoxically associated with a slow pulse. After 3 to 4 days most patients improve and their symptoms disappear. However, 15% of patients will enter a toxic stage. Fever reappears and several organ systems are affected. Jaundice and abdominal pain may develop rapidly. Bleeding can occur from the mouth, nose, eyes, rectum, and stomach. Myocardial injury and shock may occur. Renal involvement ranges from asymptomatic proteinuria to renal failure. Case-fatality rate is as high as 50%. The definitive diagnosis is made by a viral culture of blood or tissue specimens, or by identifying a viral antigen or nucleic acid in tissues using immunohistochemistry, enzyme-linked immunosorbent assay, or PCR. Detection of yellow fever IgM antibody with confirmation of 4-fold rise in neutralizing antibody titers between acute and convalescent serum samples is also diagnostic.

Vaccine Information

A live, attenuated vaccine (17D) was developed in 1936 by means of serial passage of the wild-type virus in chicken-embryo tissue. The 17D vaccine induces long-lasting neutralizing antibodies in about 99% of those who are vaccinated.[55] A single dose of vaccination provides protection for 10 years and probably for life.[56] It is part of a routine immunization program for children 9 months and older in endemic countries as recommended by WHO; however, vaccination coverage in many countries remains suboptimal.

Indications for Vaccination

Persons aged 9 months and older who are traveling to or living in areas of tropical Africa and South America where the disease is endemic should be vaccinated. These areas are listed on the WHO Web site (www.who.int) and the CDC Travelers' Health Web site (www.cdc.gov/travel).[57] Vaccination is also recommended for travel to countries that do not officially report the disease but that lie in the yellow fever endemic zone. To prevent importing yellow fever into a country where it was never reported, certain countries require that persons, even if only in transit, have valid ICVPs if they were in countries known or thought to have yellow fever. Such requirements might be enforced strictly for persons traveling from Africa or South America to Asia, where yellow fever does not exist but *Aedes* mosquito vectors are present.

Although this vaccine is not recommended for infants younger than 9 months, vaccination for infants 6 to 8 months of age should be considered if exposure to yellow fever is unavoidable. Due to the risk of vaccine-associated encephalitis, infants younger than 6 months should not receive yellow fever vaccine. Laboratory workers who might be exposed to yellow fever virus should be vaccinated.

Administration

Yellow fever vaccine is given subcutaneously at a dose of 0.5 mL. The International Health Regulations require revaccination every 10 years; however, the yellow fever vaccine immunity may persist up to 35 years and probably for life.[58]

Side Effects

Side effects to 17D yellow fever vaccine are usually mild, including headache, myalgia, low-grade fevers, or other minor symptoms for 5 to 10 days. Immediate hypersensitivity reactions, characterized by urticaria or wheezing, are very uncommon and occur principally among persons with a history of allergies to eggs. Gelatin in yellow fever vaccine has been implicated as a cause of allergic reaction to the vaccine.

Yellow fever vaccine–associated neurotropic disease among children has been the most common serious adverse event associated with yellow fever vaccines. The presentation is similar to viral encephalitis. The majority occur among children younger than 6 months. However the occurrence of vaccine-associated neurotropic disease does not appear to be confined to infants. The risk for vaccine-associated neurotropic disease has been estimated as fewer than 1 per 8 million persons.

In 2001, yellow fever vaccine–associated viscerotropic disease was described among recipients of different yellow fever vaccines.[59,60] It manifests with fever, hypotension, respiratory failure, elevated hepatocellular enzymes, hyperbilirubinemia, lymphocytopenia, thrombocytopenia, and death. This serious adverse reaction probably occurs as a clinical spectrum of disease severity, from moderate illness with focal organ dysfunction to severe disease with overt multiple organ system failure and death. Vaccine-type yellow fever virus was isolated from the blood of these patients. Persons are most at risk for yellow fever vaccine–associated viscerotropic disease after their first vaccination. Accurately measuring the incidence of this rare vaccine-associated viscerotropic disease is impossible because adequate prospective data are unavailable; however, crude estimates of the reported frequency are around 2.4 per 1 million doses. Those older than 65 years seem to have the highest risk of serious adverse events from vaccination.[61]

Because of recent reports of yellow fever deaths among unvaccinated travelers to areas endemic for yellow fever, and of reports of vaccine-associated viscerotropic disease, physicians should be careful to administer yellow fever vaccine only to persons truly at risk for exposure to yellow fever.

Precautions and Contraindications

Vaccinating infants younger than 9 months should be avoided because of the risk of vaccine-associated neurotropic disease. In addition, travel to countries in yellow fever endemic zones or to countries experiencing an epidemic should also be avoided. However, the ACIP and WHO recognize that situations occur in which vaccination of an infant 6 to 8 months might be considered, such as residence in or unavoidable travel to a yellow fever endemic or epidemic area. The decision to immunize must balance the infant's risk for exposure with the risk for vaccine-associated encephalitis. Physicians who consider vaccinating infants younger than 9 months should contact their state health department or the CDC for further advice. Yellow fever vaccine should never be administered to infants younger than 6 months.

Persons 65 years and older might be at increased risk for systemic adverse events after vaccination compared with younger persons. Nevertheless, yellow fever remains a key cause of illness and death in South America and Africa where potential yellow fever transmission zones have expanded to urban areas with substantial populations of susceptible humans and the *Aedes* vector mosquito. In addition, unvaccinated travelers to endemic areas have contracted fatal yellow fever. Consequently, despite these rare adverse events, yellow fever vaccination of travelers to high-risk areas should be encouraged as a key prevention strategy.

The safety of yellow fever vaccination during pregnancy has not been established, and the vaccine should be administered only if travel to an endemic area is unavoidable and if an increased risk for exposure exists. If vaccination of a pregnant woman is deemed necessary, serologic testing through the state health department or CDC to document an immune response to the vaccine can be considered because the sero-conversion rate for pregnant women has been reported to be lower than observed for other adults.[62] Vaccination of nursing mothers should be avoided because of the theoretical risk for transmitting the vaccine virus to the breastfed infant. Nursing mothers can be vaccinated when travel to high-risk yellow fever endemic areas cannot be avoided or postponed.

Infection with yellow fever vaccine virus poses a theoretical risk for encephalitis to patients with symptomatic HIV or AIDS, or malignancy, and those whose immunologic responses are suppressed by corticosteroids, chemotherapy, or radiation; these patients should not be vaccinated. If travel to a yellow fever–infected zone is necessary, patients should be instructed in methods for avoiding vector mosquitoes. In addition, their physician should provide them with vaccination waiver letters.

Asymptomatic HIV-infected persons who have established laboratory evidence of adequate immune system function and who cannot avoid potential exposure to yellow fever virus should be offered the choice of vaccination. Measurement of their neutralizing antibody response to vaccination should be considered before travel. If international travel requirements are the only reason to vaccinate an asymptomatic HIV-infected person, rather than an increased risk for infection, efforts should be made to obtain a waiver letter from the traveler's physician.

Yellow fever vaccine is produced in chick embryos and should not be administered to persons hypersensitive to eggs; typically, persons who are able to eat eggs or egg products can receive the vaccine. If vaccination is considered essential because of a high risk of exposure, an intradermal test dose can be administered under close medical supervision for those with a questionable history of egg hypersensitivity.

No data exist about possible interference between yellow fever vaccine and other vaccines. Because yellow fever vaccine is live, it should be given simultaneously or at least 1 month apart from other live vaccines. No alteration of the immunologic response to yellow fever vaccine was detected when given simultaneously with intramuscular immunoglobulin. Although chloroquine inhibits replication of yellow fever virus in vitro, it does not adversely affect antibody responses to yellow fever vaccine among humans receiving antimalarial prophylaxis.[63]

■ ACCELERATED IMMUNIZATION SCHEDULES FOR PEDIATRIC TRAVELERS

Routine pediatric vaccination may need to be accelerated before the standard primary vaccine series can be completed when travel of young infants is imminent. Table 13-6 lists the recommended minimum amount of time between doses. The minimum interval is required to produce an immunologic response; however, longer intervals are preferred.

■ KEY POINTS

- Most international travelers need a combination of routine and travel-specific immunizations.
- To determine which vaccines are needed for the traveler
  — Review the traveler's itinerary.
  — Determine the traveler's medical status.
  — Review the traveler's immunization record.
  — Determine vaccine requirements to enter the country.
- Factors that complicate the immunization of the traveler include
  — Number of vaccines and their particular schedules
  — Length of time until departure
  — Incompatibility of vaccines with other vaccines and medications
  — Traveler's health status, including allergies
  — Traveler's interest and personal or financial concerns
- International Certification of Vaccination or Prophylaxis or certificate of vaccination against yellow fever is required for travelers entering countries endemic to yellow fever or for travelers arriving from endemic areas, even if only in transit.
- Hepatitis A vaccine is indicated for persons traveling to countries that have high or intermediate hepatitis A endemicity.
- *Japanese encephalitis:* Only Vero cell culture–derived vaccine (Ixiaro [JE-VC]) is available in the United States and is approved only for use in persons aged 17 years or older. Vaccine should be offered to persons spending a month or longer in endemic areas during the transmission season, especially if travel includes rural areas.
- *Meningococcal vaccines:* These vaccines are recommended for travelers visiting the parts of sub-Saharan Africa known as the meningitis belt during the dry season. The government of Saudi Arabia requires a certificate of vaccination with tetravalent meningococcal vaccine for all travelers to Mecca during the annual Hajj.

Table 13-6. Acceleration of Routine Childhood Immunization

VACCINE	EARLIEST AGE FOR FIRST DOSE	MINIMUM INTERVAL BETWEEN DOSES
DTaP	6 weeks	4 weeks Minimum interval between DTaP dose 3 and DTaP dose 4 is 6 months. Minimum age for DTaP dose 4 and DTaP dose 5 is 12 months and 4 years.
IPV	6 weeks	4 weeks
Oral poliovirus	Birth	4 weeks
Hib	6 weeks	4 weeks Minimum interval between Hib dose 3 and Hib dose 4 is 8 weeks. Minimum age for Hib dose 4 is 12 months.
HepB	Birth	Minimum interval between HepB dose 1 and HepB dose 2 is 4 weeks. Minimum interval between HepB dose 2 and HepB dose 3 is 8 weeks (with 16 weeks between HepB dose 1 and HepB dose 3).
PCV	6 weeks	4 weeks Minimum interval between PCV dose 3 and PCV dose 4 is 8 weeks. Minimum age for PCV dose 4 is 12 months.
Rotavirus (mono-valent and penta-valent)	6 weeks[64]	4 weeks
MMR	6 months. However, all doses given before 12 months of age should not be counted as part of the complete series.	4 weeks
Varicella	12 months	3 months for children aged 12 years and younger, and 4 weeks for persons aged 13 years and older[65]
Hepatitis A	12 months	6 months

Abbreviations: DTaP, diphtheria, tetanus, and acellular pertussis; HepB, hepatitis B; Hib, *Haemophilus influenzae* type b; IPV, inactivated poliovirus; MMR, measles, mumps, and rubella; PCV, pneumococcal conjugate vaccine.

Adapted from American Academy of Pediatrics. *Red Book: 2009 Report of the Committee on Infectious Diseases*. Pickering LK, Baker CJ, Kimberlin DW, Long SS, eds. 28th ed. Elk Grove Village, IL: American Academy of Pediatrics; 2009:29–31

- *Rabies vaccine:* Pre-exposure prophylaxis is recommended for anyone at increased risk of exposure to the rabies virus.
- *Typhoid vaccines:* The protective immunity with Vi-capsular polysaccharide typhoid vaccines is only 55% over 3 years. An overall protective efficacy of live, attenuated oral typhoid vaccine is 67% to 80% up to 7 years. All available vaccines are effective only against *S typhi* and not against *S paratyphi*, particularly *S paratyphi A,* which is increasing in the Indian subcontinent. The parenteral Vi polysaccharide vaccine does not stimulate mucosal immunity. A unique phenomenon of typhoid vaccine immunity is that it can be overcome by a high inoculum dose and thus, other protective measures must be followed despite vaccination.
- *Yellow fever:* A single dose of vaccination provides protection for 10 years and probably for life. Vaccine is recommended for persons aged 9 months and older who are traveling to or living in areas of tropical Africa and South America where the disease is endemic.

■ REFERENCES

1. World Health Organization. *International Travel and Health.* 2008
2. Shapiro CN, Margolis HS. Worldwide epidemiology of hepatitis A virus infection. *J Hepatol.* 1993;18(Suppl 2):S11–S14
3. Soucie JM, Robertson BH, Bell BP, McCaustland KA, Evatt BL. Hepatitis A virus infections associated with clotting factor concentrate in the United States. *Transfusion.* 1998;38(6):573–579
4. Benjamin RJ. Nucleic acid testing: update and applications. *Semin Hematol.* 2001;38 (4 Suppl 9):11–16
5. Krugman S, Ward R, Giles JP, Bodansky O, Jacobs AM. Infectious hepatitis: detection of virus during the incubation period and in clinically inapparent infection. *N Engl J Med.* 1959;261:729–734
6. Yotsuyanagi H, Koike K, Yasuda K, et al. Prolonged fecal excretion of hepatitis A virus in adult patients with hepatitis A as determined by polymerase chain reaction. *Hepatology.* 1996;24(1):10–13
7. Sjogren MH, Tanno H, Fay O, et al. Hepatitis A virus in stool during clinical relapse. *Ann Intern Med.* 1987;106(2):221–226
8. Mutsch M, Spicher VM, Gut C, Steffen R. Hepatitis A virus infections in travelers, 1988–2004. *Clin Infect Dis.* 2006;42(4):490–497
9. Fiore AE, Wasley A, Bell BP. Prevention of hepatitis A through active or passive immunization: recommendations of the Advisory Committee on Immunization Practices (ACIP). *MMWR Recomm Rep.* 2006;55(RR-7):1–23
10. Rendi-Wagner P, Korinek M, Winkler B, Kundi M, Kollaritsch H, Wiedermann U. Persistence of seroprotection 10 years after primary hepatitis A vaccination in an unselected study population. *Vaccine.* 2007;25(5):927–931
11. Hammitt LL, Bulkow L, Hennessy TW, et al. Persistence of antibody to hepatitis A virus 10 years after vaccination among children and adults. *J Infect Dis.* 2008;198(12):1776–1782

12. Wiedermann G, Kundi M, Ambrosch F. Estimated persistence of anti-HAV antibodies after single dose and booster hepatitis A vaccination (0–6 schedule). *Acta Trop.* 1998;69(2):121–125

13. Update: Prevention of hepatitis A after exposure to hepatitis A virus and in international travelers. Updated recommendations of the Advisory Committee on Immunization Practices (ACIP). *MMWR Morb Mortal Wkly Rep.* 2007;56(41):1080–1084

14. Greenwood CS, Greenwood NP, Fischer PR. Immunization issues in pediatric travelers. *Expert Rev Vaccines.* 2008;7:651–661

15. Fischer M, Lindsey N, Staples JE, Hills S. Japanese encephalitis vaccines: recommendations of the Advisory Committee on Immunization Practices (ACIP). *MMWR Recomm Rep.* 2010;59:1–27

16. Centers for Disease Control and Prevention. Update on Japanese encephalitis for children—United States. MMWR. 2011;60(10):664–665

17. World Health Organization. Japanese encephalitis vaccines. Weekly Epidemiological Record. 2006;81(34/35):325–340

18. Inactivated Japanese encephalitis virus vaccine. Recommendations of the Advisory Committee on Immunization Practices (ACIP). *MMWR Recomm Rep.* 1993;42(RR-1):1–15

19. Japanese encephalitis vaccine and adverse effects among travelers. *Canada Dis Wkly Rep.* 1991;17(32):173–177

20. Bilukha OO, Rosenstein N. Prevention and control of meningococcal disease. Recommendations of the Advisory Committee on Immunization Practices (ACIP). *MMWR Recomm Rep.* 2005;54(RR-7):1–21

21. Raghunathan PL, Bernhardt SA, Rosenstein NE. Opportunities for control of meningococcal disease in the United States. *Annu Rev Med.* 2004;55:333–353

22. Rosenstein NE, Perkins BA, Stephens DS, et al. The changing epidemiology of meningococcal disease in the United States, 1992–1996. *J Infect Dis.* 1999;180(6):1894–1901

23. Dull PM, Abdelwahab J, Sacchi CT, et al. Neisseria meningitidis serogroup W-135 carriage among US travelers to the 2001 Hajj. *J Infect Dis.* 2005;191(1):33–39

24. Raghunathan PL, Jones JD, Tiendrebeogo SR, et al. Predictors of immunity after a major serogroup W-135 meningococcal disease epidemic, Burkina Faso, 2002. *J Infect Dis.* 2006;193(5):607–616

25. Trotter CL, Greenwood BM. Meningococcal carriage in the African meningitis belt. *Lancet Infect Dis.* 2007;7(12):797–803

26. Gold R, Lepow ML, Goldschneider I, Draper TF, Gotshlich EC. Kinetics of antibody production to group A and group C meningococcal polysaccharide vaccines administered during the first six years of life: prospects for routine immunization of infants and children. *J Infect Dis.* 1979;140(5):690–697

27. Peltola H, Kayhty H, Kuronen T, Haque N, Sarna S, Makela PH. Meningococcus group A vaccine in children three months to five years of age. Adverse reactions and immunogenicity related to endotoxin content and molecular weight of the polysaccharide. *J Pediatr.* 1978;92(5):818–822

28. Pinner RW, Onyango F, Perkins BA, et al. Epidemic meningococcal disease in Nairobi, Kenya, 1989. The Kenya/Centers for Disease Control (CDC) Meningitis Study Group. *J Infect Dis.* 1992;166(2):359–364

29. Rosenstein N, Levine O, Taylor JP, et al. Efficacy of meningococcal vaccine and barriers to vaccination. *JAMA.* 1998;279(6):435–439

30. Cochi SL, Markowitz LE, Joshi DD, et al. Control of epidemic group A meningococcal meningitis in Nepal. *Int J Epidemiol.* 1987;16(1):91–97

31. Ambrosch F, Wiedermann G, Crooy P, George AM. Immunogenicity and side-effects of a new tetravalent meningococcal polysaccharide vaccine. *Bull WHO.* 1983;61(2):317–323

32. Zangwill KM, Stout RW, Carlone GM, et al. Duration of antibody response after meningococcal polysaccharide vaccination in US Air Force personnel. *J Infect Dis.* 1994;169(4):847–852

33. Keyserling H, Papa T, Koranyi K, et al. Safety, immunogenicity, and immune memory of a novel meningococcal (groups A, C, Y, and W-135) polysaccharide diphtheria toxoid conjugate vaccine (MCV-4) in healthy adolescents. *Arch Pediatr Adolesc Med.* 2005;159(10):907–913

34. Centers for Disease Control and Prevention. License of a meningococcal conjugate vaccine (Menveo) and guidance for use: Advisory Committee on Immunization Practices. *MMWR.* 2010;59(09):273

35. Revised recommendations of the Advisory Committee on Immunization Practices to vaccinate all persons aged 11-18 years with meningococcal conjugate vaccine. *MMWR Morb Mortal Wkly Rep.* 2007;56(31):794–795

36. American Academy of Pediatrics. *Red Book: 2009 Report of the Committee on Infectious Diseases.* 28th ed. Elk Grove Village, IL: American Academy of Pediatrics; 2009

37. Update: Guillain-Barre syndrome among recipients of Menactra meningococcal conjugate vaccine—United States, June 2005–September 2006. *MMWR Morb Mortal Wkly Rep.* 2006;55(41):1120–1124

38. World Health Organization. Rabies vaccines WHO position paper. *Wkly Epidemiol Rec.* 2007:425–435

39. Wilde H, Tipkong P, Khawplod P. Economic issues in postexposure rabies treatment. *J Travel Med.* 1999;6(4):238–242

40. Winkler WG, Fashinell TR, Leffingwell L, Howard P, Conomy P. Airborne rabies transmission in a laboratory worker. *JAMA.* 1973;226:1219–1221

41. Fishbein DB, Yenne KM, Dreesen DW, Teplis CF, Mehta N, Briggs DJ. Risk factors for systemic hypersensitivity reactions after booster vaccinations with human diploid cell rabies vaccine: a nationwide prospective study. *Vaccine.* 1993;11(14):1390–1394

42. Angell SY, Cetron MS. Health disparities among travelers visiting friends and relatives abroad. *Ann Intern Med.* 2005;142(1):67–72

43. Basnyat B, Maskey AP, Zimmerman MD, Murdoch DR. Enteric (typhoid) fever in travelers. *Clin Infect Dis.* 2005;41(10):1467–1472

44. Tankhiwale SS, Agrawal G, Jalgaonkar SV. An unusually high occurrence of Salmonella enterica serotype paratyphi A in patients with enteric fever. *Indian J Med Res.* 2003;117:10–12

45. Acharya IL, Lowe CU, Thapa R, et al. Prevention of typhoid fever in Nepal with the Vi capsular polysaccharide of Salmonella typhi. A preliminary report. *N Engl J Med.* 1987;317(18):1101–1104

46. Klugman KP, Gilbertson IT, Koornhof HJ, et al. Protective activity of Vi capsular polysaccharide vaccine against typhoid fever. *Lancet.* 1987;2(8569):1165–1169

47. Klugman KP, Koornhof HJ, Robbins JB, Le Cam NN. Immunogenicity, efficacy and serological correlate of protection of Salmonella typhi Vi capsular polysaccharide vaccine three years after immunization. *Vaccine.* 1996;14(5):435–438

48. Kossaczka Z, Lin FY, Ho VA, et al. Safety and immunogenicity of Vi conjugate vaccines for typhoid fever in adults, teenagers, and 2- to 4-year-old children in Vietnam. *Infect Immun.* 1999;67(11):5806–5810

49. Lin FY, Ho VA, Khiem HB, et al. The efficacy of a Salmonella typhi Vi conjugate vaccine in two- to-five-year-old children. *N Engl J Med.* 2001;344(17):1263–1269

50. Levine MM, Ferreccio C, Abrego P, Martin OS, Ortiz E, Cryz S. Duration of efficacy of Ty21a, attenuated Salmonella typhi live oral vaccine. *Vaccine.* 1999;17(Suppl 2): S22–S27

51. Levine MM, Ferreccio C, Cryz S, Ortiz E. Comparison of enteric-coated capsules and liquid formulation of Ty21a typhoid vaccine in randomised controlled field trial. *Lancet.* 1990;336(8720):891–894

52. Levine MM, Ferreccio C, Black RE, Tacket CO, Germanier R. Progress in vaccines against typhoid fever. *Rev Infect Dis.* 1989;11(Suppl 3):S552–S567

53. Guzman CA, Borsutzky S, Griot-Wenk M, et al. Vaccines against typhoid fever. *Vaccine.* 2006;24(18):3804–3811

54. Centers for Disease Control and Prevention. Typhoid immunization recommendations of the Advisory Committee on Immunization Practices. MMWR. 1994;43(RR14):1–7

55. Monath TP. Dengue and yellow fever—challenges for the development and use of vaccines. *N Engl J Med.* 2007;357(22):2222–2225

56. Niedrig M, Lademann M, Emmerich P, Lafrenz M. Assessment of IgG antibodies against yellow fever virus after vaccination with 17D by different assays: neutralization test, haemagglutination inhibition test, immunofluorescence assay and ELISA. *Trop Med Int Health.* 1999;4(12):867–871

57. Cetron MS, Marfin AA, Julian KG, et al. Yellow fever vaccine. Recommendations of the Advisory Committee on Immunization Practices (ACIP), 2002. *MMWR Recomm Rep.* 2002;51(RR-17):1–11

58. Poland JD, Calisher CH, Monath TP, Downs WG, Murphy K. Persistence of neutralizing antibody 30-35 years after immunization with 17D yellow fever vaccine. *Bull WHO.* 1981;59(6):895–900

59. Centers for Disease Control and Prevention. Fever, jaundice, and multiple organ system failure associated with 17D-derived yellow fever vaccination, 1996-2001. *MMWR Morb Mortal Wkly Rep.* 2001;50(30):643–645

60. Martin M, Tsai TF, Cropp B, et al. Fever and multisystem organ failure associated with 17D-204 yellow fever vaccination: a report of four cases. *Lancet.* 2001;358(9276):98–104

61. Martin M, Weld LH, Tsai TF, et al. Advanced age a risk factor for illness temporally associated with yellow fever vaccination. *Emerg Infect Dis.* 2001;7(6):945–951

62. Nasidi A, Monath TP, Vandenberg J, et al. Yellow fever vaccination and pregnancy: a four-year prospective study. *Trans R Soc Trop Med Hyg.* 1993;87(3):337–339

63. Barry M, Patterson JE, Tirrell S, Cullen MR, Shope RE. The effect of chloroquine prophylaxis on yellow fever vaccine antibody response: comparison of plaque reduction neutralization test and enzyme-linked immunosorbent assay. *Am J Trop Med Hyg.* 1991;44(1):79–82

64. Cortese MM, Parashar UD. Prevention of rotavirus gastroenteritis among infants and children: recommendations of the Advisory Committee on Immunization Practices (ACIP). *MMWR Recomm Rep.* 2009;58(RR-2):1–25

65. Marin M, Guris D, Chaves SS, Schmid S, Seward JF. Prevention of varicella: recommendations of the Advisory Committee on Immunization Practices (ACIP). *MMWR Recomm Rep.* 2007;56(RR-4):1–40

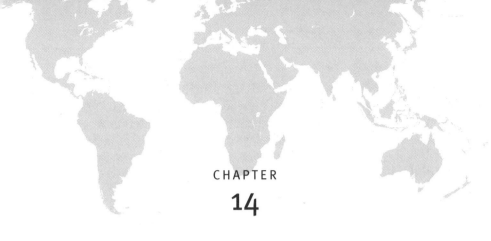

CHAPTER

14

Traveler's Diarrhea

Jocelyn Y. Ang, MD, FAAP
Ambika Mathur, PhD

■ INTRODUCTION

Children often accompany adults as they travel overseas for pleasure, business, or employment. Unfortunately, during travel, children can encounter several enteric pathogens, some of which are associated with traveler's diarrhea (TD), the most frequent condition among travelers, especially to lower-income countries.[1] Although TD is generally self-limiting, it is a frustrating condition and negatively affects the travel experience. Data on etiology, incidence, and management of TD in children are limited. This chapter reviews recommendations addressing prevention, prophylaxis, and self-treatment of TD. These recommendations are not standardized in children and are largely based on expert opinion extrapolated from studies on TD in adults.

■ DEFINITION

Definitions of TD in the literature are varied. In adults, classic TD is defined as 3 or more loose stools per day along with other symptoms (eg, nausea, vomiting, abdominal pain or cramps, fever, blood in stool).[2] Stool frequency and consistency vary during different periods in childhood.[3] Stool frequency can range from a mean of 3 times per day at 4 weeks of age to 1 time a day at 42 months of age.[3] In babies, stool consistency can be soft and liquidy.[3] Therefore, TD, as defined by the 1985 National Institutes of Health consensus report as a syndrome lasting for 2 to 3 days and characterized by a 2-fold or greater increase in the frequency of unformed stools, is more applicable for pediatric TD.[4] *Persistent* TD refers to the condition when it lasts longer than 14 days, while chronic diarrhea is used when it occurs for a period longer than 30 days.[5,6]

■ EPIDEMIOLOGY

The incidence of TD varies in relationship to the numerous risk factors present and can be as high as 60%.[2] Risk factors for TD include host factors (age, dietary behavior, country of origin, genetic) and environmental (destination).[2] Travel destination is the leading risk factor, with countries in Asia (except Singapore), Africa, Latin America, and parts of the Middle East considered high risk because incidence rates can range from 20% to 90%.[2] China, South Africa, Israel, southern Europe, and some Caribbean islands are considered intermediate risk areas with incidence rates ranging from greater than 8% to less than 20%.[2] Low-risk areas include most of the industrialized countries, where incidence rates are lower than 8%.[2] The second most frequent risk of TD is travel in summer and during the monsoon or rainy seasons.[7,8]

Studies on the incidence of TD in children are lacking. A study by Pitzinger et al[9] evaluated 363 children (birth to 20 years of age) who recently traveled to the tropics and subtropics from Switzerland to determine the incidence and characteristics of TD in children. Within 2 weeks of travel, the overall incidence of TD was 31%. The highest rate was seen in young children (birth to 2 years of age) at 40%, followed by adolescents (15 to 20 years of age) at 36%. Incidence rates of 8.5% and 22% were found among children aged 3 to 6 years and 7 to 14 years, respectively. Traveler's diarrhea incidence rates varied by location and were 67% for North Africa; 61% for India; 27% to 31% for East Africa, Southeast Asia, and Latin America; and 17% for West Africa.

Another study of TD in 174 Portuguese children (aged 2 months to 16 years) visiting tropical countries found a lower TD attack rate of 21.8% and lower rates by world regions: 31.5% for India; 26.9% in southern Africa; 22.2% in West Africa; and 6.7% in Latin America compared with Pitzinger et al.[9,10]

■ RISK FACTORS FOR TRAVELER'S DIARRHEA

In addition to environmental risk factors by destination, age, gastrointestinal conditions, and genetic susceptibility to enteric infections can also influence susceptibility to TD.

Age

Traveler's diarrhea is observed with higher frequency among toddlers, which is probably because of their immature immune system combined with their active environmental exploration (particularly oral exploration).[9] Traveler's diarrhea is also observed more frequently among young adults, possibly because of their more adventurous lifestyles and lower vigilance in avoiding contaminated food and water.[2,7,9]

Gastrointestinal Conditions

Individuals with underlying gastrointestinal disorders and those receiving antacids, H_2 blockers, and proton pump inhibitors are at increased risk for TD.[7]

Genetic Susceptibility to Enteric Infections

Recently, with the advent of genomic testing, genetic basis for host susceptibility to infectious diseases including TD was demonstrated. Only a few studies have been published about this association. Genetic variability in inflammatory response has been associated with increased risk for TD.[11-14] Subjects with polymorphism in the lactoferrin gene,[13] osteoprotegerin gene,[14] and promoter region of interleukin (IL)-8[11] and IL-10[12] were found to be associated with increased risk of TD from different pathogens.

Lactoferrin is a glycoprotein found in milk, mucosal secretions (ie, tears, saliva, and intestinal mucus), and secondary granules of neutrophils.[15] Multiple activities of lactoferrin (antimicrobial,[16] anti-inflammatory,[17] and immunomodulatory[18]) have been described. Fecal lactoferrin is a marker of intestinal inflammation in patients with diarrhea. Lactoferrin concentrations have been found to be elevated in stool specimens obtained from travelers with diarrhea.[19,20] A study investigating the effect of a single nucleotide polymorphism (SNP) in the human lactoferrin gene and the susceptibility to TD was conducted among North American adult travelers to Mexico.[13] The study found that an SNP in the lactoferrin gene (the T/T genotype in position codon 632) in these individuals with TD was associated with susceptibility to diarrhea.[13] Although lactoferrin levels in stools were higher in those subjects with pathogen-confirmed diarrhea, fecal lactoferrin levels did not correlate with the SNP genotype.

In a study among travelers with enteroaggregative *Escherichia coli*, subjects with an SNP in the promoter region of IL-8 were associated with the occurrence of diarrhea and increased levels of fecal IL-8 suggestive of cytokine-mediated intestinal inflammation.[11]

Osteoprotegerin is an immunoregulatory gene that is a member of the tumor necrosis factor receptor superfamily. It is reported to be up-regulated in human intestinal cells after infection with enteropathogens.[21] An SNP in the gene encoding osteoprotegerin was found to be associated with increased susceptibility to TD with various *E coli* pathogens among North American travelers to Mexico.[14]

Symptomatic enterotoxigenic *E coli* (ETEC) diarrhea were more common in travelers with an SNP in IL-10 promoter gene where they produced higher levels of IL-10.[12]

Additional studies are needed to better understand the contribution of genetic host factors and susceptibility to enteric pathogens.

■ ETIOLOGY

The etiology of TD in children is not adequately studied. According to an update on pediatric diarrheal illness in developing countries,[22] rotavirus and diarrheagenic *E coli* are the most common pathogens associated with acute diarrhea in children. Diarrheagenic *E coli* include enteropathogenic (EPEC), ETEC, Shiga toxin producing, enteroaggregative, and enteroinvasive. Enteroaggregative *E coli*, EPEC, and ETEC cause endemic diarrhea and are seen in children younger than 2 years. Enteroinvasive *E coli* causes invasive diarrhea associated with fever and is indistinguishable from other enteroinvasive pathogens *(Shigella)*. Shiga toxin–producing *E coli* has been reported to cause bloody diarrhea and hemolytic uremic syndrome in children, and outbreaks have been reported in some developed and developing countries.[23–26] In poorer areas of the world, other organisms *(Shigella, Salmonella, Campylobacter, Vibrio, Aeromonas,* and *Plesiomonas)* are more commonly seen.[22] On the other hand, protozoa and helminths are seen in areas with extremely poor environmental sanitation.[22]

Bacteria are the most common causative agents (up to 70% of cases) of TD in adults, with viruses and parasites associated with the remaining cases.[27,28] Among bacterial causes, ETEC is isolated in the majority of cases (between 50% and 70%) of TD.[27] Enteroaggregative *E coli* is increasingly recognized as a cause of TD and may be responsible for up to 33% of cases.[29] Other *E coli* species, such as enteroinvasive *E coli* and enteropathogenic *E coli,* are also isolated from patients with TD.[27,30] Enterohemorrhagic *E coli* has caused outbreaks in the United States,[31] Europe,[32] and Japan,[33] with complication of hemolytic-uremic syndrome, but is rarely reported in children who traveled. Other invasive bacterial pathogens associated with TD include *Shigella, Campylobacter,* and nontyphoid *Salmonella. Aeromonas* and *Vibrio* are seen less frequently.

Shah et al[28] recently reviewed all TD studies published between 1973 and 2008 to determine the global etiology of TD by regions of the developing world. Indeed, there were regional differences among different pathogens identified. While *E coli* is responsible for the majority of TD cases identified in these areas, invasive pathogens *(Campylobacter, Shigella,* and *Salmonella)* were more commonly seen in southern Asia compared with Latin America and Africa (Figure 14-1). Knowledge concerning regional differences in causative etiologies of TD is important. This information will help guide recommendations on the appropriate use of antimicrobial agents for chemoprophylaxis treatment (where applicable) as well as the use of vaccines for TD.

Viruses, especially *Norovirus,* rotaviruses, and enteric adenoviruses, are associated with diarrhea among children in developing countries and are responsible for 2% to 25% of TD cases.[27] Parasitic infestations also occur in travelers who visit lower-income countries for prolonged periods and are usually associated with persistent diarrhea. *Giardia lamblia* is the most common parasite associated with TD,[27] especially in South and Southeast Asia.[28] *Entamoeba histolytica, Cryptosporidium parvum,* and *Cyclospora cayetanensis* are the other parasites associated with TD but are less common compared with *G lamblia.*[27]

■ CLINICAL PRESENTATION

In the majority of patients with TD, symptoms occur within the first 2 weeks of travel.[34] However, symptoms can begin even after completion of travel. Typical symptoms of TD include loose stools associated with abdominal pain, cramps with nausea, and vomiting; fever; fecal urgency; tenesmus; and passage of mucus or blood in the stool. The majority of patients have abdominal pain or cramps; about 25% of patients have fever and vomiting, while a small number (fewer than 10%) have mucoid or bloody stools.[7,9,35] Traveler's diarrhea is generally self-limited. In a single pediatric study,[9] TD started on the eighth day of travel; the average duration was 11.5 days and median duration was 3 days. Children younger than 3 years had a more prolonged illness, averaging 29.5 days, while older children and adolescents 3 to 20 years of age had a shorter duration of symptoms ranging from 2.6 to 4 days.

■ COMPLICATIONS

The primary complication observed in TD is dehydration. Young children usually suffer from a more severe and prolonged course of TD. Children have a high proportion of water per body mass and turn over 25% of total body water per day, and are therefore at a higher risk of dehydration from acute water loss associated with diarrhea than

Figure 14-1. Major Causes of Traveler's Diarrhea According to World Regions Visited

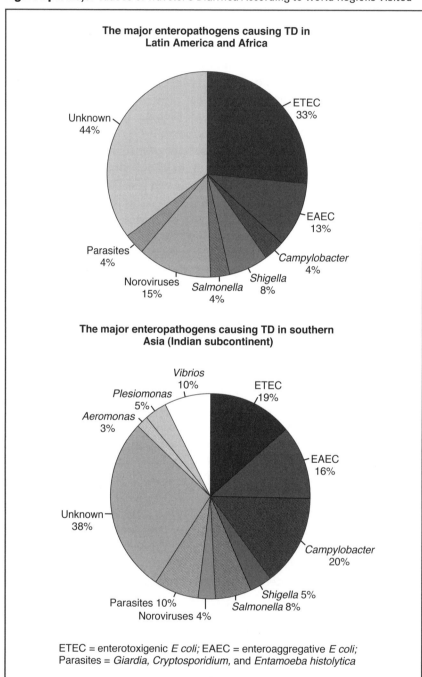

The major enteropathogens causing TD in Latin America and Africa

- ETEC 33%
- EAEC 13%
- Campylobacter 4%
- Shigella 8%
- Salmonella 4%
- Noroviruses 15%
- Parasites 4%
- Unknown 44%

The major enteropathogens causing TD in southern Asia (Indian subcontinent)

- Vibrios 10%
- Plesiomonas 5%
- Aeromonas 3%
- ETEC 19%
- EAEC 16%
- Campylobacter 20%
- Shigella 5%
- Salmonella 8%
- Noroviruses 4%
- Parasites 10%
- Unknown 38%

ETEC = enterotoxigenic *E coli*; EAEC = enteroaggregative *E coli*;
Parasites = *Giardia, Cryptosporidium,* and *Entamoeba histolytica*

Adapted with permission from Dupont HL. Systemic review: the epidemiology and clinical features of travellers' diarrhoea. *Aliment Pharmacol Ther.* 2009;30(3):187–196. © 2009 Blackwell Publishing Ltd.

adults.[7,9,35] Treatment of children with fluids with inappropriate electrolyte concentrations can result in neurologic complications such as altered sensorium, seizures, and coma.[37,38] Other complications associated with dysentery are intestinal perforation and sepsis[38] as well as diaper dermatitis (probably caused by skin breakdown from chemical composition of the stool, or superinfection with *Candida* from prolonged diarrhea and inability to change diapers frequently and keep the area dry).

Sequelae associated with TD are increasingly reported in adults. In particular, post-infectious irritable bowel syndrome (IBS-PI) is observed more frequently. The incidence of IBS-PI, characterized by persistent gastrointestinal signs and symptoms (ie, acute onset of symptoms of at least 3 months, persistent abdominal discomfort or pain, and altered bowel habits) after the initial episode of acute diarrhea, is reported to be between 4% and 32%.[39]

In children, the relationship between TD and IBS-PI is not well studied. Saps et al[40] recently investigated the development of post-infectious functional gastrointestinal disorders (FGIDs) in children aged 3 to 19 years after a documented episode of culture—proven acute bacterial gastroenteritis (AGE). The study aimed to determine the proportion of AGE cases progressing to FGIDs compared with age- and sex-matched control subjects without AGE. Questionnaires were administered to the parents to assess symptoms of FGIDs (eg, pain, diarrhea, disability) in their children at 6 months or older after the initial positive culture. Subjects with abdominal pain were additionally classified as having IBS, dyspepsia, or functional abdominal pain.

Among the 88 patients recruited (44 exposed and 44 control), 54% of the exposed subjects had *Salmonella,* 32% had *Campylobacter,* and 14% had *Shigella* AGE. Significantly more exposed patients complained of abdominal pain (36%) compared with the control group (11%) (*P*<.01). Among the 16 exposed patients who complained of abdominal pain, 14 (88%) had changes characteristics of IBS and 4 (22%) had dyspepsia (ie, nausea, bloating, and early satiety). Overall, there was a 36% prevalence of post-infectious FGIDs in the exposed group versus 11% in the control subjects. The study supports the existence of post-infectious FGIDs as an entity in children, with most patients having symptoms of IBS.

In adults, reported risk factors for IBS-PI include younger than 60 years, female, psychological factors (depression and anxiety), and severity of diarrhea.[41-43] The underlying mechanism of IBS-PI is still not well understood; however, ongoing chronic inflammation appears to play an important role, including an increase in serotonin-containing enterochromaffin cells, proinflammatory cytokines, numbers of T lymphocytes, mast cells, and intestinal permeability.[41,44] Management of IBS-PI is not standardized and can be challenging.[45] Further understanding of the pathologic mechanisms of IBS-PI is needed to develop new and effective medications to treat this disease. Identification of enteric pathogens more likely to cause IBS-PI can be important, leading to early treatment and careful follow-up. Prophylaxis for TD may need to be reconsidered as a primary means of preventing IBS-PI if agents most likely to cause IBS-PI are identified.

In addition to IBS-PI, inflammatory bowel disease (Crohn disease or ulcerative colitis),[46] tropical sprue,[47] and reactive arthritis[48] following TD in susceptible persons are also reported after travel.

■ PREVENTION

Because of the high rate of TD among travelers to developing countries and the potential complications associated with TD such as IBS-PI, it is important to prevent TD. Prevention of TD can be divided into 2 broad categories, dietary and non-dietary prevention.

Dietary Prevention

Consuming contaminated food and drinks is known to be the main source of enteric pathogens and can lead to TD. Although unproven, counseling families about properly selecting and preparing food and drinks appears to be the most important strategy for preventing TD.

Water Purification

Safe water should be used not just for drinking but also for brushing teeth and preparing food and formula for infants. Travelers should be reminded to buy bottled water from reliable sources.

Water can be made safe and potable by 3 standard methods (heat, filtration, and halogenation) outlined in Table 14-1.[49] Heating water is the most reliable method. Water should be boiled (100°C) for at least 1 minute to kill most pathogens (eg, bacteria, viruses, protozoa, parasites). Using a filter with a micron size of less than or equal to 0.2 µm for bacteria and less than or equal to 1 µm for parasites effectively eliminates most organisms except viruses too small to be filtered, such as hepatitis A. An additional process (halogenation) is therefore necessary and can be done before or after filtration. Halogenation, chemical disinfection with halogens, is done using iodine or chlorine. Halogenation is effective in eliminating bacteria and viruses but is considered unreliable for protozoan cysts such as *Cryptosporidia* and *Giardia*.[28,49,50] The effectiveness

Table 14-1. Water Disinfection

TECHNIQUE	BACTERIA	VIRUSES	GIARDIA OR AMEBIC CYSTS	CRYPTOSPORIDIUM
Heat	+	+	+	+
Filtration	+	+/−[a]	+	+
Halogens	+	+	+	−

+, susceptible; −, not susceptible; +/−, inconsistent.

[a]Manufacturers of most filters make no claims with regard to viruses. General Ecology, Inc., claims virus removal by use of its First Need filter. Reverse osmosis filtration can remove viruses.

Adapted from Backer H. Water disinfection for international and wilderness travelers. *Clin Infect Dis.* 2002;34(3):355–364, by permission of Oxford University Press.

of halogenation depends on contact time, temperature, pH, organic contaminants, and turbidity.[49] For example, if the water is cold, contact time should be longer. Similarly, if the water is turbid, the concentration of halogens should be increased. Chlorine preparations are more likely to be affected by these factors compared with iodine preparations.

Iodine water disinfection should be limited to a few weeks of emergency use because iodine has physiologic activity. It is not recommended in persons with uncontrolled thyroid disorder, known iodine allergy, or pregnancy because of potential effect on fetal thyroid. Chlorine and iodine are available in liquid and tablet form (Table 14-2).

The taste of halogens in water can be improved by several methods, including increasing contact time and reducing concentration, and adding a tiny pinch of vitamin C (available in most flavored drinks in powder or crystal form) after contact time by converting chlorine to chloride or iodine to iodide, which have no color or taste.

Food Safety and Personal Hygiene Precautions

The gold standard for safely consuming milk and food continues to be, "Boil it, cook it, peel it, or forget it." Consume only boiled or pasteurized milk. Avoid fresh vegetables. Encourage breastfeeding in infants to reduce the chance of contamination. Fruits that can be peeled, such as bananas and oranges, are safe to eat. Wash all other fruits with clean water and then peel with a clean knife before eating. Consume only freshly cooked food that is thoroughly prepared; avoid leftover food. Baked foods, such as bread, and hyperosmolar food, such as candy, are safe. Always wash hands with soap and water (or with a commercially available hand sanitizer if water is unavailable) prior to touching or preparing food.

Table 14-2. Iodine and Chlorine Formulations and Doses		
IODINATION TECHNIQUES ADDED TO 1 L OR QT OF WATER	YIELD 4 MG/L CONTACT (WAIT) TIME 45 MIN AT 30°C 180 MIN AT 5°C[a]	YIELD 8 MG/L CONTACT (WAIT) TIME 15 MIN AT 30°C 60 MIN AT 5°C[a]
Iodine tablets (tetraglycine hydroperiodide) (eg, Potable Aqua, Globaline)	1/2 tablet	1 tablet
2% iodine solution (tincture)	0.2 mL 5 gtts[b]	0.4 mL 10 gtts[b]
Saturated solution: iodine crystals in water (eg, Polar Pure)	13.0 mL	26.0 mL
CHLORINATION TECHNIQUES	YIELD 5 MG/L	YIELD 10 MG/L
Sodium hypochlorite Household bleach 5%	0.1 mL 2 drops	0.2 mL 4 drops
Sodium dichloroisocyanurate (eg, AquaClear)		1 tablet
Chlorine plus flocculating agent (eg, Chlor-floc)		1 tablet

[a]Very cold water requires prolonged contact time with iodine or chlorine to kill *Giardia* cysts. These contact times have been extended from the usual recommendations in cold water to account for this and for the uncertainty of residual concentration.
[b]Drops per minute.

Adapted from Centers for Disease Control and Prevention. *CDC Health Information for International Travel 2010.* Atlanta, GA: US Department of Health and Human Services, Public Health Service; 2010

Non-dietary Prevention

Reports indicate that 60% of travelers do not comply with dietary recommendations during international travel.[9,51] However, TD occurs at about the same frequency among dietary compliant and non-compliant travelers[52,53]; thus, non-dietary factors also contribute to the development of TD. Therefore, it is essential to advise travelers about non-dietary precautions, which include immunization and chemoprophylaxis, to prevent TD.

Immunization

Vaccines for prevention of ETEC-related TD are being developed because ETEC is the main cause of TD and natural development of anti-ETEC immunity is known to occur in persons living in ETEC-endemic areas. Presently, the only licensed vaccine with an indication for prevention of diarrhea due to ETEC is an oral inactivated cholera vaccine. The oral vaccine is made of inactivated whole-cell *Vibrio cholerae* strains combined with the inactivated B-subunit of cholera toxin. Because of the antigenic similarity between the B-subunit of cholera toxin and ETEC heat labile enterotoxin (LT), immunization using the oral B-subunit of cholera toxin combined with whole-cell cholera vaccine was found to be 67% and 85% protective against episodes of diarrhea caused by ETEC and *V cholerae*, respectively.[54,55] The vaccine is marketed as Dukoral in Canada and Europe and is indicated for prevention and protection against TD caused by ETEC and *V cholerae* in adults and children 2 years and older. This vaccine is not available in the United States.[54]

Another vaccine for prevention of TD is the transcutaneous purified ETEC-LT patch vaccine.[56] This vaccine utilizes the novel method of transcutaneous immunization with antigen applied to the skin through a patch; the antigens are then processed by antigen-presenting Langerhans cells and transported to the lymph node with subsequent production of anti-LT antibodies. A study on the use of the patch vaccine given twice before travel was conducted among 170 travelers (59 vaccines, 111 placebo patients) to Mexico or Guatemala.[57] The vaccine was found to be safe and immunogenic. Patch vaccine recipients were protected against moderate to severe diarrhea compared with placebo patients. Currently, this vaccine is still under investigation.

Effective oral and injectable *Salmonella typhi* vaccines are available but recommended only for travelers to areas where the risk of exposure to *S typhi* is recognized.[58] Risk for acquiring *S typhi* infection is highest for travelers to the Indian subcontinent, Latin America, the Middle East, and Africa who may have prolonged exposure to contaminated food products.

Cholera vaccine is not available in the United States; however, vaccination is not currently recommended for US travelers because of the low risk of acquiring cholera.

Chemoprophylaxis

Chemoprophylaxis can be achieved by using antimicrobial or non-antimicrobial agents. Chemoprophylaxis for TD is less preferred by many travel medicine experts because effective antimicrobial agents are available to treat TD if diarrhea develops.[59] Therefore, chemoprophylaxis for TD should only be considered in certain groups of people traveling to high-risk regions. Persons to whom chemoprophylaxis may be considered include those on a tight schedule where short-term illness may severely affect the purpose of the trip, those who have chronic medical conditions in which diarrhea may potentially complicate the underlying illness, and those who had prior TD, which may suggest genetic susceptibility to TD. Travelers should be monitored for the development of adverse events and drug resistance while receiving chemoprophylaxis; chemoprophylaxis should not be continued for more than 2 weeks.[59]

Non-antimicrobial Agents

Bismuth Subsalicylate as Chemoprophylaxis

Bismuth subsalicylate (BSS) is the primary non-antimicrobial agent studied for TD prevention. When taken as 2 oz of liquid or 2 (263 mg) tablets 4 times a day, the protection rate for TD was 62% and 65%, respectively.[60] Bismuth subsalicylate undergoes acid hydrolysis and dissociates in the mouth or stomach, which results in release of salicylate and insoluble bismuth metabolites. It causes blackening of stools and tongues from the bismuth sulfide salt metabolites, which are generally harmless. The insoluble bismuth metabolites appear to have antibacterial property.[61] The free salicylate, which has anti-secretory and anti-inflammatory properties, is absorbed.[62] Tinnitus and encephalitis rarely occur. Bismuth subsalicylate should be avoided in patients with a history of aspirin allergy as well as those taking aspirin for other reasons.

Although used in adults, BSS is not recommended as a prophylactic agent in children because the dose of BSS for TD prevention in children is currently unknown. Furthermore, frequent and prolonged BSS use may cause salicylate intoxication[63] and increased the risk of Reye syndrome in patients with concomitant influenza or chickenpox infection.[64]

Probiotics as Chemoprophylaxis

Probiotics are other non-antimicrobial prophylactic agents used to prevent TD. They act by interfering with the colonization of the gut by pathogenic organisms. Two meta-analyses on the use of probiotics for the prevention of TD yielded conflicting results.[65,66] More studies are needed on the efficacy, optimal dosing, and frequency of administration of probiotics for TD prevention. In the future, probiotics may offer a safe and effective method to prevent TD. A wide range of probiotics products (eg, capsules, liquid, powder) with varying quality are available on the market. The dose of probiotics varies in children; regardless of the preparation, the minimum daily dose is suggested to be between 5 and 10 billion colony-forming units.[67]

Antimicrobial Agents

Antibiotic prophylaxis is reported to be about 80% to 90% effective in preventing TD. Although trimethoprim-sulfamethoxazole (TMP/SMX) has been used successfully in the prevention of TD, due to widespread resistance, its use is now limited. Even though fluoroquinolones are very effective in adults, they are not routinely used in children younger than 18 years. Fluoroquinolone use in children is limited because fluoroquinolones cause arthrotoxicity in juvenile animals. Fluroquinolones have been associated with reversible musculoskeletal events in children.[68] Ciprofloxacin[69] is currently the only Food and Drug Administration–approved fluoroquinolone for use in children. Approved indications include inhalational anthrax and complicated urinary tract infections and pyelonephritis due to *Pseudomonas aeruginosa.* According to the American Academy of Pediatrics, fluoroquinolone use should be restricted to situations in which there is no safe and effective alternative treatment of an infection or to provide oral treatment when parenteral therapy is not feasible and no other effective oral agent is available.[70]

Azithromycin is used successfully in treating TD, especially in cases caused by ciprofloxacin-resistant *Campylobacter.*[71] Rifaximin, a poorly absorbed rifamycin antibiotic, recently became available; it has in vitro activity against important enteric pathogens[72] with very few adverse effects. It offered 72% to 77% protection against TD when studied among travelers to Mexico where the predominant pathogen was *E coli.*[73] Despite high concentration in the gut, it did not alter colonic flora significantly. It is unclear whether rifaximin will be effective in preventing invasive forms of TD caused by *Shigella, Salmonella,* and *Campylobacter;* more studies are needed. Rifaximin is currently indicated for treatment of TD caused by noninvasive strains of *E coli.* The use of prophylactic antibiotics for TD has the potential for development of drug-related adverse events including allergic reaction and resistant bacteria and thus is not recommended routinely. When considering all types of prophylaxis, including antimicrobial chemoprophylaxis, against TD, the risk of developing adverse events from prophylaxis should be weighed against the benefit of using prompt and effective self-treatment for TD when signs and symptoms of TD develop.

Antimicrobial chemoprophylaxis is not recommended for infants 12 months or younger. Because the safety and efficacy of chemoprophylaxis in young infants is still not known, potential adverse events may outweigh the benefit of using antimicrobial chemoprophylaxis.

■ TREATMENT

The mainstay of TD treatment in children is preventing and treating dehydration. Traveler's diarrhea treatment can be initiated by the child's caregiver or the traveler (self-treatment). Treatment can also be prescribed by a physician after appropriate evaluation.

Prevention and Treatment of Dehydration

Dehydration and electrolyte abnormalities are more commonly observed in children and infants with TD compared with adults. It is essential that preventive measures against dehydration be instituted at the very onset of diarrhea to prevent the complications discussed previously. Children with diarrhea should be started on oral rehydration solution (ORS).[74]

The World Health Organization (WHO) introduced a new ORS solution with reduced osmolarity for global use in 2002.[74] Oral rehydration solution from the WHO contains glucose (13.5 g/L), which facilitates the absorption of sodium and water in the small intestine; sodium chloride (2.6 g/L) and potassium chloride (1.5 g/L), which replace essential ions that are lost from diarrhea and vomiting; and trisodium citrate (2.9 g/L), which corrects the acidosis resulting from diarrhea and dehydration. Acute diarrhea was reportedly improved by the use of the reduced-osmolarity solutions, as evidenced by less stool output, less vomiting, and a decreased need for supplemental intravenous therapy on reduction of the sodium concentration from 90 to 75 mEq/L, the glucose concentration from 111 to 75 mmol/L, and total osmolarity from 311 to 245 mOsm/L.[74] Small packets of ORS containing glucose and sodium chloride in powder form are available commercially in most developing countries and can be reconstituted with appropriate quantities of clean water as instructed by the manufacturer to prevent hyponatremia or hypernatremia. Families should be advised to carry ORS packets and encouraged to start therapy as soon as diarrhea begins. When commercial ORS packets are not available, home-prepared sugar and salt solution can be made by adding 1 teaspoon of table salt and 8 teaspoons of sugar to 1 L of clean water (bottled or boiling water for 1–3 minutes) and given early during the diarrhea episode to prevent dehydration.[75] However, errors can occur while preparing these products. Infants who are breastfed should continue to be breastfed even if they develop TD. Oral rehydration solution packets are available in the United States from Jianas Brothers (http://rehydrate.org/resources/jianas.htm).

Antimicrobials for Treatment of Traveler's Diarrhea

Because enteric pathogens are the causative agents in most instances of TD, antibiotic treatment remains the best form of TD management. The use of antibiotics and antidiarrheal agents is shown to be safe in adults and to decrease severity and duration of the diarrhea to about 1 day.[27,76,77] Pediatric antibiotic treatment recommendations for TD are limited and elucidated from expert opinions, case reports, and the Centers for Disease Control and Prevention *Health Information for International Travel.* There is belief that the benefits of antibiotics outweigh the risks of potential side effects of antibiotics; thus, many experts believe that antibiotic treatment should be provided in pediatric patients with TD,[78] especially in patients with severe diarrhea (ie, diarrhea associated with fever or blood in stool).

Choice of Antimicrobials

The choice of antimicrobials for TD treatment depends on a number of factors—patient's age, pregnancy status, travel destination, antimicrobial susceptibility pattern of the enteropathogen, duration of diarrhea, drug allergies, and other medications used by the traveler. Antimicrobial choices for TD treatment in children are presented in Table 14-3.

Fluoroquinolones are the antibiotics of choice for treating TD in adults but are not yet approved by the Food and Drug Administration in children and adolescents younger than 18 years. Azithromycin recently gained popularity in treating TD and is the preferred agent for treating TD acquired from South Asia where invasive pathogens, including ciprofloxacin-resistant *Campylobacter,* are more prevalent. Azithromycin is considered the drug of choice in treating TD in children because of its safety, tolerability, and ease of administration. Rifaximin has been approved to treat noninvasive TD caused by *E coli* in persons 12 years and older.[79] Nitazoxanide is another agent used in the treatment of persistent TD caused by *G lamblia* and *Cryptosporidium.*[80]

Other drugs that have been used to treat TD are TMP/SMX, nalidixic acid, and furazolidone. Trimethoprim-sulfamethoxazole is currently not used because of resistance developed by multiple organisms. However, it should be considered for treatment of TD in areas where *Cyclospora* is prevalent, such as in Nepal.[81] Although nalidixic acid treats enteric pathogen, it is not widely used because newer-generation quinolones are now available and more effective. Furazolidone is mainly used for treating *Giardia* and may be effective against a broad range of enteric pathogens.[50,82]

Antidiarrheal Medications for Symptomatic Treatment

Bismuth subsalicylate and loperamide are the 2 most commonly used drugs in adults to provide symptomatic relief from TD. Bismuth subsalicylate has anti-secretory[62] and antibacterial[61] effects, while loperamide has anti-secretory and anti-motility effects.[83] A combination of the anti-peristaltic agent diphenoxylate and atropine (Lomotil) is also being used to treat TD.

Table 14-3. Antimicrobial Choices for Treatment of Traveler's Diarrhea in Children

DRUG	DOSE	PEDIATRIC PREPARATION	ANTIMICROBIAL COVERAGE	COMMENTS
Azithromycin	10 mg/kg/d for 3 d (maximum 500 mg/d)	100 mg/5 mL 200 mg/5 mL	Gram-negative enteric pathogens, Escherichia coli, Salmonella; including multidrug-resistant Shigella and quinolone-resistant Campylobacter	Ease of administration, once-daily dosing; no need to refrigerate; not FDA approved for this indication
Ciprofloxacin	20 to 30 mg/kg/d in 2 divided doses (maximum 1.5 g/d) for 1 to 3 d	250 mg/5 mL	Most gram-negative enteric pathogens, except quinolone-resistant Campylobacter from Southeast Asia (Thailand)	Not FDA approved in children younger than 18 years except for treatment of anthrax and complicated urinary tract infection
Furazolidone	6 mg/kg/d in 4 divided doses for 7 to 10 d (maximum 400 mg/d)	50 mg/15 mL	Antiprotozoal agent, active against Giardia lamblia; also an antibacterial agent, active against enteric gram-negative pathogens (E coli, Salmonella, Shigella, Vibrio cholera)	Used mainly in the treatment of giardiasis or cholera; used with caution in patients with G6PD deficiency; not recommended for infants younger than 1 year
Nalidixic acid	55 mg/kg/d in 4 divided doses (maximum adult dose 4 g/d)	250 mg/5 mL	First-generation quinolone; coverage same as quinolones (ciprofloxacin)	Not given to infants younger than 3 months; duration for TD treatment not determined, likely same as quinolones; in general, not being used because of availability of newer quinolones
Nitazoxanide	1 to 3 y: 100 mg every 12 h 4 to 11 y: 200 mg every 12 h 12 y and older: 500 g every 12 h Taken for 3 d	100 mg/5 mL	Activity against anaerobic bacteria (Clostridium difficile), protozoa (Cryptosporidium, G lamblia), tapeworms (Hymenolepis nana), and viruses (rotavirus)	FDA approved for treatment of cryptosporidiosis and giardiasis

Table 14-3. Antimicrobial Choices for Treatment of Traveler's Diarrhea in Children, continued

DRUG	DOSE	PEDIATRIC PREPARATION	ANTIMICROBIAL COVERAGE	COMMENTS
TMP/SMX	Dose based on TMP component; 5 mg/kg/d divided in 2 doses for 7 to 10 days for treatment of cyclosporidiasis (maximum dose 320 TMP/d)	40 mg TMP/200 mg SMX per 5 mL	Antibacterial agent: most enteric pathogens are resistant to TMP/SMX. Antiprotozoal agent: *Cyclospora cayetanensis, Isospora belli*	Not recommended for use in infants younger than 2 months; not FDA-labeled for treatment of protozoal diseases
Rifaximin	12 y and older: 200 mg 3 times a day for 3 days	No pediatric suspension available	Effective against *E coli* (noninvasive strains ETEC and EAEC); not effective against *Campylobacter jejuni*; effectiveness against *Salmonella* and *Shigella* not known	Poorly absorbed antibiotics; few adverse effects; FDA approved for treatment of TD from noninvasive strains of *E coli* in persons 12 y and older

Abbreviations: EAEC, enteroaggregative *Escherichia coli*; ETEC, enterotoxigenic *Escherichia coli*; FDA, Food and Drug Administration; G6PD, glucose-6-phosphate dehydrogenase; TD, traveler's diarrhea; TMP/SMX, trimethoprim-sulfamethoxazole.

Adapted from Ang IY, Mathur A. Traveler's diarrhea: updates for pediatricians. *Pediatr Ann.* 2008;37(12):814–820. Reprinted with permission from SLACK Inc.

Studies show the benefit of BSS in adults with mild to moderate epi-sodes of TD. Two tablets or 2 oz liquid preparation given every 30 min-utes for a maximum of 2 days reduces the number of unformed stools by 16%.[84] This drug is not widely available in Europe, New Zealand, or Australia.

Although 3 randomized, controlled trials[85–87] compared BSS with placebo in infants and young children with acute watery diarrhea and found that although BSS reduced the duration and severity of diar-rhea, the reduction was modest.[88] The use of BSS for treatment of diar-rhea requires frequent dosing and has potential toxicity from salicylate absorption.[63] Bismuth subsalicylate is not routinely used in the manage-ment of children with gastroenteritis.[89,90]

Loperamide use for children with acute diarrhea was reviewed in a meta-analysis.[91] The study included 13 trials with 1,788 children younger than 12 years (975 children in the loperamide group; 813 children in the placebo group). Dosing of loperamide varied—6 studies used loper-amide doses at less than or equal to 0.25 mg/kg/d, while 4 studies used doses at greater than 0.25 mg/kg/d; the maximum doses were not clear for the 3 remaining studies. The study reported benefit of loperamide use in children with acute diarrhea. Patients in the loperamide group were less likely to continue to have diarrhea at 24 hours, had a shorter dura-tion of diarrhea by 0.8 days, and had a lower count of stools at 24 hours compared with patients in the placebo group. Serious adverse events (ie, ileus, lethargy, or death) were reported in 8 out of 927 children younger than 3 years in the loperamide group and none in the placebo group. The authors concluded that loperamide may be a useful adjunct to oral rehydration and early refeeding in children older than 3 years with mild to no dehydration.

Nevertheless, according to a recent evidence-based review of self-therapy for TD by renowned travel experts, loperamide is not recom-mended in children due to lack of data addressing its efficacy and the concern for associated adverse events.[89]

Other anti-secretory agents are being developed to treat various forms of diarrhea; these drugs are still not available in the United States. Zaldaride maleate is a calmodulin inhibitor that alters the intracellular calcium transport process. Crofelemer is a chloride channel blocker. Racecadotril is an anti-secretory agent that works by inhibiting intestinal enkephalinase and thus prevents the breakdown of endogenous opioids (enkephalins), thereby reducing the secretion of water and electrolytes into the gut without interfering with motility. Zaldaride[92] and crofele-mer[93] are reported to reduce the frequency of stool output in patients with TD. Although racecadotril was found to reduce the stool output and duration of diarrhea in children,[94] it was not evaluated in TD.

■ KEY POINTS

• Traveler's diarrhea is a condition that affects children who travel just as it does adults; however, the treatment, etiology, and actual risk in children are presently ill defined.

• Traveling families should be counseled before they travel on methods to prevent and self-treat TD.

• Mild forms of TD can be effectively managed by the appropriate use of ORS; thus, families should be advised to carry ORS packets and start treatment in children as soon as diarrhea begins.

• In cases of severe diarrhea, self-treatment with antibiotics, such as azithromycin, should be considered. Caregivers should contact local health authorities if there is no improvement, especially after self-treatment with antibiotics.

• Because the majority of TD studies were conducted in adults, further studies are needed to determine the clinical and microbiological characteristics of TD exclusively in children. Additional studies are also needed to further determine the role of genetic factors and susceptibility to TD and its potential complications, such as IBS-PI, so treatment and preventive strategies can be designed to help reduce and prevent TD.

■ REFERENCES

1. Steffen R, Tornieporth N, Clemens SA, et al. Epidemiology of travelers' diarrhea: details of a global survey. *J Travel Med*. 2004;11(4):231–237

2. Steffen R. Epidemiology of traveler's diarrhea. *Clin Infect Dis*. 2005;41(Suppl 8): S536–S540

3. Steer CD, Emond AM, Golding J, Sandhu B. The variation in stool patterns from 1 to 42 months: a population-based observational study. *Arch Dis Child*. 2009;94(3):231–233

4. Travelers' diarrhea. NIH Consensus Development Conference. *JAMA*. 1985;253(18): 2700–2704

5. DuPont HL, Capsuto EG. Persistent diarrhea in travelers. *Clin Infect Dis*. 1996;22(1): 124–128

6. Taylor DN, Connor BA, Shlim DR. Chronic diarrhea in the returned traveler. *Med Clin North Am*. 1999;83(4):1033–1052

7. Cobelens FG, Leentvaar-Kuijpers A, Kleijnen J, Coutinho RA. Incidence and risk factors of diarrhoea in Dutch travellers: consequences for priorities in pre-travel health advice. *Trop Med Int Health*. 1998;3(11):896–903

8. Hoge CW, Shlim DR, Echeverria P, Rajah R, Herrmann JE, Cross JH. Epidemiology of diarrhea among expatriate residents living in a highly endemic environment. *JAMA*. 1996;275(7):533–538

9. Pitzinger B, Steffen R, Tschopp A. Incidence and clinical features of traveler's diarrhea in infants and children. *Pediatr Infect Dis J*. 1991;10(10):719–723

10. Silva FG, Figueiredo A, Varandas L. *J Travel Med.* 2009;16(1):53–54

11. Jiang ZD, Okhuysen PC, Guo DC, et al. Genetic susceptibility to enteroaggregative Escherichia coli diarrhea: polymorphism in the interleukin-8 promotor region. *J Infect Dis.* 2003;188(4):506–511

12. Flores J, DuPont HL, Lee SA, et al. Influence of host interleukin-10 polymorphisms on development of traveler's diarrhea due to heat-labile enterotoxin-producing Escherichia coli in travelers from the United States who are visiting Mexico. *Clin Vaccine Immunol.* 2008;15(8):1194–1198

13. Mohamed JA, DuPont HL, Jiang ZD, et al. A novel single-nucleotide polymorphism in the lactoferrin gene is associated with susceptibility to diarrhea in North American travelers to Mexico. *Clin Infect Dis.* 2007;44(7):945–952

14. Mohamed JA, DuPont HL, Jiang ZD, et al. A single-nucleotide polymorphism in the gene encoding osteoprotegerin, an anti-inflammatory protein produced in response to infection with diarrheagenic Escherichia coli, is associated with an increased risk of nonsecretory bacterial diarrhea in North American travelers to Mexico. *J Infect Dis.* 2009;199(4):477–485

15. Ochoa TJ, Cleary TG. Effect of lactoferrin on enteric pathogens. *Biochimie.* 2009;91(1): 30–34

16. Ellison RT 3rd, Giehl TJ, LaForce FM. Damage of the outer membrane of enteric gram-negative bacteria by lactoferrin and transferrin. *Infect Immun.* 1988;56(11):2774–2781

17. Haversen L, Ohlsson BG, Hahn-Zoric M, Hanson LA, Mattsby-Baltzer I. Lactoferrin down-regulates the LPS-induced cytokine production in monocytic cells via NF-kappa B. *Cell Immunol.* 2002;220(2):83–95

18. Kuhara T, Yamauchi K, Tamura Y, Okamura H. Oral administration of lactoferrin increases NK cell activity in mice via increased production of IL-18 and type I IFN in the small intestine. *J Interferon Cytokine Res.* 2006;26(7):489–499

19. Greenberg DE, Jiang ZD, Steffen R, Verenker MP, DuPont HL. Markers of inflammation in bacterial diarrhea among travelers, with a focus on enteroaggregative Escherichia coli pathogenicity. *J Infect Dis.* 2002;185(7):944–949

20. Bouckenooghe AR, Dupont HL, Jiang ZD, et al. Markers of enteric inflammation in enteroaggregative Escherichia coli diarrhea in travelers. *Am J Trop Med Hyg.* 2000; 62(6):711–713

21. Castellanos-Gonzalez A, Yancey LS, Wang HC, et al. Cryptosporidium infection of human intestinal epithelial cells increases expression of osteoprotegerin: a novel mechanism for evasion of host defenses. *J Infect Dis.* 2008;197(6):916–923

22. O'Ryan M, Prado V, Pickering LK. A millennium update on pediatric diarrheal illness in the developing world. *Semin Pediatr Infect Dis.* 2005;16(2):125–136

23. Rivas M, Miliwebsky E, Chinen I, et al. The epidemiology of hemolytic uremic syndrome in Argentina. Diagnosis of the etiologic agent, reservoirs and routes of transmission. Medcine (B Aires). 2006;66(Suppl 3):27–32

24. McCall BJ, Slinko VG, Smith HV, et al. An outbreak of shiga toxin-producing Escherichia coli infection associated with a school. *Common Dis Intell.* 2010;34(1):54–56

25. Centers for Disease Control and Prevention. Two multistate outbreaks of Shiga toxin-producing Escherichia coli infections linked to beef from a single slaughter facility—United States, 2008. *MMWR.* 2010;59(18):557–560

26. Espié E, Grimont F, Mariana-Kurkjian A. Surveillance of hemolytic uremic syndrome in children less than 15 years of age, a sytem to monitor O157 and non-O157

27. Diemert DJ. Prevention and self-treatment of traveler's diarrhea. *Clin Microbiol Rev.* 2006;19(3):583–594

28. Shah N, DuPont HL, Ramsey DJ. Global etiology of travelers' diarrhea: systematic review from 1973 to the present. *Am J Trop Med Hyg.* 2009;80(4):609–614

29. Adachi JA, Jiang ZD, Mathewson JJ, et al. Enteroaggregative Escherichia coli as a major etiologic agent in traveler's diarrhea in 3 regions of the world. *Clin Infect Dis.* 2001;32(12):1706–1709

30. Ogata K, Kato R, Ito K, Yamada S. Prevalence of Escherichia coli possessing the eaeA gene of enteropathogenic E. coli (EPEC) or the aggR gene of enteroaggregative E. coli (EAggEC) in traveler's diarrhea diagnosed in those returning to Tama, Tokyo from other Asian countries. *Jpn J Infect Dis.* 2002;55(1):14–18

31. Feng P, Weagant SD, Monday SR. Genetic analysis for virulence factors in Escherichia coli O104:H21 that was implicated in an outbreak of hemorrhagic colitis. *J Clin Microbiol.* 2001;39(1):24–28

32. Soderstrom A, Lindberg A, Andersson Y. EHEC O157 outbreak in Sweden from locally produced lettuce, August-September 2005. *Euro Surveill.* 2005;10(9):E050922 050921

33. Ahmed AM, Kawamoto H, Inouye K, et al. Genomic analysis of a multidrug-resistant strain of enterohaemorrhagic Escherichia coli O157:H7 causing a family outbreak in Japan. *J Med Microbiol.* 2005;54(Pt 9):867–872

34. Steffen R, van der Linde F, Gyr K, Schar M. Epidemiology of diarrhea in travelers. *JAMA.* 1983;249(9):1176–1180

35. DuPont HL, Ericsson CD. Prevention and treatment of traveler's diarrhea. *N Engl J Med.* 1993;328(25):1821–1827

36. Snell DM, Bartley C. Osmotic demyelination syndrome following rapid correction of hyponatraemia. *Anaesthesia.* 2008;63(1):92–95

37. Roh JH, Kim JH, Oh K, Kim SG, Park KW, Kim BJ. Cortical laminar necrosis caused by rapidly corrected hyponatremia. *J Neuroimag.* 2008

38. Grant HW, Hadley GP, Wiersma R, Rollins N. Surgical lessons learned from the Shigella dysenteriae type I epidemic. *J R Coll Surg Edinb.* 1998;43(3):160–162

39. Connor BA. Sequelae of traveler's diarrhea: focus on postinfectious irritable bowel syndrome. *Clin Infect Dis.* 2005;41(Suppl 8):S577–S586

40. Saps M, Pensabene L, Di Martino L, et al. Post-infectious functional gastrointestinal disorders in children. *J Pediatr.* 2008;152(6):812–816

41. Spiller RC. Role of infection in irritable bowel syndrome. *J Gastroenterol.* 2007;42 (Suppl 17):41–47

42. Marshall JK. Post-infectious irritable bowel syndrome following water contamination. *Kidney Int Suppl.* 2009;(112):S42–S43

43. Lee KJ, Kim YB, Kim JH, Kwon HC, Kim DK, Cho SW. The alteration of enterochromaffin cell, mast cell, and lamina propria T lymphocyte numbers in irritable bowel syndrome and its relationship with psychological factors. *J Gastroenterol Hepatol.* 2008;23(11):1689–1694

44. Dunlop SP, Jenkins D, Neal KR, Spiller RC. Relative importance of enterochromaffin cell hyperplasia, anxiety, and depression in postinfectious IBS. *Gastroenterology.* 2003;125(6):1651–1659

45. Hammerle CW, Surawicz CM. Updates on treatment of irritable bowel syndrome. *World J Gastroenterol.* 2008;14(17):2639–2649

46. Yanai-Kopelman D, Paz A, Rippel D, Potasman I. Inflammatory bowel disease in returning travelers. *J Travel Med.* 2000;7(6):333–335

47. Peetermans WE, Vonck A. Tropical sprue after travel to Tanzania. *J Travel Med.* 2000; 7(1):33–34

48. Yates JA, Stetz LC. Reiter's syndrome (reactive arthritis) and travelers' diarrhea. *J Travel Med.* 2006;13(1):54–56

49. Backer H. Water disinfection for international and wilderness travelers. *Clin Infect Dis.* 2002;34(3):355–364

50. Ansdell VE, Ericsson CD. Prevention and empiric treatment of traveler's diarrhea. *Med Clin North Am.* 1999;83(4):945–973

51. Mattila L, Siitonen A, Kyronseppa H, Simula II, Peltola H. Risk behavior for travelers' diarrhea among Finnish travelers. *J Travel Med.* 1995;2(2):77–84

52. Kozicki M, Steffen R, Schar M. 'Boil it, cook it, peel it or forget it': does this rule prevent travellers' diarrhoea? *Int J Epidemiol.* 1985;14(1):169–172

53. Shlim DR. Looking for evidence that personal hygiene precautions prevent traveler's diarrhea. *Clin Infect Dis.* 2005;41(Suppl 8):S531–S535

54. Sanofi Pasteur Limited. Dukoral: Oral, Inactivated Travelers' Diarrhea and Cholera Vaccine (Oral Suspension). 2007. http://www.vaccineshoppecanada.com/secure/pdfs/ca/dukoral_e.pdf. Accessed March 14, 2008

55. Jelinek T, Kollaritsch H. Vaccination with Dukoral against travelers' diarrhea (ETEC) and cholera. *Expert Rev Vaccines.* 2008;7(5):561–567

56. Glenn GM, Flyer DC, Ellingsworth LR, et al. Transcutaneous immunization with heat-labile enterotoxin: development of a needle-free vaccine patch. *Expert Rev Vaccines.* 2007;6(5):809–819

57. Frech SA, Dupont HL, Bourgeois AL, et al. Use of a patch containing heat-labile toxin from Escherichia coli against travellers' diarrhoea: a phase II, randomised, double-blind, placebo-controlled field trial. *Lancet.* 2008;371(9629):2019–2025

58. Typhoid immunization. Recommendations of the Immunization Practices Advisory Committee (ACIP). *MMWR Recomm Rep.* 1990;39(RR-10):1–5

59. DuPont HL, Ericsson CD, Farthing MJ, et al. Expert review of the evidence base for prevention of travelers' diarrhea. *J Travel Med.* 2009;16(3):149–160

60. DuPont HL. Therapy for and prevention of traveler's diarrhea. *Clin Infect Dis.* 2007;45(Suppl 1):S78–S84

61. Cornick NA, Silva M, Gorbach SL. In vitro antibacterial activity of bismuth subsalicylate. *Rev Infect Dis.* 1990;12(Suppl 1):S9–S10

62. Ericsson CD, Tannenbaum C, Charles TT. Antisecretory and antiinflammatory properties of bismuth subsalicylate. *Rev Infect Dis.* 1990;12(Suppl 1):S16–S20

63. Pickering LK, Feldman S, Ericsson CD, Cleary TG. Absorption of salicylate and bismuth from a bismuth subsalicylate–containing compound (Pepto-Bismol). *J Pediatr.* 1981;99(4):654–656

64. Hughes RJ. Dangers from hidden salicylates. *Am Pharm.* 1986;NS26(4):5

65. Takahashi O, Noguchi Y, Omata F, Tokuda Y, Fukui T. Probiotics in the prevention of traveler's diarrhea: meta-analysis. *J Clin Gastroenterol.* 2007;41(3):336–337

66. McFarland LV. Meta-analysis of probiotics for the prevention of traveler's diarrhea. *Travel Med Infect Dis.* 2007;5(2):97–105

67. Kligler B, Hanaway P, Cohrssen A. Probiotics in children. *Pediatr Clin North Am.* 2007;54(6):949–967

68. Grady R. Safety profile of quinolone antibiotics in the pediatric population. Pediatr Infect Dis. 2003;22(12)1128–1132

69. Stahmann R, Kuhner S, Shakibaer M, et al. Chondrotoxicity of ciprofloxacin in immature beagle dogs: immunohistochemistry, electron microscopy and drug plasma concentrations. Arch Toxicol. 2000;73(10–11:564–572

70. American Academy of Pediatrics. The use of systematic fluoroquinolones. Pediatrics. 2006;118(3):1287–1292

71. Tribble DR, Sanders JW, Pang LW, et al. Traveler's diarrhea in Thailand: randomized, double-blind trial comparing single-dose and 3-day azithromycin-based regimens with a 3-day levofloxacin regimen. *Clin Infect Dis*. 2007;44(3):338–346

72. Gomi H, Jiang ZD, Adachi JA, et al. In vitro antimicrobial susceptibility testing of bacterial enteropathogens causing traveler's diarrhea in four geographic regions. *Antimicrob Agents Chemother*. 2001;45(1):212–216

73. DuPont HL, Jiang ZD, Okhuysen PC, et al. Antibacterial chemoprophylaxis in the prevention of traveler's diarrhea: evaluation of poorly absorbed oral rifaximin. *Clin Infect Dis*. 2005;41(Suppl 8):S571–S576

74. King CK, Glass R, Bresee JS, Duggan C. Managing acute gastroenteritis among children: oral rehydration, maintenance, and nutritional therapy. *MMWR Recomm Rep*. 2003;52(RR-16):1–16

75. Dale J. Oral rehydration solutions in the management of acute gastroenteritis among children. *J Pediatr Health Care*. 2004;18(4):211–212

76. Ericsson CD. Travelers' diarrhea. Epidemiology, prevention, and self-treatment. *Infect Dis Clin North Am*. 1998;12(2):285–303

77. Essers B, Burnens AP, Lanfranchini FM, et al. Acute community-acquired diarrhea requiring hospital admission in Swiss children. *Clin Infect Dis*. 2000;31(1):192–196

78. Mackell S. Traveler's diarrhea in the pediatric population: etiology and impact. *Clin Infect Dis*. 2005;41(Suppl 8):S547–S552

79. Keenum AJ, Stockton MD. Rifaximin (Xifaxan) for traveler's diarrhea. *Am Fam Physician*. 2005;72(12):2525–2526

80. Anderson VR, Curran MP. Nitazoxanide: a review of its use in the treatment of gastrointestinal infections. *Drugs*. 2007;67(13):1947–1967

81. Hoge CW, Echeverria P, Rajah R, et al. Prevalence of Cyclospora species and other enteric pathogens among children less than 5 years of age in Nepal. *J Clin Microbiol*. 1995;33(11):3058–3060

82. DuPont HL, Ericsson CD, Galindo E, et al. Furazolidone versus ampicillin in the treatment of traveler's diarrhea. *Antimicrob Agents Chemother*. 1984;26(2):160–163

83. Epple HJ, Fromm M, Riecken EO, Schulzke JD. Antisecretory effect of loperamide in colon epithelial cells by inhibition of basolateral K+ conductance. *Scand J Gastroenterol*. 2001;36(7):731–737

84. Ericsson CD. Nonantimicrobial agents in the prevention and treatment of traveler's diarrhea. *Clin Infect Dis*. 2005;41(Suppl 8):S557–S563

85. Sorianobrucher H, Avendano P, Oryan M, et al. Bismuth subsalicylate in the treatment of acute diarrhea in children—a clinical study. *Pediatrics*. 1991;87(1):18–27

86. Chowdhury HR, Yunus M, Zaman K, et al. The efficacy of bismuth subsalicylate in the treatment of acute diarrhoea and the prevention of persistent diarrhoea. *Acta Paediatr*. 2001;90(6):605–610

87. Figueroa-Quintanilla D, Salazar-Lindo E, Sack RB, et al. A controlled trial of bismuth subsalicylate in infants with acute watery diarrheal disease. *N Engl J Med*. 1993;328(23):1653–1658

88. Guarino A, Bruzzese E. Which place for bismuth subsalicylate in the treatment of enteric infections? *Acta Paediatr*. 2001;90(6):601–604

89. DuPont HL, Ericsson CD, Farthing MJ, et al. Expert review of the evidence base for self-therapy of travelers' diarrhea. *J Travel Med*. 2009;16(3):161–171

90. Guarino A, Albano F, Ashkenazi S, et al. European Society for Paediatric Gastroenterology, Hepatology, and Nutrition/European Society for Paediatric Infectious Diseases evidence-based guidelines for the management of acute gastroenteritis in children in Europe: executive summary. *J Pediatr Gastroenterol Nutr.* 2008;46(5):619–621

91. Li ST, Grossman DC, Cummings P. Loperamide therapy for acute diarrhea in children: systematic review and meta-analysis. *PLoS Med.* 2007;4(3):e98

92. DuPont HL, Ericsson CD, Mathewson JJ, Marani S, Knellwolf-Cousin AL, Martinez-Sandoval FG. Zaldaride maleate, an intestinal calmodulin inhibitor, in the therapy of travelers' diarrhea. *Gastroenterology.* 1993;104(3):709–715

93. DiCesare D, DuPont HL, Mathewson JJ, et al. A double blind, randomized, placebo-controlled study of SP-303 (Provir) in the symptomatic treatment of acute diarrhea among travelers to Jamaica and Mexico. *Am J Gastroenterol.* 2002;97(10):2585–2588

94. Tormo R, Polanco I, Salazar-Lindo E, Goulet O. Acute infectious diarrhoea in children: new insights in antisecretory treatment with racecadotril. *Acta Paediatr.* 2008;97(8):1008–1015

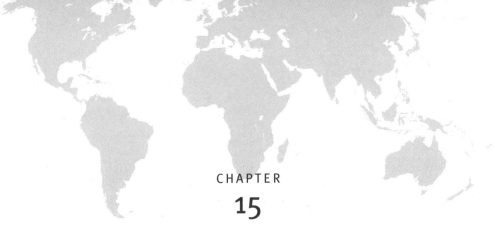

CHAPTER

15

Injury Prevention

Victor Balaban, PhD
David Sleet, PhD, FAAHB

■ INTRODUCTION

World travel has reached unprecedented proportions in the past decade, with international tourist arrivals increasing from 541 million in 1995 to more than 842 million in 2007. This figure includes just over 64 million Americans who traveled outside the United States.[1] In today's increasingly globalized world, travel itineraries are constantly expanding to include new locations previously inaccessible to most travelers, making many travel destinations accessible to new populations, including children and adolescents. The number of children who travel or live outside their home country has also increased dramatically; an estimated 1.9 million children travel overseas each year.[2]

Children are now exposed to greater injury risks while traveling as a result of the increase in the number of travelers. The majority of travelers do not encounter any serious health problems; however, injuries are one of the leading causes of death among international travelers and the leading cause of death to healthy Americans traveling overseas. Injuries cause 23% of tourist deaths, compared to infectious diseases which account for approximately 2% of deaths.[3] Exposure to unfamiliar and perhaps risky environments; differences in language and communications, product safety, vehicle standards, and rules and regulations; a carefree spirit while on holiday or vacation leading to more risk-taking behaviors; and overreliance on travel and tour operators to protect one's safety and security all contribute to the number of injuries that occur while traveling.

Injuries are not inevitable and can be prevented or controlled. Clinicians can play a critical role in helping reduce the injury risk among children and adolescents who travel by discussing travel and country risk factors and strategies to help avoid injury. Travelers should be advised about traffic and water safety, environmental risks, and personal safety. They should be prepared to develop a plan for dealing with medical emergencies and be advised on the importance of purchasing adequate medical and emergency evacuation insurance coverage. Adult caregivers should be prepared to provide closer supervision of children, be aware of basic first-aid procedures, and know how to access appropriate care, if needed, at their travel location.[4]

■ EPIDEMIOLOGY OF PEDIATRIC TRAVEL INJURIES

Epidemiology of Pediatric Injuries

Injuries account for about 40% of all child deaths throughout the world.[5] In 2004, injuries caused approximately 950,000 deaths in children and adolescents younger than 18 years.[5] Worldwide, injuries account for 6 of the 15 leading causes of death among persons 5 to 44 years of age. Unintentional injuries account for almost 90% of these cases and are the leading cause of death for children 10 to 19 years of age.[6] The majority of these injuries are the result of traffic crashes, drowning, burns (fire or scalds), falls, or poisoning. Head injuries are the single most common—and potentially most severe—type of injury sustained by children.

Injuries vary by age. Suffocation, fires, drowning, and falls are the leading causes of death among infants in many countries. Among 1- to 4-year-old children, drowning is the leading cause of injury-related death, followed by motor vehicle traffic crashes (including pedestrian injuries) and fires (as children start to move more independently). For example, drowning, road traffic injuries, and animal bites are the main causes of death in children 5 to 9 years of age in Asia.[6]

Cuts and bruises are the most frequently seen injuries in children. Arm and leg fractures are the most common nonfatal injuries requiring hospitalization in children younger than 15 years.[6]

Epidemiology of Pediatric Travel Injuries

Global data on the incidence of various pediatric injuries associated with international travel are limited. It is likely that many of the injury risks that children face while traveling are similar to the risks they face at home, but the levels of protection available overseas and access to quality medical care may be substandard or absent. Hence, closer supervision of children while traveling overseas may be warranted to prevent injuries.

Mortality

A recent analysis found that an estimated 2,276 US citizens died from injuries and violence while in foreign countries (excluding deaths in Iraq and Afghanistan) from 2003 to 2005. Motor vehicle crashes were the most common cause (34%), followed by homicide (17%) and drowning (13%). Inside the United States, motor vehicle crashes accounted for 27% of injury-related deaths, homicide 11%, and drowning 2% during 2003.[3] In a study that estimated the American tourist population using data from the World Tourist Organization, the injury mortality rate among US international travelers was higher than that among Americans residing abroad.[7]

Morbidity

Although injuries may be the most likely health hazard for international travelers, very little epidemiologic data are available on the incidence of nonfatal injuries occurring during travel.[8] Injuries are reported as the primary reason US travelers are transported back to the United States by air medical evacuation; the main nonfatal causes are motor vehicle traffic accidents (45%); falls (8%); sports injuries, including diving into shallow water (4.5%); boating incidents (2%); aircraft crashes (1.5%); and burns and electrical shocks (1%).[9]

■ COMMON PEDIATRIC TRAVEL INJURIES

Road Traffic Injuries

Mortality

Road traffic injuries are crashes involving drivers and passengers of motor vehicles, trucks, minivans, buses, motorcycles and motorbikes, and bicycles, as well as pedestrians hit by a motor vehicle. In 2004, road traffic injuries accounted for approximately 262,000 deaths among children younger than 1 year to 19 years, which accounts for almost 30% of all injury deaths among children.[6] Globally, road traffic injuries are the leading cause of death among 15- to 19-year-olds and the second leading cause among 5- to 14-year-olds. Children up to 9 years of age are more likely to be accompanied by parents when traveling, in vehicles or as pedestrians, while older children tend to travel more independently, initially as pedestrians and later as bicyclists, motorcyclists, and finally drivers and passengers. The higher rates of mortality among older children are likely a result of this increased mobility as well as their increased tendency to engage in risk-taking behaviors.[6]

Although young children do not drive motor vehicles, they do use roads as pedestrians, bicyclists, motorcyclists, and vehicle passengers.[3] Children's small stature makes them less visible and increases their injury risk on the road. Children are also more likely than adults to sustain a head or neck injury. A child's head, chest, abdomen, and limbs are still growing and relatively soft, making them physically more vulnerable to the impact of injury.[6]

Morbidity

The number of children injured or disabled each year as a result of road traffic crashes is not precisely known but is estimated at around 10 million. This estimate is based on data from health care institutions, suggesting that children make up 20% to 25% of people admitted to a hospital because of injuries from a motor vehicle crash.[6] However, community-based surveys from Asia suggest that figure could be much higher.[10]

Motor vehicle traffic injures are the 11th highest cause of death and the 10th highest cause of burden of disease in children younger than 15 years.[6] A child's head and limbs are the most common parts of the body injured in a motor vehicle crash. Injury severity varies depending on the child's age, road user, and whether protective devices (eg, seat belts) were used.

Risk Factors

Road traffic injuries are common among international travelers of all ages for a variety of reasons. In many lower-income areas of the world, unsafe roads and vehicles and an inadequate transportation infrastructure contribute to traffic crashes and injuries. Streets and roads in many countries often do not have crosswalks, signals and signs, and pedestrian refuge islands. Safely driving or crossing the road in a country where cars drive on the opposite side can be challenging and dangerous. An additional risk for crashes and injuries in developing countries includes cars, buses, and large trucks sharing the road with pedestrians, motorbikes, bicycles, rickshaws, and animals. Other factors that can increases the risk for motor vehicle crashes and injuries include

- Lack of familiarity with roads
- Use of alcohol, sleep aids, or drugs (including use among hired drivers)
- Driving on the opposite side of the road
- Poorly made or maintained vehicles that lack seat belts, air bags, child restraints, or rollover protection

- Travel fatigue and jet lag
- Poor visibility from lack of adequate lighting on the road and on the vehicle[3]
- Overcrowded buses and public transport conveyances
- Poorly constructed or designed roads, especially in mountainous terrain

Drowning

Mortality

Global data show that approximately 28% of all unintentional injury deaths among children are from drowning.[6] The overall global rate for drowning among children is 7.2 deaths per 100,000 population. Approximately 175,000 children and adolescents younger than 20 years around the world died as a result of drowning in 2004.[6] Drowning is the leading cause of injury-related deaths in children in many southeast Asian and western Pacific countries. Drowning accounts for 13% of deaths among Americans abroad and is the second leading cause of death in young travelers.[4] Drowning is also the leading cause of injury death among Americans visiting countries where water recreation is a major tourist attraction. There were 3,582 fatal unintentional drownings in the United States in 2005, an average of 10 deaths per day. An additional 710 people died in boating-related incidents, which included drowning and other causes.[3] Children 14 years and younger account for more than 25% of fatal drowning victims in the United States. In addition, drowning is the second leading cause of unintentional injury-related death among US children 1 to 14 years of age.[2]

Morbidity

There are no accurate estimates of serious nonfatal cases of drowning among children and adolescents. The World Health Organization (WHO) global estimates for nonfatal drowning among children younger than 1 year to 14 years are between 2 and 3 million each year.[6] For every child who dies from drowning in the United States, another 4 receive emergency department care.[11] Nonfatal drowning can cause brain damage that may result in long-term disabilities such as memory problems, learning disabilities, and permanent loss of basic functioning (ie, permanent vegetative state). One study also found that two thirds of quadriplegic spinal injury admissions were linked with a history of steeply diving into shallow water while on vacation.[12]

Risk Factors

The risks factors for drowning among international travelers are not clearly defined but are suspected to be related to unfamiliarity with local water currents, riptides, and changing water conditions. General risk factors for drowning in children and adolescents, whether traveling or at home, include:

- *Age and developmental stage.* Children younger than 5 years are at highest risk for drowning, followed by adolescents 15 to 19 years of age. A small child can drown in a few centimeters of water in a bucket, bath, or agricultural setting; children younger than 1 year most often drown in bathtubs, buckets, or toilets. In the US, most drowning occurs in residential swimming pools among children 1 to 4 years of age.[13]
- *Gender.* Boys drown nearly twice as often as girls.
- *Lack of lifeguards or parent/caregiver supervision.* Many swimming facilities may not have lifeguards. Studies show that lifeguards, especially those trained in attention and surveillance, can be a protective factor.[14,15] In addition, inadequate parent or caregiver supervision is an important risk factor for pediatric drowning. Most young children who drown in pools were last seen in the home, were out of sight less than 5 minutes, and were in the care of one or both parents.[16]
- *Lack of barriers.* In many countries, swimming pools, open bodies of water, wells, and rainwater collection container systems are not protected by fencing or barriers to keep children from gaining access.[17]
- *Natural water settings.* Most drowning in children older than 15 years occurs in natural water settings, such as lakes, rivers, and oceans and seas.[18] Children may not recognize hazards in an unfamiliar ocean or river. Hypothermia, rather than drowning, is the main cause of death at sea.
- *Absence of life jackets.* In 2006, the US Coast Guard received reports of 4,967 boating incidents, 3,474 injured boaters, and 710 boating deaths. Among those who drowned, 9 out of 10 were not wearing life jackets.[3]
- *Unsafe vessels.* People are regularly transported in unsafe or overcrowded boats in many countries. Capsizing boats, ferries, and launches are a particular risk during the rainy season and certain times of the year, such as national holidays, when many people are likely to crowd onto boats.[3] Vessel safety standards and their enforcement vary widely around the world.
- *Alcohol.* Alcohol use is involved in up to half of adolescent and adult deaths associated with water recreation and about 1 in 5 reported boating fatalities.[19] Alcohol can trigger hypoglycemia and cause a rapid

fall in body temperature, and it influences balance, coordination, and judgment. In addition, sun exposure and heat heighten the effects of alcohol.

- *Seizure disorders.* Drowning is the most common cause of unintentional death among children and adolescents with seizure disorders.[6]
- *Pool and spas.* Serious injuries can occur near outlets where suction is strong enough to catch small body parts or hair, trapping the head underwater. Other risks include slipping and tripping, which can lead to loss of consciousness on impact.

Burns

Mortality

Just more than 310,000 people worldwide died as a result of fire-related burns in 2004; 30% were younger than 20 years.[5] Fire-related burns are the 11th leading cause of death for children between 1 and 9 years of age. Children are at a high risk for death from burns; the global rate is 3.9 deaths per 100,000 population. Globally, infants have the highest death rate. Small children have a lower resistance to burn trauma and are less able to escape in a fire emergency. Smoke inhalation is strongly associated with mortality for children older than 3 years.

Morbidity

Little global data are available for nonfatal outcomes from burns. However, the 2004 WHO Global Burden of Disease project makes it clear that burns are an important contributor to the overall disease toll in children.[5]

While burns from fire contribute to the majority of burn-related deaths in children, scalds and contact burns are an important factor in overall morbidity and a significant cause of disability. The skin of infants and young children burns more deeply and quickly and at lower temperatures than thicker skin of adults. In addition, children's larger ratio of body surface area to volume means the size of a burn for a given volume of hot liquid will be greater than for an adult and there will be more fluid lost from the burnt area, thus complicating injury management. Chemical and electrical burns are relatively rare among children.[5]

Scald burns are the most frequent type of burn among children younger than 6 years. Typical scald burns occur when a child pulls down a container of hot fluid, such as a cup of tea or coffee, which spills on the child's face, upper extremities, and trunk. These are typically superficial second-degree burns. Despite the pain this causes the child and the parents' distress, these burns will typically heal within weeks, leaving little or no permanent damage.[5]

Burns to the palms of the hands are common among infants younger than 1 year as a result of touching cooking equipment, heaters, hot-water pipes, and cups containing hot liquid. Such contact burns may be deep and require prolonged and careful therapy during the healing phase to prevent flexure contractures because the skin on a child's palm is thinner and withdrawal reflexes are slower.[5]

Risk Factors

Fires can be a significant risk in developing countries where building codes are not present or enforced and where there may not be smoke alarms or access to emergency services.[3] Other risk factors for burn injuries in children include

- *Unsafe equipment.* Hotels and residences in many countries are not designed to accommodate the safety of small children and often have unsafe electrical appliances, plugs, wires, and other connections that increase the risk of electrical burns.[5] Bathroom faucets may use different letters or colors for hot and cold water, and hot water from the tap may be scalding (in some developed countries, plumbing standards require temperature-limiting devices to protect from accidental scald burns). In addition, equipment used for heat, light, and cooking during trekking and camping may be inherently unsafe. Heating or cooking on open fires that are not enclosed or that stand at ground level pose significant dangers to children.[17]
- *Preexisting conditions.* Disabled children have a significantly higher incidence of burn injuries than nondisabled children. Children who suffer from uncontrolled epilepsy also appear to be at greater risk for burn injuries.[5]
- *Fireworks.* Many countries celebrate religious or national festivals with fireworks, which pose a significant risk of burn injuries for children, particularly adolescent boys.[5] Fireworks manufactured in many foreign countries can be inherently dangerous and pose risks to anyone handling them. Firework displays should always be left to the professionals.
- *Environmental hazards.* Flammable substances such as gasoline, kerosene, and paraffin can combust easily and are poisonous. Most children's burns occur in the kitchen, or in areas where food is prepared. This poses a special risk to children who congregate near the fire or stove during meal preparation.

- *Sun exposure.* In addition to skin cancers, overexposure to the sun, especially in countries close to the equator, can cause severe, debilitating sunburn and sunstroke, particularly in light-skinned individuals. Unprotected skin that is exposed to sunlight can cause a variety of dermatologic problems—some acute and some cumulative. Adverse skin reactions can also occur with sun exposure and the use of some antimalarial drugs and antibiotics. Ultraviolet radiation may penetrate clear water to a depth of 1 m or more.[20]

Falls

Mortality

An estimated 424,000 people of all ages died from falls worldwide in 2004, nearly 47,000 of whom were children and youth younger than 20 years. Falls are the 12th leading cause of death among 5- to 9-year-olds and 15- to 19-year-olds.[5]

Morbidity

Global nonfatal injury statistics are not readily available. In most countries, falls are the most common type of childhood injury seen in emergency departments, accounting for 25% to 52% of assessments.[21] In addition, the Global School-based Student Health Survey identified falls as the leading cause of injury among 13- to 15-year-olds in 26 countries.[22]

Limb fractures, particularly of the forearm, are the most common type of fall-related injury in children beyond the age of infancy because they tend to protect their heads with their arm when falling.[23] Falls are also a leading cause of traumatic brain injury, especially in young children, with a significant risk of long-term consequences. Approximately one third of the 1.4 million people who suffer traumatic brain injuries in the United States are children aged 0 to 14 years who have disproportionately higher fall rates than other age groups.[6]

Risk Factors

Risk factors for falls in children include
- *Gender.* Boys are at greatest risk for fatal and nonfatal falls.
- *Family and social factors.* Falls in children are associated with single parenthood, unemployment, younger maternal age, low maternal education, caregiver stress and mental health problems, and limitations in health care access.[6]

- *Height of fall.* In general, the greater the height from which a child falls, the more severe the injury. Fall injuries from heights of more than 2 stories typically involve windows, balconies, and roofs. Falls from stairs, trees, and playground equipment are also common, as are falls into ditches, wells, shafts, and other holes in the ground.[6] Trees can be particularly hazardous, as can bunk beds, particularly in unfamiliar settings.[17]
- *Physical environment.* Safety regulations may not be enforced or even exist in many lower-income countries. As a result, there may be a variety of risks to children such as high-rise buildings without window guards, low balcony railings with enough space for young children to crawl through, or amusement park rides that are rarely inspected.[17] In addition, falls are more likely to occur with greater exposure to overcrowding and environmental hazards.[6]
- *Animals.* In recent years, studies from several developing countries have shown an increase in the number of children and young people presenting to the hospital as a result of falling from horses[6] and pets.[24]

Bites and Stings

Morbidity and Mortality

Children tend to be fascinated with animals and use poor judgment around them, and may not report minor licks and bites. Children are particularly vulnerable to dog bites as a result of their small stature and because their face is usually close to the dog's mouth. Dog bites are a potentially serious injury and a frequent cause of hospitalization; however, they are rarely fatal. Dog bite–related injuries are highest among children 5 to 9 years of age. Children are more likely than adults to be bitten on the head or neck, which can lead to more severe injuries.[6]

Animal bites in many developing countries can carry the added risk of rabies. In many areas where rabies exists, including India, China, and many parts of Africa, 40% of rabies cases occur in children. Rabies is the 10th most common cause of death from infection worldwide. There is evidence that between 30% and 60% of dog bite victims in endemic areas of canine rabies are children younger than 15 years.[6] Children who die from rabies were not treated or received inadequate postexposure treatment. Many bite victims do not receive rabies immunoglobulin due to a perennial global shortage.

Travelers to tropical, subtropical, and desert areas should be aware of the risks from venomous snake, scorpion, and spider bites and stings. All venomous bites should be considered a medical emergency requiring immediate medical attention. Aquatic animals, such as eels, stingrays, scorpion fish, jellyfish, and sea lice, can inflict serious harm. Swimming in waters populated with these organisms carries a high risk for children.

Mosquito, tick, flea, fly, and other insect bites can transmit diseases such as river blindness, dengue fever, Lyme disease, and sleeping sickness in some parts of the world. Repellents should be used in strict accordance with manufacturer instructions; the dosage must not be exceeded, especially for young children and during pregnancy.[20]

Risk Factors

In many areas where rabies exists, 40% of cases occur in children. Stray dogs are common in many developing countries. Bat caves are popular tourist attractions in many countries. Monkeys, some of which have rabies, congregate around temples and other shrines in Southeast Asia.[2,17] Swimming in unfamiliar waters, camping without repellents or protection, outdoor exposure at night, and walking in hostile and unfamiliar environments can increase bites and stings.

Poisoning

Mortality

An estimated 345,814 people of all ages died worldwide as a result of poisoning in 2004. Of this number, an estimated 45,000 were children and adolescents younger than 20 years.[5] Poisoning is the 13th leading cause of death among 15- to 19-year-olds. The global death rate from poisoning is 1.8 per 100,000 population for children younger than 20 years.[6]

Children younger than 1 year have the highest rate of fatal poisoning. The higher mortality rate in very young infants may be explained by greater susceptibility of the infant body to damage by toxins.[6]

Morbidity

Accurate global data on nonfatal outcomes of poisoning are not available. Data for 2006 from the American Association of Poison Control Centers showed that the most common poisonings among children were caused by pharmaceutical products. Inquiries relating to children younger than 6 years made up 50.9% of cases and 2.4% of total reported fatalities.[25]

Risk Factors

Common risk factors for children accidentally ingesting toxic substances include

- *Appearance.* Studies show that children prefer liquids over solids; clear liquids over dark; and small solids over large, and are more likely to ingest these.[6] Brightly colored solid medications may also be more attractive to children.
- *Storage and access.* A toxic substance within reach of a child is the most obvious risk factor for ingestion. Children may still ingest dangerous products that are stored in distinctive containers with visual warning labels (eg, skull and crossbones) because they often do not understand the meaning of these signs.[6] Some studies indicate that stickers, such as skull and crossbones and Mr. Yuk, are ineffective deterrents and can even attract children to the toxic product.[26,27]
- *Safety precautions.* No child-resistant container is the perfect deterrent. Tests show that up to 20% of children between the ages of 42 and 51 months may be able to open a child-resistant container.[28] The poison-prevention value of a tamperproof container is lost when the top is not replaced properly. Thus, child-resistant containers should never replace parent or caregiver supervision.

Data from poison control centers and hospitals[6] indicate that the most common agents involved in child poisonings include

- Over-the-counter medications, such as aspirin, ibuprofen, cough and cold remedies, iron tablets, antihistamines, and anti-inflammatory drugs
- Prescription medications, such as antidepressants, narcotics, and analgesics
- Recreational drugs, such as cannabis and cocaine
- Household products, such as bleach, disinfectants, detergents, cleaning agents, cosmetics, and vinegar
- Pesticides, including insecticides, rodenticides, and herbicides
- Poisonous plants
- Animal or insect repellent

Factors determining the severity of poisoning and its outcome in children include

- Poison type
- Dose
- Formulation
- Exposure route
- Child's age
- Presence of other poisons
- Child's nutrition status
- Presence of other diseases or injuries

■ ADVICE FOR PARENTS AND CAREGIVERS

Clinicians should advise parents that the best way to keep their children safe is to practice prevention.[3,8,17,29] Families should be encouraged to use their judgment about what types of travel are appropriate for their children. Families should be advised to

- Check the health, safety, and security information for their destinations on the Centers for Disease Control and Prevention Travelers' Health (www.cdc.gov/travel) and the US Department of State (www.travel.state.gov) Web sites.
- Consider learning basic first aid and cardiopulmonary resuscitation, as well as bringing a travel medical (first aid) kit customized to their anticipated itinerary and activities. The kit should include basic health information (eg, name, birth date, vaccination history, current medication use [with dosages noted], known medical allergies, blood type, chronic health conditions). Antiseptic solutions and lotions, bandaging supplies, and perhaps splinting material could also be included.[17]
- Educate their children. Parents should inform and educate their children in age-appropriate ways about risk factors for injuries, as well as how injuries can be prevented. Parents should always encourage their children to wear safety devices, and they should act as role models by adopting safe behaviors and using safety devices.[2,17]
- Wear MedicAlert identification if they have chronic health conditions. Such identification may help a health care professional access medical information about the traveler in event of an emergency.[17]
- Avoid unnecessary risk-taking while traveling. Understandably, many tourists travel to participate in activities that are not part of their usual routine. Doing so provides novel experiences but can also lead to situations in which the traveler is completely inexperienced (eg, driving a motorcycle for the first time). Adolescents in particular may be inclined to take risks that can lead to injury or death.[4]
- Identify doctors and hospitals in the cities they are visiting prior to departure. Names and addresses of local health care professionals at the travel destination can be obtained from a number of sources, including the International Society of Travel Medicine (www.istm.org) and International Association for Medical Assistance to Travellers (www.iamat.org). Embassies and consulates also have lists of local English-speaking physicians.[3,17,29]
- In the event of an emergency, try to take their children to the largest medical facility in the area. Such facilities are more likely to have pediatric units and trauma services. Parents should ask for the diagnosis, test results, and treatments administered before leaving the facility;

this information will be very helpful for ongoing treatment.[17] Travelers should seek medical care in a neighboring country if medical care facilities in the country they are visiting cannot provide rapid, effective, or safe medical treatment.

- Carry an international-capable cell phone for emergency contacts within the country of travel, as well as for any help needed while abroad.

Some specific recommendations that clinicians should provide to travelers for avoiding common pediatric travel injuries are described as follows:

Motor Vehicle Traffic Injuries

- Bring a child safety seat(s) from home.
- Use safety belts and child safety seats whenever possible. Safety belts reduce the risk of death in a crash by 45% to 60%, child safety seats by 54%, and infant seats by 70%.[3]
- When possible
  — Rent newer, better-maintained vehicles with safety belts and air bags.
  — Avoid riding a motorcycle or motorbike for the first time. Vacationing in a foreign land is not a safe way to learn how to ride.
  — Rent larger vehicles if possible because they provide more protection in a crash.
  — Try to ride only in taxis with functional safety belts, and ride in the rear seat.
  — Avoid driving at night or on mountainous roads (or both).
- Wear a helmet when riding a motorcycle, motorbike, bicycle, or horse. Helmets should be brought from home if they are likely to be unavailable at the travel destination.
- Consider hiring a driver who is familiar with the travel destination and language and is an expert in maneuvering through local traffic.
- Avoid riding on overcrowded, overweight, top-heavy busses or minivans, or with any driver who has consumed or is consuming alcohol.
- Visit the Web sites of the Association for Safe International Road Travel (www.asirt.org) and Make Roads Safe (www.makeroadssafe.org). These organizations have useful safety tips for international travelers, including road safety checklists and country-specific driving risks.

Drowning

- Closely supervise children around water at all times.
- Children should always wear flotation devices, such as life jackets. Appropriate water safety devices, such as life vests, may not be available abroad; families should consider bringing them from home.
- Wear protective footwear in water to avoid injury in marine environments.
- Avoid unsafe or overcrowded vessels.
- Seek advice from local sources or tour guides about potential dangers, such as currents and tides, before swimming in open water.
- Travelers who wish to participate in potentially dangerous water activities such as diving and jet skiing should only use reliable, scheduled, and official water sports services. Travelers should ensure they are thoroughly briefed by operators on safety procedures of the particular water sport in which they will be participating. Operators should ensure the safety of tourists as much as possible.[2,3,17]

Burns

- Select accommodations on the sixth floor or below (fire ladders generally cannot reach above the sixth floor) whenever possible to minimize the risk of fire-related injuries. If possible, stay in hotels with smoke alarms and preferably sprinkler systems. Carry your own battery-operated smoke alarm if you are not sure that the hotel has them. Be alert for improperly vented heating devices, which may cause poisoning from carbon monoxide. Travelers should identify 2 escape routes from buildings and remember to escape a fire by crawling under the smoke and covering their mouth with a wet cloth.[3]
- Teach children to stop, drop, and roll in the event that their clothes catch on fire.
- If a child does suffer a serious burn, she should be stabilized before being transported to a hospital. Explain to parents that
  - The overall aim of first aid is to cool the burn and prevent additional burning and contamination.
  - First aid treatment for burn injuries is best accomplished with cool, clean water.
  - Traditional treatments, such as applying butter, oil, or other substances on burns, can be harmful, as they can cause the skin to slough away, leaving lower layers exposed and susceptible to infection.[6]

- The American College of Surgeons and American Burn Association recommend that children with the following conditions be treated in a burn center[30]:
  - Partial-thickness (second-degree) burns greater than 10% of the total body surface area
  - Burns involving the face, hands, feet, genitalia, perineum, or major joints
  - Full-thickness (third-degree) burns
- To avoid scalds, always check the temperature of water coming from the tap and supervise young children bathing to reduce the chances of expelling scalding water.

Falls

- Wear a helmet when engaging in adventure activities (eg, zip lines, rock climbing, horseback riding). Bring a helmet from home if they are unlikely to be available at the travel destination.[2,3,17]
- Parents must be reminded that hotels and homes they visit may not be childproofed. There may not be gates on stairs or locks on kitchen cabinets, and there may be floor and rug hazards, accessible medications, and matches.[3,17]

Bites and Stings

- Children and their families should be counseled to avoid all stray or unfamiliar animals, insects, and rodents.
- Never leave infants or young children alone with a dog.
- Do not allow children to play with a dog unless an adult supervises.
- Children should be taught to immediately tell adults about any contact, bites, or stings from any animal or insect.
- Seek medical care immediately in the event of a bite. Thoroughly wash mammal-associated injuries with water and soap (and povidone iodine if available) and promptly assess the child to see if rabies post-exposure prophylaxis is needed.
- Avoid eating food around animals, such as dogs or monkeys, in case they jump for the food and bite the child in the process.[2,3,6,17]
- Obtain local advice on the presence of dangerous aquatic animals before swimming.
- Wear shoes when walking on the shore or water's edge.
- Seek medical advice if a bite or sting from a poisonous animal is suspected.

Poisoning

- Keep all drugs in secure containers and locations that young children cannot reach.
- Avoid taking medicine in front of children because they often copy adults.
- Do not call medicine "candy."
- Be aware of any legal or illegal drugs that guests may bring into your home. Do not let guests leave drugs where children can find them, such as in a pillbox, purse, backpack, or coat pocket.
- Do not put the next dose of medicine on the counter or table where children can reach it.
- Never leave children alone with household products or drugs. If an adult is using chemical products or taking medicine and has to do something else, such as answer the phone, children should accompany the adult.
- In the event of accidental poisoning
  - Remain calm.
  - Call a doctor or go to a hospital or clinic immediately. Carry the Poison Help number, 1-800-222-1222 (in the United States), for immediate advice on a possible poisoning incident.
  - Try to have the following information ready:
    - Victim's age and weight
    - Container or bottle of the poison, if available
    - Time of the poison exposure[2,3,6,17]

■ HEALTH INSURANCE AND MEDICAL EVACUATION ISSUES

Travel insurance is one of the most important safety nets available to travelers in the event of accidents and injuries; travel health advisers should reinforce this advice.[4] Clinicians and health advisors should recommend that travelers consider purchasing special travel insurance that includes medical evacuation or air ambulance transport if their destinations include countries where there may be difficulties accessing adequate medical care.[2,3] Such insurance generally provides worldwide, 24-hour telephone hotlines that direct callers to English-speaking physicians and hospitals, pay for treatment and hospitalization at the time of the incidence, and when medically indicated, arrange and pay for evacuation to a medical facility that can provide necessary treatment. Examples of companies that provide such insurance include Medex (www.medexassist.com) and International SOS (www.internationalsos.com).[17]

Travelers should verify insurance coverage for illnesses and accidents while abroad before departure. They should be advised to read their policies carefully to see what is covered and to check for any exclusions. In particular, travelers with known preexisting conditions who are working long-term overseas or undertaking any form of hazardous recreational or occupational activities may need to obtain a special travel insurance policy. In addition, travelers who wish to participate in potentially dangerous activities, such as skydiving, mountain climbing, scuba diving, or jet skiing, should ensure that their travel insurance will cover them in the event of accidents, as many of these activities may not be covered.[4,17]

■ PSYCHOSOCIAL EFFECTS

Children's immature abilities to understand and process immediate and long-term effects of accidents and injuries—whether their own or exposure to accidents that traumatize or injure parents or loved ones—can make them vulnerable to psychosocial effects afterward. The physical and emotional consequences of experiencing or witnessing accidents and injuries can continue long after the initial event. On every level—physical, medical, psychological, emotional, and social—children have unique needs and vulnerabilities that must be taken into account after a traumatic injury.[31,32]

Children can be at risk for a variety of psychosocial responses after a traumatic injury or accident, including post-traumatic stress disorder, anxiety, depression, somatic disturbances, learning problems, and behavioral disorders. Children's stress reactions may vary depending on age but typically include

- Reexperiencing the trauma during play, dreams, or flashbacks
  — Repeatedly acting out what happened in the disaster when playing with toys or with other children
  — Nightmares or repeated dreams about the disaster
  — Becoming distressed when exposed to reminders of the disaster
  — Acting or feeling as if the disaster is happening again
- Avoiding disaster reminders
  — Avoiding activities that remind of the disaster
  — Being unable to remember all or parts of the disaster
  — Withdrawing from other people
  — Having difficulty feeling positive emotions
- Increased arousal symptoms
  — Difficulty falling or staying asleep
  — Irritability
  — Difficulty concentrating
  — Startling more easily

- Depressive symptoms
  - General emotional numbness
  - Crying
  - Changes in appetite
  - Fatigue
  - Insomnia or not wanting to sleep alone
  - Sadness
  - Loss of interest in previously preferred activities
- Fears
  - Being left behind or separated from family
  - Thinking something will happen to a family member
  - The dark
  - Being alone
  - Believing the child caused some part of the traumatic event
- Behavioral symptoms
  - Regressive behaviors, such as acting like a younger child (eg, bed-wetting, baby talk)
  - Irritability
  - Whining
  - Clinging
  - Aggressive behaviors or angry outbursts at home or with other children
  - Hyperactive or silly behaviors
  - Dangerous risk-taking behaviors, such as high-risk sexual behavior, or use of alcohol or other drugs (in adolescents)
- Somatic symptoms
  - Headache
  - Stomachache
  - Nausea
  - Dizziness

Risk Factors

A variety of studies identified risk factors that influence response to trauma and affect recovery. Children and adolescents who experienced any of the following are more likely to experience long-term difficulties and may be at higher risk for developing psychopathology[33]:

- Injury
- Trauma (eg, disasters, sexual abuse, motor vehicle crash)
- Witnessed a traumatic event (eg, fire, shooting, drowning, beating)
- Preexisting mental health issues (eg, depression, anxiety disorders)
- Exposure to disturbing or grotesque scenes or to extreme life threats
- Social isolation

- Being very upset during and after an injury or accident
- Becoming separated from parents or caregivers
- Parents or caregivers died, were significantly injured, or are missing
- Family members or friends died
- Physical disabilities or illness

Evaluations of children who experienced or witnessed injuries or accidents should assess
- Behavioral and psychiatric symptoms, including
  — Experiences during or soon after travel that were painful, hard to reconcile, or still cause distress, anxiety, or avoidance
  — Persistent sleep disturbance or unusual fatigue
  — Excessive use of alcohol or drugs (in adolescents)
  — Behavioral or interpersonal difficulties at home or school, or with friendships or relationships
- Somatic symptoms that can also be indications of distress, including
  — Unexplained somatic symptoms, such as headache, backache, or abdominal pain, and somatic disorders, such as chronic fatigue syndrome, temporomandibular disorder, and irritable bowel syndrome
  — Rashes, itching, and skin diseases, such as psoriasis, atopic dermatitis, and urticaria, which can be exacerbated by stress

Clinicians should be aware that some children and adolescents may be reluctant to acknowledge psychiatric symptoms or distress. For example, many cultures have stigmas associated with experiencing or disclosing behaviors associated with mental illness, as well as different culturally appropriate ways of expressing grief, pain, and loss. In addition, some children and adolescents may fear being stigmatized if they are labeled with a psychiatric diagnosis.[31,33]

The returned child or adolescent traveler who is having difficulty functioning or who appears unduly depressed or distressed should be referred to appropriate treatment or counseling regardless of the type or duration of travel and whether the child appears to meet criteria for a psychiatric diagnosis.

■ KEY POINTS

- In today's increasingly globalized world, travel itineraries are constantly expanding to include new locations previously inaccessible to most travelers, making many travel destinations accessible to many new populations, including children and adolescents.
- Children are now exposed to greater injury risks while traveling as a result of the increase in the number of child and adolescent travelers (an estimated 1.9 million children travel overseas each year).

- Injuries are one of the leading causes of death among international travelers and the leading cause of death to healthy Americans traveling overseas. Injuries are still the most frequent cause of death abroad in developing countries.
- Effective prevention strategies are available, particularly for travelers with children or adolescents who find themselves in new environments and who may be more likely to be unaware of risks or complacent in exotic surroundings.
- Health care professionals can be important allies to alert the public to the known risks and especially about simple and effective preventive measures to implement during international travel.
- Clinicians can play a critical role in helping reduce the injury risk among children and adolescents who travel by discussing travel and country risk factors and strategies to help avoid injury.
- Travelers should be advised about traffic and water safety, environmental risks, and personal safety. They should be prepared to develop a plan for dealing with medical emergencies and be advised on the importance of purchasing adequate medical and emergency evacuation insurance coverage.
- Adult caregivers should be prepared to provide closer supervision of children, be aware of basic first aid procedures, and know how to access appropriate care, if needed, at their travel location.

■ REFERENCES

1. US Department of Commerce, Office of Travel and Tourism Industries. 2007 Profile of US Resident Traveler Visiting Overseas Destinations. Survey of International Air Travelers. http://www.tinet.ita.doc.gov/outreachpages/download_data_table/2007_Outbound_Profile.pdf. Accessed April 20, 2009
2. Weinberg N, Weinberg M, Maloney S. Travel with children. In: Brunette GW, Kozarsky PE, Magill AJ, Shlim DR, eds. *CDC Health Information for International Travel, 2010.* Philadelphia, PA: Elsevier: 2010
3. Sleet DA, Wallace LJD, Shlim DR. Injuries and safety. In: Brunette GW, Kozarsky PE, Magill AJ, Shlim DR, eds. *CDC Health Information for International Travel, 2010.* Philadelphia, PA: Elsevier: 2010
4. Leggat PA, Fischer PR. Accidents and repatriation. *Travel Med Infect Dis.* 2006;4:135–146.
5. World Health Organization. *Global Burden of Disease, 2004.* Geneva, Switzerland: World Health Organization; 2008. http://www.who.int/healthinfo/global_burden_disease/GBD_report_2004update_full.pdf. Accessed June 9, 2011
6. Peden M, Oyegbite K, Ozanne-Smith J, et al. *World Report on Child Injury Prevention.* Geneva, Switzerland: World Health Organization; 2008
7. Baker TD, Hargarten SW, Guptill KS. The uncounted dead—American civilians dying overseas. *Public Health Rep.* 1992;107:155–159
8. McInnes RJ, Williamson LM, Morrison A. Unintentional injury during foreign travel: a review. *J Travel Med.* 2002;9:297–307

9. Hargarten SW, Bouc GT. Emergency air medical transport of US citizen tourists: 1988–1990. *Air Med J.* 1993;12:398–402

10. Linnan M, et al. *Child Mortality and Injury in Asia: Policy and Programme Implications.* Florence, Italy: UNICEF Innocenti Research Centre; 2007. http://www.unicef-irc.org/ publications/pdf/iwp_2007_07.pdf. Accessed January 21, 2008

11. Centers for Disease Control and Prevention, National Center for Injury Prevention and Control. Web-based Injury Statistics Query and Reporting System (WISQARS) [online]. 2008. www.cdc.gov/ncipc/wisqars. Accessed May 29, 2009

12. Grundy D, Penny P, Graham L. Diving into the unknown. *BMJ.* 1991;302:670–671

13. Brenner RA, Trumble AC, Smith GS, Kessler EP, Overpeck MD. Where children drown, United States, 1995. *Pediatrics.* 2001;108(1):85–89

14. Branche CM, Stewart S, eds. *Lifeguard Effectiveness: A Report of the Working Group.* Atlanta, GA: Centers for Disease Control and Prevention, National Center for Injury Prevention and Control; 2001

15. Schwebel DC, Lindsay S, Simpson J. Brief report: a brief intervention to improve life-guard surveillance at a public swimming pool. *J Pediatr Psychol.* 2007;32(7):862–868

16. Present P. *Child Drowning Study. A Report on the Epidemiology of Drowning in Residential Pools to Children Under Age Five.* Washington, DC: Consumer Product Safety Commission; 1987

17. Neumann K. Family travel: an overview. *Travel Med Infect Dis.* 2006;4:202–217

18. Gilchrist J, Gotsch K, Ryan GW. Nonfatal and fatal drownings in recreational water settings—United States, 2001 and 2002. *MMWR.* 2004;53(21):447–452

19. Howland J, Mangione T, Hingson R, et al. Alcohol as a risk factor for drowning and other aquatic injuries. In: Watson RR, ed. *Alcohol, Cocaine, and Accidents.* Totowa, NJ: Humana Press, Inc; 1995:85–104

20. World Health Organization. *International Travel and Health.* Geneva, Switzerland: World Health Organization; 2007

21. Khambalia A, et al. Risk factors for unintentional injuries due to falls in children aged 0–6 years: a systematic review. *Inj Prev.* 2006;12:378–385

22. World Health Organization. WHO Global School Health Survey. http://www.who.int/ chp/gshs/en. Accessed May 18, 2009

23. Rennie L, et al. The epidemiology of fractures in children. *Injury.* 2007;38:913–922

24. Centers for Disease Control and Prevention. Nonfatal fall-related injuries associated with dogs and cats—United States, 2001–2006. *MMWR.* 2009;58(11):277–281

25. Bronstein AC, et al. 2006 annual report of the American Association of Poison Control Centres' National Poison Data System (NPDS). *Clin Toxicol.* 2007;45:815–917

26. Vernberg K, Culver-Dickinson P, Spyker DA. The deterrent effect of poison-warning stickers. *Am J Dis Child.* 1984;138:1018–1020

27. Fergusson DM, Horwood LJ, Beautrais AL, Shannon FT. A controlled field trial of a poisoning prevention method. *Pediatrics.* 1982;69:515–520

28. Chien C, et al. Unintentional ingestion of over the counter medications in children less than 5 years old. *J Pediatr Child Health.* 2003;39:264–269

29. Kolars JC. Rules of the road: a consumer's guide for travelers seeking health care in foreign lands. *J Travel Med.* 2002;9:198–203

30. American Burn Association. *Organization and Delivery of Burn Care: Practice Guidelines of the American Burn Association.* 2001. http://www.ameriburn.org/PracticeGuidelines2001. pdf. Accessed May 25, 2009

31. Balaban V. Psychological assessment of children in disasters and emergencies: a review. *Disasters*. 2006;30(2):178–198
32. Olofsson E, Bunketorp O, Andersson AL. Children and adolescents injured in traffic—associated psychological consequences: a literature review. *Acta Paediatrica*. 2009;98(1): 17–22
33. Balaban V. Mental health and travel. In: Brunette GW, Kozarsky PE, Magill AJ, Shlim DR, eds. *CDC Health Information for International Travel, 2010*. Philadelphia, PA: Elsevier; 2010

CHAPTER

16

Insect Bite Prevention

David R. Boulware, MD, MPH, CTropMed

■ INTRODUCTION

When one imagines the most dangerous animals in the world, images of lions stalking prey on the African Savannah, Bengal tigers silently slipping through the bush, or rampaging elephants leap to mind. Or, if one is of a certain age, fears arise of great white sharks, piranhas, venomous snakes, killer bees, or deadly jellyfish as the most deadly animals in the world—fears seemingly driven by a genre of movies from the 1970s. In reality, the world's deadliest creature is much, much smaller—it is the mosquito. The mosquito has stopped armies, caused the rise and fall of empires, and still causes an estimated 1 to 3 million deaths annually.[1]

While mosquitoes are the most obvious insect vector of infectious diseases, there are many others. Biting arthropods that are potential disease vectors include mosquitoes, ticks, mites, lice, tsetse flies, *Triatoma* (kissing) bugs, phlebotomine sand flies, fleas, *Simulium* blackflies, and *Chrysops* deerflies. The mechanism of infection varies by disease but primarily is from direct inoculation via bites. Yet in other cases, rubbing the arthropod's feces into bite wounds can cause disease, notably for *Triatoma* bugs (Chagas disease), human body louse (typhus, quintana fever), and fleas (murine typhus). Regardless, avoiding infectious vectors and bites is the best prevention for vector-borne disease.

Malaria and mosquitoes are typically the primary focus for insect bite prevention, as malaria is the leading killer of children younger than 5 years in sub-Saharan Africa. Before the World Health Organization (WHO) Roll Back Malaria Partnership, an estimated 1 in 17 persons worldwide died of a mosquito-borne illness.[2] Caution and perspective are warranted because although mosquitoes are insects, not all insects are mosquitoes. Results from mosquito studies cannot be generalized to all biting insects. Table 16-1 lists the primary flying insects that serve as vectors for human disease.

Interventions for insect avoidance can be summarized into interventions on public and individual levels. While many of the interventions are one in the same, one must realize that what will work for an individual often may fail to protect a population. Thus, the intended goal affects the choice of intervention. In general, interventions that require an individual's active compliance with use, such as frequently applying insect repellent, will fail to protect the population from disease. Individual personal protective measures to prevent vector-to-human contact, while effective, are often the least reliable means of disease control because they require considerable motivation, perseverance, and financial resources to maintain ongoing effectiveness.

■ PRINCIPALS OF PUBLIC HEALTH INTERVENTIONS

From a public health perspective, the 3 critical components for consideration in vector-borne disease (Figure 16-1) are the necessity of having a

1. *Reservoir* of disease
2. *Susceptible host*
3. Competent *vector* with contact between the reservoir and susceptible host

The appropriate public health intervention may vary depending on specifics of each of these factors for a given disease.

Disease Reservoir

Every infectious disease has a reservoir. Zoonotic diseases, by definition, cross the species barrier. Eliminating the reservoir of disease is often impossible when zoonotic diseases cross species. However, when the reservoir is only humans, such as the smallpox epidemic in 1977, eradication is possible. The current list of diseases with only human reservoirs that could potentially be eradicated are poliomyelitis, dracunculiasis, mumps, rubella, lymphatic filariasis, and trichuriasis (whipworm). Dracunculiasis (guinea worm) is notable as there is neither an effective drug nor a vaccination. Disease eradication is possible by physically removing the reservoir and preventing new infections to susceptible hosts by filtering drinking water and treating water supplies. Although reservoir eradication can be the most effective method to confront

Table 16-1. Summary of the Principal Flying Insect Vectors for Human Disease Transmission

DISEASE	PRINCIPAL VECTOR[a]	GEOGRAPHY	LOCALE	BITING TIME
Malaria	*Anopheles* (approximately 45 competent vectors)	Tropics worldwide	Temperature: 16°C to 33°C Altitude: < 2,000 m	Dusk to dawn primarily
Dengue	*Aedes aegypti* *Aedes albopictus*	Tropics, subtropic areas Tropics, subtropics	Urban	Daytime
Yellow fever	*Aedes aegypti* *Aedes africanus* *Haemagogus*	Tropic/subtropics Africa South America	Urban Forest/jungle Forest/jungle	Daytime
Chikungunya	*Aedes aegypti* *Aedes albopictus*	Tropic/subtropics	Urban	Daytime
Viral encephalitis				
• Japanese encephalitis	*Culex tritaeniorhynchus*	Asia	Pig is preferred feeding source.	Night
• West Nile encephalitis	*Culex pipiens, Culex univittatus;* also *Aedes, Anopheles*	Worldwide	Varies and is indoors	Night
• Eastern equine encephalitis	*Coquillettidia perturbans, Aedes sollicitans, Aedes taeniorhynchus, Culiseta,* other *Culex, Aedes*	Western hemisphere	Freshwater hardwood swamps	Various
• Western equine encephalitis	*Culex tarsalis, Aedes dorsalis, Aedes melanimon*	Western hemisphere	Warm, moist environments	Various
• La Crosse encephalitis	*Aedes triseriatus*	North America	Deciduous forest	Daytime
• St. Louis encephalitis	*Culex (Culex nigripalpus, Culex pipiens, Culex quinquefasciatus, Culex tarsalis)*	Western hemisphere	Various	Night
• Murray Valley encephalitis	*Culex annulirostris*	Australia	River valleys	Dusk and dawn
• Venezuelan equine encephalitis	*Culex (Melanoconion),* approximately 40 species implicated	Latin America	Wetlands	Varies

Table 16-1. Summary of the Principal Flying Insect Vectors for Human Disease Transmission, continued

DISEASE	PRINCIPAL VECTOR[a]	GEOGRAPHY	LOCALE	BITING TIME
Filariasis • Lymphatic filariasis (*Wuchereria bancrofti, Brugia malayi, B timori*)	Multiple mosquito species, including *Anopheles, Aedes, Culex, Coquillettidia, Mansonia*	Africa Asia Indonesia	Various	Dependent on local vector; most at midnight
• *Mansonella*	*Culicoides* (midges or no-see-ums) (*Simulium* blackflies for *M ozzardi*)	Africa, South America Latin America	Various, often near banana plantations	Midnight
• Loa loa	*Chrysops silicea* and *C dimidiata* (deerflies)	Africa	Rain forest	Bright sunlight
• Onchocerciasis	*Simulium* (blackflies)	Africa, foci in Latin America	Savannah or forest; do not enter homes	Day
Leishmaniasis	*Phlebotomus* and *Lutzomyia* (sandflies)	Africa, South Asia, Latin America, Mediterranean foci		Dusk and night
Tularemia	*Chrysops discalis* (deerfly) and also ticks	Western North America	Shady areas	Daytime
Trypanosoma • Acute sleeping sickness *T bruci v rhodesiense*	*Glossina* (tsetse flies)	East Africa	Savannah	Daytime, bright sunlight
• Chronic sleeping sickness *T bruci v gambiense*		West Africa	Waterside	Daytime, bright sunlight

[a]Mosquito vectors unless otherwise stated.

Figure 16-1. Vector-Borne Disease Prevention Strategies

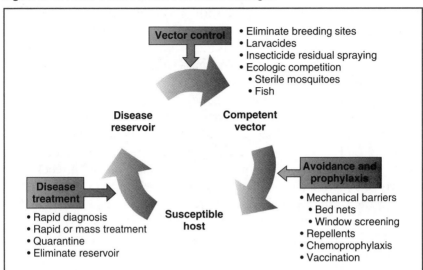

disease, most vector-borne diseases are not amenable to eliminating the disease reservoir.

Elimination of Susceptible Hosts

Elimination of susceptible hosts is another method of preventing vector-borne disease. Vaccination is the primary method to decrease susceptible hosts. Three basic necessities are generally needed for vaccine development. The first is the experiment of nature, as natural infection should convey a long-lasting natural immunity following recovery from primary infection. Second, the type of immune response needed for protection must be known. A third essential necessity is an organization willing to fund and support vaccine development. Unfortunately, many vector-borne diseases are limited in their geographic scope or are neglected diseases with minimal research interest and minimal financial reward for private enterprises. Where there is global interest, such as with malaria, the challenge remains great. Diseases, such as malaria, without natural long-lasting immunity and in which reinfection frequently occurs are not easy vaccine candidates for development. The goal of current malaria vaccine development is to reduce disease severity and prevent mortality, not prevent infection. Such pragmatic goals can improve global health, but the complete elimination of susceptible hosts is often near impossible.

Vector Control

Vector control is the third public health prevention method. When neither the reservoir nor susceptible hosts can be eliminated, the focus of public health interventions turns to disrupting the vector-mediated transmission of disease. This is the primary and only strategy available for most vector-borne diseases. Successful public health interventions often require targeting more than one aspect of transmission. Appreciating the ecology and life cycle of vectors is challenging yet allows targeting multiple stages of the vector's life cycle to interrupt transmission. For vector-borne disease, the classic strategies are to remove breeding sites, kill the ova or larvae, kill the vector, or repel the vector, or community-wide measures to develop physical separation between the vector and susceptible host. For mosquitoes, successful prevention techniques are often multifaceted to target multiple stages of the mosquito life cycle and behavior, which is further tailored to the local vector-causing disease.

■ BREEDING SITE REMOVAL

Mosquito breeding is confined to water collection that is amenable to drainage, such as swamps, marshes, rain pools, stagnant sewage, or water cisterns. Removing breeding sites for ova and larvae is the most effective method of mosquito control. Some interventions may be possible with simple engineering by creating better drainage to prevent standing water. In cases of sizable wetlands, drainage is not possible without significant adverse ecologic impact.

Historically, eliminating breeding sites was the primary method of mosquito control. After Walter Reed proved that the *Aedes ageypti* mosquito transmitted yellow fever, William C. Gorgas famously eliminated yellow fever from Havana in 30 days even though it had been in Cuba for 300 years. Gorgas' approach was 2-fold. First, *Aedes ageypti* breading sites in Havana were aggressively eliminated by enacting fines for property owners harboring breeding sites. The transmission cycle was then interrupted by isolating yellow fever–infected patients in the hospital with screening and netting. This created a physical separation between the reservoir and vector, which rapidly eliminated yellow fever.

This tradition continues today with mosquito-control officers removing breeding site districts in Havana. Breeding site elimination requires significant, sustained, and well-coordinated public health efforts. The urban nature of *Aedes ageypti,* coupled with the ubiquitous use of plastic containers and used tires, creates an infinite amount of suitable breeding sites for this and *Aedes albopictus* species. However, each species of mosquito has unique behaviors, breeding patterns, and ecologic niches. Knowledge of the vector and its habits is essential to eliminate breeding sites.

■ LARVAL CONTROL

Larval control methods historically used oils and hydrocarbons to coat the surface of stagnant water to prevent mosquito larvae from developing. This required frequent application and adversely affected the environment. More bio-ecologically friendly approaches now focus on products with minimal adverse environmental effect. While there are a significant number of larvicides and insecticides, the WHO recommends the addition of 1 bacterial larvicide and 4 insecticide chemical compounds to drinking water as larvicides: *Bacillus thuringiensis israelensis,* methoprene, pyriproxyfen, temephos, and novaluron. These have been assessed by the WHO International Programme on Chemical Safety and are believed to be safe for use in potable drinking water. A summary of the larval control compounds and their activity is provided in Table 16-2.

Bacillus thuringiensis israelensis is a natural soil gram-positive bacterium used in breeding sites to disrupt larval progression. It produces δ-endotoxins that are toxic to mosquito larvae gut epithelium by forming pores that lead to cell lysis. This disrupts mosquito larvae gut epithelium, leading to sepsis from enteric *Enterococcus* and *Enterobacter* species present in the larval midguts.[3] *Bacillus thuringiensis israelensis* is a highly effective intervention with no apparent adverse ecologic effect. It has

Table 16-2. Larval Control Measures

LARVAL CONTROL METHOD	MECHANISM	TARGET
Bacillus thuringiensis israelensis	Crystal δ-endotoxin, gut disruption, enteric bacterial infection, death	Mosquitoes and blackfly larvae
Methoprene	Juvenile hormone analog, stops development	Mosquito pupa
Pyriproxyfen	Juvenile hormone analog, stops development	Mosquito pupa
Temephos	Nonsystemic organophosphate	Flea, mosquito, blackfly, or sand fly larvae
Novaluron	Inhibits chitin synthesis, prevents molting	Mosquito larvae

been incorporated into bioengineered crops to resist pests and decrease chemical pesticide usage.[4]

Another method is methoprene, which disrupts the mosquito's biological life cycle by keeping larval mosquitoes from fully developing into adults. Methoprene mimics the juvenile hormone found naturally in immature mosquitoes.[5] The juvenile hormone must be absent for a mosquito pupa to molt to an adult. Pyriproxyfen acts by similar mechanisms, as a juvenile hormone analog, and was the first WHO-recommended product for application to drinking water, particularly to control *Aedes ageypti* populations to decrease dengue. Pyriproxyfen is also used in many countries on citrus fruit to decrease agricultural pests.[6]

Temephos is a nonsystemic organophosphate larvicide used to treat water infested with flea, mosquito, blackfly, or sand fly larvae. Temephos is the primary larvicide used in the guinea worm (dracunculiasis) eradication program and the WHO Onchocerciasis Control Programme.[7] While temephos has a very short persistence in the water (approximately 2 hours), it does have toxicity for freshwater aquatic invertebrates, saltwater shrimp, oysters, and some species of fish (notably rainbow trout and salmon). Use in all geographic areas is not possible and depends on local aquatic species present.

Lastly, novaluron is a benzoylphenyl urea insecticide that acts as an insect growth regulator to inhibit chitin synthesis. This affects the molting stages of larvae development because chitin is a necessary component of the cytoskeleton. Prior field studies demonstrated effectiveness at suppressing immature mosquito larvae and pupa for 3 to 7 weeks after a single application in polluted water and without any adverse effect on freshwater fish or aquatic plants.[8] Novaluron is the most recent of the larvicides, registered in the United States in 2004 and the European Union in 2007.

■ KILLING ADULT VECTORS

Insecticides have been used since the 1940s for mosquito control. The most infamous insecticide is DDT, which was first synthesized in 1874. The insecticide properties of DDT were not discovered until 1939 by Paul Hermann Müller, who was subsequently awarded the 1948 Nobel Prize in Physiology or Medicine. DDT is active against a wide variety of arthropods, including mosquitoes, fleas, and lice. In World War II, environmental spraying reduced malaria in the South Pacific theatre as well as eliminated typhus spread by lice. More extensive widespread environmental spraying occurred in the 1950s and 1960s for mosquito control. DDT was the cornerstone of the WHO malaria eradication program from

1955 to 1969; however, with extensive indiscriminate use, resistance in mosquitoes developed in the 1960s and toxicity in wildlife occurred. DDT is concentrated up the food chain with avian species, notably the American bald eagle, being dramatically affected with increased fragility of its eggs. It was banned in the United States in 1972, but worldwide use continued. Three of the major mosquito vectors for human disease are displayed in Figure 16-2.

Indoor Residual Spraying

Indoor residual spraying (IRS) is the application of long-acting insecticides inside domestic housing. The objective of IRS is to reduce the morbidity and mortality of malaria and other mosquito-borne infectious diseases. The primary effects of IRS toward curtailing malaria transmission include reducing the life span of vector mosquitoes so that mosquitoes can no longer transmit malaria parasites from one person to another, and reducing the density of the vector mosquitoes. In some situations, IRS can lead to the elimination of locally important malaria vectors.

With IRS, insecticide is sprayed on the internal walls and roofs of houses to kill the adult vector mosquitoes that land on treated surfaces. Typically, after feeding, mosquitoes land on nearby surfaces to rest and digest their blood meal. While resting, the mosquitoes pick up the insecticide and are poisoned by the neurotoxic effects. *Anopheles* species have a predilection toward landing on vertical surfaces; thus, indoor walls are a target for IRS treatment. Most insecticides act through acetylcholine esterase inhibition; however, development of resistance is possible with transient instead of fatal neurotoxicity. As well, some mosquitoes can exhibit behavioristic avoidance in which they alter their behavior and avoid landing on treated surfaces.

Figure 16-2. Principal Mosquitoes Responsible for Human Disease

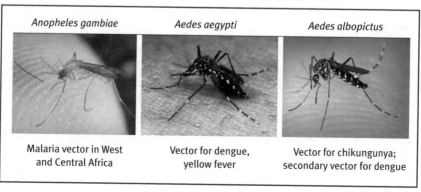

Anopheles gambiae	*Aedes aegypti*	*Aedes albopictus*
Malaria vector in West and Central Africa	Vector for dengue, yellow fever	Vector for chikungunya; secondary vector for dengue

The majority of IRS systems use an insecticide, with DDT controversially being one of these. During DDT use in the United States, approximately 600 million kg were used over 25 years. In contrast, the current estimate is that 4 to 5 million kg of DDT are used annually for targeted IRS programs worldwide, primarily in Africa and India. DDT is less expensive than some other organophosphate and carbamate insecticides, such as malathion; however, DDT is approximately the same cost or more than synthetic pyrethroids, such as deltamethrin and permethrin, which require less frequent applications than DDT and thus a lesser amount for IRS treatment.[9]

Example of Public Health Interventions

A historical example of a public health intervention is the WHO Malaria Eradication Programme (1955–1969), which focused on vector control with DDT and reducing the reservoir by treating infected persons with chloroquine. Although ultimately unsuccessful, temporary gains were achieved where the program was implemented. Notably, this program was never implemented in sub-Saharan Africa or other regions; thus, country-by-country implementation created a patchwork of implementers. After the malaria eradication program was discontinued, the incidence of malaria rapidly increased in many regions.

Several lessons are learned from this program. Interventions must be sustained or the premature discontinuation will result in disease resurgence. Multiple interventions are often necessary; relying on a single agent (eg, DDT and chloroquine) will eventually generate resistance and fail. While vectors may align with climate, ecosystem, and altitude, vectors rarely align with geopolitical map lines. Thus, implementation strategies for reducing disease burden need to encompass the geographic boundaries of the disease and vector, not political boundaries. Filariasis control programs are a good example of projects defined by disease boundaries and not solely by geopolitical borders. As programs span countries, lack of political leadership can greatly hamper control programs (eg, polio).

A representative public health program that uses a multitiered strategy is the current Roll Back Malaria Partnership, launched in November 1998. Roll Back Malaria has 4 pillars (Table 16-3) and a goal to decrease malaria-related mortality. The mechanisms to achieve this goal are multi-focused to decrease vector transmission, as well as to implement rapid effective treatment, which decreases the disease reservoir.

| Table 16-3. World Health Organization Roll Back Malaria Partnership ||
ROLL BACK MALARIA PARTNERSHIP PILLARS	PUBLIC HEALTH STRATEGY
1. Prevention, with an emphasis on insecticide-treated nets	Vector avoidance
2. Rapid diagnosis and treatment	Reservoir reduction
3. Rapid response to malaria epidemics	Reservoir reduction/susceptible host
4. Treatment of pregnant women	Susceptible host

■ COMMUNITY-WIDE PREVENTION MEASURES

Improving local living conditions is often an effective intervention for preventing some vector-borne diseases. Simple interventions, such as screened windows and doors, decrease mosquito-to-human contact. The marked reduction in malaria in the United States during the 1920s and 1930s was principally caused by improvement in housing and living conditions in the southern part of the country. For diseases such as American trypanosomiasis (Chagas disease), replacing thatched roofs and dirt floors is a highly effective intervention to decrease *Triatoma* infestation and reduce vector-to-human contact.[10,11]

Community-wide surveillance of disease is necessary. Promptly identifying and treating newly infected persons eliminates disease reservoirs. For diseases with obvious stigmata, such as yellow fever, smallpox, or measles, surveillance for new disease is straightforward. For malaria, it is essential not only to have access to medical care but to have public health surveillance in place. In many resource-limited areas, access to care and public health are inadequate. Historically, standard approaches used passive surveillance and reporting at the national level. Not surprisingly, such approaches are slow and largely depend on the effectiveness of the local ministry of health. In resource-limited areas, the ability to generate a timely response is difficult.

With increased technology (eg, cell phones) and mobile populations (eg, travelers), novel approaches for disease surveillance may be more successful. The penetration of cell phones into broad portions of all populations creates a ubiquitous information platform. In many countries in sub-Saharan Africa, cell phone companies are the single most profitable business. The ability to implement programs will likely need novel public-private partnerships. Harnessing this technology with newer generation smartphones may be an innovative approach to disseminate field epidemiology reporting in a rapid manner. As part of the WHO Roll Back Malaria Partnership, rapidly identifying malaria outbreaks is a pillar of the program.

Personal Protective Measures

Methods of personal protection are quite effective, when used. There are a variety of behavioral interventions known to reduce insect bites for an individual (Box 16-1). Since the 1950s in North America mosquitoes were viewed as pests that cause annoyance or discomfort but rarely disease. With the emergence of West Nile virus, the North American general population has more recognition of the dangers of mosquito-borne illness. While mosquito avoidance is traditionally recommended in regions with malaria, one must recognize that other mosquito- and tick-borne illnesses are worldwide. For example, *Aedes aegypti,* the vector for dengue fever, is an urban daytime-biting mosquito expanding in geographic range since the 1960s.[12] Tick-borne disease also occurs worldwide, with increasing incidence of Lyme disease in North America. Exposure in recreational populations is frequent. In one prospective cohort study of Appalachian Trail backpackers in North America, nearly 5% acquired a vector-borne illness, principally Lyme disease.

Box 16-1. Behavioral Recommendations for Mosquito Avoidance

- Avoid peak biting periods.
  - *Anopheles* species feed before and after sunset and again before dawn (malaria vector).
  - *Aedes aegypti* feed throughout the day (dengue, yellow fever vector).
  - *Ochlerotatus triseriatus,* eastern tree hole mosquito. Females feed any time (LaCrosse encephalitis vector).
  - *Culex pipiens* species feed throughout the evening and night (West Nile virus, St. Louis virus, Sindbis virus, Rift Valley fever, Bancroftian filariasis vector).
  - *Culex tritaeniorhynchus* feeds primarily on pigs, with a short average flight span of less than 2 km (Japanese encephalitis vector).
- Stay in well-screened housing.
  - Window screens should be in good state of repair.
  - Doors and window should be tight-fitting.
- Minimize exposed skin with long-sleeved shirts and long trousers.
- Light-colored clothing is less attractive for mosquitoes.[13] Tuck trouser legs into boots or socks, especially in tick regions.
- Avoid blue-colored clothing in tsetse fly areas.
- Use insecticide-treated mosquito netting when sleeping outdoors or in poorly or unscreened buildings.
- Use insecticide-treated mosquito netting on children younger than 2 years at all times.
- Indoor residual spraying is a primary vector control intervention to create spatial protection against mosquitoes for a living unit.
- Outdoor spraying with insecticidal fog or mist (often permethrin) is effective only for 7 days or fewer. Permethrin is degraded by ultraviolet light.
- Insect light electrocuting devices ("bug zappers") do not reduce biting mosquitoes.

Repellents

Preventive measures, including the use of repellents (Box 16-2), are simple and effective. There are many natural and synthetic compounds that act as insect repellents. Not all repellents act against all insects; the effectiveness of repellents may vary by mosquito species. Even when standard, safe, effective repellents exist, one must appreciate that lack of individual compliance jeopardizes repellents' effectiveness. In a plethora of studies, including American travelers to Africa, soldiers,[14] aid workers,[15] and Boy Scouts,[16] antimosquito measures were employed by less than half, even when recommended in disease endemic areas. Though repellents are protective for an individual, repellent use often does not correlate with reduced incidence of vector-borne disease in a population.[14,15] This is because of 2 factors. First, most repellents require frequent application (eg, every 4 to 6 hours), and erratic application will not protect individuals. Second, personal repellents simply shift vector-feeding behaviors to other unprotected persons. Thus, while an individual may be protected, those individuals not using a repellent in the immediate vicinity are at higher risk of acquiring mosquito bites.

DEET

While insect repellents will not work for the population, they are very effective for a compliant individual willing to reapply every 4 to 6 hours. Consider DEET to be the first choice among insect repellents. DEET has

---

Box 16-2. General Suggestions for Repellents

- Apply DEET sparingly on exposed skin.
- Do not use repellent under clothing.
- Do not use DEET on the hands of young children (ie, those putting their hands in their mouth).
- Have parents or older children apply DEET to young children.
- Avoid applying to areas around the eyes and mouth.
- Do not use DEET over cuts, wounds, or broken skin.
- Wash treated skin with soap and water after returning indoors.
- Do not use on clothing. DEET is a plasticizer and will dissolve many synthetics.
- Do not use combination DEET-and-sunscreen protection as application frequency and amount differ.
- Avoid spraying in enclosed areas.
- Do not use DEET near food.
- Use caution with newer synthetic insect repellents (toxicity in children is unknown; efficacy against variety of insects is unknown).
- Picaridin at 20% concentration is likely fairly equivalent to 20% DEET, though with less of a safety record in children.
- Picaridin at 9% to 10% is a reasonable substitute for DEET where the risk of serious disease is low (eg, North America) or exposure is short (< 2 hours).

been extensively tested over 50 years and performs reliably under a wide variety of real-world conditions.[17] DEET concentrations up to approximately 30% have increasing repellent, but DEET does not provide additional protection above 30%.[18] In a field trial, the percent protective efficacy of extended-duration 32% DEET against *Anopheles stephensi* at 0, 3, 6, 9, and 12 hours was 100%, 99.3%, 92.8%, 79.7%, and 66.3% for females and 100%, 100%, 97.6%, 91.9%, and 77.5% for males.[19] In a field trial, extended-duration 35% DEET provided more than 10 hours of protection against the daytime biting *Aedes* mosquito.[20] In an arm box study, 23.8% DEET offered complete protection for 6 hours compared with a soybean oil–based repellent, which protected for an average of 1.5 hours.[18] In another study, a mosquito-repellent soap (20% DEET with 0.5% permethrin) was compared with a placebo soap. Cases of falciparum malaria occurred in 3.7% (23 of 618) of those in the repellent soap group compared with 8.9% (47 of 530) of the placebo group.[21]

■ SAFETY DATA ON CHILDREN

DEET

The skin absorption of DEET in relation to age has not been studied specifically. However, data from similar substances suggest that skin absorption should not differ above 2 months of age. DEET is not water soluble, but unlike many sunscreens it does not wash off. Sunscreens require more frequent application and in greater concentration than DEET. Thus, combined sunscreen-and-DEET products should not be used. Repeated excessive DEET application increases the risk of toxicity. The American Academy of Pediatrics Council on Environmental Health states that DEET concentrations of 10% appear to be equally safe in children as concentrations of 30% when used according to the directions on product labels.[22] Specifically, reapplication is generally recommended for most repellent products every 4 to 6 hours, and repellents should not be used on abraded or non-intact skin. DEET is not recommended for use on children younger than 2 months.

Picaridin

Picaridin (also known as icaridin and KBR 3023; trade names Bayrepel and Saltidin) is a new mosquito repellent that has similar efficacy at 19.2% concentration compared with 20% DEET over 9 hours.[23] The name picaridin is used in the United States, but the repellent was renamed icaridin by the WHO. The most attractive feature of picaridin is its lack of an odor; it may be an option for those unwilling to use DEET. The originally marketed US commercial formulations did not use the proven 19.2% concentration but rather lesser concentrations of 5% to 10%. Efficacy of 9.3% picaridin is less, with complete protection for only 2 hours.[23] While this may be adequate protection in low biting-pressure areas with few mosquitoes, such as suburban North America, the protection is suboptimal when extended duration of protection is desired. Picaridin also repels ticks but to a lesser extent and duration than DEET, with only 56% protection at 2 hours.[24] Long-term safety data are unknown, as picaridin has been distributed only since 1988. Safety data in children are limited.

There is accumulating evidence of efficacy for picaridin from in vitro laboratory studies and field trials. In arm box studies, *Aedes aegypti* and *Anopheles stephensi* mosquitoes, as well as the sand fly *Phlebotomus papatasi*, were repelled by DEET and picaridin. Each reduced bites by about 50%.[25] Another in vitro assay testing DEET and picaridin against *Aedes aegypti* and *Anopheles stephensi* at a fixed dose of 24 nmol/cm^2 showed a significant repellent effect for both compounds.[26] In comparative laboratory tests with *Aedes aegypti* and *Anopheles gambiae*, the effective dose for 90% repellence was not significantly different for *Anopheles gambiae*, whereas picaridin was slightly more potent than DEET against *Aedes aegypti*.[27] Conversely, in a different laboratory assay assessing the fixed-dose repellency and dose-response curve, DEET was more effective than picaridin against *Aedes aegypti* but equally effective against *Anopheles stephensi*.[28]

While arm box studies are good at assessing repellents' efficacy, field trials are better at assessing the real-world efficacy under a variety of temperatures and humidity levels. One important factor to consider is the mosquito-biting pressure present at a study location. In a Brazilian study, picaridin at 10% to 20% concentrations had an average protection of 6 hours against *Aedes aegypti* in a very low mosquito-biting pressure area of 3 bites per hour.[29] A field trial comparing the performance of picaridin and DEET against *Anopheles gambiae* showed similar activity, with the 95% effective repellency dosages for DEET and picaridin being 94 and 81.8 µg/cm^2, respectively.[30] A field trial comparing 19.2% picaridin, 20% DEET in ethanol, and 35% DEET gel against *Culex annulirostris*, *Anopheles meraukensis*, and *Anopheles bancrofti* reported Picaridin and 35% DEET gel provided more than 95% protection for only 1 hour. In contrast, all 3 repellents provided good protection against *Culex annulirostris*, with picaridin providing more than 95% protection for 5 hours and both DEET products providing more than 95% protection for at least 7 hours.[31] In a field trial against black salt marsh mosquitoes *(Ochlerotatus taeniorhynchus)* in the Florida Everglades, the mean complete protection times were 5.4 hours for picaridin and 5.6 hours for DEET.[32] Field trials against rain forest mosquitoes in northern Queensland, Australia, found that 19.2% picaridin compared favorably with 35% DEET, providing at least 8 hours of greater than 95% protection, while a lower concentration of 9.3% picaridin was inferior.[33] In a study comparing picaridin (5% and 12%) and DEET (7.5% and 15%), all 4 showed high-level efficacy against day-biting *Aedes albopictus* and night-biting *Culex quinquefasciatus;* however, for protection against night-biting *Anopheles,* the higher concentrations of both repellents were clearly superior to lower concentrations.[34] Field trials comparing 9.3% picaridin, 10% DEET, and 80% DEET found more than 95% protection against all mosquitoes for 2 hours, 7 hours, and more than 8 hours, respectively. Although picaridin performed worse than DEET overall, picaridin did provide more than 95% protection for 5 hours against *Culex annulirostris* but not *Ochlerotatus normanesis* or *Anophiles meraukensis.*[35]

Picaridin repellence of 19.2% concentration in field trials generally appears equivalent to recommended DEET concentrations. A second key finding is that picaridin has dose-dependent repellence activity, and that the 19.2% formulation is superior to the 9.3% formulation. Picaridin is widely used in Germany as a mosquito repellent, but data regarding other arthropods are scant. The efficacy of picaridin against the vector of African tick fever *(Amblyomma hebraeum)* at 2 hours was 56% compared with DEET efficacy of 84%.[36] In a study of lone star ticks *Amblyomma americanum,* 10% and 20% formulations of picaridin had protection for 12 hours.[37] In vitro studies and laboratory arm box studies cannot fully substitute for field trials.

Permethrin Passive Protection

Passive methods to reduce mosquito exposures are more likely to be consistently effective. Three primary examples exist: The first is IRS; the second is sleeping under a bed net, which is ideally pretreated with permethrin; and the third is to soak or spray pretravel clothes with 0.5% permethrin. Permethrin binds to clothing and is still effective after up to 10 washings.[38] Treating clothes or objects, such as tents, not only protects the individual but also offers nearly 50% protection to others in the immediate vicinity.[16] Permethrin-treated clothing alone has a 70% mosquito reduction rate and in combination with DEET, a 99% effectiveness against ticks and mosquitoes.[39,40] DEET still is highly recommended, but such a recommendation is tempered by the real-world practicality that fewer than 50% of individuals will consistently comply.[14-16]

It is important to note that permethrin is not a repellent but an insecticide that causes toxicity to the mosquito by acting as an acetylcholine-esterase inhibitor. However, permethrin is not approved by the Food and Drug Administration for chronic application to the skin and should not be used topically. Permethrin, a semi-synthetic insecticide derived from the chrysanthemum flower, is shown to reduce the incidence of blood-sucking arthropod attachment and mosquito bites for more than 6 weeks after a single application to clothing. Treating bed nets and clothing with permethrin can be used as an adjunctive measure in addition to repellents. Pyrethroids are stable in heat and humidity and through a number of wash cycles. Washing permethrin-treated uniforms reduces permethrin concentration by 60%, but the concentration is not reduced further after subsequent washings (up to 20 times).[41]

One interesting aspect of permethrin use is the ability to provide passive prophylaxis in the immediate vicinity by treating other objects. A randomized, double-blind, controlled trial of 0.4% permethrin used to treat canvas tents at a Boy Scouts summer camp showed that permethrin-treated campsites had 44% fewer bites ($P<0.001$) over an 8-week period after a single permethrin application.[16] Two previous pilot studies examined permethrin-treated tents. Eight volunteers sleeping inside a permethrin-treated tent had an 84% to 94% reduction of mosquito bites.[42] Even those sleeping outside of a treated tent had a 43% to 82% reduction of mosquito bites.[42] The duration of effectiveness of tent treatment is at least 6 to 12 months.[43,44]

In a field trial in a malaria endemic area, treating bedsheets with permethrin, alphacypermethrin, or deltamethrin reduced the incidence of bites, but deltamethrin caused more skin irritation.[45] In one field trial, deltamethrin-treated bed nets significantly reduced the incidence of malaria transmitted by *Anopheles culicifacies*.[46]

■ DEET AND PERMETHRIN

Permethrin-treated clothes are more effective when used with a repellent applied to exposed skin for preventing mosquito bites. The combination of permethrin on clothing and DEET on skin results in a formidable barrier that provides 99.9% protection against mosquito bites, even under conditions in which unprotected subjects received an average of 1,188 bites per hour.[14] The US military uses a DEET-based repellent and permethrin-treated clothing to prevent arthropod-borne disease. Permethrin and DEET have shown efficacy, alone and in combination, against *Aedes taeniorhynchus*. In a field trial, combined use was most effective (average of 1.5 bites per 9-hour day), compared with 53.5 and

98.5 bites with only treated clothing or DEET, respectively.[47] Against tsetse flies, the combination of permethrin-impregnated clothing and controlled-release DEET provided 91% mean protection but was not significantly better (P>0.05) than DEET alone.[48]

■ NEW REPELLENTS

Use caution when considering the use of newer synthetic insect repellents. The rationale for this recommendation is that DEET has a 60-year track record of known efficacy and toxicity, and not all insects are the same. Testing methods are important because some repellents will perform well in low biting-pressure situations, but as mosquito bites and landings increase (more than 60 per hour), efficacy and duration of protection may decrease dramatically. Oddly, some of the marketed, commercially available concentrations of new repellents do not match their field-tested concentrations. This is particularly true for the 9.3% picaridin marketed in North America.

Until more field testing of new synthetic agents is completed for a wide variety of arthropods, do not substitute any of the following agents for DEET:
- α-permethrin
- Deltamethrin (useful for pyrethroid resistance)
- DEPA (N,N-diethyl phenylacetamide)
- 1-(3-cyclohexen-1-yl-carbonyl)-2-methylpiperidine (AI3-37220)
- Metofluthrin
- Picaridin at 5% to 10% concentrations (Some caution should exist for advocating picaridin use in locales where there is a prolonged exposure [more than 2 hours] and serious risk of vector-borne disease.)

The rationale for not widely substituting, where vector-borne diseases exist, is 4-fold. First, isolated tests against a single insect or species may not predict protection against a variety of insects or different species of the same insect. Second, while various botanical and essential oils show promise as repellents, field testing under high-biting conditions is needed. Third, the active moiety of a new repellent is not always well characterized, and minor manufacturing differences may make significant differences. For example, AI3-37220 has multiple optical stereo-isomers that have 2-fold differences in mosquito repellency.[49] Thus, minor manufacturing differences could significantly alter the repellence. Fourth, human toxicity data are limited on many of the newer compounds, particularly in children. Overall, there remains significant consumer appeal for natural alternatives to chemical repellents, so testing of promising agents will likely continue in the future.

Existing Evidence on Newer Repellents

DEPA showed repellence against *Aedes aegypti* for 6 to 8 hours in the laboratory. Under field conditions, there was no significant difference between DEPA and DEET at 0.25 and 0.5 mg/cm^2 against blackflies and mosquitoes.[50] In a study comparing the repellent AI3-37220 25% in ethanol with a formulation containing 35% DEET, both provided greater than 95% protection against *Anopheles kiliensis* for 2 hours.[51] Metofluthrin-impregnated multilayer paper strips reduced bites from *Culex quinquefasciatus, Anopheles balabacensis,* and *Anopheles sundaicus.* The device is simple and does not require electricity.[52] In one study, 2% α-terpinene was superior to DEET against *Culex pipiens*.[53] In another study, neem oil and DEPA showed similar repellent activity against *Phlebotomus papatasi* (sand fly), a vector of leishmaniasis.[54] Fifteen controlled trials of slow-burning mosquito coils showed a reduction in the number of bites; however, none of the trials used malaria prevention as an outcome.[55]

Repellency data on essential oils are limited but not very promising compared with synthetic repellents. Essential oils should not be recommended for use where vector-borne disease exists. In a study of the mosquito repellent activity of 38 essential oils, undiluted oils of *Cymbopogon nardus* (citronella), *Pogostemon cablin* (patchouli), *Syzygium aromaticum* (clove), and *Zanthoxylum limonella* (makaen) provided at least 2 hours of repellent effect. Diluted oils showed little effect. Clove oil was the most effective overall but is a potential contact allergen.[56] Oils of lemon eucalyptus *(Eucalyptus maculata citrodion),* rue *(Ruta chalepensis),* oleoresin of pyrethrum *(Chrysanthemum cinerariaefolium),* and neem *(Azadirachta indica)* all show some repellent action. Oil of lemon eucalyptus, DEET, and pyrethrum were more effective than rue and neem ($P<0.05$) in one study.[57] A eucalyptus-based repellent containing 30% p-menthane-diol provided 97% protection against an *Anopheles* mosquito for 4 hours, similar to DEET.[58] Andiroba oil 100% *(Carapa guianensis)* was superior to soybean oil but inferior to 50% DEET as a repellent for *Aedes*. The first and third bites occurred at 60 and 101 seconds with soy oil and at 56 and 142 seconds with Andiroba oil. There were no bites within 1 hour in the DEET group.[59] Cocoa oil has shown some protection against *Simulium damnosum*.[60] Regarding ticks, in a field trial, lemon eucalyptus extract reduced *Ixodes ricinus* tick bites. While the repellent was used, the median number of attached ticks decreased from 1.5 to 0.5 ($P<0.05$).[61] One of the critical considerations in assessing insect repellents' effectiveness is the biting pressure in which a study is conducted.

■ KEY POINTS

- Fundamental methods of decreasing vector-borne disease include decreasing the disease reservoir, decreasing susceptible hosts, and decreasing the vector or contact with the vector.
- Vector control requires sustained efforts, financial resources, and public health infrastructure.
- Insect repellents are effective for an individual if used; however, they are not effective on a population level.
- In children older than 2 months, DEET less than 30% is likely the preferred insect repellent.
  - — DEET has a long safety record.
  - — Combination sunscreen-and-DEET products should not be used.
- Picaridin 19.2% has similar efficacy as 20% DEET.
  - — Dose-dependent activity up to at least 19.2%
  - — Limited safety data in children

■ REFERENCES

1. Snow RW, Guerra CA, Noor AM, Myint HY, Hay SI. The global distribution of clinical episodes of Plasmodium falciparum malaria. *Nature*. 2005;434:214–217
2. World Health Organization. *Africa Malaria Report 2003*. Geneva, Switzerland: World Health Organization; 2003 http://www.rbm.who.int/amd2003/amr2003/amr_toc.htm. Accessed March 2, 2004
3. Broderick NA, Raffa KF, Handelsman J. Midgut bacteria required for Bacillus thuringiensis insecticidal activity. *Proc Natl Acad Sci USA*. 2006;103:15196–15196
4. Vaeck M, Reynaerts A, Höfte H, et al. Transgenic plants protected from insect attack. *Nature*. 1987;328:33–37
5. Henrick CA. Methoprene. *J Am Mosq Control Assoc*. 2007;23(S2):225–239
6. Payá P, Oliva J, Zafrilla P, Cámara MA, Barba A. Bioavailability of insect growth regulator residues in citrus. *Ecotoxicology*. 2009;18:1137–1142
7. Traoré S, Wilson MD, Sima A, et al. The elimination of the onchocerciasis vector from the island of Bioko as a result of larviciding by the WHO African Programme for Onchocerciasis Control. *Acta Trop*. 2009;111:211–218
8. Tawatsin A, Thavara U, Bhakdeenuan P, et al. Field evaluation of novaluron, a chitin synthesis inhibitor larvicide, against mosquito larvae in polluted water in urban areas of Bangkok, Thailand. *Southeast Asian J Trop Med Public Health*. 2007;38:434–441
9. Sadasivaiah S, Tozan Y, Breman JG. Dichlorodiphenyltrichloroethane (DDT) for indoor residual spraying in Africa: how can it be used for malaria control? *Am J Trop Med Hyg*. 2007;77(S6):249–263
10. Campbell-Lendrum DH, Angulo VM, Esteban L, et al. House-level risk factors for triatomine infestation in Colombia. *Int J Epidemiol*. 2007;36:866–872
11. Zeledón R, Vargas LG. The role of dirt floors and of firewood in rural dwellings in the epidemiology of Chagas' disease in Costa Rica. *Am J Trop Med Hyg*. 1984;33:232–235
12. Petersen LR, Marfin AA. Shifting epidemiology of flaviviridae. *J Travel Med*. 2005;12:S3–S11
13. Allan SA, Kline D. Evaluation of various attributes of gravid female traps for collection of Culex in Florida. *Culex J Vector Ecol*. 2004;29(2):285–294

14. Frances SP, Auliff AM, Edstein MD, Cooper RD. Survey of personal protection measures against mosquitoes among Australian defense force personnel deployed to East Timor. *Mil Med.* 2003;168:227–230

15. O'Leary DR, Rigau-Perez JG, Hayes EB, Vorndam AV, Clark GG, Gubler DJ. Assessment of dengue risk in relief workers in Puerto Rico after Hurricane Georges, 1998. *Am J Trop Med Hygiene.* 2002;66:35–39

16. Boulware DR. Passive prophylaxis with permethrin treated tents reduces mosquito bites among North American summer campers. *Wilderness Environ Med.* 2005;16:9–15

17. Qiu H, Jun HW, McCall JW. Pharmacokinetics, formulation, and safety of insect repellent N,N-diethyl-3-methylbenzamide (deet): a review. *J Am Mosq Control Assoc.* 1998;14:12–27

18. Fradin MS, Day JF. Comparative efficacy of insect repellents against mosquito bites. *N Engl J Med.* 2002;347:13–18

19. Golenda CF, Solberg VB, Burge R, Gambel JM, Wirtz RA. Gender-related efficacy difference to an extended duration formulation of topical N,N-diethyl-m-toluamide (DEET). *Am J Trop Med Hyg.* 1999;60:654–657

20. Schreck CE, McGovern TP. Repellents and other personal protection strategies against Aedes albopictus. *J Am Mosq Control Assoc.* 1989;5:247–250

21. Rowland M, Downey G, Rab A, et al. DEET mosquito repellent provides personal protection against malaria: a household randomized trial in an Afghan refugee camp in Pakistan. *Trop Med Int Health.* 2004;9:335–342

22. American Academy of Pediatrics Committee on Environmental Health. *AAP News.* June 2003

23. Frances SP, Van Dung N, Beebe NW, Debboun M. Field evaluation of repellent formulations against daytime and nighttime biting mosquitoes in a tropical rainforest in northern Australia. *J Med Entomol.* 2002;39:541–544

24. Pretorius AM, Jensenius M, Clarke F, Ringertz SH. Repellent efficacy of DEET and KBR 3023 against Amblyomma hebraeum (Acari: Ixodidae). *J Med Entomol.* 2003;40:245–248

25. Klun JA, Khrimian A, Debboun M. Repellent and deterrent effects of SS220, Picaridin, and Deet suppress human blood feeding by Aedes aegypti, Anopheles stephensi, and Phlebotomus papatasi. *J Med Entomol.* 2006;43:34–39

26. Klun JA, Kramer M, Debboun M. A new in vitro bioassay system for discovery of novel human-use mosquito repellents. *J Am Mosq Control Assoc.* 2005;21:64–70

27. Badolo A, Ilboudo-Sanogo E, Ouédraogo AP, Costantini C. Evaluation of the sensitivity of Aedes aegypti and Anopheles gambiae complex mosquitoes to two insect repellents: DEET and KBR 3023. *Trop Med Int Health.* 2004;9:330–334

28. Klun JA, Khrimian A, Margaryan A, Kramer M, Debboun M. Synthesis and repellent efficacy of a new chiral piperidine analog: comparison with Deet and Bayrepel activity in human-volunteer laboratory assays against Aedes aegypti and Anopheles stephensi. *J Med Entomol.* 2003;40:293–299

29. Naucke TJ, Kröpke R, Benner G, et al. Field evaluation of the efficacy of proprietary repellent formulations with IR3535 and picaridin against Aedes aegypti. *Parasitol Res.* 2007;101:169–177

30. Costantini C, Badolo A, Ilboudo-Sanogo E. Field evaluation of the efficacy and persistence of insect repellents DEET, IR3535, and KBR 3023 against Anopheles gambiae complex and other Afrotropical vector mosquitoes. *Trans R Soc Trop Med Hyg.* 2004;98:644–652

31. Frances SP, Waterson DG, Beebe NW, Cooper RD. Field evaluation of repellent formulations containing deet and picaridin against mosquitoes in Northern Territory, Australia. *J Med Entomol.* 2004;41:414–417

32. Barnard DR, Bernier UR, Posey KH, Xue RD. Repellency of IR3535, KBR3023, paramenthane-3,8-diol, and deet to black salt marsh mosquitoes (Diptera: Culicidae) in the Everglades National Park. *J Med Entomol.* 2002;39:895–899

33. Frances SP, Van Dung N, Beebe NW, Debboun M. Field evaluation of repellent formulations against daytime and nighttime biting mosquitoes in a tropical rainforest in northern Australia. *J Med Entomol.* 2002;39:541–544

34. Yap HH, Jahangir K, Zairi J. Field efficacy of four insect repellent products against vector mosquitoes in a tropical environment. *J Am Mosq Control Assoc.* 2000;16:241–244

35. Frances SP, Waterson DG, Beebe NW, Cooper RD. Field evaluation of commercial repellent formulations against mosquitoes (Diptera: Culicidae) in Northern Territory, Australia. *J Am Mosq Control Assoc.* 2005;21:480–482

36. Pretorius AM, Jensenius M, Clarke F, Ringertz SH. Repellent efficacy of DEET and KBR 3023 against Amblyomma hebraeum (Acari: Ixodidae). *J Med Entomol.* 2003;40:245–248

37. Carroll JF, Benante JP, Klun JA, et al. Twelve-hour duration testing of cream formulations of three repellents against Amblyomma americanum. *Med Vet Entomol.* 2008;22:144–151

38. Fryauff DJ, Shoukry MA, Hanafi HA, Choi YM, Kamel KE, Schreck CE. Contact toxicity of permethrin-impregnated military uniforms to Culex pipiens and Phlebotomus papatasi: effects of laundering and time of exposure. *J Am Mosq Control Assoc.* 1996;12:84–90

39. Lillie TH, Schreck CE, Rahe AJ. Effectiveness of personal protection against mosquitoes in Alaska. *J Med Entomol.* 1988;25:475–478

40. Schreck CE, Snoddy EL, Spielman A. Pressurized sprays of permethrin or deet on military clothing for personal protection against Ixodes dammini (Acari: Ixodidae). *J Med Entomol.* 1986;23:396–399

41. Miller RJ, Wing J, Cope SE, Klavons JA, Kline DL. Repellency of permethrin-treated battle-dress uniforms during Operation Tandem Thrust 2001. *J Am Mosq Control Assoc.* 2004;20:462–464

42. Heal JD, Surgeoner GA, Lindsay LR. Permethrin as a tent treatment for protection against field populations of Aedes mosquitoes. *J Am Mosq Control Assoc.* 1995;11:99–102

43. Bouma MJ, Parvez SD, Nesbit R, Sondorp HE. Rapid decomposition of permethrin in the outer fly of an experimental tent in Pakistan. *J Am Mosq Control Assoc.* 1996;12:125–129

44. Schreck CE. Permethrin and dimethyl phthalate as tent fabric treatments against Aedes aegypti. *J Am Mosq Control Assoc.* 1991;7:533–535

45. Graham K, Mohammad N, Rehman H, Farhan M, Kamal M, Rowland M. Comparison of three pyrethroid treatments of top-sheets for malaria control in emergencies: entomological and user acceptance studies in an Afghan refugee camp in Pakistan. *Med Vet Entomol.* 2002;16:199–206

46. Yadav RS, Sampath RR, Sharma VP. Deltamethrin treated bednets for control of malaria transmitted by Anopheles culicifacies (Diptera: Culicidae) in India. *J Med Entomol.* 2001;38:613–622

47. Schreck CE, Haile DG, Kline DL. The effectiveness of permethrin and deet, alone or in combination, for protection against Aedes taeniorhynchus. *Am J Trop Med Hyg.* 1984;33:725–730

48. Sholdt LL, Schreck CE, Mwangelwa MI, Nondo J, Siachinji VJ. Evaluations of permethrin-impregnated clothing and three topical repellent formulations of deet against tsetse flies in Zambia. *Med Vet Entomol.* 1989;3:153–158

49. Klunc JA, Maa D, Gupta R. Optically active arthropod repellents for use against disease vectors. *J Med Entomol.* 2000;37:182–186

50. Kalyanasundaram M, Mathew N. N,N-diethyl phenylacetamide (DEPA): a safe and effective repellent for personal protection against hematophagous arthropods. *J Med Entomol.* 2006;43:518–525

51. Frances SP, Cooper RD, Popat S, Beebe NW. Field evaluation of repellents containing deet and AI3-37220 against Anopheles koliensis in Papua New Guinea. *J Am Mosq Control Assoc.* 2001;17:42–44

52. Kawada H, Maekawa Y, Tsuda Y, Takagi M. Trial of spatial repellency of metofluthrin-impregnated paper strip against Anopheles and Culex in shelters without walls in Lombok, Indonesia. *J Am Mosq Control Assoc.* 2004;20:434–437

53. Choi WS, Park BS, Ku SK, Lee SE. Repellent activities of essential oils and monoterpenes against Culex pipiens pallens. *J Am Mosq Control Assoc.* 2002;18:348–351

54. Srinivasan R, Kalyanasundaram M. Relative efficacy of DEPA and neem oil for repellent activity against Phlebotomus papatasi, the vector of leishmaniasis. *J Commun Dis.* 2001;33:180–184

55. Lawrance CE, Croft AM. Do mosquito coils prevent malaria? A systematic review of trials. *J Travel Med.* 2004;11:92–96

56. Trongtokit Y, Rongsriyam Y, Komalamisra N, Apiwathnasorn C. Comparative repellency of 38 essential oils against mosquito bites. *Phytother Res.* 2005;19:303–309

57. Hadis M, Lulu M, Mekonnen Y, Asfaw T. Field trials on the repellent activity of four plant products against mainly Mansonia population in western Ethiopia. *Phytother Res.* 2003;17:202–205

58. Moore SJ, Lenglet A, Hill N. Field evaluation of three plant-based insect repellents against malaria vectors in Vaca Diez Province, the Bolivian Amazon. *J Am Mosq Control Assoc.* 2002;18:107–110

59. Miot HA, Batistella RF, Batista K de A, et al. Comparative study of the topical effectiveness of the Andiroba oil (Carapa guianensis) and DEET 50% as repellent for Aedes sp. *Rev Inst Med Trop Sao Paulo.* 2004;46:253–256

60. Pitroipa X, Sankara D, Konan L, Sylla M, Doannio JM, Traore S. [Evaluation of cocoa oil for individual protection against Simulium damnosum s.i.]. *Med Trop (Mars).* 2002;62:511–516

61. Gardulf A, Wohlfart I, Gustafson R. A prospective cross-over field trial shows protection of lemon eucalyptus extract against tick bites. *J Med Entomol.* 2004;41:1064–1067

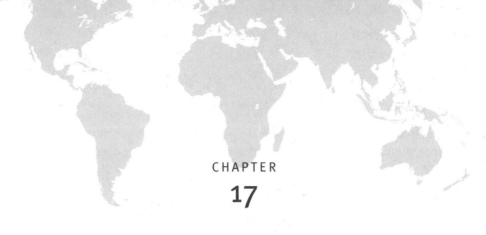

CHAPTER

17

The Ill-Returned Traveler

Andrea P. Summer, MD, MSCR, FAAP
Gregory Juckett, MD, MPH

■ INTRODUCTION

Children commonly accompany their parents to international destinations—an estimated 1.9 million children travel overseas annually.[1] The purpose of parents' travel may be leisure, business, mission work, or visiting friends and relatives. When children return ill after international travel, they typically present to their primary physician's office or to the emergency department. Evaluating and managing illness in the returned pediatric traveler is often a challenging process because of the extensive list of possible infectious etiologies that must be considered. Routine as well as destination-specific pathogens are common, the epidemiology of which is influenced by age-specific variation in immunity and behavior. When fever is one of the presenting complaints, urgent evaluation is mandatory to identify and promptly treat potentially life-threatening infections such as malaria.

Research on illnesses in returning pediatric travelers is limited. Routine respiratory viral infections are usually the most commonly diagnosed problem, followed by diarrheal illness, malaria, typhoid fever, and dengue fever.[2,3] A recent prospective controlled study revealed that diarrhea and abdominal pain are the most frequent complaints of children and adults.[4] When evaluating an ill-returning traveler, it is important to obtain a comprehensive history and perform a detailed physical examination to promptly identify more serious infections and narrow differential diagnoses. Approaching the evaluation in a systematic fashion helps ensure a timely and cost-effective workup.

■ HISTORY

When taking the history of a returned traveler, document details about the trip, including the destination(s) and activities. Box 17-1 lists topics about which questions can be asked to help obtain specific details about the trip. It is important to ask if pretravel medical advice was sought and to determine if the child is up-to-date on routine vaccines or whether the child received the recommended destination-specific vaccines. Many travelers visiting friends and relatives do not receive pretravel consultation and destination-specific vaccines and thus lack protection during their travel. Keep in mind that adherence may be reported incorrectly. It is also important to determine if bed nets and other personal protective measures, such as insect repellents, were regularly used.

Gathering these details about the trip allows the practitioner to determine exposures that may have led to the present illness. Exposures to consider typically include those related to food and water, the environment, insects, contact with animals, and various activities. Table 17-1 lists possible exposures with their corresponding risks for particular infections. The risk of certain infections varies by age group secondary to age-dependent immunity and behavior. Children younger than 2 years have a relatively immature immune system, which increases their risk for routine and travel-related infections. As children become older and more mobile, they often spend more time outdoors, where they may come into contact with various pathogens, vectors, or animals. Furthermore, adolescents who engage in a variety of high-risk activities may be susceptible to infections related to intravenous drug use, sexual contact, body piercing, and tattooing.

Comparing the time of exposure with the incubation periods of specific pathogens and the patient's specific symptom sequence enables the practitioner to narrow the list of potential diagnoses. Many resources are available that summarize incubation periods for a variety of travel-related infections. Table 17-2 provides an abbreviated list of common infections with typical incubation periods. GIDEON (www.gideononline. com), a very useful diagnostic travel program, formulates an extensive differential diagnosis based on patient symptoms, destination, and reported exposures.

Box 17-1. Trip Specifics

Destination(s)
Travel dates/duration of trip
Rural versus urban location
Type of lodging (eg, upscale hotel, budget hotel, tent, private homes)
Type of activities

Table 17-1. Example Exposures and Corresponding Risk for Certain Infections

EXPOSURE	INFECTION RISK
INGESTION	
Untreated water	Hepatitis A and E, enteric bacteria, amebiasis, *Giardia*
Unpasteurized dairy	Brucellosis, salmonellosis, listeriosis
Undercooked meat	Cysticercosis, trichinosis, enteric bacteria
BITES	
Mosquito	Malaria, yellow fever, dengue, filariasis, other arboviruses
Sandfly	Bartonellosis, leishmaniasis
Tsetse fly	African trypanosomiasis
Tick	Rickettsioses, Q fever, borreliosis, ehrlichiosis/anaplasmosis, tularemia
Flea	Plague, tungiasis
Reduviids	American trypanosomiasis (Chagas disease)
Blackfly	Onchocerciasis
Mites	Scrub typhus
Lice	Epidemic typhus, trench fever
Mammal	Rabies, tularemia, bacterial cellulitis, rat-bite fever
ACTIVITY EXPOSURE	
Freshwater contact	Schistosomiasis, leptospirosis
African game parks	African trypanosomiasis, malaria, rickettsial diseases (eg, Africa tick bite fever), botfly
Caves	Histoplasmosis, Marburg virus
Rivers	Leptospirosis, onchocerciasis
Barefoot (sand, dirt, mud)	Strongyloides, hookworm, cutaneous larva migrans
Body fluid exposure	Hepatitis B or C, HIV, syphilis, chlamydia, gonorrhea

From Summer A, Stauffer WM. Evaluation of the sick child following travel to the tropics. *Pediatr Ann.* 2008;37(12):821–826. Reprinted with permission from SLACK Inc.

Table 17-2. Typical Incubation Periods for Certain Travel-Related Infections		
SHORT (<14 D)	MEDIUM (≤2 TO 6 WK)	LONG (>4 TO 6 WK)
Arboviruses	Amebiasis	American trypanosomiasis
Babesiosis	Babesiosis	Enteric protozoa/helminths
Dengue	Brucellosis	Fascioliasis
Enteric bacteria	Hepatitis A, E	Filariasis
Leptospirosis	Leptospirosis	Hepatitis B, C
Malaria	Malaria	HIV
Meningococcal disease	Melioidosis	Leishmaniasis
Plague	Schistosomiasis	Malaria
Polio	Strongyloides	Strongyloides
Rickettsial disease	Trichinosis	Trichinosis
SARS	Tuberculosis	Typhoid fever
Strongyloides	Tungiasis	Tuberculosis

Abbreviation: SARS, severe acute respiratory syndrome.

From Summer A, Stauffer WM. Evaluation of the sick child following travel to the tropics. *Pediatr Ann.* 2008;37(12):821–826. Reprinted with permission from SLACK Inc.

■ PHYSICAL EXAMINATION

A thorough physical examination may provide additional clues to the diagnostic process. Carefully review vital signs for evidence of severe systemic illness such as fever, tachycardia, tachypnea, or hypotension, which can be associated with a life-threatening infection such as malaria. A child with fever and relative bradycardia may have an infection with an intracellular pathogen such as *Salmonella typhi* or *Babesia*. Respiratory findings such as wheezing and rales are commonly associated with viral or bacterial infections but may also occur with more exotic pulmonary infections. The presence of a hemorrhagic rash is worrisome for serious infections such as meningococcemia, rickettsial, yellow fever, or other hemorrhagic fevers. Altered mentation, meningismus, or a focal neurologic deficit should prompt an immediate evaluation for central nervous system infections.

Developing a Differential Diagnosis by Signs and Symptoms

All presenting symptoms should be recorded even if they initially appear unrelated. Fever, reported in up to 25% to 30% of cases, is of special concern.[5] Documenting the timing and sequence of symptoms relative to potential exposures is imperative. When fever is part of the symptomatology, initial efforts should focus on identifying and treating potentially life-threatening infections. Once life-threatening infections are eliminated, a systematic approach may be used to determine appropriate laboratory and imaging studies.

Life-Threatening Infections

Malaria

Travelers presenting with fever who visited a malaria endemic area must be assumed to have malaria until proven otherwise. In humans, malaria is caused by 1 of 5 protozoan *Plasmodium* species, which is transmitted by the bite of an infected female *Anopheles* mosquito: *P falciparum, P vivax, P ovale, P malariae,* or *P knowlesi.* Malaria transmission occurs in much of Africa (highest rates of transmission), Asia, Central and South America, Hispaniola, and the South Pacific. Africa is also where *P falciparum,* the most lethal and drug-resistant species, predominates.[1] *P vivax,* which is associated with a relapsing course but is typically not fatal, is the most prevalent species in Asia. Malaria usually presents with nonspecific symptoms, especially in children. Symptoms such as fever, chills, myalgias, fatigue, and headache are often present. Classically described periodic fever patterns are not helpful for diagnosis as they are seldom noted until the infection has been present for many days. In young children, respiratory and gastrointestinal symptoms may also occur, which can easily confuse the evaluation and lead to mistaken diagnoses of gastroenteritis or respiratory infections. A febrile child with travel to a malaria-endemic region should always have malaria excluded even in the presence of other symptoms, such as gastroenteritis.

Laboratory findings in children with malaria are also nonspecific but often include thrombocytopenia, neutropenia, and an elevated C-reactive protein. Anemia commonly occurs but may be due to a variety of other causes, including nutritional deficiencies. Hyperbilirubinemia and mildly elevated liver enzymes may also be observed, especially in children with severe or chronic infection. Hypoglycemia, hyponatremia, and acidosis are indicative of a severe disease. Other indicators of severe malaria include impaired consciousness and respiratory distress, which are shown to be associated with a high risk of death.[6,7] Cerebral malaria can occur in children infected with *P falciparum* and leads to a spectrum of neurologic symptoms ranging from mildly depressed sensorium to deep coma. Focal motor deficits and opisthotonic posturing may be observed. Mortality rates vary depending on available resources and timeliness of treatment but range from 7% to 50%.

Diagnosing malaria is traditionally accomplished with thick and thin blood smears, the sensitivity and specificity of which depend on the parasitemia level and laboratory personnel experience. Alternative, non-microscopic methods, such as rapid antigen tests and polymerase chain reaction (PCR)-based methods, are being used more commonly. Rapid antigen tests are generally fast and easy to use and have high sensitivity and specificity, especially for *P falciparum*.[8,9] When rapid diagnostic methods are not available, presumptive treatment should always be initiated until the diagnosis can be confirmed.

Bacterial Etiologies

Potentially life-threatening bacterial infections can also occur in pediatric travelers, most notably typhoid fever and meningococcemia. Vaccines are available for these infectious diseases, none of which are fully protective. Typhoid fever is caused by the bacterium *S typhi* and is transmitted by the fecal-oral route. The highest incidence of typhoid fever occurs in south-central and southeast Asia.[10] Regions of medium incidence include the rest of Asia, as well as less-developed areas in Africa, Latin America, and the Caribbean. Approximately 400 cases of typhoid fever occur annually in the United States, the majority of which are reported in travelers.[1] Clinically, typhoid presents with fever, headache, abdominal pain, constipation, diarrhea, and rash. Diagnosis is made by isolating the causative organism in blood or stool, but neither method is very sensitive. Treatment options include a third-generation cephalosporin, fluoroquinolones, and azithromycin; however, emerging antibiotic resistance, especially to fluoroquinolones, is increasingly reported.[11]

Travelers to sub-Saharan Africa, as well as those who participate in the Hajj pilgrimage in Saudi Arabia, may be at risk for meningococcal disease. Attack rates of the serogroup A meningococcal strain peak annually during the dry season within the "meningitis belt" of Africa, which extends from Mali to Ethiopia.[12,13] Serogroup W-135 has caused epidemic disease in West Africa and in Hajj visitors.[14] Clinical signs and symptoms of meningitis most often include fever, headache, nausea, vomiting, and stiff neck. These symptoms can rapidly progress and result in death if they are not recognized and treated promptly with antibiotics.

Immediately administering antibiotics is justified, even before performing a lumbar puncture, unless it can be performed without delay. Meningococcal meningitis is characterized by typical cerebrospinal fluid (CSF) findings (eg, high white blood cell count, low glucose) and confirmed by isolating the causative agent in blood or CSF. The slightly increased risk of negative cultures from early antibiotic administration is more than offset by decreased risk of mortality. Meningococcal infections are typically treated with ceftriaxone or penicillin G (in cases in which the isolate is proven susceptible).

Dengue Fever

Dengue fever, a mosquito-borne flavivirus infection, is prevalent in warm-weather climates in rural and urban areas of Asia, Africa, and the Americas. The infection is carried by the *Aedes aegypti* mosquito and has a short incubation period (3 to 14 days). Symptoms often include fever, headache, myalgias, arthralgias, and rash. Muscle aches can be so severe that the infection is sometimes referred to as *breakbone fever*. Diagnosis is clinical and may be confirmed through dengue-specific antibody tests. Treatment is supportive care. Patients should be monitored for bleeding complications that may occur in dengue hemorrhagic fever or dengue shock syndrome. These complications rarely occur in travelers but are important to recognize because they may progress to disseminated intravascular coagulation and hemodynamic instability. Cases of dengue fever have increased considerably over the past several years, which is possibly caused by climate change.[15,16]

Other Febrile Illnesses

Routine Infections

Once potentially life-threatening infections are eliminated, other causes of febrile illness should be considered. Several studies show that routine viral and bacterial infections are commonly reported in travelers of all ages, especially children. A child presenting with fever and focal findings (eg, rhinorrhea, cough, sore throat) would most likely have a common upper respiratory viral infection. In a prospective study that followed nearly 800 Americans who traveled to lower-income countries, 26% experienced cough, sore throat, congestion, or earache, and 46% reported diarrhea for an average of 3.7 days.[17] For these travelers, risk of illness was most strongly correlated with travel duration; each additional day of travel increased the chance of illness by 3% to 4%.

Exotic Infections

Travelers may be at risk of rickettsial diseases if they engage in recreational activities that expose them to arthropods associated with these intracellular pathogens. The rickettsioses are traditionally divided into 3 main groups: spotted fevers, typhus, and scrub typhus. Clinical symptoms vary but often include fever, headache, myalgias, arthralgias, and rash. Rickettsial infections have been reported more commonly over the past couple of decades and are most often diagnosed by serology, although culture and PCR tests are sometimes used.[18] Treatment is usually with a tetracycline antibiotic, even in children.

Schistosomiasis, a parasitic infection caused by *Schistosoma* blood flukes, results from wading or swimming in infected freshwater. *Schistosoma* infection occurs widely throughout the tropics, especially in Africa, and appears to be becoming more common in travelers.[19,20] Acute infections are generally asymptomatic but occasionally can present with a constellation of findings known as Katayama fever (ie, fever, abdominal pain, fatigue, headache, myalgias, diarrhea, and cough). In a study by the GeoSentinel Global Surveillance Network, the most commonly reported symptoms were fever, fatigue, and gastrointestinal and genitourinary.[21] Furthermore, travelers with schistosomiasis who presented within 6 months after travel had more respiratory symptoms than those who presented later. Diagnosis can be made by identifying *Schistosoma* eggs in stool or urine or by antibody detection. Praziquantel is the preferred drug for all *Schistosoma* infections.

Leptospirosis, caused by spirochetes of the genus *Leptospira,* is distributed worldwide, with a higher incidence in tropical areas, and is becoming increasingly more common in travelers.[22] Human infection occurs through direct contact with urine or tissues of carrier animals, typically during recreational water exposure in contaminated rivers or lakes. Symptoms are variable and nonspecific early in the illness but may progress to jaundice, renal failure, and hemorrhagic manifestations. Diagnosis is usually by serology. Treatment options include penicillin antibiotics and doxycycline.

Chikungunya fever, a tropical arbovirus similar to dengue, is also reported in travelers. Symptoms are usually flu-like, with severe joint pain that can persist for months following infection.[23] Diagnosis is by serology and treatment is supportive.

African trypanosomiasis, or African sleeping sickness, is another rare but important cause of fever in travelers. There are 2 forms, East and West African, of this protozoal infection, both of which are transmitted by the bite of the tsetse fly. Most cases in travelers are acquired in East

African game parks.[24,25] Symptoms usually include fever, rash, fatigue, and lymphadenopathy; altered mental status or coma may also occur as the disease progresses. Diagnosis can be confirmed by identifying motile trypanosomes in the blood or CSF. Treatment includes a course of anti-trypanosomal therapy with the specific regimen depending on the infecting species and stage of infection.

Respiratory Infections

Respiratory infections commonly develop in travelers of all ages, with estimates ranging from 10% to 20%. Air travel alone is associated with an increased risk of respiratory infections and is shown to be related to the proximity of the traveler to an infected passenger.[26] The spectrum of clinical presentation varies from mild upper respiratory tract infections to life-threatening pneumonias. In a review conducted by the GeoSentinel Global Surveillance Network, which comprises 25 globally dispersed clinics, nonspecific upper respiratory infection was the most common diagnosis, with pharyngitis, otitis media, and sinusitis occurring significantly more often in younger persons.[27] In a study that examined the etiology of respiratory infections in travelers, influenza virus was detected in 38% of those with respiratory symptoms, followed by rhinovirus, adenovirus, and respiratory syncytial virus.[28]

Tuberculosis and more exotic pulmonary infections must also be considered, especially if the history is concerning for exposures to rodents (eg, tularemia, plague), bird or bat droppings (eg, histoplasmosis), or undercooked crustaceans (eg, paragonimiasis). Furthermore, travelers to the Far East, especially Thailand, are at risk of acquiring melioidosis, an infection caused by the bacterium *Burkholderia pseudomallei*. The incubation period is variable, ranging from a few days to many years. Clinical presentation also varies but typically includes the abrupt onset of headache, myalgias, fever, and rigor after several days of cough, shortness of breath, and occasional hemoptysis. Chest radiographs may reveal consolidation of the upper lobes and cavitation, which closely mimics tuberculosis. Treatment is usually accomplished with third-generation cephalosporins, broad-spectrum penicillins, or imipenem.

Gastrointestinal Illness

Gastrointestinal symptoms, especially diarrhea, occur frequently during and after travel.[29] When children present with complaints of diarrhea after travel it is helpful to determine whether the diarrhea is acute or chronic (longer than 2 weeks' duration). An invasive organism should be considered if the child also has fever, bloody stools, abdominal pain, and tenesmus. Diarrhea of longer duration accompanied by weight loss and malabsorptive symptoms may be secondary to a protozoan infection such as *Giardia lamblia* or *Cryptosporidium*. The etiology of traveler's diarrhea in children is not well studied, but data from a few small studies suggest that bacterial pathogens are common.[30] Viral etiologies (eg, rotavirus) are thought to be an important source of traveler's diarrhea in the youngest children. The most commonly identified bacterial agents include enterotoxigenic and enteroaggregative *Escherichia coli*, *Salmonella* and *Shigella* species, and *Campylobacter*. Diarrhea caused by *E coli* O157:H7 has not been reported in pediatric travelers.

Laboratory studies for children with traveler's diarrhea should initially include routine stool cultures even though they fail to detect diarrhea caused by pathogenic *E coli*. In cases of chronic diarrhea, *Giardia* and *Cryptosporidium* antigen tests should also be obtained, as well as a stool ova and parasite examination and special stains for *Cyclospora* and *Isospora*.[31] The most commonly used treatment in children for bacterial pathogens is azithromycin. Targeted therapy is used for most protozoal and helminth infections.

Many workups of post-travel diarrhea fail to demonstrate any specific organism and are currently thought to be caused by post–traveler's diarrhea irritable bowel. Temporary lactose intolerance may contribute to patient discomfort. Most of these cases eventually resolve with probiotics and dietary modification.

Another fairly common gastrointestinal ailment in travelers is viral hepatitis, which typically presents with flu-like symptoms and nausea followed by jaundice, abdominal pain, malaise, and vomiting. Hepatitis A and E, both widely endemic viruses readily transmitted by the fecal-oral route, are the types of hepatitis most often reported in travelers.[32,33] Hepatitis A is often minimally symptomatic in younger children but can be transmitted to older children and adults, who usually develop a more severe disease. A highly efficacious and safe hepatitis A vaccine is routinely given to toddlers (older than 1 year) as part of the routine immunization series and is also recommended for anyone traveling to the developing world.[34] Treatment for hepatitis A and E is supportive care.

Dermatologic Manifestations

Skin problems in a returning traveler are often related to environmental factors, allergic reactions, infestations, and infections.[35] Key questions should focus on the characteristic primary lesion (eg, macule, papule, vesicle, petechiae), exposure history (including medications), tenderness of the primary lesion (suggesting infection) versus pruritus (suggesting allergy), the presence or absence of accompanying systemic symptoms, and the rash's duration and evolution. Many rashes are related to allergic reactions to recent therapy.

As might be expected, many skin problems in tropical climates stem from sun or other environmental exposures. Polymorphous light eruption (sun allergy), appearing as a variable maculopapular eruption, is a sensitivity reaction to intense ultraviolet A light in an unacclimated individual. Rash and pruritus occur soon after exposure. Sunburn, and its unpleasant aftermath, also complicates many tropical vacations but is easily preventable with some forethought. Miliaria or prickly heat usually resolves in returned travelers but its more chronic form, miliaria profunda, may follow prolonged exposure to hot, humid conditions.

Allergic and photosensitivity reactions to medications or plants are routinely encountered. Photosensitivity reactions often occur on exposed ankles and the tops of sandal-clad feet. Doxycycline, popular for malaria prophylaxis, is a common offender, but hydrochlorothiazide and ciprofloxacin also cause many reactions. Lemon or lime juice may cause an impressive photodermatitis if it drips onto skin while at the beach. Exposure to a variety of tropical plants provokes an allergic contact dermatitis resembling poison ivy. Exposure to unpeeled mangos, the rind of which cross-reacts with poison ivy, frequently causes a persistent itchy rash around the lips. Other offenders are Caribbean poisonwood, cashew nut fruits, and Asian lacquerware (Japanese lacquer tree).[36] Any prolonged self-treatment with potentially sensitizing creams (eg, Neosporin, topical diphenhydramine) or topical anesthetics (eg, benzocaine) can seriously extend rash duration.

Infectious rashes related to overseas exposures are often found in returning travelers. Impetigo and various bacterial pyodermas are most common in children. Herpes labialis or cold sores follow intense ultraviolet A exposure. Fungal infections, especially athlete's foot and tinea cruris, are frequent in older travelers. The most common parasitic infection by far (25% of all rashes in returning travelers in one series) is cutaneous larva migrans or creeping eruption from exposure to dog hookworm on beaches.[35] However, cutaneous myiasis from human botflies will also occasionally present as a post-vacation boil. Children often acquire scabies, head lice, or even chigoes *(Tunga penetrans)* while abroad if they have contact with local children or wear improper footwear.

Marine exposures produce their own set of rashes. Sea lice from jellyfish larvae usually produce an itchy rash beneath the bathing suit, whereas swimmer's itch, from avian cercaria, affects exposed skin. A history of freshwater swimmer's itch in the tropics may well be the first sign of infection with human schistosomiasis. Fire coral produces long-lasting areas of hyperpigmentation long after the sting subsides.

Neurologic Illness

The returned traveler presenting with neurologic symptoms, especially when accompanied by fever, is always a cause for concern. A patient complaining of headache, neck pain or stiffness, fever, and photophobia must be rapidly evaluated for meningitis or encephalitis. To rule out life-threatening infections, initial management should include obtaining CSF for laboratory studies and initiating empiric antibiotic, antiparasitic, or antiviral therapy as appropriate. Possible bacterial etiologies include *Neisseria meningitidis, Streptococcal pneumoniae,* and *Listeria monocytogenes* (immunocompromised patients), and *Haemophilus influenzae* type b in incompletely immunized children younger than 5 years. A variety of encephalitic viruses can be transmitted by the bite of arthropod vectors such as mosquitoes, ticks, and fleas. Dengue fever, discussed previously, is the arboviral infection most often acquired by travelers. Japanese encephalitis (JE) is a mosquito-borne flavivirus infection that is common in parts of Asia and occasionally reported among travelers.[37] Infection severity varies, with many JE cases being asymptomatic. Central nervous system (CNS) manifestations of more serious infections may include seizures, delirium, ataxia, and cranial nerve palsies. Diagnosis can be achieved through detection of virus-specific antibodies in the CSF. Characteristic findings on magnetic resonance imaging (MRI) include abnormal intensity signals in the thalami, basal ganglia, and brain stem.[38] Severe infections have a high mortality rate, especially in children, and high rates of post-infectious neurologic sequelae.[39]

A wide variety of parasitic infections can impact the CNS, including *Taenia solium, Schistosoma, Strongyloides stercoralis,* and *Toxocara canis.* Any new onset seizure should prompt an investigation (including a head MRI scan) to exclude neurocysticercosis from the ingestion of pork tapeworm eggs. Transmission methods of CNS parasites vary from ingestion to direct contact with skin or mucous membranes. Symptoms are usually related to a host inflammatory response induced by the parasite larvae or eggs within the brain or spinal cord.[40] Eosinophilic meningoencephalitis is characterized by a pleocytosis with 10% or more eosinophils in the CSF and can result from several parasitic infections; *Angiostrongylus cantonensis* or *Gnathostoma spinigerum* are 2 of the more common causes.[41] Treatment is targeted antihelminthic therapy.

Lymphadenopathy

Lymphadenopathy suggests the presence of a systemic infection that could range from a transient acute illness (eg, herpes simplex virus, pyoderma, tonsillitis, cat scratch disease, mononucleosis) to a much more serious or chronic condition (eg, scrofula, acute retroviral syndrome). Localizing symptoms often point to the primary cause of the lymphadenitis, but fever and malaise are far less helpful. A careful medication history is also important because certain drugs (eg, phenytoin) produce enlarged lymph nodes, often in the absence of rash.

Generalized lymphadenopathy should prompt a workup to exclude HIV infection, hepatitis B, syphilis, cancer, and lymphoma. A typical investigation should include complete blood cell count (CBC), tuberculosis skin test (purified protein derivative), tests for HIV infection, rapid plasma reagin, hepatitis B surface antigen, chest radiography, and sedimentation rate. A more challenging situation is when a traveler complains of new enlarged lymph nodes without any obvious source of infection. In such cases, it is reasonable to biopsy persistent nodes that would otherwise remain unexplained.[42]

■ LABORATORY EVALUATION

The initial laboratory investigation of an ill-returning traveler often includes a CBC with differential, blood films or rapid antigen test for malaria (if patient traveled to a malaria endemic destination), blood culture, liver transaminases, electrolytes, urinalysis, and a sedimentation rate. Lumbar puncture for CSF evaluation is indicated for patients with meningeal signs or altered sensorium, especially if fever is present. Serologic testing for specific pathogens such as schistosomes, dengue fever, hepatitis, and rickettsia may be useful but may often only be available at reference laboratories, delaying results. Also, cross-reactivity can occur between helminths. Evaluation of stool is recommended when diarrhea is the predominant symptom, especially in cases of bloody or persistent diarrhea. Diagnostic imaging should be based on specific findings in the history or physical examination. More invasive diagnostic tests, such as colonoscopy or bronchoscopy, are rarely needed; however, biopsy of skin lesions may be useful in cases in which a laboratory evaluation is inconclusive. If the patient is severely ill, presumptive treatment should be initiated immediately and continued until results of diagnostic testing are available.

Eosinophilia in a returned traveler is usually caused by an allergic response to infections, drug reactions, connective tissue diseases, or more rarely, malignancies. Eosinophilia may be mild (500 to 1,000 cells/mm^3), moderate (1,000 to 3,000 cells/mm^3) or severe (greater than 3,000 cells/mm^3). A newly acquired tissue-invading helminth infection (eg, Löffler syndrome in early ascaris infection) should always be suspected; however, this finding is usually a transient phenomenon with intestinal parasites and resolves once the worms reach the gut. Fortunately, empiric dosing with albendazole is usually curative (stool ova and parasite examination results may be negative at this early stage). On the other hand, most tissue helminths, such as *Strongyloides* and trichinosis, produce significant, persistent eosinophilia in immunocompetent patients. Protozoal infections, unlike those caused by helminths, seldom cause eosinophilia. Eosinophilia is frequently found in drug hypersensitivity reactions. An allergic rash and the history of recent drug use (often an antibiotic) suggest this diagnosis.

A basic evaluation for unexplained eosinophilia should include a CBC with differential, stool ova and parasite examination with acid-fast staining, urinalysis, and chest radiograph. If these results are normal, further evaluation for connective tissue diseases and malignancies may be necessary. Depending on prior exposure, skin snips for onchocercosis and *Strongyloides, Schistosoma,* and filarial serologies may even be justified. It is common to have negative workup results, in which case stable patients may be given a trial of albendazole therapy or merely followed for 3 to 6 months to see if the condition resolves.[43]

■ MANAGEMENT

Treatment options are dictated by the specific pathogen. Aggressive therapy must be initiated for potentially life-threatening infections, including empiric treatment with antibiotics and antimalarials in toxic-appearing children who visited a malaria endemic destination. Routine infections should be approached in the same manner as with the non-traveler. Empiric therapy with azithromycin is reasonable for cases of pediatric traveler's diarrhea assumed to be caused by the most common bacterial pathogens. In situations in which a more exotic infection is suspected, consultation with a specialist in infectious diseases or travel medicine is recommended.

■ KEY POINTS

- Travel to exotic locations has become much more common among children.
- The evaluation of the ill-returned traveler usually includes a comprehensive history, careful examination, and focused laboratory panel.
- Fever in a returned traveler should prompt immediate evaluation for potentially life-threatening infections.
- Referral to a specialist in infectious or tropical diseases is recommended in cases in which the child is severely ill or when the diagnosis is not apparent after an initial thorough evaluation.

■ REFERENCES

1. Arguin PM, Reed C, eds. *CDC Health Information for International Travel.* 2008 ed. Philadelphia, PA: Elsevier Mosby; 2008
2. Klein JL, Millman GC. Prospective, hospital based study of fever in children in the United Kingdom who had recently spent time in the tropics. *BMJ.* 1998;316(7142): 1425–1426
3. Greenwood Z, et al. Gastrointestinal infection among international travelers globally. *J Travel Med.* 2008;15(4):221–228
4. Newman-Klee C, et al. Incidence and types of illness when traveling to the tropics: a prospective controlled study of children and their parents. *Am J Trop Med Hyg.* 2007;77(4):764–769
5. Wilson ME, et al. Fever in returned travelers: results from the GeoSentinel Surveillance Network. *Clin Infect Dis.* 2007;44(12):1560–1568
6. Marsh K, et al. Indicators of life-threatening malaria in African children. *N Engl J Med.* 1995;332(21):1399–1404
7. English M, et al. Deep breathing in children with severe malaria: indicator of metabolic acidosis and poor outcome. *Am J Trop Med Hyg.* 1996;55(5):521–524
8. Moody A. Rapid diagnostic tests for malaria parasites. *Clin Microbiol Rev.* 2002;15(1): 66–78
9. Proux S, et al. Paracheck-Pf: a new, inexpensive and reliable rapid test for P. falciparum malaria. *Trop Med Int Health.* 2001;6(2):99–101
10. Crump JA, Luby SP, Mintz ED. The global burden of typhoid fever. *Bull WHO.* 2004; 82(5):346–353
11. Crump JA, et al. Clinical response and outcome of infection with Salmonella enterica serotype Typhi with decreased susceptibility to fluoroquinolones: a United States foodnet multicenter retrospective cohort study. *Antimicrob Agents Chemother.* 2008;52(4):1278–1284
12. Leimkugel J, et al. Clonal waves of Neisseria colonisation and disease in the African meningitis belt: eight-year longitudinal study in northern Ghana. *PLoS Med.* 2007; 4(3):e101
13. Teyssou R, Muros-Le Rouzic E. Meningitis epidemics in Africa: a brief overview. *Vaccine.* 2007;25(Suppl 1):A3–A7
14. Taha MK, et al. Neisseria meningitidis serogroups W135 and A were equally prevalent among meningitis cases occurring at the end of the 2001 epidemics in Burkina Faso and Niger. *J Clin Microbiol.* 2002;40(3):1083–1084

15. Kyle JL, Harris E. Global spread and persistence of dengue. *Annu Rev Microbiol.* 2008; 62:71–92

16. Schwartz E, et al. Seasonality, annual trends, and characteristics of dengue among ill returned travelers, 1997–2006. *Emerg Infect Dis.* 2008;14(7):1081–1088

17. Hill DR. Health problems in a large cohort of Americans traveling to developing countries. *J Travel Med.* 2000;7(5):259–266

18. Jensenius M, Fournier PE, Raoult D. Rickettsioses and the international traveler. *Clin Infect Dis.* 2004;39(10):1493–1499

19. Meltzer E, et al. Schistosomiasis among travelers: new aspects of an old disease. *Emerg Infect Dis.* 2006;12(11):1696–1700

20. Leshem E, et al. Acute schistosomiasis outbreak: clinical features and economic impact. *Clin Infect Dis.* 2008;47(12):1499–1506

21. Nicolls DJ, et al. Characteristics of schistosomiasis in travelers reported to the GeoSentinel Surveillance Network 1997–2008. *Am J Trop Med Hyg.* 2008;79(5):729–734

22. Pappas G, et al. The globalization of leptospirosis: worldwide incidence trends. *Int J Infect Dis.* 2008;12(4):351–357

23. Taubitz W, et al. Chikungunya fever in travelers: clinical presentation and course. *Clin Infect Dis.* 2007;45(1):e1–e4

24. Jelinek T, et al. Cluster of African trypanosomiasis in travelers to Tanzanian national parks. *Emerg Infect Dis.* 2002;8(6):634–635

25. Sinha A, et al. African trypanosomiasis in two travelers from the United States. *Clin Infect Dis.* 1999;29(4):840–844

26. Leder K, Newman D. Respiratory infections during air travel. *Intern Med J.* 2005;35(1): 50–55

27. Leder K, et al. Respiratory tract infections in travelers: a review of the GeoSentinel surveillance network. *Clin Infect Dis.* 2003;36(4):399–406

28. Camps M, et al. Incidence of respiratory viruses among travelers with a febrile syndrome returning from tropical and subtropical areas. *J Med Virol.* 2008;80(4):711–715

29. Kolars JC, Fischer PR. Evaluation of diarrhea in the returned traveler. *Prim Care.* 2002; 29(4):931–945

30. Mackell S. Traveler's diarrhea in the pediatric population: etiology and impact. *Clin Infect Dis.* 2005;41(Suppl 8):S547–S552

31. Regnath T, Klemm T, Ignatius R. Rapid and accurate detection of Giardia lamblia and Cryptosporidium spp. antigens in human fecal specimens by new commercially available qualitative immunochromatographic assays. *Eur J Clin Microbiol Infect Dis.* 2006;25(12):807–809

32. Gosselin C, et al. Comparison of trip characteristics of children and adults with travel-acquired hepatitis A infection. *Pediatr Infect Dis J.* 2006;25(12):1184–1186

33. Piper-Jenks N, Horowitz HW, Schwartz E. Risk of hepatitis E infection to travelers. *J Travel Med.* 2000;7(4):194–199

34. Update: Prevention of hepatitis A after exposure to hepatitis A virus and in international travelers. Updated recommendations of the Advisory Committee on Immunization Practices (ACIP). *MMWR Morb Mortal Wkly Rep.* 2007;56(41):1080–1084

35. Caumes E, et al. Dermatoses associated with travel to tropical countries: a prospective study of the diagnosis and management of 269 patients presenting to a tropical disease unit. *Clin Infect Dis.* 1995;20(3):542–548

36. Lovell CR. Phytodermatitis. *Clin Dermatol.* 1997;15(4):607–613

37. Japanese encephalitis in a U.S. traveler returning from Thailand, 2004. *MMWR Morb Mortal Wkly Rep.* 2005;54(5):123–125

38. Shoji H, et al. Magnetic resonance imaging findings in Japanese encephalitis. White matter lesions. *J Neuroimaging*. 1994;4(4):206–211

39. Kumar R, et al. Clinical features in children hospitalized during the 2005 epidemic of Japanese encephalitis in Uttar Pradesh, India. *Clin Infect Dis*. 2006;43(2):123–131

40. Ferrari TC, Moreira PR, Cunha AS. Clinical characterization of neuroschistosomiasis due to Schistosoma mansoni and its treatment. *Acta Trop*. 2008;108(2-3):89–97

41. Graeff-Teixeira C, da Silva AC, Yoshimura K. Update on eosinophilic meningoencephalitis and its clinical relevance. *Clin Microbiol Rev*. 2009;22(2):322–348

42. Ferrer R. Lymphadenopathy: differential diagnosis and evaluation. *Am Fam Physician*. 1998;58(6):1313–1320

43. Weller PF. Eosinophilia in travelers. *Med Clin North Am*. 1992;76(6):1413–1432

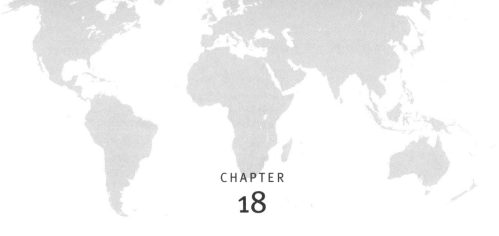

CHAPTER
18

International Adoption

Carol Cohen Weitzman, MD, FAAP

■ INTRODUCTION

As of 2009, approximately 13,000 children each year are adopted into
the United States from countries around the world who experience
varied caregiver arrangements, losses, separations, and emotional,
nutritional, and social deprivation. Together, the child and adoptive
family must forge a new relationship that supports the child's transition
and adaptation to the new home and promotes healthy development.
The child's and family's success in adapting to these changes in care
are influenced by a complex interaction between innate, individual capabilities and external resources. The pediatric provider can play a critical
role in providing continuity of care, family guidance, and support for
the physical, neurodevelopmental, and emotional needs of the child.

■ EPIDEMIOLOGY OF INTERNATIONAL ADOPTION

It is estimated that as of 2004, 1.6 million children younger than
18 years live with adoptive parents and that 2.5% of US families have
an adopted child. Approximately 127,000 children are adopted in the
United States each year; contribution of international adoption rose
from approximately 5% to 15% of this total (Figure 18-1).[1] The total
number of children adopted each year from other countries fluctuates
and peaked in 2004 at approximately 23,000. In 2009, this number
decreased to approximately 12,700 children and seems to be following
this trend (Figure 18-2).[2] The reasons for this shift include greater efforts
within countries to adopt children internally, allegations of adoption

Figure 18-1. Percent of All Adoptions in the United States by Type

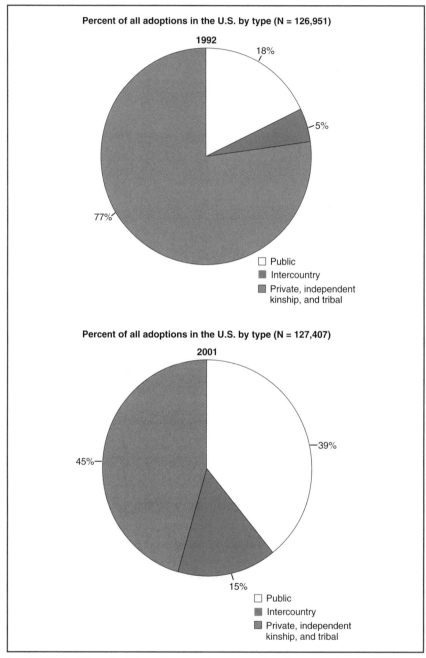

From Child Welfare Information Gateway. How many children were adopted in 2000 and 2001?—Highlights. August 2004. http://www.childwelfare.gov/pubs/s_adoptedhighlights.pdf. Accessed June 22, 2011

Figure 18-2. Adoptions to the United States

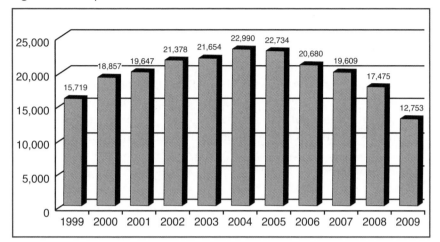

From US Department of State. Intercountry Adoption. Statistics. Adoptions by Year.
http://adoption.state.gov/about_us/statistics.php. Accessed July 6, 2011

procedure fraud in foreign countries, changing political climates, and difficulty with implementing the Hague convention.

The demographics of adoption also shifted over the last few decades and vary considerably by birth country. In 1986, children were primarily adopted from Korea and South and Central America. These children tended to be very young, from foster care, and without significant medical and developmental challenges.[3] As of 2008, the greatest number of children was adopted from Guatemala and China, followed by Russia, Ethiopia, and Korea—children from more than 18 countries were entering the United States.[2] Currently, most children adopted internationally are females younger than 4 years.[1] This skewing can be explained by the large proportions of girls adopted from China. The demographic of adoption will probably continue to change with time, and that makes caring for internationally adopted children challenging.

Family demographics also shifted with increasing numbers of children being adopted into transracial, transcultural, single-parent, and same-sex families.[4] Overall, parents of international adoptees tend to be white, married, well-educated, and economically stable.[3,5] Some of these characteristics are most likely due to requirements by the foreign country and the high cost of international adoption, but issues such as cultural norms and stigma around adoption may also play a part. Current estimates suggest that there are 5 to 6 adoption seekers for every completed adoption.

■ ADOPTION PROCESS FOR FAMILIES

The process of adopting a child from another country is characterized by long waits, uncertainty and confusion, high costs, paperwork, and bureaucracy. Families choose to adopt for many reasons; adoption is frequently the culmination of failed pregnancies, infertility, and loss of the imagined child, as well as for humanitarian reasons and to enlarge a family. Understanding these possible events can help give pediatric providers greater insight into parents' experiences, expectations, and motivations leading up to the adoption. The following section provides a brief overview of the complex steps that families must follow to complete an adoption.

Agency Selection

There is variability in the quality between agencies and the services they offer. Fees may vary among agencies as well as experience and reliability. Agencies must currently be accredited through the Council on Accreditation or the Colorado Department of Human Services to provide adoption services for Hague adoption cases.

Eligibility

There are a number of US and foreign country requirements that parents must fulfill to be deemed eligible to adopt a child.
- *US requirements:* Each family must complete a home study, which typically involves at least one home visit by a social worker. Home study requirements vary per state. During this visit, the physical, mental, and emotional capabilities of the prospective parents are assessed, as well as family demographics, financial resources, criminal history, and any history of abuse or violence.
- *Country requirements:* Requirements for prospective parents vary enormously among countries and are easily accessible on the US Department of State Office of Children's Issues Web site (www. adoption.state.gov). There are often specific age, income, marital, and health requirements. Some countries have highly specific requirements, such as a maximal allowed body mass index, and many countries do not permit adoption by same-sex couples.

Paperwork

There are various forms required by state and federal agencies and by the intended adoptive country that need to be filed before a family can be approved for adoption. Documents that families must complete can be lengthy, confusing, and time-consuming. The US Citizenship and

Immigration Services is the agency that determines whether a child is eligible to immigrate to the United States.

Financial Resources

Costs for adoption vary between countries, but the National Adoption Information Clearinghouse estimates the cost of international adoption to range between $7,000 and $30,000. This figure includes home study expenses, dossier and immigration processing and court costs, and foreign and domestic agency fees or donations. This figure does not include travel fees, which can be costly, particularly if a family needs to make more than one trip to the child's country, as is the case in Russia.

Waiting

The waiting time to adopt varies between countries and can be as long as 3 to 5 years (current estimate to adopt a child from China). This waiting period is often frustrating, demoralizing, and fraught with anxiety and uncertainty.

■ HAGUE CONVENTION

Safeguarding the rights of children is an important aspect of international adoption and controversy around the world as to whether international adoption is beneficial to children. The United Nations Convention on the Rights of the Child (UNCRC) emphasizes "the right of the child to preserve his or her identity including nationality, name and family relations."[3] The UNCRC stresses that international adoption should be viewed as the last option, except for institutional care, after all efforts to place a child with existing family members or within the child's community are exhausted.

The Hague Convention on Protection of Children and Cooperation in Respect of Intercountry Adoption was drafted in 1993 to recognize the legitimacy of international adoption and to establish a set of minimum requirements and procedures to ensure that children are not exploited, trafficked, abducted, or sold. The Hague convention was ratified by the United States in 2007 and implemented in 2008. The Department of State is the US central authority for adoption. More than 75 countries ratified the Hague convention. Many countries where children are commonly adopted, such as Russia and South Korea, are still non-Hague countries and regulations differ depending on whether a country is Hague compliant. One important distinction is that parents prospectively adopting from Hague-compliant countries must now complete at least 10 hours of pre-adoption training and education.

■ PRE-ADOPTION CARE OF CHILDREN

The caregiving environment for children around the world prior to adoption varies greatly, from care in a loving and stable foster home to an impoverished orphanage or conditions of extreme poverty that is bereft of the very basic necessities children require to grow and thrive. Currently, more than half of all adoptees spent some of their early life in institutional care. The quality of care in these settings is highly variable, but there is generally an inadequate caregiver-to-child ratio. Nutrition and health care may be inadequate and children are exposed to a high turnover of caregivers who often have limited training in child development.

Some international adoptees experienced abuse and neglect in the homes of their biological family or within an orphanage, although this is rarely reported on the records that prospective parents receive. Children may also have sustained some neurobiological insult as a result of poor prenatal care and nutrition, and prenatal substance abuse with a high prevalence of alcohol abuse in Russia and Eastern Europe. Acute and chronic medical problems are common and include infections, such as HIV, hepatitis, and tuberculosis (TB), malnutrition, parasitic infestations and inadequate immunizations to developmental delays, speech and language disorders, disrupted emotional development or behavior, abnormal stress responses, and attachment disorders. These risk factors place these children at a higher risk for medical, behavioral, developmental, and mental health issues.[6]

Pediatric providers are often called on to assist families prior to adopting a child for assistance with evaluating a referral for a child they are contemplating adopting. Prospective parents may have already accepted a referral but are looking for information to assist them with planning. Some prospective parents will not receive a referral until they arrive in the foreign country, such as in Ukraine and parts of Russia and Eastern Europe. Once there, they will need assistance understanding what to look for and have a referred child's record reviewed. Irrespective of the specific reasons that prospective families call on pediatricians, this contact with parents prior to adoption presents an important opportunity to provide support and valuable information about potential risks, possible adverse outcomes, and appropriate expectations of the child.

■ PRE-ADOPTION MEDICAL RECORDS

Medical records for children in other countries are highly variable and often contain inaccuracies, omissions, and unfamiliar diagnoses.[7] There are a number of international adoption clinics across the country with specialists that regularly review these types of records and are familiar with the information that is typically available and the potential pitfalls. The American Academy of Pediatrics (AAP) recently launched the Council on Foster Care, Adoption, & Kinship Care Web site at www. aap.org/sections/adoption/index.html; pediatricians who specialize in services for adopted children can be searched for by state. Table 18-1 lists information that may be included on a pre-adoption record. In addition, some countries provide videotaped footage of the child; although, the quality varies widely. In some countries, such as China, children are always found after abandonment, so some of the information listed in

Table 18-1. Information to Look for in Pre-adoption Medical Records	
Basic Demographics	• Date of birth • Date of placement • Information about birth family and siblings • Use of alcohol or drugs by birth mother • Age of birth mother and birth father • Prior pregnancies
Birth Information	• Birth weight • Hospital birth • Prenatal care • Gestational age • Apgar scores • Complications
Child's Social History	• Age at placement • Reason for placement • Number of placements
Child's Medical History	• Hospitalizations • Medications • Laboratory and other evaluations • Chronic and acute illnesses • Vaccinations
Growth	• Birth growth parameters • Current growth parameters including height, weight, and head circumference
Laboratory Studies	• HIV • Syphilis • Hepatitis B • Hepatitis C
Developmental Status	• Language • Cognition • Motor • Personal-social • Behavior

Table 18-1 is never available, such as information about birth parents and siblings. The presence or absence of information contained in the record does not ensure its accuracy. There are a number of caveats to bear in mind when evaluating a prospective child's record.

Birth Information

The prevalence of low birth weight is approximately 10% to 40% in developing countries[8] and prematurity rates are reported on records as high as 25%.[9] Maternal alcohol use tends to be severely underreported on records despite high rates of alcohol abuse in parts of Eastern Europe. Additional risk factors that may be seen on a record include parental mental health or cognitive issues, history of sexually transmitted infections, poverty, single or teenaged birth mother, and involuntary termination due to abuse or neglect.[10]

Child's Social History

The longer a child spends in institutional care, the greater the risk for adverse developmental, behavioral, and mental health issues. In addition, the greater the number of placements and disruptions, the higher the likelihood that the child will have greater difficulty establishing intimate and secure relationships. It is often tempting to minimize the risks seen on medical records to a child's outcome, but this should be avoided. Such children may be more vulnerable as they are often placed in understaffed and impoverished orphanages after being removed from a neglectful or abusive home. If there is a maternal history of alcohol consumption or if the child is from Russia or Eastern Europe or other countries, such as Korea, Guatemala, and the Philippines, it is critical to carefully evaluate the child's record for growth failure and developmental delay, and to examine pictures and videos for facial features consistent with fetal alcohol syndrome.

Child's Medical History

It is not unusual to see diagnoses that are unfamiliar to US physicians, particularly in Eastern European records. Sorting out which have meaning and which do not requires some familiarity with foreign medical records. Diagnoses, such as perinatal encephalopathy, are common in Russian records and usually carry little risk for adverse outcomes of the child.[8]

Growth

It is not unusual to see growth delays in children reared in impoverished settings and orphanages. The rule is that for every 3 months a child spends in a neglectful situation, that child loses 1 month of linear growth[11]; however, this rule may no longer apply as an increase in the quality of nutritional care has been seen. Microcephaly is also more commonly seen in children who were institutionalized.[8]

Laboratory Studies

It is extremely rare for a child with HIV disease to escape detection because testing across the world is fairly reliable. Timing of testing is important and it is always possible that a child recently infected with HIV may not have positive laboratory studies. Parents need to be informed that the quality of testing varies around the world and that there is an inherent risk of under-detection.

Developmental Status

Developmental delay is the rule rather than the exception for children in institutional care, and most children are reported to have some delays.[9] Videotapes and photographs can be helpful in corroborating narrative reports and examining the quality of development across domains. It is helpful to parents who will be making more than one trip to the child's country if the pediatric provider gives them specific guidance about what to look for. It is important to bear in mind that videotapes may be misleading because children may be evaluated in unfamiliar settings by people they never met.

■ ADOPTION OF OLDER CHILDREN AND CHILDREN WITH SPECIAL NEEDS

As waiting times for adoption continue to grow, there are an increasing number of older children and children with special health care needs being adopted. Countries like China have a well-established program of placing children with "medically and surgically correctable" diagnoses, which can encompass a wide range of disorders. Pediatric providers can help families understand the effect these disorders have on children and help plan for their ongoing needs. Common disorders include cleft lip and palate, clubfoot, limb abnormalities, colo-rectal malformations, and minor cardiac defects, such as a ventricular septal defect.

In addition, these older children are at a much higher risk for adverse developmental, behavioral, emotional, and cognitive outcomes.

■ PEDIATRIC PROVIDER'S ROLE PRIOR TO ADOPTION

Working with families prior to the adoption is an important opportunity for pediatricians to provide support and guidance during this highly vulnerable and often frightening period. Pediatricians can work with families to help clarify their goals and more fully understand what challenges they can accept and what their limitations may be. Families should be encouraged to openly discuss these questions with the pediatrician, their agency, and among themselves so that the best possible fit can be made between a waiting child and prospective parents. Box 18-1 provides a list of items that parents can consider bringing with them when they travel to meet the child.

■ AFTER THE ADOPTION

The placement of a child in an adoptive home is often the culmination of an unpredictable long wait and exhausting journey that brings excitement and uncertainty about the future. In many ways, it is similar to the pregnancy and birth of a biological child. However, with adoption, there exists an adoptive triad consisting of the child, the birth parent(s), and the adoptive parent(s), who are each forever present if only in the psychological sense.[12] The adopted child must blend life experiences and feelings toward the adoptive family with the reality of a birth family that may exist in another country. Confusion over identity, fantasies about birth parents and their reasons for relinquishing the child, and feelings of rejection may arise and influence the child's sense of belonging and self-esteem. An open and accepting family attitude toward adoption is shown to be predictive of a child's positive adjustment to these psychological issues. The pediatrician has the opportunity to help and support families as they navigate this journey and it assumes different dimensions and contours.

Common Behaviors

For internationally adopted children, the transition to their new home signifies a radical shift from everything familiar and predictable, which includes different sensory input, such as scents, textures, climate, and tastes, as well as new routines, culture, relationships, and language. Even the child's name may change. Further, children experience a significant loss during this transition even if the prior living arrangement was suboptimal. This seismic shift often exacerbates underlying problems for children who often already have poorly developed regulatory capacities and limited ability to manage transitions well.

Box 18-1. Items for Parents to Consider Bringing When Traveling to Meet Child

MEDICATIONS
- Acetaminophen
- Diphenhydramine (eg, Benadryl)
- Ibuprofen
- Cortisone cream or ointment
- Bacitracin ointment
- Antifungal cream or powder (eg, Lotrimin)
- Pedialyte or other oral rehydration solutions or powders
- Anesthetic teething gel

SUPPLIES
- Band-Aids
- Gauze pads
- Alcohol pads
- Hand sanitizer
- Thermometer
- Tweezers
- Disinfectant (eg, Betadine pads)
- Insect repellent
- Sunscreen, if appropriate
- Water purification system, if necessary

ITEMS FOR THE CHILD
- Sweets and treats to soothe or engage the child
- Age-appropriate toys

ITEMS IF ADOPTING AN INFANT
- Foods and formula for babies
- Diapers
- Baby-feeding essentials (eg, bottles, baby spoons, sippy cups)
- Pacifiers
- Diaper rash ointment
- Baby soap and baby shampoo
- Baby wipes
- Bibs
- Baby fingernail and toenail clippers

ITEMS FOR THE ORPHANAGE
- Gifts for orphanage director, orphanage staff, adoption facilitators, translators, etc
- Donation of medical supplies, clothing, or toys to the orphanage

Adapted with permission from Adoption ARK. Travel packing tips. http://www.adoptionark.org/public/pag55.aspx. Accessed June 16, 2011

There may be greater ambivalence about adoption for older children even if they endorsed it.[13] If they lived in difficult family situations or experienced many unstable and changing living environments prior to adoption, older adoptees may be anxious about another transition, instability, and loss. They will have conscious memories that they may or may not be willing to share and distorted expectations about what adoption may represent. For many older adoptees, there may be a reluctance or an inability to allow themselves to be vulnerable within relationships and they may initially resort to more primitive defenses to protect themselves.

Box 18-2[14] shows some of the common behaviors seen in international adoptees shortly after adoption. Many of these behaviors tend to quickly abate after adoption[13,15;] however, they may persist in some children.[16]

First Visit With the Pediatric Provider

The first visit with the pediatric provider should optimally occur within the first week after adoption. Although the family may still be jet-lagged, this visit offers an opportunity to assess the early adjustment of the child, parents, and any siblings and to identify any potential areas of significant concern. Box 18-3[17] outlines a strategy for surveilling

---

Box 18-2. Common Behaviors Seen After Adoption

- Sleep disturbances
  - Difficulty falling asleep
  - Frequent awakenings
  - Nightmares
  - Reluctance to sleep alone
- Eating disturbances
  - Overeating
  - Poor appetite regulation
  - Hoarding of food
  - Poor appetite
  - Food refusal
- Developmental regression
  - Loss of toileting skills
  - Regression in language, attention, and adaptive skills
- Mood lability or instability
  - Temper tantrums
  - Irritability
  - Impulsivity
- Apathy and withdrawal
- Hypervigilance and exaggerated fear response
- Indiscriminate sociability
- Self-stimulating behaviors
  - Excessive masturbation
  - Rocking
  - Repetitive movements
- Aggression
- Relationship disturbances
  - Avoidance of eye contact
  - Dislike of physical touch

Adapted from Berman B, Weitzman C. Foster care and adoption. In: Rudolph C, Rudolph A, First L, Gershon A, eds. *Rudolph's Pediatrics.* 22nd ed. New York, NY: McGraw Hill; 2011. Reprinted with permission from The McGraw-Hill Companies.

Box 18-3. Supportive Role of the Pediatrician in the Care of the Adoptive Child

- Prior to adoption
  - Preview information on the child, eg, medical records, prenatal information, family history, videotapes.
  - Advise on supplies to take to pick up the child, eg, medicines, formula.
  - Advise on vaccines, medicines for parents traveling to a foreign country.
  - Plan for evaluation of the child on return.
  - Refer family to support group for international adoption.
  - Deliver anticipatory guidance to new parents.
- Immediate visit (first week)
  - Obtain available records including prenatal and birth history, growth curves, immunization records, hospitalizations, results of health screening (eg, lead, anemia), and medications.
  - Evaluate/treat acute illnesses.
  - Measure baseline growth/check nutritional status of the child.
  - Address any immediate concerns the family may have.
  - Assess immediate family coping and adjustment.
  - Provide support.
- Comprehensive examination (4–6 weeks)
  - Complete PE: check for congenital anomalies, chronic conditions, and nutritional disorders.
  - Screenings: vision, hearing, and dental.
  - Update immunizations.
  - Recheck newborn screening if child is younger than 3 months.
  - Screening medical tests when appropriate to include: CBC, lead, iron (look for hemoglobinopathies), urinalysis, TB (PPD), stool O+P for parasitic infections, HepB+C, HIV, syphilis, malaria (if appropriate).
  - Developmental evaluation: gross and fine motor, communication, adaptive and cognitive skills, initial behavior/coping responses.
  - Developmental screen for language, autism spectrum disorders, learning/attentional difficulties if appropriate.
  - Anticipatory guidance: refer to support groups, appropriate literature.
- Periodic surveillance
  - Examine children in sensitive and compassionate settings.

Abbreviations: CBC, complete blood cell count; HepB+C, hepatitis B and hepatitis C; HIV, human immunodeficiency virus; O+P, ova and parasites; PE, physical examination; PPD, purified protein derivative; TB, tuberculosis.

Adapted from Berman B, Weitzman C. Foster care and adoption. In: Rudolph C, Rudolph A, First L, Gershon A, eds. *Rudolph's Pediatrics*. 22nd ed. New York, NY: McGraw Hill; 2011. Reprinted with permission from The McGraw-Hill Companies.

the adopted child that allows the pediatric provider to be an effective advocate, a source of support and information for parents, and a careful monitor of the child's and family's well-being.[14,18–20]

Parental Adjustment

Parents may experience post-adoption depression or even remorse.[13,21] Although this phenomenon is well-described after the birth of a child, it is less well understood and may not even be accepted after an adoption.

Parents are often reluctant to talk about this because they may feel shame, embarrassment, and doubt, particularly after all the effort and cost expended to adopt the child. Children may have greater medical, developmental, or behavioral issues than anticipated. They may behave in a rejecting manner to the adoptive parents, making them feel personally inadequate as parents. Parents may feel undeserving of parenthood and inadequate in their abilities to ease the child's transition. Mothers, in particular, who gave up careers to raise the child, may feel conflicted and guilty and that they lost a vital part of their lives.

Many adoptive parents are reluctant to discuss these feelings and often report that friends and family do not understand the complex feelings associated with adoption. Families may not wish to pursue counseling after so much scrutiny prior to adoption; they may just want to get on with being a family. Pediatricians can ask parents one of the following open-ended questions, which may help them feel comfortable exploring such topics: "In what ways has the experience of adoption differed from what you anticipated?" or "What is the most unexpected or challenging part of adoption?"

The Medical Evaluation

Many internationally adopted children are exposed to a number of infectious agents in their countries of origin, particularly if they were living within the crowded conditions of an orphanage. The AAP recommends that internationally adopted children be evaluated within 2 weeks of arriving in the United States. United States immigration law requires that internationally adopted children begin immunizations, if necessary, within 30 days of arriving in the United States.[22]

Box 18-4 displays the most common infectious diseases seen in internationally adopted children.[17] Even if children were screened for these diseases in their native country, it is recommended that testing be repeated after adoption. Screening to identify infectious diseases is important to promote the long-term health of the child and to prevent transmission to family members and other close contacts. International adoptee transmission of vaccine-preventable diseases (eg, hepatitis A, hepatitis B, measles) to US caregivers and TB transmission to community contacts emphasizes the importance of screening and appropriate follow-up of test results after adoption.[23]

The AAP developed recommendations for screening internationally adopted children (Table 18-2).[22,23] In addition to these tests, urinalysis, thyroid stimulating hormone level, and vision and hearing screenings are also recommended.[17] Screening for Cytomegalovirus is not indicated, as rates in adoptees are comparable to rates in US children in child care;

Box 18-4. Infectious Diseases in International Adoptees

- Viral
  - Varicella-zoster virus
  - Hepatitis B virus
  - Hepatitis C virus
  - Measles virus
  - HIV
- Bacterial
  - *Mycobacterium tuberculosis* (active or latent)
  - Syphilis
  - Gastroenteritis
  - Urinary tract infection
- Parasitic
  - Intestinal protozoa (*Giardia lamblia, Dientamoeba fragilis*)
  - Ectoparasites (scabies, head lice)
  - Intestinal nematodes (*Strongyloides stercoralis, Trichuris trichiura, Ascaris lumbricoides,* hookworm); visceral larva migrans (*Toxocara*)

From Murray TS, Groth ME, Weitzman C, Cappello M. Epidemiology and management of infectious diseases in international adoptees. *Clin Microbiol Rev.* 2005;18(3):510–520. Reprinted with permission from American Society for Microbiology.

screening does not distinguish between congenital infection and asymptomatic shedding.

Recommended Screening Tests for Internationally Adopted Children

Tuberculosis

Rates of positive skin tests in international adoptees range from 3% to 19% due to the high rates of TB in countries from which children are adopted.[23] Most experts agree that an area of induration equal to or greater than 10 mm is considered positive for international adoptees, with 5 to 9 mm considered positive if a child is immunocompromised, had definite exposure to a person with TB, or has signs or symptoms of TB disease, including an abnormal chest radiograph. The risk of a false-positive purified protein derivative (PPD) skin test associated with prior bacille Calmette-Guérin immunization is considered low if the skin test is placed at least 1 year following the vaccine.

False-negative results may be caused by a number of factors, including malnutrition, concurrent inflammatory or rheumatologic disease, underlying immune deficiency, inactive antigen, or poor technique when placing the PPD test. Most TB cases in internationally adopted children are asymptomatic and classified as latent TB infection. Retesting should be considered 3 months after adoption at which point some of the factors contributing to a false negative, such as malnutrition, may have resolved. In addition, if the child was exposed to TB shortly before adoption, retesting will detect an evolving profile.

Table 18-2. American Academy of Pediatrics–Recommended Screening Tests for Internationally Adopted Children

TEST	POPULATION TO BE SCREENED	ADDITIONAL TESTING OR CONSIDERATIONS
Tuberculin skin test	All adoptees	Consider repeating in 2 to 3 months or when nutritional status is improved if negative on initial screen. Retesting will also detect an evolving infection.
Hepatitis serology Hepatitis B surface antigen (HBsAg) Hepatitis B surface antibody (HBsAb) Hepatitis B core antibody (HBcAb)	All adoptees	Consider repeating in 6 months.
Hepatitis C	Adoptees from China, Russia, Eastern Europe, and Southeast Asia Adoptees with risk factors for infection	Consider repeating in 6 months if negative on initial screen.
Syphilis serology	Non-treponemal tests for all adoptees	Children with positive test results and those diagnosed or treated in their birth country need additional testing.
Non-treponemal test (RPR, VDRL, ART)	Treponemal tests if non-treponemal tests are reactive	
Treponemal test (MHA-TP, FTA-ABS)	If clinical signs or symptoms of syphilis are present	
Stool examination for ova and parasites (3 specimens) Stool specimen for antigen for *Giardia lamblia* and *Cryptosporidium parvum* (1 specimen)	All adoptees	Repeat in those with persistent symptoms.
HIV 1 and 2 ELISA (consider DNA PCR in infants)	All adoptees	Consider repeating in 6 months if negative on initial screen.

Abbreviations: ART, automated reagin test; ELISA, enzyme-linked immunosorbent assay; FTA-ABS, fluorescent treponemal antibody absorption; HIV, human immunodeficiency virus; MHA-TP, micro-hemagglutination test for *Treponema pallidum*; PCR, polymerase chain reaction; RPR, rapid plasma reagin; VDRL, Venereal Disease Research Laboratory.

Adapted from Barnett E. Immunizations and infectious disease screening for internationally adopted children. *Pediatr Clin N Am.* 2005;52(5):1287–1309, with permission from Elsevier.

Hepatitis B

Approximately 5% to 7% of international adoptees are infected with hepatitis B; this percentage may be higher if children are coming from countries that do not routinely immunize against hepatitis B. Recent adoptees that do not have hepatitis B surface antibody on the initial screen should undergo repeat testing for hepatitis B in 2 to 3 months to rule out infection immediately prior to adoption. Children with hepatitis B should be vaccinated against hepatitis A. Children infected with hepatitis B will require further evaluation beyond routine screening tests and should be referred to an expert in managing hepatitis. It is critical that family members and close contacts are immunized against hepatitis B to prevent further infection.

Hepatitis C

Hepatitis C is rarely seen in internationally adopted children, although there are increasing numbers of women infected around the world. Current recommendations for testing include screening at the time of adoption and rescreening consideration 6 months later.[23] The recommended test is hepatitis C antibodies. Maternal antibodies can persist up to 15 months; in these cases, confirmatory polymerase chain reaction (PCR) testing should be done.

Syphilis

Most children with congenital syphilis are asymptomatic. The Venereal Disease Research Laboratory (VDRL) and rapid plasma reagin (RPR) tests are highly sensitive, although false-positive results may occur in individuals with rheumatologic or inflammatory conditions. All positive non-treponemal tests (VDRL or RPR) must be confirmed using the fluorescent treponemal antibody absorption test, which is more specific. Non-treponemal tests become nonreactive over time whereas treponemal tests tend to stay positive for life. If the child is reported as being treated in the country of origin, the child requires close follow-up to detect falling titers. Infected children should undergo lumbar puncture for VDRL testing of the cerebrospinal fluid to rule out neurosyphilis, as well as a complete blood cell count, liver function tests, long-bone radiographs, and vision and hearing screening.[17,23,24]

Human Immunodeficiency Virus

Although the rates of HIV infection are quite high in some countries from where children are adopted, the prevalence of HIV in international adoptees is quite low. This suggests that screening for this disease around the world is effective and, therefore, HIV does not represent a major risk for adoptees. Infants, who may have persistent maternal antibodies, need additional testing if it was not done in their country of origin. Two negative DNA PCR tests at or beyond 1 month of age and a third test performed at 4 months of age or older confirm a negative HIV status. When HIV antibody testing is used in children older than 6 months, 2 negative antibody tests performed at an interval of at least 1 month can confirm a negative HIV status.[25]

Evaluating Immunization Status

There are a number of challenges in interpreting the vaccination records of children from other countries. Multiple studies show that many international adoptees have incomplete vaccination records, inappropriate timing of vaccinations, or inadequate protection against disease despite appropriate vaccination records.[7,26,27] The reasons for the latter might include
- Falsified records
- Improper vaccine storage
- Use of outdated vaccines
- Use of diluted vaccines
- Poor immune response because of reasons such as malnutrition

Based on these findings, the AAP recommends[22]
1. Repeat all vaccine doses when immunization records are assumed to be unreliable.
2. Accept as valid those immunizations for which there is documentation of vaccines doses administered according to current US vaccine schedules.
3. Judiciously use serologic testing to assess a child's immunity to vaccine-preventable diseases and make decisions about what vaccines to administer based on these results.

Determining the most appropriate strategy toward interpreting vaccination records and planning immunizations need to be made collaboratively with parents. Obtaining multiple titers and delaying vaccination may not be cost-effective or practical, but many parents are wary of over-vaccinating their children. Careful discussion may be needed to contrast vaccination practice in the United States and the rationale behind it with the adoptive child's vaccination record. In addition, parents need to be made aware that an unrecorded vaccination given shortly before adoption could result in a transient elevation of antibody or titer to a specific vaccine but may not confer lasting immunity. The goal is to choose a route that minimizes excess distress for the child in obtaining multiple blood draws, is the most cost-effective, and likely most importantly, confers the greatest assurance of long-term protection to the child and community from serious preventable illnesses.

The Developmental Evaluation

Anywhere from 50% to 90% of internationally adopted children from many countries around the world exhibit developmental delays at the time of their initial evaluation, and a significant proportion are delayed in multiple areas (eg, language, cognition, motor skills).[28-30] It is often difficult to prognosticate a child's development based on early presentation shortly after adoption. Many children begin to show remarkable catch-up shortly after adoption and many unknown biological, genetic, and experiential influences on development are unknown. Approximately 4 to 6 weeks after adoption, when the child and family are recovered from jet lag and have had time to begin adjusting, it is useful to obtain a baseline assessment of the adopted child's current level of developmental functioning across domains, including social-emotional and adaptive skills. It is important to provide an interpreter who speaks the child's native language during this assessment. The limitations to obtaining an accurate assessment include

• Using measures normed on American children
• Administering tests in English
• Using materials that are unfamiliar and culturally foreign to the child
• Assessing the child during a period of intense adjustment

The value of assessing a child early is to help the family understand the child's baseline functioning, which may help interpret some of the behaviors displayed and help obtain appropriate intervention services. It is important that pediatricians are cautious not to underreact or overreact to a child's developmental delays and behavior problems. It is equally harmful to prematurely intervene or become alarmed, or wait too long to refer a child for services with the belief that he simply needs more time to catch up. It is often helpful to refer children to an international adoption clinic or a developmental-behavioral pediatrician who is familiar with this population and is skilled in assessing a child's behavior and development. During the developmental screening and assessment, it is important to prepare parents for the fact that the child is likely to show delays for a myriad of reasons and that these delays are not an indicator of long-term disability. Without this knowledge, parents' anxiety, uncertainty, ambivalence, and fear may be unnecessarily heightened.

■ LONG-TERM CONSEQUENCES

Reportedly, adopted children are more frequently referred for mental health concerns[6,31] than their non-adopted peers; however, international adoptees show less problems overall than domestic adoptees.[32] This discrepancy may be because international adoptees are younger at the time of adoption than domestic adoptees, especially those adopted from foster care. The higher adoptee referral rate may be attributed to a number of factors, including heightened vigilance for problems by adoptive parents with greater resources and awareness of mental health services in addition to higher rates of true problems.

Behavior and Emotion

Multiple studies indicate that international adoptees have a greater incidence of behavioral difficulties that include internalizing (ie, withdrawal, anxiety, depression, and mood disorders) and externalizing problems (eg, acting out, aggression, opposition), impairments in peer relations, and attention disorders.[6,16,32–36] However, a large meta-analysis that reviewed approximately 100 studies on adoption suggested that the effect size was small.[32] Many studies robustly indicate that the most important predictor of behavioral problems is the length of institutionalization and the severity of early deprivation[6,37,38]; however, other studies do not demonstrate adoption age as an important predictor.[32] Many studies indicate that although many of the behavior problems improve, they also often persist long after adoption,[39] but considerable heterogeneity exists within adoptees. New information suggests that a threshold response may occur (particularly for children who experienced harsh and highly depriving early environments) where, after a certain period of deprivation, there may be some damaging effects that become more difficult to reverse. Despite this robust evidence suggesting that internationally adopted children are at higher risk for behavior and emotional problems, a recent meta-analysis indicated that these children did not have poorer self-esteem.[40]

Cognition

Similar to behavior and emotion studies, the length and severity of early deprivation is the strongest predictor of cognitive impairments in internationally adopted children.[6,30,37,41–43] Studies show that catch-up in cognitive attainments can occur many years after adoption, although significant catch-up seen more than 2 years after adoption are in children who exhibited the greatest level of initial impairment.[42] Children adopted at young ages, who are female, and who have been reared in foster care in their country of origin are most likely to show the least amount of delays at adoption and the greatest capacity for full developmental catch-up. Studies suggest that early evidence of poor nutritional status does not predict later cognitive functioning.[43] Similar to findings related to behavior and emotion, there is some suggestion that a sensitive period in cognitive development or threshold may exist, after which it becomes more difficult to fully reverse the effects of severe early adversity.[41] Recent literature suggests that even in children functioning within the normal intelligence range, high rates of specific neurocognitive deficits in areas such as memory, executive function, and language may be seen, with length of early institutional care exerting the greatest influence.[35,44]

Attachment

Studies examining attachment in internationally adopted children echo the patterns seen in behavioral and cognitive domains where length of deprivation highly predicts the presence and persistence of an attachment disturbance.[6,37,45,46] However, once again there is considerable variability seen in attachment difficulties in internationally adopted children, with those with the most institutional care having more atypical and disorganized attachment patterns. Recent evidence suggests that approximately 20% of currently institutionalized children have some attachment strategy, suggesting some coherent method of gaining proximity and support from a preferred caregiver during times of stress and perceived threat; however, only a fraction of their strategies are well-developed.[46,47]

The most common pattern seen in internationally adopted children is indiscriminate sociability characterized by superficial relationships with others, approaching strangers without discrimination, a tendency to wander off from a parent without checking back, and a willingness to go off with a stranger. Indiscriminate sociability tends to be highly persistent over time, particularly in older adoptees, but the relationship between parents' assessments of attachment security diverge over time, suggesting that indiscriminate sociability may not represent an attachment disorder.[48]

Identity Development

Understanding adoption is an unfolding process that occurs over a lifetime and plays a role in the development of all adoptees' identity. Although each child and family will metabolize the experience of adoption differently, there are some predictable patterns (Table 18-3).[49,50]

Table 18-3. Identity Development in Adoption

AGE	COMMON RESPONSES	RECOMMENDATIONS
Toddlers	Often enjoy adoption story but lack complex understanding of adoption	• Many books available to use as aids to discuss adoption • Adoption often viewed by children as highly positive during this period
Preschoolers	Children begin to notice differences and ask questions about these differences.	• Important not to overinterpret these questions as a marker of distress. • Children may have distortions in their understanding of adoption. • Older adoptees may have conscious memories of events but may be reluctant to talk about them.
School-aged children	Adoption may be first perceived as problematic even if adoption was years earlier.	• Begin to first understand experience of loss. • Problem behaviors may emerge. • Fantasies of reunion with birth parent may emerge. • Child may begin an "internal" search.
Adolescence	May see emergence of "identity crisis"	• May see prolongation of reunion fantasies • May blame adoptive parents and self for adoption losses • May experience fear of repeating adoptive parent's possible mistakes and desire to undo these mistakes • May initiate a physical search for birth parent(s)

Adoption may come in and out of focus for children and families, particularly at nodal points such as life transitions, adoption anniversaries, or as a child enters a new developmental stage. It is important that pediatric providers continue to routinely ask about the role that adoption is playing for the child and parent at different points so that intervention and support can be provided if necessary. It is critical for pediatric providers to understand that a psychological or physical search does not necessarily imply psychopathology or distress and that the experience of mourning and loss may represent an important and healthy developmental step for a child. However, if a child is struggling with behavioral and emotional challenges, along with changes in functioning and school performance, this may represent more than a healthy component of identity development, and additional evaluation may be warranted.

■ FOLLOW-UP VISITS AND SURVEILLANCE

The risks and rewards of international adoption can be great for families, and pediatricians can play a special role. Pediatricians need to follow internationally adopted children intensively over the first year after adoption to monitor development, health, growth, and family adjustment and adaptation. In addition, it is important to detect the emergence of atypical or maladaptive behaviors that may come into greater focus after an initial honeymoon period. Frequent visits will also ensure that children receive appropriate medical, developmental, and educational services, and that families feel supported so they can develop into a cohesive and loving family.

■ KEY POINTS

- More than 100,000 children are adopted in the United States each year; approximately 5% to 15% of children are adopted from other countries.
- The overall number of children entering the United States from other countries is decreasing; a larger proportion of international adoptees have major or minor special health care needs.
- More than half of all international adoptees spent part or all of their early life in institutional care.
- Pre-adoption medical records are often scant but may provide important information about risks to health, development, and behavior.
- The length of time in institutional care is the greatest predictor of adverse cognitive, behavioral, developmental, and mental health outcomes.
- Shortly after international adoptions it is common to see regulatory disturbances; mood instability; challenges in relationships, including indiscriminate sociability; and developmental regression.
- The AAP developed recommendations for screening international adoptees for infectious diseases and illness, which include obtaining assessments after adoption for TB, HIV, syphilis, and hepatitis.
- Revaccination, acceptance of prior records, or serologic testing may be necessary to ensure that an adoptee's immunization status is appropriate.
- Between 50% and 90% of adoptees exhibit some developmental delay at the time of adoption.
- International adoptees may face long-term problems related to behavior and mental health, cognition, and attachment primarily characterized by indiscriminate sociability.

• Most international adoptees do not show poorer self-esteem when compared with non-adopted peers.
• Identity development is a lifelong task for adoptees and often follows some predictable patterns.
• Pediatricians are in a position to monitor the overall well-being of internationally adopted children and to assess for the emergence of atypical or maladaptive patterns of behavior or development.

■ REFERENCES

1. Child Welfare Information Gateway. How Many Children Were Adopted in 2000 and 2001? Highlights. 2004. http://www.childwelfare.gov/pubs/s_adoptedhighlights.cfm
2. Adoptions to the United States. http://adoption.state.gov/about_us/statistics.php
3. Johnson DE. International adoption: what is fact, what is fiction, and what is the future? *Pediatr Clin North Am.* 2005;52(5):1221–1246
4. American Academy of Pediatrics Committee on Psychosocial Aspects of Child and Family Health. Coparent or second-parent adoption by same-sex parents. *Pediatrics.* 2002;109(2):339–340
5. Hellerstedt WL, Madsen NJ, Gunnar MR, Grotevant HD, Lee RM, Johnson DE. The International Adoption Project: population-based surveillance of Minnesota parents who adopted children internationally. *Matern Child Health J.* 2008;12(2):162–171
6. Weitzman C, Albers L. Long-term developmental, behavioral, and attachment outcomes after international adoption. *Pediatr Clin North Am.* 2005;52(5):1395–1419
7. Albers L, Johnson D, Hostetter M, Iverson S, Miller L. Health of children adopted from the former Soviet Union and Eastern Europe. Comparison with preadoptive medical records. *JAMA.* 1997;278(11):922–924
8. Chambers J. Preadoption opportunities for pediatric providers. *Pediatr Clin North Am.* 2005;52:1247–1269
9. Jenista J. Pre-adoption review of medical records. *Pediatr Ann.* 2000;29(4):212–215
10. Jenista J. Findings from foreign medical records. *Adoption Med News.* 1999;10:1–6
11. Johnson DE, Miller LC, Iverson S. The health of children adopted from Romania. *JAMA.* 1992;268:3446–3451
12. Schulman I, ed. *The Future of Children: Adoption.* Vol 3. Los Altos, CA: The David and Lucille Packard Foundation; 1993
13. Miller LC. Immediate behavioral and developmental considerations for internationally adopted children transitioning to families. *Pediatr Clin North Am.* 2005;52(5): 1311–1330
14. Berman B, Weitzman C. Foster care and adoption. In: Rudolph C, Rudolph A, eds. *Rudolph's Pediatrics.* 22nd ed. New York, NY: McGraw Hill. In press
15. Fisher L, Ames EW, Chisholm K, Savoie L. Problems reported by parents of Romanian orphans adopted to British Columbia. *J Behav Develop.* 1997;20:67–83
16. Beckett C, Bredenkamp D, Castle J, Groothues C, O'Connor TG, Rutter M. Behavior patterns associated with institutional deprivation: a study of children adopted from Romania. *J Dev Behav Pediatr.* 2002;23(5):297–303
17. Murray TS, Groth ME, Weitzman C, Cappello M. Epidemiology and management of infectious diseases in international adoptees. *Clin Microbiol Rev.* 2005;18(3):510–520
18. Szilagyi M. The pediatrician and the child in foster care. *Pediatr Rev.* 1998;19(2):39–50
19. Borchers D. Families and adoption: the pediatrician's role in supporting communication. *Pediatrics.* 2003;112(6 Pt 1):1437–1441

20. American Academy of Pediatrics Committee on Early Childhood, Adoption, and Dependent Care. Developmental issues for young children in foster care. *Pediatrics.* 2000;106(5):1145–1150

21. Weitzman CC, Avni-Singer R. Building the bonds of adoption: from separation and deprivation toward integration and continuity. *Zero Three.* 2005;25(6):14–20

22. American Academy of Pediatrics. Medical evaluation of internationally adopted children for infectious diseases. In: Pickering LK, Baker CJ, Kimberlin DW, Long SS, eds. *Red Book: 2009 Report of the Committee on Infectious Diseases.* 28th ed. Elk Grove Village, IL: American Academy of Pediatrics; 2009:177–184

23. Barnett E. Immunizations and infectious disease screening for internationally adopted children. *Pediatr Clin North Am.* 2005;52(5):1287–1309

24. American Academy of Pediatrics. Syphilis. In: Pickering LK, Baker CJ, Kimberlin DW, Long SS, eds. *Red Book: 2009 Report of the Committee on Infectious Diseases.* 28th ed. Elk Grove Village, IL: American Academy of Pediatrics; 2009: 638–651

25. American Academy of Pediatrics. Human immunodeficiency virus infecton. In: Pickering LK, Baker CJ, Kimberlin DW, Long SS, eds. *Red Book: 2009 Report of the Committee on Infectious Diseases.* 28th ed. Elk Grove Village, IL: American Academy of Pediatrics; 2009:380–400

26. Miller L, Comfort K, Kelly N. Immunization status of internationally adopted children. *Pediatrics.* 2001;108:1050–1051

27. Schulte J, Maloney S, Aronson J, Saiman L. Evaluating acceptability and completeness of overseas immunization records of internationally adopted children. *Pediatrics.* 2002;109:e22

28. Nalven L. Strategies for addressing long-term issues after institutionalization. *Pediatr Clin North Am.* 2005;52(5):1421–1444

29. Rutter M, for the English and Romanian Adoptees Study Team. Developmental catch-up and deficit, following adoption after severe global early privation. *J Child Psychol Psychiatry.* 1998;39(4):465–476

30. O'Conner T, Rutter M, Beckett C, et al, for the English and Romanian Adoptees Study Team. The effects of global severe privation on cognitive competence: extension and longitudinal follow-up. *Child Dev.* 2000;71(2):376–390

31. Verhulst FC, Althaus M, Versluis-den Bieman HJ. Problem behavior in international adoptees: I. An epidemiological study. *J Am Acad Child Adolesc Psychiatry.* 1990;29(1):94–103

32. Juffer F, van Ijzendoorn MH. Behavior problems and mental health referrals of international adoptees: a meta-analysis. *JAMA.* 2005;293(20):2501–2515

33. Bimmel N, Juffer F, van IMH, Bakermans-Kranenburg MJ. Problem behavior of internationally adopted adolescents: a review and meta-analysis. *Harv Rev Psychiatry.* 2003;11(2):64–77

34. Kreppner JM, O'Connor TG, Rutter M. Can inattention/overactivity be an institutional deprivation syndrome? *J Abnorm Child Psychol.* 2001;29(6):513–528

35. Colvert E, Rutter M, Kreppner J, et al. Do theory of mind and executive function deficits underlie the adverse outcomes associated with profound early deprivation? Findings from the English and Romanian adoptees study. *J Abnorm Child Psychol.* 2008;36(7):1057–1068

36. Gunnar MR, van Dulmen MH, International Adoption Project T. Behavior problems in postinstitutionalized internationally adopted children. *Dev Psychopathol.* 2007;19(1):129–148

37. MacLean K. The impact of institutionalization on child development. *Dev Psychopathol.* 2003;15(4):853–884

38. Verhulst FC, Althaus M, Versluis-den Bieman HJ. Problem behavior in international adoptees: II. Age at placement. *J Am Acad Child Adolesc Psychiatry.* 1990;29(1):104–111

39. Tieman W, Van Der Ende J, Verhulst FC. Psychiatric disorders in young adult intercountry adoptees: an epidemiological study. *Am J Psychiatry.* 2005;162(3):592–598

40. Juffer F, van Ijzendoorn MH. Adoptees do not lack self-esteem: a meta-analysis of studies on self-esteem of transracial, international, and domestic adoptees. *Psychol Bull.* 2007;133(6):1067–1083

41. Nelson CA 3rd, Zeanah CH, Fox NA, Marshall PJ, Smyke AT, Guthrie D. Cognitive recovery in socially deprived young children: the Bucharest Early Intervention Project. *Science.* 2007;318(5858):1937–1940

42. Beckett C, Maughan B, Rutter M, et al. Scholastic attainment following severe early institutional deprivation: a study of children adopted from Romania. *J Abnorm Child Psychol.* 2007;35(6):1063–1073

43. Beckett C, Maughan B, Rutter M, et al. Do the effects of early severe deprivation on cognition persist into early adolescence? Findings from the English and Romanian adoptees study. *Child Dev.* 2006;77(3):696–711

44. Behen ME, Helder E, Rothermel R, Solomon K, Chugani HT. Incidence of specific absolute neurocognitive impairment in globally intact children with histories of early severe deprivation. *Child Neuropsychology.* 2008;14(5):453–469

45. O'Connor TG, Marvin RS, Rutter M, Olrick JT, Britner PA. Child-parent attachment following early institutional deprivation. *Dev Psychopathol.* 2003;15(1):19–38

46. Zeanah CH, Smyke AT, Dumitrescu A. Attachment disturbances in young children. II: indiscriminate behavior and institutional care. *J Am Acad Child Adolesc Psychiatry.* 2002;41(8):983–989

47. Zeanah CH, Smyke AT, Koga SF, Carlson E. Attachment in institutionalized and community children in Romania. *Child Dev.* 2005;76(5):1015–1028

48. Zeanah CH. Disturbances of attachment in young children adopted from institutions. *J Dev Behav Pediatr.* 2000;21(3):230–236

49. Brodzinsky DM, Schechter MD, Henig RM. *Being Adopted: The Lifelong Search for Self.* New York, NY: Double Day; 1992

50. Brodzinsky DM, Palacios J, eds. *Psychological Issues in Adoption: Research and Practice.* Westport, CT: Praeger; 2005

CHAPTER

19

Care of Immigrants

Elizabeth D. Barnett, MD

■ INTRODUCTION

The number of foreign-born individuals in the United States has never been higher. Taking care of immigrant families is no longer an occasional event for pediatricians in the United States but rather a standard part of pediatric practice. Despite the prevalence of such patients, it is clear that health disparities continue to exist for foreign-born individuals. Caring for immigrant patients can be accomplished by acknowledging that there is a body of knowledge for the field of immigrant medicine and that best practices can be defined and put into practice. Providing patient-centered care in a multicultural environment can be accomplished by acknowledging and respecting cultural differences and learning about the differences in diseases from the country of origin and race and ethnicity; this practice should be expected of every health care professional working in the 21st-century global health environment.[1]

■ IMPROVING THE HEALTH OF NEW AMERICANS

The Minnesota Immigrant Health Task Force, a 2-year citizen advisory group, developed a group of action steps to improve the health of new Americans.[2] These steps (summarized in Box 19-1) are worth reviewing, as they apply to any immigrant group and address many of the issues involved in health disparities in immigrants.

Box 19-1. Steps to Improve the Health of New Americans

1. Provide equal access to health care.
2. Improve health care organizations' capacity to provide care to immigrant populations.
3. Recognize different health care costs for immigrants and provide equitable payment.
4. Develop clinical guidelines and best practices for immigrant patients.
5. Diversify the health care workforce.
6. Use trained interpreters.
7. Use community health workers.
8. Train and educate health care professionals and immigrant patients.

From Ohmans P. Action steps to improve the health of new Americans. In: Walker PF, Barnett ED, eds. *Immigrant Medicine.* Philadelphia, PA: WB Saunders; 2007:27–35, with permission from Elsevier.

Health care providers cannot accomplish the action steps alone; input from policy makers, administrators, academic researchers and educators, and advocates for immigrants and their families is also necessary for success.

■ ADDRESSING LANGUAGE AND CULTURAL BARRIERS

Health professionals should be comfortable working with interpreters when taking care of immigrant families. Although the ideal situation is to have a bilingual or multilingual provider for every encounter, the reality is that too many languages are spoken and there are too few providers who speak them to ensure a language-concordant provider for every encounter. Health providers are responsible for ensuring that children with limited proficiency in English and their parents or guardians have meaningful access to health services.[3] Health care organizations are also required to ensure the competence of the language assistance provided. Using family members, especially young children and friends, as interpreters is discouraged unless the patient specifically requests this and declines a professional interpreter. In many cases, patients who bring family members or friends to interpret will understand the need for professional interpreters when it is explained to them. These same patients may request that their friends be present during the encounter as an additional level of interpretation.

Linguistic access can be provided in many ways, such as through bilingual health care providers, professional in-person interpreters, and telephone interpreters. The growth of medically trained telephone interpreters has substantially increased in recent years. Access to telephone interpreters is especially valuable in settings where a large number of immigrants are seen or where many different languages, especially rare languages, are spoken.

Providing trained interpreters is, of course, just one part of providing culturally competent care. Health care professionals caring for immigrants must also be sensitive to and, ideally, knowledgeable about different concepts of healing systems outside the United States. General principles of cultural competence include awareness of one's own cultural beliefs, displaying attitudes that convey respect and engender trust, developing verbal and nonverbal communication skills that facilitate mutual understanding, and developing multicultural communication skills.[4,5]

Attending school is one of the first sustained activities immigrant children have within US culture. Health care professionals have a role in helping immigrant families access optimal education for their children. It is helpful if pediatricians understand the services that local schools provide for children with limited English proficiency.[6]

■ PUBLIC HEALTH ASPECTS OF MEDICAL SCREENING FOR IMMIGRANTS AND REFUGEES IN THE UNITED STATES

Foreign-born individuals arrive in the United States in many different ways and with highly variable exposure to medical services in their countries of origin or while in transit. Thus, US health care professionals must be prepared to face a wide spectrum of health problems. A pediatrician cannot assume that a specific process of screening or immunization was done prior to departure unless written or electronic documentation is available. Screening requirements vary depending on immigration status, and they change frequently. In reality, a small number of immigrants will have received comprehensive screening and immunization before entering the United States and be able to provide documentation of it. Additional information about the current screening requirements can be found at www.cdc.gov/ncpdcid/dgmq/index-new-sites.html.

Individuals admitted to the United States as refugees are entitled to a health assessment on arrival; however, the process is elective for states of entry and the refugee. Each state decides what it is able to provide to refugees settling in the state. Some states provide a minimal health assessment, while others provide comprehensive services including screening, immunizations, an introduction to the US health care system, and help transitioning to the US primary care health system.[7] Health care professionals are encouraged to find out what exists in their areas, states, or local health department to help immigrants with health care transition.

Medical Screening for Immigrants and Refugees

The goals of health screening on arrival to the United States include identifying contagious conditions (eg, infectious tuberculosis) that could pose a risk to the US population, providing a comprehensive health assessment to identify symptomatic and asymptomatic health conditions, providing needed immunizations, and serving as an introduction to US health services. Table 19-1 lists health assessment components.[8]

Obtaining a complete history will depend on establishing rapport with patients and their families. Some immigrants may be disinclined to reveal aspects of their past until they are able to establish a degree of trust in the provider. Elements of the history should include details of the countries lived in, living conditions, and route to the United States. Specific attention should be paid to current health concerns, such as pain or chronic health problems. The health care provider should ask about symptoms of diseases that might be absent or less common in the United States, such as fevers with malaria, jaundice with hepatitis, itching with filarial diseases, or night sweats, cough, or weight loss associated with tuberculosis (TB). Social history should include family

---

Table 19-1. Components of Health Assessment for New Immigrants

- History
- Physical examination
- Hearing and vision screening
- Dental evaluation
- Mental health assessment
- Tuberculin skin testing
- Laboratory screening
  - CBC with differential
  - Hepatitis B serology (testing for infection and existing immunity)
  - Lead level
  - Urinalysis
  - Stool for ova and parasites
  - Malaria smear or other testing (when indicated by history)
- Immunizations according to ACIP recommendations
- Other laboratory testing based on information gained from history and physical examination
  - HIV testing
  - RPR
  - Hepatitis C testing
  - Hepatitis A testing (those with hepatitis B or C infection; vaccine candidates where prevalence of hepatitis A is high enough in the country of origin so that testing may be cost-effective compared with cost of immunizing)

Abbreviations: ACIP, Advisory Committee on Immunization Practices; CBC, complete blood cell count; HIV, human immunodeficiency virus; RPR, rapid plasma reagin.

From Seybolt L, Barnett ED, Stauffer W. US medical screening for immigrants and refugees: clinical issues. In: Walker PF, Barnett ED, eds. *Immigrant Medicine*. Philadelphia, PA: WB Saunders; 135–150, with permission from Elsevier.

structure, information about literacy and school attendance, languages spoken, and exposure to trauma or torture. Obtaining complete information may take a number of visits as the relationship develops between the provider and the patient and family.

The physical examination should be complete and include special focus on conditions that may be more common in certain immigrant groups, such as dental disease, untreated heart conditions, hepatosplenomegaly, ritual scarification, or growth or developmental problems. Growth parameters should be measured and plotted; particular attention should be paid to whether there might be a discrepancy between the patient's true age and what is reported on the immigration documents. Pelvic examination is almost never appropriate during an initial health assessment unless there is a specific medical indication.

Mental health screening is regarded as an important aspect of an initial health assessment[9] but may not always be possible to accomplish in the first visit.[10] The first few months after arriving in the United States, a family's goals center around obtaining appropriate housing, enrolling children in school, finding employment, and learning English if necessary; having an assessment of conditions, such as post-traumatic stress disorder (PTSD) and depression, may not be a priority for them. It is helpful to ask about symptoms of hyperarousal, avoidance, and difficulties with memory and concentration. The patient may not offer these symptoms unless sensitive questions are asked and rapport is established. Such symptoms may not even manifest until the individual enters school or another environment where they interfere with appropriate functioning.

Depression or PTSD in parents may affect children; evaluating and treating parents may be critical in these circumstances. Assessing family function and the resettlement process can include asking if the adults in the family found employment or are learning English and if the children are enrolled in school, as well as assessing the general interfamily interactions during the encounter.

Laboratory Screening of New Immigrants

Tuberculosis

There is strong evidence to support screening all new immigrants for TB. An increasing proportion of TB cases in the United States are in foreign-born individuals; beginning in 2002 foreign-born individuals accounted for more than 50% of US TB cases.[11] The overseas screening process for refugees was enhanced recently to include TB skin tests (TSTs) and sputum cultures for certain individuals, such as those considered at an increased risk (ie, high-risk groups, a family member with TB, signs or symptoms of TB); previously, only chest radiographs were done. One significant challenge is ensuring that overseas screening records are available to the providers seeing these patients on arrival in the United States. Currently, unless overseas records are available, a TST should be placed on all new arrivals, even those with chest radiographs interpreted as showing evidence of prior TB.

Receipt of bacille Calmette-Guérin (BCG) vaccine is not a contraindication to TST, and the skin test should be interpreted without regard to BCG vaccination. Individuals with positive skin tests should be evaluated for any evidence of active TB, especially for manifestations of extrapulmonary TB. If none are found, the individual is a candidate for treatment for latent TB infection (LTBI) and should be managed by TB programs or health professionals familiar with the management and follow-up of TB and LTBI, and adverse events of antituberculosis medications. Some experts, particularly those who care for internationally adopted children, recommend repeating the TST 3 to 6 months after the first.[12] This may be especially important when the new arrival is malnourished or ill at the time of the initial health assessment, or there is other reason to suspect that response to the initial TST may not be optimal.

Blood-based assays were developed in the past decade as an alternative to skin testing for diagnosing TB. These tests are based on the release of interferon gamma in response to TB antigens and have the advantage of being more specific for *Mycobacterium tuberculosis* than TSTs. Although recommended by the Centers for Disease Control and Prevention (CDC) as being interchangeable with TSTs for use in TB screening, they have not proved easy enough to obtain to replace the use of TSTs at this time, and data about its use in children are only recently becoming available.[13]

Hepatitis B
All immigrants should be considered for testing for hepatitis B infection, especially those arriving from areas where prevalence of hepatitis B surface antigen is 2% or more (eg, parts of Asia and Africa). The consequences of missing hepatitis B infection are significant not only for the individual patient but for potential contacts as well. Some health professionals will also choose to test for hepatitis B immunity to determine the need for vaccine. Individuals infected with hepatitis B should be referred to an appropriate specialist for further evaluation of infection status and assessment of treatment options. Individuals found to have hepatitis B surface antibody should have their immunization records reviewed, as it

is common for immigrants to receive a single dose of hepatitis B vaccine prior to arriving in the United States to satisfy immigration requirements. The antibody test may be positive if tested on arrival, but immunity may not be durable unless the individual completes the 3-dose series. The use of hepatitis B core antibody is controversial when testing immigrant children but is felt to have value when assessing adults for prior hepatitis B infection.[14]

Complete Blood Cell Count

A blood cell count with differential can identify anemia, thrombocytopenia, and eosinophilia, all of which may have important implications in immigrants. Anemia may be caused by iron deficiency, hemoglobinopathy, or glucose-6-phosphate dehydrogenase deficiency. Thrombocytopenia may be associated with malaria. Eosinophilia is often associated with parasitic infection and should be addressed with appropriate serologic testing for parasitic diseases along with stool testing for ova and parasites or with empiric treatment for appropriate parasites.

Parasitic Diseases

Testing stool for ova and parasites is appropriate for many, but not all, immigrant populations. Stool testing alone is not sufficient for patients with eosinophilia; these patients also need an evaluation with serology or other appropriate tests for parasites, such as strongyloidiasis, schistosomiasis, or filarial diseases. The CDC recently published guidelines for evaluating refugees for parasites; these guidelines are available at www.cdc.gov/ncpdcid/dgmq/index-new-sites.html. Routine screening for malaria is not indicated for most immigrants. Most clinicians would focus on signs and symptoms when taking the medical history and screen those with compatible findings (eg, fevers, splenomegaly, thrombocytopenia).

Sexually Transmitted Infections

Some experts recommend testing all immigrants for syphilis and HIV. Others limit their testing to those with compatible signs or symptoms. Currently, some refugees and immigrants are tested before arriving in the United States, but testing for HIV is no longer required as a condition of immigration. US-based health professionals may want to review documentation of these results and be aware that there may be additional exposure between testing and arriving in the United States. Testing for other sexually transmitted infections may be based on information obtained during the history and physical examination.

Hepatitis C

Routine testing for hepatitis C is not recommended at this time for all immigrants, although it is often performed for internationally adopted children. Screening guidelines for the US population may be used to assess whether immigrants are candidates for testing.

Immunizations

Immigrants should be immunized according to current US recommendations. In most circumstances written documentation of immunizations given outside the United States may be accepted as valid if the vaccine name and month and year it was administered are listed. Immunization records of internationally adopted children are under increased scrutiny; the American Academy of Pediatrics (AAP) permits repeating all immunizations or using serologic testing for antibody to vaccine-preventable diseases to guide administration of needed vaccines. The AAP *Red Book* and yearly immunization schedules developed by the Advisory Committee on Immunization Practices are excellent references. Detailed discussion of immunization issues for immigrants can be found in the article, "Immunization for immigrants."[15]

Immunization records from outside the United States should be reviewed and the vaccines documented in the child's immunization record. Specific issues to look for include a measles-containing vaccine given before 1 year of age (these children need 2 additional doses after 1 year of age); reversal of day and year; and incomplete hepatitis B vaccine series (be sure to complete the series even if screening shows that the child has measurable hepatitis B surface antibody). For school-aged children, measuring antibody to varicella may be cost-effective compared with empiric immunization, especially if a history of varicella is obtained in the patient's child or sibling.

■ PREVENTIVE HEALTH CARE FOR IMMIGRANT CHILDREN

Immigrant children should receive the same preventive care as US-born children; however, immigrant children have additional barriers when accessing this care. Immigrant children have higher rates of lacking insurance. Language barriers can make it more difficult for immigrant children to access care, which may lead to a lack of awareness of services, difficulty understanding recommendations, and difficulty navigating the complexity of the health and health insurance systems.

The stresses of relocation as well as those associated with uncertain or undocumented immigration status may also affect ability to take advantage of what the health care system offers. Children of immigrant families are the fastest growing segment of the US pediatric population. Outreach into communities as well as health care professionals' cognizance of immigrant children's needs are necessary for addressing the barriers to care for these children.[16]

■ KEY POINTS

• Be prepared to provide qualified medical interpreters and an introduction to the US health care system to families new to the United States.
• Be prepared to test new immigrants for TB and hepatitis B infection.
• Become familiar with common screening tests that may be beneficial for immigrant populations.
• Provide time during multiple visits with families new to the United States to develop a relationship that will lead to increased trust and sharing of health information.
• Become familiar with catch-up immunization schedules for children of all ages.
• Be prepared to hear stories of resilience, strength, and courage from immigrant families and to be rewarded by the experience of caring for new Americans.

■ REFERENCES

1. Walker PF, Barnett ED. An introduction to the field of refugee and immigrant healthcare. In: Walker PF, Barnett ED, eds. *Immigrant Medicine*. Philadelphia, PA: Saunders Elsevier; 2007:1–9

2. Ohmans P. Action steps to improve the health of new Americans. In: Walker PF, Barnett ED, eds. *Immigrant Medicine*. Philadelphia, PA: Saunders Elsevier; 2007:27–35

3. Berg C, Van Dyke S. Communicating with limited English proficient patients: interpreter services. In: Walker PF, Barnett ED, eds. *Immigrant Medicine*. Philadelphia, PA: Saunders Elsevier; 2007:57–67

4. Culhane-Pera KA, Borkan JM. Multicultural medicine. In: Walker PF, Barnett ED, eds. *Immigrant Medicine*. Philadelphia, PA: Saunders Elsevier; 2007:69–81

5. Green AR, Betancourt JR. Cultural competence: a patient-based approach to caring for immigrants. In: Walker PF, Barnett ED, eds. *Immigrant Medicine*. Philadelphia, PA: Saunders Elsevier; 2007:83–97

6. Augustyn M. School readiness and bilingual education. In: Walker PF, Barnett ED, eds. *Immigrant Medicine*. Philadelphia, PA: Saunders Elsevier; 2007:693–698

7. Cochran J, O'Fallon A, Geltman PL. US medical screening for immigrants and refugees: public health issues. In: Walker PF, Barnett ED, eds. *Immigrant Medicine*. Philadelphia, PA: Saunders Elsevier; 2007:123–134

8. Seybolt L, Barnett ED, Stauffer W. US medical screening for immigrants and refugees: clinical issues. In: Walker PF, Barnett ED, eds. *Immigrant Medicine*. Philadelphia, PA: Saunders Elsevier; 2007:135–150

9. Eisenman DP. Screening for mental health problems and history of torture. In: Walker PF, Barnett ED, eds. *Immigrant Medicine*. Philadelphia, PA: Saunders Elsevier; 2007:633–638

10. Ellis BH, Betancourt TS. Children and adolescents. In: Walker PF, Barnett ED, eds. *Immigrant Medicine*. Philadelphia, PA: Saunders Elsevier; 2007:673–680

11. Bloom BR. Tuberculosis—the global view. *N Engl J Med*. 2002;346:1434–1435

12. Trehan I, Meinzen-Derr JK, Jamison L, et al. Tuberculosis screening in internationally adopted children: the need for initial and repeat testing. *Pediatrics*. 2008;122(1):e7–e14

13. Cruz AT, Geltemeyer AM, Starke JR, et al. Comparing the tuberculin skin test and T-SPOT.TB blood test in children. *Pediatrics*. 2010;127:e31–e38

14. Armstrong GL, Goldstein ST. Hepatitis B: global epidemiology, diagnosis, and prevention. In: Walker PF, Barnett ED, eds. *Immigrant Medicine*. Philadelphia, PA: Saunders Elsevier; 2007:321–341

15. Barnett ED. Immunization for immigrants. In: Walker PF, Barnett ED, eds. *Immigrant Medicine*. Philadelphia, PA: Saunders Elsevier; 2007:151–170

16. Mody R. Preventive healthcare in children. In: Walker PF, Barnett ED, eds. *Immigrant Medicine*. Philadelphia, PA: Saunders Elsevier; 2007:515–535

SECTION 3

Practicing Pediatrics in Resource-Limited Countries

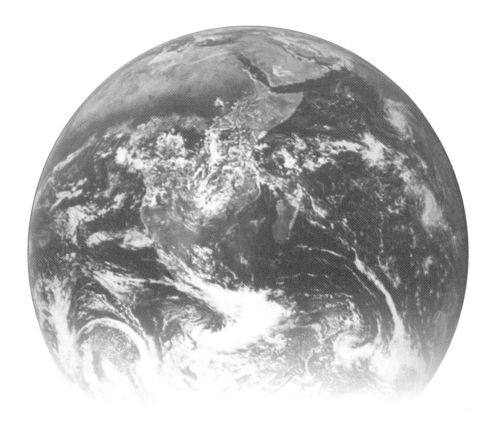

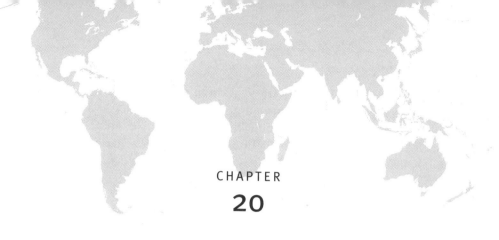

CHAPTER

20

Newborn Care

Tina Slusher, MD, FAAP
Corryn Greenwood, MD, FAAP
Margaret Nakakeeto-Kijjambu, MBChB, MMed
Clydette Powell, MD, MPH, FAAP
Yvonne Vaucher, MD, MPH

■ INTRODUCTION

Newborns account for approximately 40% of deaths in children younger than 5 years.[1] Ninety-eight percent of these 4 million neonatal deaths occur in the developing world.[1] In addition, many newborns who survive to childhood suffer lifelong problems. Many of these problems are potentially preventable by simple interventions and early treatment.
- Neurologic disability from severe perinatal asphyxia resulting from prolonged labor and a difficult delivery without a skilled attendant
- Deafness from neonatal jaundice in a neonate born near a clinic without phototherapy units and transport to a referral hospital
- Severe developmental delay after inappropriate treatment of neonatal meningitis with oral antibiotics after only 3 days of parental treatment
- Severe growth retardation in a premature newborn who is fed inappropriately diluted cow's milk

■ NEONATAL RESUSCITATION

The following section is adapted from Textbook of Neonatal Resuscitation, 6th Edition.[2]

Neonatal resuscitation is one of the most important tools in saving newborn lives and preventing birth asphyxia and its sequelae. Numerous studies across the world demonstrate decreases in neonatal mortality or birth asphyxia with the introduction of neonatal resuscitation programs. One study in China by Zhu and colleagues reported an almost 3-fold reduction in the perinatal neonatal mortality rate after a neonatal resuscitation program was introduced.[3] In Uganda, O'Hare et al reported significantly improved Apgar scores, decreased asphyxia incidences, and survival of newborns greater than 2 kg.[4] Deorari et al in India reported a significant decrease in asphyxia-related deaths.[5] Turkey saw a decrease in neonatal mortality rates of 41 to 29 per 1,000 live births between 1998 and 2003 after introducing the Neonatal Resuscitation Program (NRP).[6]

Other studies show that minimal neonatal resuscitation skills can be taught effectively to various health care practitioners in the developing world.[7-10] As so clearly pointed out by Singhal[11] and stated explicitly by Choudry,[6] neonatal resuscitation needs to be carried out in "practically all settings where asphyxiated babies are born," which as we know includes homes, communities, churches, health centers, and hospitals providing all levels of care. The appeal of the current NRP is that it is possible to effectively teach the minimal steps of resuscitation at each of these levels.

Supplies and steps of neonatal resuscitation are adapted from *Textbook of Neonatal Resuscitation*, 6th Edition,[2] to be used in lower resource settings. A relatively new simplified method of teaching the NRP is *Simply NRP*,[12] which provides low-technology simulation tools. Helping Babies Breathe[13] is a program for neonatal resuscitation in low-resource settings.

Basic Supplies for Neonatal Resuscitation

Neonatal resuscitation can be done with minimal equipment and supplies. Equipment, supplies, and instructions should be tailored to the clinic or hospital, as well as to the training and experience of the facility's personnel. Basic supplies are limited to

1. A warm place for the newborn. This can be as simple as a warm room with closed windows and overhead fans turned off or a table under an overhead warmer or bulb.
2. Two clean cloths. One cloth is to dry the neonate and one is to wrap or swaddle the baby after drying. It is important to cover the newborn's head and leave his chest and abdomen exposed should he need active resuscitation.

3. Something with which to suction the baby's airway. This can be a simple bulb aspirator, a mucus extractor, a DeLee suction trap, or a suction machine powered by foot, battery, or wall electricity. A simple bulb aspirator often works better than a small suction catheter, especially if intubation is unnecessary or not possible. Any suction device needs to be cleaned effectively and appropriately between patients to avoid infection.

4. A self-inflating bag and mask. The bag and mask need to be checked after each use to ensure they are still functional and that all parts are clean and working properly. Mouth-to-mouth resuscitation by mothers or family members is sometimes appropriately taught in community-based resuscitation programs.[10] Concerns about health care practitioners acquiring infections limit the applicability of mouth-to-mouth resuscitation in clinic and hospital settings. Reuseable bags are preferred over disposable bags. Reuseable bags need to be cleaned according to directions.

5. A clock. Although a clock is not essential, one that is easy to read helps time interventions and making other time-related decisions.

Resuscitation Steps

The inverted pyramid (Figure 20-1) is a concise summary of resuscitation and is helpful in teaching. It emphasizes the point that the first steps in resuscitation are the most likely to be successful and, therefore, are the steps on which teaching should be concentrated. Progress toward the apex of the resuscitation triangle will depend on resources and staff skill levels. Infection control should always be observed throughout resuscitation.

At the time of birth, 3 questions should be asked: Is the baby term? Is the baby breathing? Does the baby have good tone? Term, healthy, vigorous newborns who are crying or breathing well do not need resuscitation and should be dried and placed on the mother's chest and covered with a clean dry cloth or blanket.[14,15] These same newborns also do not need suctioning. Those newborns who are not crying or breathing well will need resuscitation. The first block of the resuscitation triangle includes

1. *Warm.* Place the newborn in the warmest place in the room that still allows access. Turn off fans and close windows.

2. *Position.* Position the newborn's head in a neutral or sniffing position—not hyper-flexed or hyperextended.

3. *Suction only if needed.* Suction the baby's mouth first, then the nose. Suctioning the nose first increases the chance that the baby will get angry, attempt to cry, and aspirate what is in the mouth

Figure 20-1. Inverted Neonatal Resuscitation Pyramid

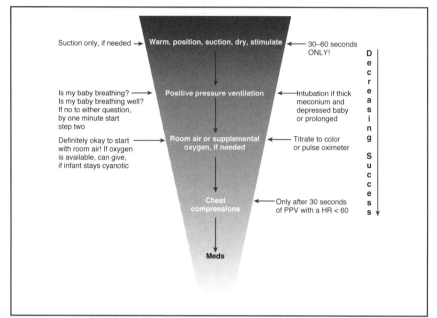

Modified from American Academy of Pediatrics, American Heart Association. *Textbook of Neonatal Resuscitation.* 6th ed. Kattwinkel J, ed. Elk Grove Village, IL: American Academy of Pediatrics; 2011

(eg, amniotic fluid, meconium). One tool that NRP uses to teach this is that M comes before N in the alphabet, just as *m*outh comes before *n*ose in neonatal resuscitation. Suction gently and avoid suctioning too deeply, especially when using a suction catheter. If a physician or health care practitioner is not available during a resuscitation of a depressed newborn with thick meconium, the nurse or midwife should be instructed to suction the mouth and nose as best as possible with the device on hand (eg, bulb, mucus extraction, large suction catheter) and then proceed with resuscitation as usual. Vigorous term newborns do not need suctioning. Suctioning can unnecessarily cause bradycardia and trauma and should therefore be avoided. See page 432 for instructions about thick meconium in a depressed newborn when a skilled provider who can intubate is available.

4. *Dry.* Dry the newborn and get rid of the wet cloth. Leaving the wet cloth on makes the newborn colder, which can make resuscitation more difficult, especially if premature.

5. *Stimulate.* Stress safe stimulation methods, which primarily include flicking the baby's feet and rubbing her back. Strongly discourage unsafe methods, such as holding the baby upside down and slapping her bottom; putting alcohol, pepper, or other substances in her nose; putting her in cold water; or compressing her abdomen or chest. Emphasize limiting stimulation time, as the newborn with primary apnea will respond rapidly. Neonates in secondary apnea will not respond to stimulation regardless of duration. If stimulation is not immediately effective, proceed to positive-pressure ventilation.

6. *Emphasize the need to respond and work quickly.* The first 5 steps should take no more than 30 to 60 seconds. A newborn who is not breathing or not breathing well by 1 minute of life should receive positive-pressure ventilation. Practice the timing with obstetric and pediatric staff until it happens without thought. Emphasize that more than 1 step can be carried out simultaneously if more than 1 person is available to assist with resuscitation.

Ventilation is the most important step in newborn resuscitation and likely to be successful in any baby who still has a heart rate.[16] Heart rate comes up almost immediately in newborns who are immediately and adequately ventilated. The majority of resuscitated newborns do not need chest compressions or medications. Teach and practice good hand position. If the chest is not rising or not rising well, quickly figure out the problem. Possibilities, in order of likelihood, include

1. Ineffective seal between the mask and face. This usually responds to repositioning the practitioner's hand on the mask or the newborn's face, or repositioning the newborn's head.
2. Secretions. Repeat suctioning.
3. Bad bag or mask. Replace.

Supplemental oxygen is not routinely needed at the beginning of a resuscitation. Most term neonates with respiratory depression at birth will respond to adequate ventilation with room air. Oxygen is toxic, especially in high concentrations when tissues become oversaturated, and may be harmful in neonatal resuscitation[2,17,18]; however, studies are ongoing. Current NRP training states that it is acceptable to begin the step of resuscitation without oxygen.[2,16] If available, oxygen should be titrated to keep the neonate pink and oxygen saturations normal. Therefore, if the practitioner begins without oxygen and the neonate remains blue (or desaturated), oxygen should be added, if available. If the neonate is pink (or well saturated) and oxygen is being used, it should be weaned rapidly as long as the neonate remains pink (well saturated). It is normal for the pre-ductal oxygen saturation (ie, right hand) to take up to 5 minutes to get to 80% to 85% oxygen saturation and up to 10 minutes to get to 85% to 95% oxygen saturation.[2]

These oxygen instructions are for the delivery room; decisions addressing which newborns should be placed on oxygen in the nursery and what saturations are appropriate are made at the time of transfer to the nursery, when indicated.

Heart rate should be checked after 30 seconds of positive-pressure ventilation. Chest compressions should not be done until after 30 seconds of effective positive-pressure ventilation. Effective ventilation means the chest is moving—not too much and not too little. Heart rate can be estimated by counting the umbilical cord pulsations for 6 seconds or by counting heart rate for 6 seconds and multiplying by 10 (ie, if the 6-second heart rate is 4, the baby's heart rate is about 40 beats per minute [BPM]). An increasing heart rate is the best sign of effective ventilation in a newborn. Positive-pressure ventilation should be continued until the heart rate is greater than 100 BPM, the baby is breathing effectively, or resuscitation efforts are stopped.

Chest compressions are indicated if heart rate remains less than 60 BPM after 30 seconds of effective ventilation. They should be done at a rate of 3 compressions to 1 ventilation, compressing the chest about one third of the chest's diameter. Encircling the baby's chest with 2 hands, using fingers to provide a hard surface for compressions, is the most effective and preferred way for providers to perform compressions (Figure 20-2). However, the baby can be placed on a hard surface and compressed with 2 fingers (Figure 20-3); this method is best for single rescuers providing ventilation and cardiac compressions.

Figure 20-2. Thumb Compressions

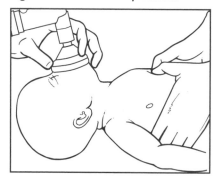

From American Academy of Pediatrics, American Heart Association. *Textbook of Neonatal Resuscitation.* 6th ed. Kattwinkel J, ed. Elk Grove Village, IL: American Academy of Pediatrics; 2011:137

Figure 20-3. Two-Finger Compressions

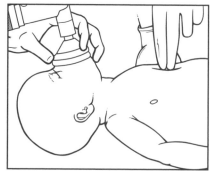

From American Academy of Pediatrics, American Heart Association. *Textbook of Neonatal Resuscitation.* 6th ed. Kattwinkel J, ed. Elk Grove Village, IL: American Academy of Pediatrics; 2011:137

Medications are not generally needed in neonatal resuscitation and, according to Wyllie and Niermeyer, are "probably justifiable in less than 0.1% of births."[19] The single most important resuscitation medication is *epinephrine* (still called adrenaline in many countries). Epinephrine increases the strength and rate of cardiac contraction and may increase blood flow to the head and coronary arteries. The only concentration routinely available in many countries is 1:1,000, which is usually supplied in a 1-mL vial; this is too concentrated to give to a neonate by intravenous (IV) or intraosseous (IO) infusion and needs to be diluted 1:10 to make a concentration of 1:10,000 (Table 20-1).

An umbilical venous catheter (UVC) may be placed to facilitate medication and fluid administration. The procedure for placement includes

1. Retrieve needed supplies.
   a. A sterile tube that can be inserted into the umbilical vein; any sterile tube that is the correct size can be used (often a 5-6 feeding tube).
   b. A tie for the umbilical stump, which can be tightened if there is bleeding.
   c. A sterile blade or scalpel.
   d. Sterile cloth or drapes (the inside wrapper of a glove package can be used in an emergency).
   e. Soap or cleaning solution for the cord and abdomen.
   f. Hemostat to hold the cord before cutting.
2. Elevate the cord off of the abdomen, clean the cord, and drape the abdomen.

Table 20-1. Dilution Options to Make 1:10,000 Epinephrine, Depending on Syringe Size

Epinephrine 1:1,000	Sterile Water or NSS	Total Concentration of 1:10,000
0.1 mL	0.9 mL	1 mL
0.2 mL	1.8 mL	2 mL
0.3 mL	2.7 mL	3 mL
0.5 mL	4.5 mL	5 mL
1 mL	9 mL	10 mL

Abbreviations: BPM, beats per minute; IO, intraosseous; IV, intravenous; NSS, normal saline solution; UVC, umbilical venous catheter.

Epinephrine can be repeated every 5 minutes if the heart rate remains less than 60 BPM.

The dose for a neonate is 0.1 to 0.3 mL/kg IV/IO (weight is estimated to the nearest 0.5 kg to make math simpler). Follow dose with a flush of sterile water or NSS. If IV cannot be quickly started, consider a UVC or IO.

3. Place the clean tie or umbilical tape on the skin at the cord's base and tighten slightly.
4. Cut the cord with a sterile blade or scalpel.
5. Insert the catheter into the larger umbilical vein just until there is good blood flow—if it is inserted more than 2 to 4 cm, it is probably in too far. Administering medication into the liver can be dangerous; it can be avoided by inserting the catheter just until good blood flow is obtained. If the UVC is to be left in, it can be replaced and positioned above the liver, confirming position with a radiograph (as described in neonatal textbooks).
6. Medication can be administered and blood samples obtained through this catheter.

If bleeding is suspected and the newborn is not responding to resuscitation, a 10 mL/kg bolus of normal saline solution (NSS) or lactated Ringer solution can be given over 5 to 10 minutes and repeated if needed.

Other medications, such as sodium bicarbonate, calcium, atropine, and narcotic antagonists, are rarely indicated and rarely effective in neonatal resuscitation in the delivery room.

Indications for Intubation

Intubation is indicated at the delivery of a depressed newborn with thick meconium when a provider is available who can effectively perform the intubation. In this situation, the provider should intubate and suction the newborn before stimulating or providing positive-pressure ventilation. It is best to suction with a device attached directly to the endotracheal tube (ETT) or to intubate directly with a large suction catheter (14FR). Small suction catheters inserted through small ETTs are ineffective in suctioning out significant amounts of thick meconium. Devices to attach a 3 or 3.5 ETT can often be made out of available tubing if commercial devices are not available. Intubation is no longer recommended for vigorous newborns with meconium-stained amniotic fluid.

Intubation is not necessary in a standard neonatal resuscitation, as ventilation can be provided even for extended times with a bag and mask. However, if the health care practitioner is skilled in intubation, the newborn may be electively intubated at any point, especially if resuscitation may be prolonged. If prolonged bag-and-mask ventilation is going to be provided, it is often helpful to pass a small nasogastric tube to keep the stomach deflated. It is possible to provide effective bag-and-mask ventilation with a small nasogastric tube in place.

Discontinuing Resuscitation Efforts

It is appropriate to discontinue resuscitation when a newborn has a heart rate above 100 BPM and good respiratory effort. If heart rate is below 100 BPM, ventilation should continue regardless of the respiratory effort unless the decision is made to discontinue all resuscitation efforts.

It is not always clear when unsuccessful resuscitative efforts should be discontinued. Generally, if there are no signs of life at 10 to 20 minutes after delivery, it is appropriate to discontinue resuscitation. Sometimes the more difficult decision is what to do when a newborn's heart rate is greater than 100 BPM but there is no respiratory effort and the newborn is in a setting without a ventilator. In this situation it is important to rule out reversible causes of apnea or agonal respirations, such as narcotic overdose. If there are no reversible causes identified and no mechanical ventilation is possible, it may be appropriate to stop resuscitation efforts at some point, which will vary depending on the specifics of the situation. This decision is made after carefully considering many factors, including the clinic's or hospital's resources and discussion with parents.

■ FLUIDS AND NUTRITION

Appropriate fluids and nutrition are extremely important for the survival of a sick and premature neonate. This can be especially challenging in environments without IV pumps, microdrip (giving) sets, and total parental nutrition.

Fluid Requirements

Fluid requirements for term newborns are 60 to 80 mL/kg/day on day 1 of life and increasing by about 20 mL/kg/day thereafter, up to 120 to 160 mL/kg/day. Factors that increase fluid requirements, such as phototherapy and overhead warmers, or decrease fluid requirements, such as congestive heart failure and renal insufficiency, must be considered when calculating fluid requirements. Term newborns may lose 5% to 10% of their birth weight in the first week before caloric intake is adequate. Most healthy term newborns regain their birth weight by day 7. Premature newborns generally require more fluid per kg per day. The more premature the baby, the higher the insensible fluid loss through the skin and the more total fluids required. Fluid requirements for the premature newborn start at the upper end of the fluid requirements for term newborns and also increase by about 20 mL/kg/day, with the maximum titrated to achieve adequate hydration without fluid overload. Generally, fluid requirements for premature newborns are a maximum of

150 to 160 mL/kg/day, but extremely premature babies with birth weight less than 1 kg may require more than 200 mL/kg/day to maintain hydration because of excessive insensible fluid loss through their thin skin. Keeping premature newborns inside a humidified incubator or placing them under a small tent of plastic wrap decreases their insensible loss and total fluid requirements. Premature newborns may lose up to 15% of their birth weight, which is proportionally more than term newborns, and take longer to regain their birth weight. It is helpful to plot their weight on a graph (Figure 20-4) every 1 to 3 days to ensure that initial weight loss and subsequent weight gain are appropriate.

Figure 20-4. Expected Neonatal Weight Changes Based on Birth Weight

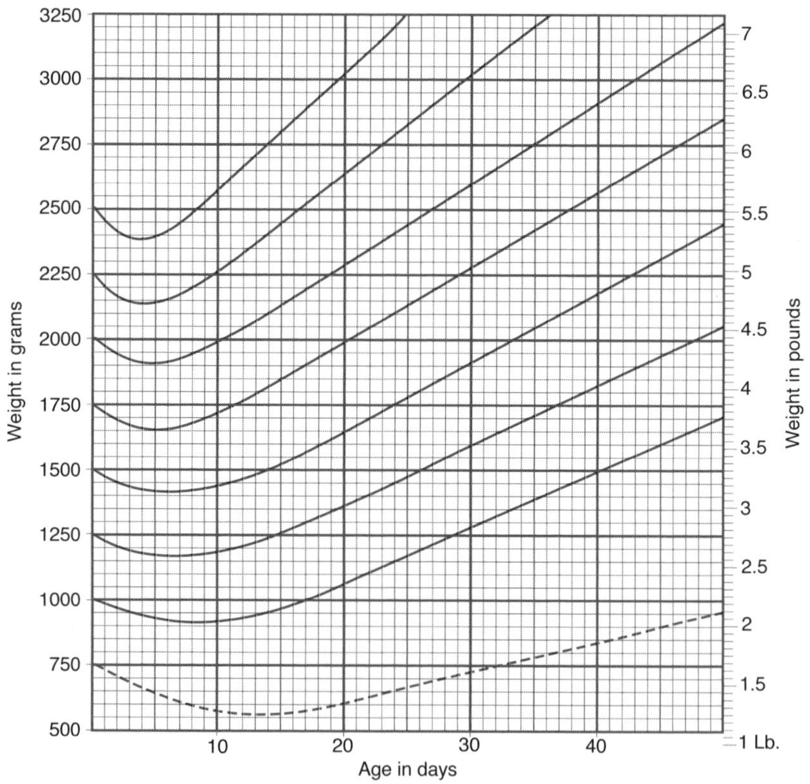

This growth chart is shown because it represents adequate growth without the availability of total parental nutrition, high-calorie formulas, or breast milk fortifiers. Newer growth charts reflect nutritional support not available in most of the developing world.

From Dancis J, O'Connell JR, Holt LE. A grid for recording the weight of premature infants. *J Pediatr.* 1948;33(11):570–572, with permission from Elsevier.

Types of Intravenous Fluids

The appropriate type of fluid also varies by day of life and birth weight or gestational age of the newborn. Dextrose 10% in water (D10W) is generally the recommended fluid on the first 1 to 2 days of life for newborns weighing 1 kg or more. Those weighing less than 1 kg should start on dextrose 5% in water (D5W). Neonates small for gestational age (SGA) and those of diabetic mothers may require a higher glucose infusion rate based on weight to maintain normoglycemia (blood glucose >40–45 mg/dL). Fluid intake per day should be calculated based on birth weight until birth weight is regained.

Electrolytes in intravenous fluid (IVF) are not needed in the first 3 days of life. Sodium (2 to 4 mEq/kg/day) should be added after day 3. Most hospitals are limited to standard IVF mixtures. An approximation can be obtained by adding 25 mL of NSS or Ringer solution (lactated Ringer may be used if Ringer solution is unavailable) to 100 mL of D10W or D5W, which provides about 3 to 4 mEq of sodium per 100 mL. Another option is to add additional glucose to D5¼ NSS if available (Box 20-1).

Potassium (1 to 2 mEq/kg/day) should also be added around the third or fourth day if the newborn is not tolerating enteric feeds and has adequate urine output. Adding 10 mEq of potassium per 1,000 mL of IVF and providing 1 mEq per 100 mL is practical and maintains normal serum potassium in most newborns. Deviation from this should only occur when clinically indicated. Add potassium to IVFs very carefully to avoid mistakes that can be fatal. Develop a check-and-balance system when adding potassium, such as having 2 nurses check the amount added. In addition, unless it is absolutely necessary to alter the amount of potassium added, add exactly the same standard amount of potassium to the same volume of IVFs. If enteral feeds (by mouth or nasogastric tube) are being advanced appropriately, consider not adding potassium to IVFs at all to avoid potential errors. Ringer and lactated Ringer solution have the advantage of providing an appropriate amount of potassium as well as a very small amount of calcium (Box 20-1).

Other additives are generally not necessary. Calcium infiltrations can result in severe burns when given via peripheral IV. If the patient has symptomatic hypocalcemia with life-threatening conditions, such as seizures, arrhythmias, or hypotension, and a central line is not available, it is safest to slowly give diluted calcium boluses under direct observation in a newly placed peripheral IV line. Be sure the IV line is patent before beginning the calcium infusion. For nonlife-threatening situations, IV or oral calcium gluconate is preferable. *Give calcium by mouth whenever*

Box 20-1. Preparing Standard Glucose and Electrolyte Solutions

TYPES OF SOLUTIONS

Dextrose 50% in water (D50W)

Dextrose 10% in water (D10W)[a]

Ringer Lactate
  Sodium: 130 mEq/L
  Potassium: 4 mEq/L
  Calcium: 2.7 mEq/L (equivalent number of CamEq as 0.6 mg/mL calcium gluconate)
  Chloride: 109 mEq/L
  Lactate: 28 mEq/L

Ringer Solution
  Sodium: 147 mEq/L
  Potassium: 4 mEq/L
  Calcium: 4 mEq/L (equivalent number of CamEq as 0.9 mg/mL calcium gluconate)
  Chloride: 156 mEq/L

D5 $^1/_4$ NSS (0.225% sodium chloride)
  Sodium: 34 mEq/L
  Chloride: 34 mEq/L

$^1/_2$ NSS (0.45% sodium chloride)
  Sodium: 77 mEq/L

PREPARATION OF SPECIAL SOLUTIONS

To make D10 $^1/_4$ NSS from D5 $^1/_4$ NSS and D50W
  1. Remove 50 mL from 500-mL bag of D5 $^1/_4$ NSS.
  2. Add back 50 mL of D50W.

  When infused at 100 mL/kg/d, provides
  • GIR: 7 mg/kg/min
  • NaCl: 3.6 mEq/kg/d

To make D7.5 $^1/_4$ NSS from D5 $^1/_4$ NS and D50W
  1. Remove 25 mL from 500-mL bag of $^1/_4$ NS.
  2. Add back 25 mL of D50W.

  When infused at 100 mL/kg/d, provides
  • GIR: 5.2 mg/kg/min
  • NaCl: 3.8 mEq/kg/d

To make D7.5 $^1/_4$ NSS from D10W and NSS
  1. Remove 62.5 mL from a 250-mL bag of D10W.[b]
  2. Add back 62.5 ml NSS to the 250-mL bag of D10W.

  Or

  1. Remove 250 mL from a 1-L bag of D10W.
  2. Add back 250 mL NSS to the 1-L bag of D10W.

  When infused at 100 mL/kg/d, provides
  • GIR: 5.2 mg/kg/min
  • NaCl: 4 mEq/kg/d

Box 20-1. Preparing Standard Glucose and Electrolyte Solutions, continued

PREPARATION OF SPECIAL SOLUTIONS, CONTINUED

To make D7.5 electrolyte solution

1. Remove 62.5 mL from a 250-mL bag of D10W.
2. Add back 62.5 mL of Ringer solution to the 250-mL bag of D10W.

Or

1. Remove 250 mL from a 1-L bag of D10W.
2. Add back 50 mL of Ringer solution to the 1-L bag of D10W.

When infused at 100 mL/kg/d, provides (rounded to the nearest whole number where possible)

- GIR: 5 mg/kg/min
- Na: 4 mEq/kg/d
- K: 0.1 mEq/kg/d
- Ca: 0.1 mEq/kg/d (equivalent to 86 mg/kg/d calcium gluconate—a small dose)
- Chloride: 4 mEq/kg/d

To make D10 lactated Ringer

1. Remove 200 mL from a 1-L bag of lactated Ringer.
2. Add back 200 mL of D50 to the 1-L bag of lactated Ringer.

The resulting solution will have 80% of the original lactated Ringer.

When infused at 100 mL/kg/d, provides (rounded to the nearest whole number where possible)

- GIR: 7 mg/kg/min
- Na: 10 mEq/kg/d
- K: 0.3 mEq/kg/d
- Ca: 0.2 mEq/kg/d (equivalent to 43 mg/kg/d calcium gluconate—a very small dose)
- Chloride: 9 mEq/kg/d
- Lactate: 2 mEq/kg/d

To make D10 $^1/_2$ NSS

1. Remove 200 mL of $^1/_2$ NSS from a 1-L bag of $^1/_2$ NSS.
2. Add back 200 mL of D50 to the 1-L bag of $^1/_2$ NSS.

If infused at 100 mL/kg/d, provides

- GIR: 7 mg/kg/min
- NaCl: 6 mEq/kg/day

Abbreviations: GIR, glucose infusion rate; NSS, normal saline solution.

[a]Other permutations using D5W instead of D10W will result in electrolyte solutions with dextrose concentrations less than 5%.
[b]Save removed D10W in sterile, capped syringes for later (eg, for D10 boluses or for "y-ing" into maintenance intravenous fluids to increase GIR).

possible because it is the safest route. The IV calcium gluconate preparation is well tolerated orally. Calcium carbonate antacid can also be given. Calcium glubionate syrup, an oral calcium preparation, is not recommended in newborns as it is hyperosmolar and often causes diarrhea. Although calcium chloride is preferred in life-threatening situations because it does not require conversion in the liver, calcium gluconate, the only form of IV calcium available in many hospitals, is also effective.

Nutrition

Total parental nutrition is seldom available in nurseries in low-resource settings; therefore, early enteral nutrition is essential and should be started as soon as possible after birth.

Term newborns generally require about 110 to 120 cal/kg/day (180 mL/kg/day) enterally to gain weight appropriately. Adequate weight gain is about 20 to 30 g/day or about 10 to 15 g/kg/day after the first 3 to 5 days.[20,21] Most healthy, term, breastfeeding newborns regain their birth weight by days 7 through 10. If a term newborn has not regained his birth weight by then, an explanation should be sought and the newborn followed closely. Changes in breastfeeding technique, higher calorie feeds, or supplementation may be needed. The newborn stomach is small, holding only approximately 5 mL/kg immediately after birth; therefore, appropriate initial feeding volumes for term newborns are 5 to 20 mL per feed on the first day and 10 to 45 mL per feed on the second day after birth. Feeds in excess of this often result in emesis.

Premature neonates born before 35 weeks' gestation generally require about 120 kcal/kg/day to gain weight optimally. Adequate weight gain is 15 to 20 g/day or about 13 to 15 g/kg/day. As with term newborns, the optimal and best-tolerated feeding is maternal human milk. Because of weak suck, limited stamina, and incoordination, preterm newborns born before 35 weeks' gestation are unable to take full nipple feeds or breastfeed exclusively. Although some will appear to be breastfeeding well, actual milk transfer is low. These preterm newborns require some or all feedings every 2 to 3 hours by nasogastric gavage (5FR) tubes or, in more physiologically mature preterm newborns, by cup or spoon.

Feeding Advancement

In preterm newborns, begin feeds slowly at 20 mL/kg/day on day 1 if clinically stable. Intravenous fluids need to be given to maintain adequate hydration until 60 to 80 mL/kg/day of enteral feeding is reached. Advance feedings slowly by 20 mL/kg/day to reach full feeds at 7 to 10 days of age unless signs of feeding intolerance occur. One suggested systematic method of increasing feeds is included in Table 20-2. The gavage tube is aspirated and the gastric residual measured prior to each feed. Small residuals (2 mL or less) of clear gastric fluid or undigested milk are normal and can be refed without changing feeding volume or schedule. Brown-tinged residuals usually indicate old blood in the stomach and, in the absence of any other sign of gastrointestinal problems (see "Necrotizing Enterocolitis" on page 440), are not an indication to

	INITIAL VOLUME OF FEEDINGS (ML)	INTERVAL BETWEEN FEEDING (H)	VOLUME OF INCREMENT (mL)	FREQUENCY OF CHANGE
WEIGHT (G)				
<1,000	0.5–1.0	2	0.5–1.0	Every 24 h
1,000–1,500	1.0–2.0	2	1.0–2.0	Every 12 h
1,500–2,000	2.0–3.0	2–3	2.0–4.0	Every 12 h
2,000–2,500	4.0–5.0	3	4.0–7.0	Every 8 h
>2,500	10.0	3	10–15	Every 3 h

Table 20-2. Premature Newborn Nutrition: Suggested Feeding

Adapted with permission from Zlotkin SH, Perman M. Feeding the preterm infant. In: Jeejeebhoy KN, ed. *Current Therapy in Nutrition*. Toronto, Ontario, Canada: BC Decker, Inc.; 1988

stop enteric feedings. This is important to emphasize to nursery staff as it is a frequent cause of stopping feeds for fear of necrotizing enterocolitis (NEC) but in fact, if all else is well, it is better to feed maternal breast milk than not to neutralize stomach acid. Steady weight gain of 15 to 20 g/day is a sign of adequate enteric intake. When newborns are taking oral feeds, IVFs need to be decreased proportionally as feeding volume is increased to avoid fluid overload.

Delay initial feedings if there is severe respiratory distress, shock with poor perfusion to the gut, or a condition requiring surgical intervention (eg, duodenal atresia, gastroschisis, omphalocele, or imperforate anus; diaphragmatic hernia; esophageal atresia or fistula), in which case surgical correction of the underlying problem is indicated before starting enteral feeds. Start feeding when the clinical condition is stable and when signs of gastrointestinal motility have returned (eg, bowel sounds, passing stool, not excessive or bilious residuals).

Feeding Intolerance

Signs of feeding intolerance include persistent or increasing gastric residuals, emesis, abdominal distention, and abnormal stool. Abdominal distention without any other abnormalities may resolve after stooling. Small but persistent non-bilious gastric residuals may indicate slow gastric emptying and, if so, will resolve after temporarily decreasing feeding volume. Consider decreasing feeding by about 25% of the previous amount and holding at that level for 2 to 6 feeds, then slowly increasing again. Sepsis is often associated with an ileus, increased residuals, decreased or absent bowel sounds, and abdominal distention.

Feeds should be held when signs of feeding intolerance occur. How long feeds are held depends on the clinical stability of the neonate and seriousness of the problem. Bilious emesis or gastric residuals, bloody stools, or a definitely abnormal bowel radiograph all indicate significant gastrointestinal (GI) pathology, necessitating withholding feedings until several days after all abnormalities resolve.

Gastrointestinal bleeding that is not maternal in origin can be treated with ranitidine IV or enterally. Ranitidine[22] oral dose is 2 mg/kg/dose every 8 hours; IV dose is 0.5 mg/kg/dose every 12 hours slow push (premature) or 1.5 mg/kg/dose every 8 hours slow push (term). Any baby who is bleeding should get vitamin K_1.

Necrotizing Enterocolitis

Persistent vomiting; gastric residuals that are bilious, progressively increasing, or greater than 20% of the preceding feeding volume; abdominal distention, especially if progressive and severe and with visible bowel loops; bloody stools; and clinical instability or acute deterioration are all signs of NEC. A brown or bloody gastric aspirate alone is not a sign of NEC. If a radiograph can be obtained, look for distended, thickened bowel loops; air bubbles in the bowel wall (pneumatosis cystoides intestinalis); portal air in the liver; and free air in the abdomen (pneumoperitoneum), which are all signs of NEC. Newborns with possible, presumed, or definite NEC or surgical abdomen will need to be placed on nasogastric drainage and broad-spectrum antibiotics with close clinical follow-up, complete blood cell count (CBC), and serial abdominal films. Newborns with perforations are unlikely to survive without total parental nutrition and intensive care that is usually not available in many nurseries in the developing world. The decision to proceed with surgery will depend on the available resources and prognosis with surgery.

Human Milk Feeding

Human milk feeding is optimal for almost all newborns. The World Health Organization (WHO) currently recommends exclusive human milk feeding (no other fluids, teas, or foods) for the first 6 months of life, after which complementary feeds are added to breastfeeding, which should continue for at least 18 to 24 months.[23] The many benefits of breast milk include improved tolerance of feeds, fewer respiratory and GI infections, decreased incidence of sudden infant death syndrome, and lower infant and early childhood mortality.[24-29]

For the premature newborn, additional benefits include fewer infections, less necrotizing enterocolitis, and enhanced neurocognitive outcome.[29-31] The WHO and United Nations Children's Fund (UNICEF) strongly support exclusive breastfeeding through the Ten Steps to Successful Breastfeeding of the Baby Friendly Hospital Initiative.[32] In many cultures, mothers discard colostrum, delay the first breastfeeding for hours or days, or give various fluids and teas in the first few days after birth, all of which increase the risk of neonatal morbidity and mortality.

Stress the importance to medical staff and mothers about putting the newborn to the breast within the first hour after birth and giving colostrum, which contains a large amount of immunoglobulin (IgA), lymphocytes, vitamin A, and lactoferrin, all of which protect the baby from infection.[33,34] Many mothers are concerned that they have too little milk in the first few days after birth; reassure them that this is normal. A healthy, breastfed term newborn receives only 30 to 40 mL/kg/day on day 1. Volume gradually increases over the next few days as the mother's milk "comes in." Lactogenesis may be delayed, especially if mothers are ill or after cesarean delivery. Newborns should breastfeed on demand every 2 to 3 hours (10 to 12 times a day) during the first week. Intake is adequate if the newborn is passing urine and stool several times per day by day 3. Stools should be soft and yellow by day 4. Newborns whose human milk intake is insufficient because of low milk volume or inadequate milk transfer in the first several days after birth often present with dehydration, fever, or jaundice.

The caloric density of human milk in normal healthy mothers varies from 14 kcal/oz to 35 kcal/oz, with a mean of 21 kcal/oz,[35] depending on fat content, which is largely independent of the mother's nutritional intake or status except in extreme circumstances. This mean caloric content is from a historic article by Lemmons et al, in which the authors found a caloric content of almost 22 kcal/oz in term and preterm newborns.[36] Healthy babies compensate for the caloric density of their mother's milk by altering the volume they consume. When caloric density is low, newborns compensate by feeding longer and more frequently, taking in more milk than newborns of mothers with high-caloric (high-fat) milk. It can be very helpful to determine the caloric content of the mother's milk by measuring fat and calculating the percentage of cream in a sample of breast milk (creamatocrit). The creamatocrit can be easily determined, even in developing countries, by putting a sample of breast milk in a capillary tube and spinning it is a centrifuge. When it spins down, a layer of fat or cream will appear at the top of the capillary tube, which can be placed on a hematocrit reader to view the percentage of fat. The percentage of fat determines the caloric content of the sample (Figure 20-5 and Table 20-3).

Figure 20-5. Creamatocrit Procedure

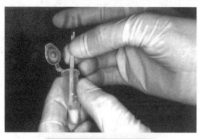

1. Mother empties her breast into container, which is shaken well for 5 seconds.
2. From this sample, pour about ½ mL into a sample cup.
3. Mix sample by shaking again for 5 seconds.
4. Fill 2 non-heparinized microhematocrit capillary tubes with milk.

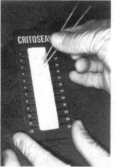

5. Seal capillary tubes at one end with Critoseal.

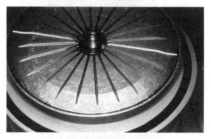

6. Place tubes with sealed end to the outside of the centrifuge, in a counterbalanced position.

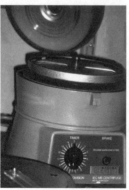

7. Screw lid in place.
8. Close top of centrifuge.
9. Set timer for 5 minutes.
10. When spinning stops, remove tubes from centrifuge.

Figure 20-5. Creamatocrit Procedure, continued

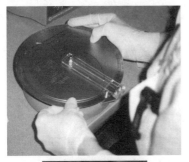

11. Place tubes on hematocrit reader with Critoseal end at top.
12. Place the intersection of sealant and milk at the cross point of the curved line.

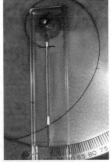

13. Rotate upper disc so that bottom of curved line intersects *bottom* point of milk in the capillary tube.

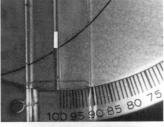

14. Set lower percentage disc at 100%.

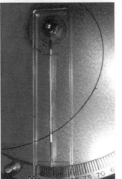

15. Rotate percentage disc until curve line intersects cream layer of milk.
16. Subtract this percentage (usually 85% to 95%) from 100%. The result is the creamatocrit (usually 5% to 15%).

Adapted from Griffin TL, Meier PP, Bradford LP, et al. Mothers' performing creamatocrit measures in the NICU: accuracy, reactions, and cost. *J Obstet Gynecol Neonatal Nurs.* 2000;29(3):249–257; *Br Med J.* 1978;1(6119):1018–1020; and © Rush Mothers' Milk Club Special Care Nursery, Rush Children's Hospital, 1653 W Congress Pkwy, Chicago, IL 60612.

Table 20-3. Nutritional Value of Human Milk Based on Creamatocrit Value										
CREAMA-TOCRIT PERCENTAGE	3	4	5	6	7	8	9	10	11	12
g fat/mL	0.017	0.023	0.03	0.037	0.044	0.051	0.058	0.064	0.071	0.078
cal/mL	0.49	0.56	0.62	0.69	0.76	0.82	0.89	0.96	1.02	1.09
cal/oz	15.7	17.8	20	22.1	24.3	26.4	28.5	30.7	32.8	34.9
% of cal – fat	22	37	44	48.2	52.1	56	58.2	60.4	62.6	64

Based on regression equations in Lucas A, Gibbons JA, Lyster RL, Baum JD. Creamatocrit: simple clinical technique for estimating fat concentration and energy value of human milk. *Br Med J.* 1978;1(6119):1018–1020

Achieving adequate intake and weight gain in breastfed premature and sick newborns can be challenging. When babies cannot obtain adequate intake by directly breastfeeding, as is the case with sick term and many premature newborns, mothers must express their milk every 2 to 3 hours for each feed. Hand expression is the most widely used method in developing countries. If done frequently, hand expression usually yields an adequate volume for premature newborns. Although these babies may take only a very small volume per feed in the first few weeks, it is important for mothers to express their milk frequently and completely empty their breasts at each expression to build up and maintain an adequate milk supply (at least 500 mL/day) as soon as possible after delivery. Although newer hand pumps and battery or electric pumps may yield higher volumes, most mothers can produce adequate amounts of milk using hand expression, as recently shown in Uganda.[37] When volume cannot be increased to compensate for low caloric intake, higher calorie hindmilk is one of the most practical and best-tolerated methods of improving weight gain without adding formula-feeding in newborns who are unable to breastfeed. The first milk (foremilk) a mother expresses appears thin—low-fat or "skim" milk. As she continues to express milk during a pumping session it becomes visually thicker as fat content increases—"whole" milk (hindmilk). The last milk or "cream" expressed has the highest fat content. Hindmilk is well tolerated even at a very high caloric content. If hindmilk is unavailable, an alternative is adding small amounts of vegetable oil (eg, corn, sunflower, olive), which contains 8 kcal/mL, to fortify mother's milk.

Health care workers and mothers can be taught to modify the caloric content of human milk to achieve appropriate growth and weight gain. Mothers can also be easily taught to express and set aside the foremilk before collecting the hindmilk.[38] If hindmilk volume is too low for the newborn at a given feeding, it can be topped off with foremilk. Foremilk, which is not used immediately, can be frozen and given later as needed. If the mother is temporarily too ill to feed her baby at the breast or go to the special-care baby nursery to feed her baby, staff or her family can help her express milk, which can then be given to the newborn.

Low Milk Volume

Ensure good breastfeeding technique for healthy term newborns with proper positioning and latching. If the baby has a good suck and there is adequate milk transfer, the mother can breastfeed more frequently to increase her milk production. She can also try hand expression with breast compression, massage, and pumping to increase milk production, as described by Morton et al in premature newborns.[39] Sometimes mothers with an overabundant supply of milk may be feeding only the low-fat foremilk. In this case, mothers can be instructed to express and discard some of the foremilk before feeding so the newborn receives more of the higher-fat hindmilk, which improves feeding satisfaction and reduces intake and frequency of feeding, thereby reducing the mother's overabundant milk supply. For premature newborns who are being fed expressed breast milk or for term newborns with poor suck and milk transfer, the mother should be encouraged to completely empty her breast at each expression or at each feed to increase her milk supply and include high-calorie hindmilk during the feeding.

If all of these measures fail to adequately improve milk production, the mother, in conjunction with her physician, can consider beginning metoclopramide or domperidone tablets to stimulate milk production. Both drugs will double milk supply providing the mother pumps frequently (ie, every 2 to 3 hours). Mothers should discuss using these drugs with their physicians before taking either. They should be screened for potential risks (eg, depression, prolonged Q-T intervals) and advised that these are off-label uses for these drugs and made aware of possible side effects.

Metoclopramide increases prolactin, thereby increasing milk supply. One dosage regimen that decreases potential sleepiness in mothers is 10 mg once on day 1; 10 mg twice on day 2; 10 mg 3 times daily on days 3 through 10; 10 mg twice daily on day 11; and 10 mg once on day 12.[40] Another suggested dosing regimen is 10 mg 3 times daily for 7 to 10 days[40] and a subsequent taper of 10 mg per week until off the drug.[41] If the metoclopramide effectively increases milk supply but milk production drops off after stopping, the dosage regimen can be repeated. Metoclopramide is widely available, even in low-resource settings. It is occasionally associated with side effects, such as fatigue, dizziness, dystonia, seizures, and depression.[40]

Domperidone also increases milk production, probably by increasing prolactin levels.[42] It is available outside the United States, where it is the preferred medication prescribed for low milk supply because it appears more effective and has fewer side effects than metoclopramide.[40] Domperidone can be taken as two 10-mg tablets (20 mg total) 3 or 4 times a day for 3 to 8 weeks or until the mother's milk supply is adequate.[43] There is no need to slowly increase or decrease domperidone.

Encourage the mother to drink non-caffeinated fluids, rest, and eat well. Mothers should drink fluids when thirsty to replace fluid lost through breastfeeding; excess fluid intake does not increase milk volume. Milk composition and volume are little influenced by diet except in conditions of severe deprivation. Make mothers comfortable and decrease anxiety as much as possible. If these measures are unsuccessful in achieving a sufficient milk supply, the milk may be supplemented with formula or animal milks.

Feeding Options for HIV-Exposed Newborns

Newborns of mothers who are HIV positive have a high risk of dying of illness such as diarrhea, especially if feeding options other than breast milk are not "acceptable, feasible, affordable, sustainable and safe" (AFASS).[26,44] Because of the increased risk of dying of infection associated with replacement feedings in the developing world, breastfeeding is often the best option for many of these mothers. HIV-positive mothers of newborns in low-resource settings should be given the option to exclusively breastfeed or use replacement feedings with formula or other milks. However, per WHO and UNICEF recommendations, if replacement feedings with formula are not AFASS, exclusive breastfeeding for 6 months is the only viable option.[45,46] This should always be discussed with the mother and her choice supported.

In the first 6 months of life, mixed feedings should be avoided because they are associated with the greatest risk of HIV transmission through human milk.[47,48] The mother should be counseled about the pros and cons of available feeding options so she can make the most informed choice for her baby's feeding. Cultural and social stigma can play a major role in determining which choice is appropriate for a mother. Whatever the mother's choice, she should be fully supported to make it as safe as possible for her baby. If the mother elects to breast-feed, duration of exclusive breastfeeding will vary depending on the mother's health, milk supply, and availability and adequacy of feeding alternatives. The baby should be transitioned any time alternate feeding is AFASS. Per WHO, Joint United Nations Programme on HIV/AIDS (UNAIDS), and UNICEF recommendations, if formula-feeding is still not AFASS at 6 months, complementary feeding along with breastfeeding should continue and the mother, baby, and situation should be frequently reevaluated.[49] Oral medications prescribed for any reason should still be given. As supported by the Kesho Bora study, the WHO now recommends providing antiretroviral prophylaxis (to mother or child) for the entire duration of breastfeeding.[50]

Current recommendations from the WHO on the use of antiretrovirals in mothers who are HIV positive and who do not meet criteria from treatment with antiretrovirals for themselves and who choose to breast-feed are as follows: option A consists of daily nevirapine to the newborn; option B consists of triple antiretroviral drugs provided to a pregnant woman starting from as early as 14 weeks' gestation, continuing until 1 week after all exposure to human milk has ended (Table 20-4).[51] In both options, the mother should receive antiretroviral therapy from 14 weeks' gestation through 1 week after delivery. If the mother chooses not to breastfeed, the baby should receive daily nevirapine or zidovudine (AZT) for 4 to 6 weeks after delivery. These recommendations are subject to change and should be verified on a regular basis with sources such as the WHO.

Commercially prepared infant formula, diluted correctly, should be used when AFASS. Other options, especially if option A and B are not possible, might include heat-treated[52] or boiled human milk from an HIV-positive mother or a homemade formula properly prepared and with correct micronutrient supplementation.[53] Commercial formulas are generally a safer option and preferred whenever possible over other homemade formulas, especially in infants younger than 6 months.

Feeding Methods and Transitioning to the Breast

Newborns weighing less than 1,200 to 1,500 g and those too weak or immature to effectively breastfeed should be given their mother's expressed milk via nasogastric tube. An alternative to nasogastric tube with gavage feedings would be a cup and spoon. However, if a cup and spoon are used, babies should be allowed to lap the milk up—the milk should not be poured down their throats. Before each feed the provider should ensure that the tube is still in the stomach and gastric residual

Table 20-4. Antiretroviral Prophylaxis Options Recommended for HIV-Infected Pregnant Women Who Do Not Need Treatment for Their Own Health

OPTION A: MATERNAL AZT	OPTION B: MATERNAL TRIPLE ARV PROPHYLAXIS
MOTHER • Antepartum AZT (from as early as 14 weeks' gestation) • Sd-NVP at onset of labor[a] • AZT + 3TC during labor and delivery[a] • AZT + 3TC for 7 days postpartum[a]	**MOTHER** Triple ARV from 14 weeks until 1 week after all exposure to breast milk has ended • AZT + 3TC + LPV/r • AZT + 3TC + ABC • AZT + 3TC + EFV • TDF + 3TC (or FTC) + EFV
INFANT *Breastfeeding* • Sd-NVP at birth plus daily NVP from birth until 1 week after all exposure to breast milk has ended *Non-breastfeeding* • Sd-NVP at birth plus AZT or NVP from birth until 4 to 6 weeks	**INFANT** *Breastfeeding* • AZT or NVP from birth until 4 to 6 weeks *Non-breastfeeding* • AZT or NVP from birth until 4 to 6 weeks

Abbreviations: ABC, abacavir; ARV, antiretroviral; AZT, zidovudine; EFV, efavirenz; FTC, emtricitabine; LPV/r, lopinavir/ritonavir; NVP, nevirapine; Sd-NVP, single-dose nevirapine; TDF, tenofovir disoproxil fumarate; 3TC, lamivudine.

[a]Sd-NVP and AZT+3TC can be omitted if mother receives > 4 weeks of AZT antepartum.

From World Health Organization. *Rapid Advice: Use of Antiviral Drugs for Treating Pregnant Women and Preventing HIV Infection in Infants.* 2010 rev ed. Geneva, Switzerland: World Health Organization; 2010

should be aspirated and measured. The appropriate feeding volume should be placed in a syringe and allowed to drip in by gravity. Because of the type of syringes available in some developing countries, feeds may need to be pushed slowly rather than dripped in. The tube should be flushed with 0.5 to 1 mL of sterile water after feedings. Healthy premature newborns between 1,250 and 1,500 g may be given the opportunity, if alert and interested, to "practice" breastfeeding at each feeding, recognizing that actual milk transfer is usually negligible and that growth will depend on receiving sufficient supplemental feeds with expressed milk. Some healthy newborns who are about 30 weeks' gestation and older can begin supplemental feeds with a cup.[54]

Babies who are neurologically intact and clinically stable may be offered feedings at the breast beginning at approximately 1,500 g. Most babies at this weight will also need to be supplemented with expressed milk. If the baby is not sucking well or is losing excessive weight, supplement with expressed milk via cup, spoon, or nasogastric tube. Initially begin supplementing with 25% of the newborn's required feeding volume and adjust to a supplemental volume that allows for a weight gain of 15 g/kg/day.

Newborns who weigh more than 1,800 g and are neurologically intact should begin feedings at the breast and be observed carefully for sucking adequacy and weight gain. If they fail to gain weight appropriately, they may need to be supplemented with expressed human milk using a cup or spoon as they learn to feed at the breast. Adequate weight gain is the best sign of adequate intake. Effectiveness of feeding in all methods and appropriateness of weight gain must be followed closely in these premature, low birth weight babies.

Holding the baby in skin-to-skin (STS) care has numerous benefits, including increasing maternal milk volume and duration of breastfeeding.[55,56]

Iron, Multivitamin Supplements, and Blood Transfusion Recommendations

When the premature newborn is about 2 to 4 weeks of age and is tolerating near or full feeds, she should begin on supplemental iron at approximately 3 mg/kg/day of elemental iron. Iron preparations from different manufacturers and in different countries vary, so the actual elemental iron content of the preparation needs to be verified and the iron dosed accordingly. Multivitamins, including vitamin D (400 IU/day), should also be started with iron supplementation in all premature newborns. Check dosing recommendations on the package; however, about a half dose is generally suggested for term newborns until their weight exceeds 2 kg.

Hematocrit should be monitored every 1 to 2 weeks in the growing premature baby. Term and preterm newborns all become anemic after birth, reaching a nadir at 4 to 6 weeks of life. Hematocrit may be as low as 25% or less in preterm newborns. Anemia is physiologic because of decreased erythropoietin and red cell production (not iron deficiency) and is usually well tolerated by most babies. Supplemental iron does not correct anemia but rather increases iron stores and prevents iron deficiency anemia at 4 to 6 months after neonatal iron stores are depleted by increased red cell production. Transfusion is not routinely recommended to correct anemia unless the baby is symptomatic with acute blood loss, respiratory distress, or otherwise unexplained apnea and bradycardia, persistent tachycardia, tachypnea, or poor feeding (Box 20-2).

Box 20-2. General Transfusion Guidelines

1. Transfuse if hematocrit is less than 35% in babies with severe cardiopulmonary disease.
2. Transfuse if less than 30% and
   - Mild to moderate cardiopulmonary disease
   - Significant apnea
   - Symptomatic anemia (weight gain less than 10 g/kg/day at full caloric intake and heart rate greater than 180 beats per minute for more than 24 hours)
   - Undergoing major surgery
3. Transfuse if hematocrit is less than 21%: asymptomatic associated with a low reticulocyte count.

Blood must be screened for at least HIV and hepatitis B, and if possible, hepatitis C.

From Gomella TL, Cunningham MD, Eyal FG, et al. Blood abnormalities. *Neonatology: Management, Procedures, On-Call Problems, Diseases, and Drugs.* 5th ed. New York, NY: McGraw-Hill; 2004: 332–353

Breastfeeding and Medications

Almost all maternal medications are compatible with breastfeeding. In general, all maternal antibiotics are compatible with breastfeeding. Very few medications (eg, antimetabolites, radioactive compounds, drugs of abuse) are absolutely contraindicated in breastfeeding. Mothers should not breastfeed while on chloramphenicol but can of course resume breastfeeding 24 hours after completing the drug.[41] Most other "contraindications" are relative. In almost all circumstances the benefits of breastfeeding in lower-income countries far outweigh any associated risks. Check reputable sources such as Hale *(Medications and Mothers' Milk)* or American Academy of Pediatrics (AAP) recommendations for information if a mother is taking medication.[41,57] *Physicians' Desk Reference* has very limited value in determining if a medication is compatible with breastfeeding.[58] If a medication is contraindicated but is only going to be needed for a limited time, have the mother express her milk while giving the baby formula and resume breastfeeding when the medication is stopped and metabolized. Formula-feedings may be indicated if the contraindicated drug will be needed long term.

Expressed human milk feeding is medically indicated in some mothers, such as those with untreated active tuberculosis (TB) or active herpes lesions on the breast.[59] For detailed recommendations on breastfeeding and infection, check a source such as the AAP *Red Book.* Some medical conditions resolve over time, and it may be possible for the mother to formula-feed while she expresses milk and then resume with breastfeeding.

Mastitis is generally not a contraindication to breastfeeding.

Some mothers choose to formula-feed even though they do not have a contraindication to breastfeeding. If the mother made an informed decision, she should be supported. Carefully explain the importance of cleaning feeding utensils well. Encourage cup feeding instead of bottle-feeding with nipples. Cups can be successfully used[20] and are safer and easier to clean than bottles, reducing the risk of bacterial contamination. The cup should be placed against the lower lip and milk should be lapped up from the cup—it should not be poured into the mouth.[20] Explain the need for clean water. Lastly, explain the importance of measuring formula carefully and not diluting it inappropriately to make it last longer. Inappropriate formula dilution, whether to save money or out of ignorance about proper dilution, is a common problem in developing countries.

■ THERMAL REGULATION

Keeping neonates warm, especially premature neonates, is essential to their survival. This task can be challenging, even in warm climates. The incidence of hypothermia is high in developing countries, where up to 85% of normal newborns are hypothermic (axillary temperature lower than 36.5°C) within the first 24 hours after birth because of excessive heat loss. Climate, seasonal changes, cultural and hospital practices, and place of delivery all influence this incidence.[60] Newborns lose body heat very quickly after birth from evaporation (because they are wet), conduction (from being placed on cold surfaces), convection (from being exposed to drafts), and radiation (from being placed in proximity to colder surfaces in the surrounding environment).[60-62] Newborn body temperature is maintained by insulation from subcutaneous fat, heat generation from motor and metabolic activity, and metabolism of brown fat. The premature newborn has decreased subcutaneous and brown fat, limited energy stores, and larger head-to-body surface area; thus, the premature newborn can become hypothermic quickly without an external heat source. Hypothermia is also associated with sepsis in term and preterm neonates, especially when the initial occurrence is after 24 hours of age.[60] Knowledge and practices by health care professionals in developing countries concerning thermal control are often inadequate but are potentially remediable with education.[63]

Hypothermia

Normothermia is critical to maintaining physiologic stability. Normal temperature for neonates is 36.5°C to 37.5°C rectally. Axillary temperatures may be 0.5°C to 1.0°C lower. World Health Organization guidelines define hypothermia as mild (36°C to 36.5°C), moderate (32°C to 35.9°C), and severe (lower than 32°C).[62]

Hyperthermia (above 37.5°C) is also dangerous and is associated with over-wrapping, an excessively high ambient temperature, dehydration, or infection. The hyperthermic baby may be tachypneic, tachycardic, flushed, sweaty, and very warm to the touch. Severe hyperthermia is life-threatening (above 42°C).[62]

Understanding the dangers of hypothermia and recognizing them promptly is vital to reducing this common, potentially life-threatening problem. Hypothermia is associated with multiple metabolic, cardiorespiratory, and neurologic derangements, including lethargy, poor feeding, poor weight gain, reduced motor activity, peripheral edema, cold skin, hypoglycemia, hypoxia, respiratory distress, apnea, bradycardia, acidosis, necrotizing enterocolitis, thrombocytopenia, coagulopathy, and death.[64–69] Although it may be beneficial to maintain a state of controlled hypothermia in some instances (eg, term newborns with hypoxic-ischemic encephalopathy[70,71]), hypothermia, especially when prolonged, is clearly harmful for a premature newborn.[72,73]

Presently, the only accurate way to detect hypothermia is with a thermometer. Touch is not a reliable way to identify mild to moderate hypothermia.[74] A premature or sick baby's temperature must be read with a thermometer at least once a day to identify hypothermia and intervene appropriately. Ideally, an incubated newborn's temperature should be measured at least every 4 to 6 hours.[62] The hypothermic neonate must be rewarmed and followed closely with frequent temperatures checks at least every 2 to 4 hours until normothermia is restored.[62]

Preventing Hypothermia

As highlighted in the WHO pamphlet, *Thermal Protection of the Newborn: A Practical Guide*,[62] preventing hypothermia is essential. Maintaining normothermia in a baby begins at birth; the delivery room must be kept warm and draft free. The newborn must be dried immediately on delivery, or wet wrappings should be removed as quickly as possible to rewrap in warm, dry cloth. Placing a hat (preferably wool) on the newborn will decrease heat loss from the head, which, being relatively large in the neonate, radiates a substantial amount of heat. Whenever possible, the naked baby should be placed in STS contact on the mother's chest immediately after birth. Skin-to-skin contact also facilitates early initiation of breastfeeding, which provides an energy source for heat production.

The first bath should not be given until at least 6 hours (up to 24 hours later) when the baby is stable and warm. The vernix has anti-infective properties and does not need to be removed.[69,75] The newborn can be cleaned quite thoroughly with clean, dry towels prior to 24 hours of age.

Hypothermia can further be avoided when the mother and her newborn are transported together in STS contact, versus transportation of mother and newborn separately or when the newborn is transferred elsewhere for care.[62] The mother and her newborn should be cared for in a warm room. Premature newborns should be kept in continuous STS care before and after discharge whenever possible (Figure 20-6).

Where STS care is not possible, additional options for keeping the newborn warm post-delivery include placing him in plastic wrap or plastic bags (which reduces evaporative heat loss[2,76]), on heated mattresses,[62] in homemade or commercial isolettes, or under overhead warmers.[62] Local technology determines what resources are available. Maintaining normothermia in premature newborns is usually impossible without an external heat source. The ambient temperature required to maintain normothermia varies according to birth weight, postnatal age, humidity, and whether the baby is dressed (Figure 20-7).

Figure 20-6. Skin-to-Skin Contact (Kangaroo Mother Care)

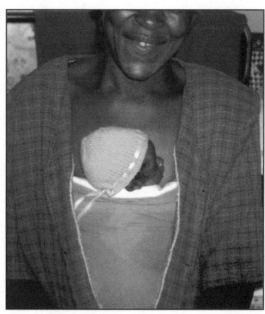

Courtesy of Tina Slusher, MD.

Skin-to-Skin Care

Skin-to-skin care, also known as kangaroo mother care, involves placing the naked newborn prone, head upright, on the mother's (or other caregiver's) chest in direct STS contact. When in direct STS contact, the mother's body heat will keep the baby warm. It was found that very low birth weight (VLBW) newborns maintained their temperature better in STS care than in conventional isolettes.[77] In Ethiopia, Worku and Kassie found that STS was associated with a much lower death rate than when conventional methods of care (usually including an artificial warming system) were used.[78] Place a hat on the newborn to prevent heat

Figure 20-7. Neutral Thermal Environment

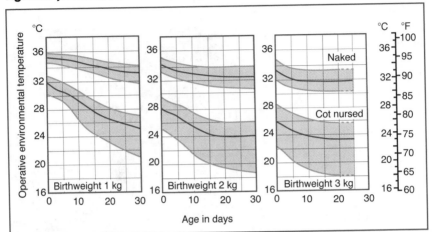

The usual ranges of environmental temperatures needed to provide warmth for newborns weighing 1 to 3 kg at birth in a draft-free uniform temperature surrounding at 50% relative humidity. Upper curves represent naked newborns. Lower curves represent swaddled, "cot-nursed" babies. Thick lines represent usual "optimal" temperature, and shaded areas are the angle within which to maintain normal temperature without increasing heat production or evaporated loss by more than 25%.

From Hey EN. The care of babies in incubators. In: Gairdner D, et al. *Recent Advances in Pediatrics.* 4th ed. London, UK: Churchill Livingstone; 1971

loss from the head and a wrapper or cloth around but not between the newborn and mother.

Continuous STS care is at least as effective as an isolette in preventing and treating hypothermia.[79] Every hour the baby is kept in STS contact raises her temperature about 1°C. The advantages of STS care as a method of keeping premature newborns warm include increased exclusive breastfeeding, decreased nosocomial infections, improved weight gain,[60,80] and decreased apnea.[80] It is especially useful in health care facilities without consistent power and while transporting premature newborns to a higher level of care.[62] It is effective and often the only available method for rewarming hypothermic newborns.

Homemade Incubators

Low-cost homemade incubators can be created from locally available materials and have the additional advantage of being easier to maintain and repair than commercial incubators. Ambient conditions inside the incubator should be continuously monitored; temperature can be controlled by adjusting the number of illuminated lightbulbs, and humidity is provided by placing a small bowl of water (changed and cleaned every 1 to 2 days) in the compartment containing the light-bulbs. Phototherapy can be installed on the top and sides of the incuba-tor. Remember to position the phototherapy unit as close as possible to the incubator for maximum phototherapy. Glass can be substituted if Plexiglas is unavailable, although it is not ideal because it can overheat or break; use Plexiglas whenever possible (figures 20-8, 20-9, and 20-10).

Figure 20-8. Blueprints for Isolette

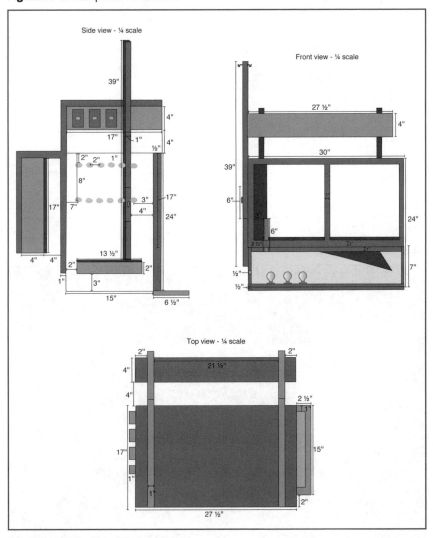

Adapted from Adrian Michael Slusher, BSME.

Figure 20-9. Components of a Homemade Isolette

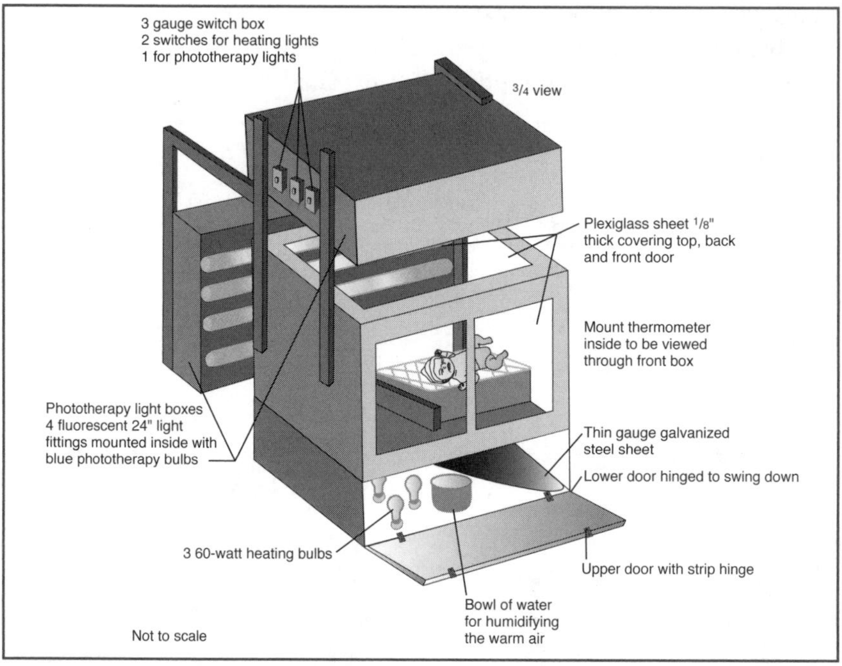

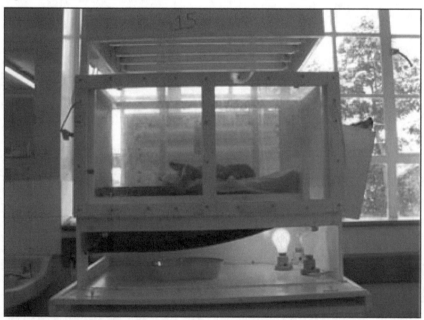

3 gauge switch box
2 switches for heating lights
1 for phototherapy lights

³/₄ view

Plexiglass sheet ¹/₈"
thick covering top, back
and front door

Mount thermometer
inside to be viewed
through front box

Phototherapy light boxes
4 fluorescent 24" light
fittings mounted inside with
blue phototherapy bulbs

Thin gauge galvanized
steel sheet

Lower door hinged to swing down

3 60-watt heating bulbs

Upper door with strip hinge

Not to scale

Bowl of water
for humidifying
the warm air

Adapted from Adrian Michael Slusher, BSME.

Figure 20-10. Homemade Isolette

With permission from Carol Spears, MD.

Commercial Incubators

Commercial incubators are expensive and often costly to repair, but they have the advantage of more accurate ambient temperature control and the ability to servo-control the baby's temperature.

Commercial Overhead Warmers

Commercial overhead warmers, while effective at warming newborns, are expensive and costly to repair, and increase evaporation of water through the newborn's skin. Their primary advantage is to allow direct visualization of immediate access to the baby. An overhead warmer can be especially valuable when performing a procedure on the newborn, or where the baby's condition requires frequent interventions (eg, positive-pressure ventilation for apnea). If a skin probe is not used, the newborn must be monitored frequently to ensure normothermia. Without a skin probe, the baby's temperature should be checked at least every 30 to 60 minutes.

Homemade Overhead Warmers

Homemade overhead warmers can be built using heat lamps, but the amount of heat generated is more difficult to control.

Other Methods

Hot water bottles and warming pads should not be used, if possible, because the newborn can be burned by these devices. However, they may be the only means available to provide warmth.[62] If used, the newborn should be well wrapped in blankets to protect him from accidental direct contact with the heat source and to help retain warmth gained. Monitor the newborn's temperature closely to avoid hyperthermia. Unwrap the newborn frequently and check carefully for erythema or burns of the skin.

Bundling the newborn loosely, allowing spaces for air between the layers of cloth, should be encouraged because this practice actually increases heat retention, while tight swaddling has the opposite effect and should be discouraged.[62] Keep the head covered, ideally with a wool hat.[60] Used alone, bundling and covering of the head will not be effective if the baby cannot generate enough heat to maintain or increase body temperature, as is often the case in premature, especially VLBW, newborns. An exogenous heat source, such as a warm incubator or STS care, is required to restore or maintain normothermia.

■ PREVENTIVE CARE

Cord Care

Cutting the cord with a clean, sharp instrument as well as clamping or tying it with a clean clamp or tie are the first steps in appropriate cord care.[81] Studies in the developed world suggest that no cord care is actually necessary and that the cord separates quicker without antiseptics.[82] However, whether these studies are applicable in the developing world, where umbilical sepsis is more common, is unknown.[81–83] If the cord is soiled, cleaning with soap and water is appropriate.[81] If mothers insist on putting something on the cord, it is better to choose a benign option, such as triple dye, instead of more dangerous practices, such as applying cow dung, plant material, or mentholated products. Alcohol is less optimal because it does not help dry the stump and actually delays cord separation.[81] The cord stump does not require covering with cloth and will dry up quicker if left exposed to the air.[81]

Delayed Cord Clamping

Several studies support delay in clamping the cord until it stops pulsating or about 1 minute. Although there is no consensus among health care practitioners about the practice of delayed cord clamping,[84] available data do support the practice of delayed cord clamping as a means of reducing anemia, increasing iron stores,[85,86] and reducing intraventricular hemorrhage (IVH).[86] The potential effect of reducing anemia and IVH is especially important in premature newborns. Decreasing baseline anemia could also significantly affect parts of lower-income countries where the incidence of malaria is high.[85] Delayed cord clamping or possibly milking is especially helpful in premature newborns. In one study, milking the cord in premature newborns had a similar result to delayed cord clamping.[87] In another study in premature newborns, milking the cord led to a decreased need for transfusions and respiratory and cardiac support.[88] In a small study by Grajeda et al, neither hyperviscosity from polycythemia nor hyperbilirubinemia were found to be problematic[89]; however, larger studies to look at both these potential problems need to be done.

Eye Prophylaxis

Several different regimens are beneficial in reducing the incidence of ophthalmia neonatorum, a preventable cause of blindness most often caused by gonococcal or chlamydial infection. Predominant organisms have changed over time; thus, prophylactic regimens have also changed.

Eyelids should be cleaned immediately after birth and followed by applying one of several potential antimicrobials within 1 hour of birth.[90] Potential antimicrobials include 1% silver nitrate, 1% tetracycline ointment, 2.5% povidone-iodine, or 0.5% erythromycin ointment.[90–92] Povidone-iodine can be locally prepared.[90,92] Silver nitrate application may cause chemical conjunctivitis[90] with swelling, erythema, and a purulent discharge, which may be confused with infectious conjunctivitis.

Vitamin K$_1$

Vitamin K deficiency is a preventable cause of bleeding in the neonate.[93] Vitamin K$_1$ should be given to neonates at birth to prevent hemorrhagic disease, which is not infrequent in developing countries where vitamin K prophylaxis is not routinely given. Term newborns should receive 1 mg intramuscular (IM) and preterm newborns should receive 0.5 mg IM.[64] Avoid vitamin K$_3$; it is associated with jaundice in neonates.[94,95]

Hepatitis B Vaccination

Hepatitis B is a leading cause of preventable cirrhosis and liver cancer. It is acquired primarily by vertical transmission during delivery and by child-to-child transmission.[96] The WHO Expanded Programme on Immunization schedule recommends hepatitis B vaccination at birth; at 6 and 14 weeks in countries where perinatal transmission of hepatitis B is high, such as Southeast Asia[96]; and at 6, 10, and 14 weeks in countries where perinatal transmission of hepatitis B is lower, such as countries in sub-Saharan Africa.[96] Some countries have developed other schedules that can be used per their country-specific guidelines; however, the first does at birth should be given as soon as possible after birth where the perinatal transmission is high. All IM injections, including vaccinations, should be given in the upper outer thigh, *not* the buttock, to avoid sciatic nerve damage.

HIV Prophylaxis

HIV prophylaxis is extremely important in babies born to mothers who are HIV infected. Regimens vary from a single dose of nevirapine to the mother at presentation of labor and to the neonate immediately after birth, to much more complicated treatment combinations. Studies are ongoing to determine which regimens are effective and affordable in resource-poor countries. Recommended regimens are in flux and vary from country to country. Providers should refer to the country-specific regimen or WHO[51] or similar source to determine what HIV prophylaxis to use and frequently check for updates (see "Feeding Options for HIV-Exposed Newborns" on page 446).

Vitamin A

Studies described in a review by Bhutta et al suggest some benefit from neonatal vitamin A supplementation.[97] In addition, a recent Cochrane review by Darlow and Graham did show a reduction in death and oxygen needs in VLBW newborns.[98] However, a recent study by Gogia and Sachdev failed to show a reduction in mortality with neonatal vitamin A supplementation in India.[99] Further studies are needed to determine whether vitamin A supplements should be routinely recommended to neonates in the developing world.

■ NEONATAL DERMATOLOGY

Skin care is an under-recognized opportunity to positively affect newborn health. The skin is an important source of potential infection, especially in preterm newborns. There have been multiple studies looking at how preventive skin care with barriers, oils, or lotions can reduce the incidence of nosocomial infections and prevent potential nutritional conditions such as essential fatty acid deficiency. In addition, skin care may serve as a means to augment maternal-newborn bonding and reduce hypothermia.[100] These interventions appear to be cost-effective, especially if the products are inexpensive and readily available. Such interventions may prevent the need for more expensive treatments, such as prolonged antibiotics.

Newborn Skin

Preterm newborn skin differs from term newborn skin—it is less mature and has less protective vernix. The immaturity causes the skin to be thinner and more prone to injury or tearing when compared with term newborn skin. In addition, all babies born in developing countries can be at risk for malnutrition, which affects skin health.

A study done by Darmstadt et al[101] using a hairless mouse found that transepithelial water loss was reduced when sunflower oil was used; this effect lasted for 5 hours. Conversely, water loss increased when other oils, such as olive, mustard seed, and soybean, were used.

Vernix caseosa, the cheesy substance found on newborn skin, can be viewed by some cultures as "dirty," and usual practice may prompt immediate removal. However, recent evidence found vernix to be an excellent skin cleanser[102] with intrinsic antimicrobial properties.[75,103] Currently, the WHO does not recommend removing vernix, instead recommending delaying a healthy newborn's first bath until at least 6 hours of age.[104]

Skin care regimens can also be harmful to newborns. In Asian countries, mustard oil, a potentially toxic substance, is often rubbed on babies' skin. If a skin regimen is adopted, it is imperative that the substance will not create harm to the newborn. Studies done in higher-income and lower-income countries using a petroleum-based ointment show mixed results; some studies showed a reduction in infection, while others, particularly those done in the United States, demonstrated a trend toward more coagulase-negative *Staphylococcus* infection.[97] However, this may be a reflection of the developed country's population bias with more access to central lines and, thus, a larger risk of infection.

Mentholated compounds found in many rubs and powders in lower-income countries are also harmful to newborns with glucose-6-phosphate dehydrogenase (G6PD) deficiency by causing hemolysis; they can be associated with severe neonatal jaundice and acute bilirubin encephalopathy.[105] Rubs containing these compounds should never be applied to babies in the neonatal period.

In addition to skin care with oils or emollients, studies have been done with antimicrobial solutions to help reduce floral colonization of newborns and, thus, potentially reduce infection. Preliminary evidence demonstrates that this temporarily reduces skin colonization and appears to be safe. A randomized trial in Nepal demonstrated that antimicrobial solutions reduced mortality in babies with birth weights less than 2,500 g, but this effect has not been described in term newborns.[106]

Rashes

Common Benign Rashes

The neonatal period is a common time for benign skin eruptions. The incidence of these very common rashes depends on the newborn's ethnic background; however, these rashes are common in newborns around the world. It is important that the clinician be able to differentiate these common rashes from more concerning rashes of diseases such as neonatal herpes.

Erythema Toxicum

Erythema toxicum is a common benign skin eruption that appears within the first few days of life and can occur intermittently within the first 1 or 2 weeks. It is characterized by white to yellow papules, measuring 1 to 2 mm, surrounded by erythema. It can be found on the entire body but is mainly seen on the head and trunk. The lesions are self-limited and treatment is not required. The hallmark characteristic of erythema toxicum is the intermittent migratory nature. If a lesion was unroofed and the fluid examined under a microscope, eosinophils would be found; however, this is not necessary for diagnosis. The etiology of this rash is not well understood.

Transient Pustular Melanosis

Transient pustular melanosis is often confused with erythema toxicum; however, it can be easily discerned with time. Pustules, often present at birth (not typically present at birth in erythema toxicum), appear in the first stage. These pustular lesions are present for approximately 3 days, in which they then rupture; central hyperpigmentation with a "collarette of scale" on the periphery follows. The scale resolves and a hyperpigmented macule remains, often for several months. Neutrophils predominate if unroofed in the pustular stage and examined under a microscope.

Milia

Milia are very common small, white papules typically found on a newborn's face. These papules are caused by inclusion cysts and will exfoliate spontaneously. Milia are also often confused with sebaceous gland hyperplasia, which is classically found on the nose.

Sebaceous Gland Hyperplasia

Sebaceous gland hyperplasia consists of yellow papules on the nasal follicles from the effect of maternal androgens. These papules will resolve without treatment, usually within the first few months of life.

Epstein Pearls

Epstein pearls are commonly seen as white papules on the roof of the mouth caused by trapped epithelial cells. These are similar to milia and only vary in placement. These are incidental findings of no clinical significance and do not require treatment.

Neonatal Acne

Neonatal acne may be pustular or comedonal. The etiology is related to the activity of maternal hormones manifesting on the newborn's skin, as well as from occlusive skin products. Two weeks is the typical age of onset, with most lesions occurring on the face and chest. The course is self-limited and no treatment is required. Because of the risk of infection and scarring, lesion manipulation is discouraged.

Miliaria

Miliaria is a benign rash commonly seen in warm climates or on tightly swaddled babies. This rash appears as dew-like papules on the skin and should resolve quickly once the baby is taken out of the warm environment.

Seborrheic Dermatitis

Seborrheic dermatitis is another benign rash of infancy that is characterized by a greasy scale on the scalp, posterior to the ears, and on the face. Like other lesions, treatment is not indicated. This condition will resolve over a period of months. If available, hydrocortisone may be applied to non-facial affected areas.

Pathologic Rashes

Herpes Simplex

Neonatal herpes simplex should be strongly considered with a newborn who has grouped vesicles on an erythematous base. Typically, the onset of vesicles is approximately at 1 week of life, although babies can be born with these lesions. Not only is the skin involved, but the mucous membranes (eg, eyes, mouth, rectum) can be also involved. This infection is more common when the mother is having a primary herpes outbreak during pregnancy; however, the majority of infected mothers do not have any history of herpes simplex virus infection. Herpes simplex virus infections typically have 3 presentations: localized to skin, eyes, and mouth; localized central nervous system (CNS) disease (may not have vesicles); or widely disseminated disease. Herpes simplex is treated with acyclovir. Systemic disease is often fatal despite treatment.

Petechiae

Disseminated petechial lesions typically imply congenital infections, such as the TORCH infections (toxoplasmosis, other [eg, syphilis], rubella, cytomegalovirus, herpes). Newborns may also have hepatosplenomegaly or jaundice. Alloimmune thrombocytopenia should also be considered. However, isolated petechial lesions are often due to birth trauma.

Staphylococcal Pustules

Staphylococcal pustules are common in neonates in the developing world. They are generally diagnosed clinically; however, a Gram stain can be done if there is doubt as to their etiology. The Gram stain will reveal gram-positive cocci. If the newborn is nontoxic, the pustules can be treated by cleaning with clean soapy water, which ruptures the pustules, and short-course antibiotics. An oral antibiotic, such as cloxacillin, is appropriate if the newborn is nontoxic, afebrile, eating well, and not in any way systemically sick. Methicillin-resistant *Staphylococcus aureus* should be treated with other antibiotics depending on sensitivities.

Syphilis

Congenitally acquired syphilis may be asymptomatic in the neonatal period. If symptomatic, newborns may have low birth weight, thrombocytopenia, petechiae, hepatosplenomegaly, or respiratory distress. Skin findings may include desquamation, especially of the hands and feet; bullous skin lesions; or copper-colored maculopapular lesions.[107] The maculopapular lesions are typically found on the hands, soles, and diaper area. Skin lesions and nasal discharge are extremely contagious. Practice universal precaution, including wearing gloves and washing hands well. Congenital syphilis is treated with IV or IM penicillin for 10 to 14 days.

■ BIRTH ASPHYXIA

Worldwide, intrapartum asphyxia is responsible for approximately 1.2 million neonatal deaths, 1.6 million stillbirths, 25% of all neonatal mortality and stillbirths, and 8% of all childhood deaths.[108–111] The contribution of asphyxia to neonatal death is similar to prematurity or infection. The incidence of asphyxia is much higher in lower-income countries. The true incidence of asphyxia is unknown because more than 50% of deliveries worldwide occur in the home, outside of the health care system. Because morbidity and mortality data are usually based on hospital or health care center deliveries, newborns who die shortly after a home birth are much less likely to be registered in the health system or have the reason for their death determined.[112]

Birth asphyxia is a clinical term denoting a series of antenatal and postnatal events that occur when there is significant tissue hypoxia and ischemia prior to delivery. In developed countries, the definition requires evidence of fetal distress, acidosis, and the need for resuscitation at birth and end-organ injury. A simpler definition often used in developing countries is "failure to breath at birth." This definition is less specific, as it includes all other causes of respiratory depression at birth, such as the effects of maternal medication or sepsis.

Asphyxia is associated with the depletion of energy supplies and increased production of cytotoxic free radicals resulting in cellular injury or death and multi-organ dysfunction. The initial fetal response to hypoxia and ischemia is to redistribute fetal blood flow from nonessential (ie, skin, kidneys, GI tract) to vital organs (ie, brain, heart, adrenals). Reflex heart rate decelerations (fetal distress), decreased respiratory activity, body movement, and muscle tone reflect ongoing hypoxia and ischemia. Fetal hypoxia results in rapid gasping, followed by primary apnea, and then by slow gasping followed by secondary apnea, hence the failure to breathe after delivery.

Whereas primary apnea responds quickly to resuscitation with oxygen and stimulation, secondary apnea requires more vigorous resuscitation with positive-pressure ventilation. The duration of intrapartum asphyxia can be roughly judged from birth to the first gasp and the onset of regular respiratory effort (Table 20-5). The reflex passage of meconium into amniotic fluid before birth can be another sign of fetal hypoxia. An Apgar score of 6 or less at 5 minutes is suggestive of some degree of birth asphyxia. Clinical problems caused by asphyxia evolve over several days and reflect the organs most often injured (ie, brain, kidneys, and lungs). These clinical problems include abnormal muscle tone, change in consciousness, seizures, oliguria or anuria, meconium aspiration, surfactant deficiency, pulmonary hemorrhage, persistent fetal circulation, hypotension, and necrotizing enterocolitis. Although most organ systems recover with time and appropriate medical support, brain injury is more likely to lead to permanent sequelae.

Preventing and Recognizing Intrapartum Hypoxia and Ischemia

Preventing and recognizing intrapartum hypoxia and ischemia is the key to reducing the incidence of birth asphyxia. Antepartum and intrapartum risk factors that predispose the fetus to birth asphyxia include a multitude of fetal or maternal problems that critically compromise placental function or blood flow to the fetus, thereby decreasing oxygen delivery (Table 20-6). Problems common to mothers in developing countries that contribute to an increased risk of asphyxia through an increased risk of prematurity and intrauterine growth restriction include

Table 20-5. Time to Onset of Respirations After Resuscitation and Duration of Intrauterine Asphyxia		
Duration of Asphyxia (min)	Time to First Gasp (min)	Time to Regular Breathing (min)
10	2	10
12	9	21
15	14	30

Adapted from Adamsons K Jr, Behrman R, Dawes GS, James LS, Koford C. Resuscitation by positive pressure ventilation and trishydroxymethylaminomethane of rhesus monkeys asphyxiated at birth. *J Pediatr.* 1964;65:807–818

Table 20-6. Factors Predisposing to Birth Asphyxia

MATERNAL	PLACENTAL/ UMBILICAL CORD	FETAL
Preeclampsia/ hypertension	Infarction	Preterm/post-term
Diabetes	Intravascular thrombosis	IUGR/SGA
Trauma	Chronic bleeding	Multiple gestation
Chorioamnionitis	Previa	Anemia/hemolytic disease
Severe anemia	Prolonged/obstructed labor	Congenital/chromosomal abnormalities
Severe malnutrition	Abruption	Birth trauma
Chronic hypoxemia	Nuchal cord/cord prolapse	Abnormal presentation
Chronic infection (eg, HIV, malaria, TB)	Uterine rupture	Hydrops fetalis

Abbreviations: HIV, human immunodeficiency virus; IUGR, intrauterine growth retardation; SGA, small for gestational age; TB, tuberculosis.

malnutrition, malaria, HIV, TB, syphilis, anemia, and living at a high altitude.[113-115] Recognizing fetal and maternal risk factors, maternal infection treatment, fetal distress intervention, urgent cesarean delivery, and maternal transfer to a higher level of care will all reduce the incidence of birth asphyxia.

When birth asphyxia occurs, it is essential to have the appropriate personnel and resources immediately available for resuscitation at delivery. Unfortunately, cost, transport difficulties, inadequate health center facilities, untrained staff, limited resources at health care facilities, and sociocultural barriers encourage delivery at home with unskilled birth attendants.[115] Even without advanced skills in resuscitation, vigorous drying and stimulating the apneic newborn are effective if the degree of depression is mild (ie, primary apnea). More severely depressed term newborns with secondary apnea usually respond to effective ventilation using a self-inflating bag-valve mask and room air. Although resuscitation with oxygen has long been the accepted standard of care, term newborns resuscitated with 100% oxygen actually have more delayed onset of respiratory effort, lower Apgar scores, and increased mortality.[116,117] Therefore, per American Academy of Pediatrics recommendations,[2] it is appropriate to begin initial resuscitation with room air and titrate oxygen in as needed, ideally using pulse oximetry.

Hypoxic-Ischemic Encephalopathy

Hypoxic-ischemic encephalopathy (HIE) is the neurologic consequence of hypoxic-ischemic damage to the brain associated with birth asphyxia. Hypoxic-ischemic encephalopathy is usually the proximate cause of death in asphyxiated newborns and, for surviving babies, a major cause of lifelong neurologic disability. Disability is an especially serious problem in most lower-income countries where resources for care or rehabilitation of neurodevelopmentally impaired children are minimal or not available. Consequently, the entire social, economic, and emotional burden of impaired survival falls completely on the individual child's family.

The CNS response to asphyxia depends on the severity and duration of hypoxia and ischemia as well as the gestational age of the fetus. Before 36 weeks the periventricular white matter is most susceptible to injury; after 36 weeks the deep gray matter of the basal ganglia and cortical gray matter are at greater risk. Abrupt, complete asphyxia (eg, placental abruption, cord prolapse) is more likely to injure the central gray matter (eg, thalamus) and brain stem. Prolonged, partial asphyxia (eg, uteroplacental insufficiency) is more likely to injure the watershed regions of the cerebral hemispheres.

Hypoxic-ischemic brain injury results in the release of excitatory neurotransmitters, secondary cytotoxic and vasogenic cerebral edema, and neuronal necrosis. These abnormalities are clinically reflected by an increased intracranial pressure manifest by increasing head circumference; a full, bulging fontanel; changes in levels of consciousness; increased or decreased muscle tone; changes in reflex activity; and seizures. Despite markedly increased intracranial pressure, newborns rarely develop brain stem herniation because they can decompress via their open fontanelles and suture. Classification systems can be used to grade the severity of HIE as mild, moderate, or severe (Table 20-7). Mild HIE is characterized by a hyperalert or hyperexcitable state with normal motor tone; moderate HIE is characterized by a mildly depressed state with hypotonia; and severe HIE is characterized by stupor with flaccidity. Moderate and severe HIE are associated with electroencephalogram (EEG) abnormalities and clinical seizures.

Maternal Fever and Neonatal Hyperthermia

Maternal fever and neonatal hyperthermia exacerbate asphyxial brain injury. Carefully controlled hypothermia is being used to treat post-asphyxial brain injury in developed countries with evidence of decreased mortality and improved neurodevelopmental outcome, particularly in

Table 20-7. Severity and Outcome of Hypoxic-Ischemic Encephalopathy in the Full-term Newborn

SEVERITY	LOC	SEIZURES	PRIMITIVE REFLEXES	BRAIN STEM DYSFUNCTION	ELEVATED ICP	DURATION	POOR OUTCOME[a] %
Mild	↑ irritability, hyperalertness	Rare, jitteriness	Exaggerated	Rare	Rare	<24 h	0
Moderate	Lethargy	Variable	Suppressed	Rare	Rare	>24 h (variable)	20–40
Severe	Stupor or coma	Common	Absent	Common	Variable	>5 d	100

Abbreviations: ICP, intracranial pressure; LOC, loss of consciousness.

[a]Poor outcome is defined as the presence of mental retardation, cerebral palsy, or seizures.

From McDonald MG, Mullett MD, Seshia MMK. *Avery's Neonatology Pathophysiology & Management of the Newborn.* 6th ed. Phildelphia, PA: Lippincott Williams & Wilkins; 2005:1388

newborns with moderate HIE.[118] Models using this treatment in developing countries are being explored.[119] Mild hypothermia (35.0°C to 36.5°C) may be beneficial. Certainly, overheating and hyperthermia should be avoided. Basic neuroprotective care includes treating the underlying condition (eg, infection) whenever possible, maintaining physiologically normal levels of oxygen saturation (95% or higher), glucose, electrolytes, and maintaining an adequate blood volume and perfusion. Hypoglycemia should be avoided because it exacerbates brain injury.[120] Although cerebral edema is common, steroids are not indicated because there is no beneficial evidence in HIE. The use of dexamethasone in particular may worsen long-term outcome.[120]

Seizures

Asphyxia is the most common cause of neonatal seizures, which may be very difficult to control. Seizures usually occur within the first 48 hours after the hypoxic-ischemic insult, may be focal or generalized, and take many different, sometimes subtle, clinical forms, including tonic posturing, clonic and myoclonic movements, eye deviation, repetitive sucking, tongue thrusting, eye blinking, purposeless movements, or apnea. Post-asphyxial seizures, unlike tremors or jitteriness, cannot be suppressed by gentle restraint or limb flexion. Associated intracranial bleeding and trauma and metabolic abnormalities, such as hypoglycemia and hypocalcemia, can also precipitate seizures. Hypoxic-ischemic encephalopathy–induced seizures usually resolve within the first week as acute injury and the cerebral edema subside. Seizures are associated with worse long-term outcome. Clinical seizures should be treated aggressively—ongoing seizure activity appears to worsen brain injury. Phenobarbital is a very effective anticonvulsant and has the advantage of being inexpensive and widely available. The major risk at high doses is apnea. Other anticonvulsants, including phenytoin and fosphenytoin, and benzodiazepines, such as diazepam, can be considered for seizures persisting after giving phenobarbital. For dosing of phenobarbital and other anticonvulsants, see pages 500 and 501.

A newborn's neurologic status may be difficult to accurately assess until many days after phenobarbital is discontinued because the half-life of the drug is very long (2 to 5 days). Anticonvulsant medications for post-asphyxial seizures can usually be discontinued before discharge home.

Neurodevelopmental Sequelae

Neurodevelopmental sequelae of HIE include spastic cerebral palsy, mental retardation, seizures, microcephaly, and hearing deficit. Apgar score alone is a poor predictor of long-term outcome, although newborns whose Apgar scores are 3 or less for 20 minutes or more are unlikely to recover without disability. Neonates with low Apgar scores at 1 and 5 minutes, but without evidence of neonatal encephalopathy, usually develop normally. However, a large cohort study of term newborns reported that newborns who required resuscitation at birth but were asymptomatic thereafter did have an increased risk of lower IQ scores at 8 years of age.[121] Long-term outcome correlates with the time until onset of spontaneous respirations, as the magnitude of delay in breathing reflects the severity of the underlying brain injury. Prolonged apnea for more than 30 minutes after delivery in term newborns is associated with irreversible brain damage.[120]

Using the severity of HIE as a guide, newborns with mild HIE survive and generally recover fully. About 20% of survivors with moderate HIE develop mild to moderate long-term neurologic sequelae. Those without neurologic sequelae generally have IQ scores slightly lower than healthy newborns but are still within the normal range.[122] Almost all newborns with severe HIE die in the neonatal period without intensive care. Those who do survive have severe neurodevelopmental disability. Despite the advent of sophisticated neuroimaging, the neurologic examination at the time of discharge remains the best predictor of outcome. Neonates who have normal neurologic examination results by 5 to 7 days of age can be expected to develop normally.

■ HYPOGLYCEMIA

Incidence

The incidence of hypoglycemia in higher-income countries is estimated to be approximately 10%. The exact definition of hypoglycemia is controversial; however, it is defined as a plasma glucose below 40 to 45 mg/dL.[64] It is likely that the incidence of neonatal hypoglycemia is substantially greater in lower-income countries because of factors such as maternal malnutrition (secondary to poor nutritional intake or diseases such as malaria), fetal malnutrition, asphyxia, and cold stress. In Nepal, approximately 58% of uncomplicated deliveries had evidence of hypoglycemia when screened.[123] Independent risk factors associated with hypoglycemia included hypothermia, young maternal age, low birth weight, and sampling soon after birth. It is likely that the incidence of hypoglycemia is higher in sick or premature newborns. Small for gestational age newborns are more common in developing countries and are more likely to become hypoglycemic than their normally grown counterparts. Studies in India[124] found that 25% of SGA newborns became hypoglycemic, especially when feeding was delayed. Mothers who received dextrose-containing fluids during labor had an increased incidence of delivering a newborn with hypoglycemia. Babies fed early had less hypoglycemia.

Definition

Hypoglycemia is most likely to occur in the first few hours after birth. In the term, otherwise healthy neonate, the physiologic nadir of blood glucose typically occurs 2 to 3 hours after delivery. This normal process reflects the transition from dependence on maternal glucose delivery in the uterine environment to dependence on the newborn's own ability to mobilize glucose stores and stimulate glucose production. Blood glucose levels of 40 to 50 mg/dL (2.2 to 2.7 mmol/L) in the first few hours of life are normal. Levels below 35 mg/dL (approximately 2.0 mmol/L) are generally regarded as abnormally low.[125] Newborns with low glucose stores in utero (eg, SGA) or whose stores were depleted during the delivery process (eg, fetal distress, asphyxia) are especially prone to early hypoglycemia. The level or duration of hypoglycemia resulting in neurologic injury is not known; it is preferable to err on the side of caution with early treatment and close follow-up.

Screening and Prevention

Screening glucose measurements in otherwise healthy, asymptomatic term newborns (without risk factors for hypoglycemia) is not recommended, as it may capture the physiologic nadir and lead to unnecessary treatment and interfere with maternal-newborn bonding and breastfeeding. Early (within 30 minutes of birth) and frequent breastfeeding every 2 to 3 hours on demand is the most important intervention to maintain normal blood glucose levels in healthy newborns. However, many cultures delay breastfeeding and give nonnutritive teas and other liquids for 1 to 3 days after birth. Small for gestational age babies whose feeds are delayed are at an especially high risk for hypoglycemia.[124] Hypoglycemia can also be prevented by reducing cold stress (see "Hypothermia" on page 451).

Risk Factors and Signs and Symptoms

Risk factors for transient hypoglycemia are shown in Table 20-8. Newborns may or may not demonstrate nonspecific signs of hypoglycemia shown in Box 20-3. Screening at-risk or symptomatic newborns for hypoglycemia with test strips is generally not available in developing countries. Therefore, treatment is usually empiric, based on clinical setting and presentation.

Treatment

There are several options for treating suspected or documented hypoglycemia depending on the newborn and supplies available. Breastfeeding (preferred) or formula-feeding is the first step. Fat and

Table 20-8. Risk Factors for Transient Neonatal Hypoglycemia

MATERNAL	FETAL/NEONATAL
Diabetes mellitus	Hypothermia
Excessive intrapartum glucose delivery	Birth asphyxia
Maternal medications (eg, terbutaline, oral hypoglycemic agents)	Infection
	Prematurity
	Intrauterine growth restriction Small for gestational age
	Large for gestational age
	Polycythemia, hyperviscosity

Box 20-3. Clinical Signs Associated With Hypoglycemia[a]	
Abnormal cry	Irritability
Jitteriness/tremors	Hypotonia, limpness
Lethargy, stupor	Seizures
Apnea, cyanotic spells	Grunting, tachypnea
Poor feeding	Hypothermia
Tachycardia, sweating	Pallor

[a]Clinical signs should be alleviated with concomitant correction of plasma glucose levels.

protein from the enteral feed provide substrate for ongoing glucose production. Oral sugar water (D5W [5 g/100 mL] 10 mL/kg) may be used if breastfeeding or formula is not available but should not be used routinely. Frequent breastfeeding should be encouraged. If oral feeding is not feasible, cup or gavage feeding (orogastric or nasogastric tube) of expressed human milk or formula may be used. The feeding target for the newborn on the first day of life is approximately 40 to 60 mL/kg/day, which can be divided into small bolus feeds every 2 to 3 hours.

Immediate treatment is indicated if glucose is very low (ie, less than 25 mg/dL) or if the neonate is symptomatic. If IV glucose is available, give a small initial bolus of 200 mg/kg (2 mL/kg of D10W or 4 mL/kg of D5W) followed by a glucose infusion rate of 5 to 7 mg/kg/minute (approximately 80 to 100 mL/kg/day of D10W), which can be calculated using the following formula:

Glucose infusion rate (mg/kg/minute) = (% dextrose concentration × total mL/kg/day)/144

Dextrose is typically supplied as D50W, which must be diluted to make a concentration of D10W (ie, 2 mL of D50W added to 8 mL of sterile water or NSS). Hyperosmolar D25 or D50 should not be used in neonates.[126] Hyperosmolar glucose in neonates has increased potential for rebound hypoglycemia, risk of sclerosing vein, and potential risk of intracranial hemorrhage in premature newborns.[126]

As enteral feeds are established, persistent hypoglycemia should not be an issue unless there is an underlying metabolic problem such as hyperinsulinism, endocrine abnormality, or inborn errors of metabolism.

■ JAUNDICE

Neonatal jaundice is common, affecting more than 60% of term and almost all premature newborns. Generally, neonatal jaundice is benign and does not needs specific treatment other than observation and follow-up if it worsens. However, it may be associated with significant morbidity.[127–134] Although appropriate population-based studies to determine true incidence of severe jaundice, acute bilirubin encephalopathy, and kernicterus have not been done, these conditions are leading causes of neonatal morbidity and mortality in many nurseries in the developing world.[127–134] According to AAP recommendations, *acute bilirubin encephalopathy* is defined as the acute changes seen in the neonatal period secondary to severe jaundice, such as tone abnormalities, opisthotonus, and abnormal cry, while *kernicterus* is reserved for chronic sequelae seen beyond the neonatal period, such as choreoathetoid cerebral palsy, deafness, and dental enamel dysplasia.[131]

Diagnosis

Every newborn should be monitored for jaundice while in the hospital.[131] A definitive plan should be in place to appropriately assess and follow up with jaundiced infants.[131] A transcutaneous or serum bilirubin should be checked if the newborn is jaundiced in the first 24 hours of life, is more jaundiced than appears appropriate for her age, or the level of jaundice is difficult to ascertain.[131] Ideally every baby will have bilirubin checked before discharge from neonatal hospitalization.[135] A transcutaneous bilirubin (TCB) can be done first if that device is available.[131,135] If TCB is elevated, the newborn has any jaundice in the first 24 hours of life, or the newborn appears more than mildly to moderately jaundiced beyond the first 24 hours of life, and a TCB is not available, a total serum bilirubin (TSB) should be determined. The natural cephalocaudal progression of jaundice and tools, such as the Kramer scale (modified) (see Figure 20-11) and icterometer, has been used to try to quantify the degree of jaundice.[136–139]

All these measures would be helpful in community health centers. However, these tools are at best used as screening tools, as any clinical assessment of jaundice is fraught with inaccuracies, even among expert health care workers.[140] Whenever possible the visual assessment of more than mild to moderate jaundice should be followed by a TCB or TSB to determine if or what treatment is needed. A TCB or TSB is always indicated for any jaundice noted in the first day of life and for jaundice involving the newborn's palms or soles because levels are highest when jaundice reaches the palms or soles.[136] If possible, micromethods for

Figure 20-11. Kramer Scale (Modified)

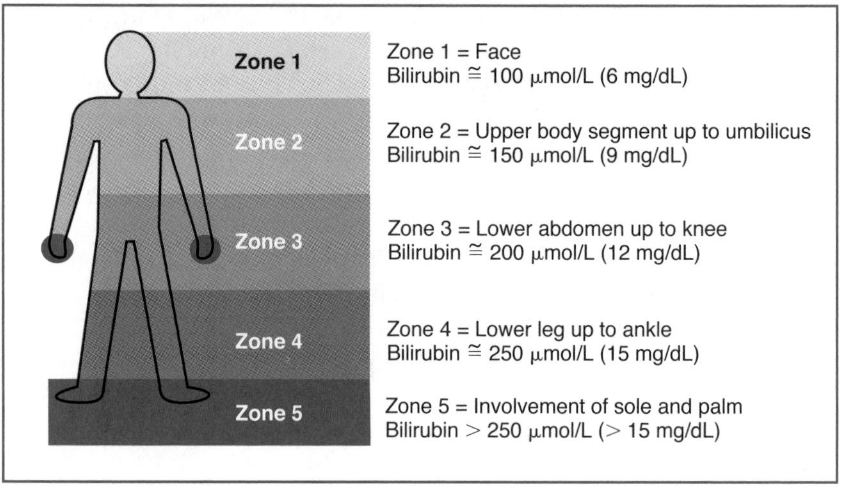

Zone 1 = Face
Bilirubin $\cong$ 100 μmol/L (6 mg/dL)

Zone 2 = Upper body segment up to umbilicus
Bilirubin $\cong$ 150 μmol/L (9 mg/dL)

Zone 3 = Lower abdomen up to knee
Bilirubin $\cong$ 200 μmol/L (12 mg/dL)

Zone 4 = Lower leg up to ankle
Bilirubin $\cong$ 250 μmol/L (15 mg/dL)

Zone 5 = Involvement of sole and palm
Bilirubin > 250 μmol/L (> 15 mg/dL)

Modified from Kramer LI. Advancement of dermal icterus in the jaundiced newborn. *Amer J Dis Child.* 1969;118(3):454–458, with permission from the American Medical Association.

determining serum bilirubin concentrations should be used. Standard laboratory equipment often requires large blood samples and this can be a problem when obtaining multiple samples in small neonates. The cost of the device and disposables, durability, and accuracy of the results in pigmented newborns must be considered when choosing a device for measuring TCBs in developing countries.

Any newborn presenting with severe neonatal jaundice should be evaluated for acute bilirubin encephalopathy, looking for the stages noted per Volpe[141] in Box 20-4. In addition, neonates with severe acute bilirubin encephalopathy will often display a characteristic *kernicteric facies* (Figure 20-12) even after the jaundice resolves (as seen in Figure 20-12). As noted by Slusher et al, the kernicteric facies consists of paresis of upward gaze often referred to as the setting sun sign; eyelid retraction; facial dystonia that makes the newborn appear "stunned, scared or anxious"; and sometimes dysconjugate gaze.[142]

Etiology

The etiology of moderate to severe jaundice should be determined. Whenever possible, the workup should include total and direct bilirubin, a CBC with peripheral smear looking for hemolysis and evidence of infection, maternal and newborn blood type, direct Coombs test, and G6PD deficiency screening in populations with significant rates of G6PD deficiency.[64] A sepsis evaluation should also be done if clinically

Box 20-4. Major Clinical Features of Acute Bilirubin Encephalopathy

INITIAL PHASE
Slight stupor (lethargic, sleepy)
Slight hypotonia, paucity of movement
Poor sucking, slightly high-pitched cry

INTERMEDIATE PHASE
Moderate stupor—irritability
Tone variable—usually increased, some
  with retrocollis-opisthotonos
Minimal feeding, high-pitched cry

ADVANCED PHASE
Deep stupor to coma
Tone usually increased, pronounced
  retrocollis-opisthotonos
No feeding, shrill cry

From Volpe JJ. Bilirubin and brain injury. In: *Neurology of the Newborn*. 4th ed. Philadelphia, PA: WB Saunders; 2008:635–637, with permission from Elsevier.

Figure 20-12. Kernicteric Facies

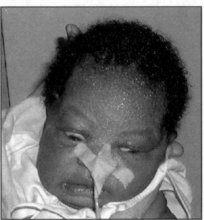

Courtesy of Tina Slusher, MD.

indicated.[64] The etiology of jaundice may be increased production of bilirubin (eg, hemolytic disease, polycythemia) or a decreased rate of excretion (eg, newborn of a diabetic mother, prematurity, poor feeding and intake).[64]

Etiology alone does not determine the need for treatment but can help guide decisions about the frequency of bilirubin checks, likelihood of the neonate progressing to severe jaundice with an increased risk of acute bilirubin encephalopathy, and risk to future siblings. Unless clinically indicated, direct bilirubin does not need to be repeated if it is not elevated on the initial bilirubin check.

Treatment

Treatment should be based on guidelines such as the one published by the AAP for newborns with a gestational age of 35 weeks or older where the age of the newborn and associated risk factors, such as ongoing hemolysis, sepsis, asphyxia, and prematurity, are taken into consideration.[131] Clear guidelines are not yet determined and there is more clinician variability in determining the level at which treatment is needed for newborns younger than 35 weeks' gestation (Table 20-9).

Newborns with significant jaundice should be treated with effective phototherapy. The most effective or intensive phototherapy available should be used. Intensive phototherapy per AAP guidelines involves

Table 20-9. Guidelines for the Use of Phototherapy and Exchange Transfusions in Low Birth Weight Neonates Based on Birth Weight

TOTAL BILIRUBIN LEVEL (MG/DL[a])

BIRTH WEIGHT (G)	PHOTOTHERAPY[b]	EXCHANGE TRANSFUSION[c]
≤1,500	5–8 (85–140)	13–16 (220–275)
1,500–1,999	8–12 (140–200)	16–18 (275–300)
2,000–2,499	11–14 (190–240)	18–20 (300–340)

Note that these guidelines reflect ranges used in neonatal intensive care units. They cannot take into account all possible situations. Lower bilirubin concentrations should be used for newborns who are sick (eg, sepsis, acidosis, hypoalbuminemia) or who have hemolytic disease.

[a]Consider initiating therapy at these levels. Range allows discretion based on clinical conditions or other circumstances. Note that bilirubin levels refer to total serum bilirubin concentrations. Direct or conjugated bilirubin levels should not be subtracted from the total.
[b]Used at these levels and in therapeutic doses, phototherapy should, with few exceptions, eliminate the need for exchange transfusions.
[c]Levels for exchange transfusion assume that bilirubin continues to rise or remains at these level despite intensive phototherapy.

From Maisels M. Jaundice. In: MacDonald M, Mullett M, Seshia MMK, eds. *Avery's Neonatology Pathophysiology & Management of the Newborn.* 6th ed. Philadelphia, PA: Lippincott, Williams & Wilkins; 2005

irradiance levels of at least 30 μW/cm^2 per nm in the visible blue-green (430 to 490 nm) range.[131] As noted by Jirapaet,[143] many things can and should be done to maximize phototherapy even when newer phototherapy devices are not available. Lights should be placed as close as possible to the newborn without overheating him (<15 cm above the baby [unless the baby overheats at this level] or as stated by the manufacture).[131,144] Bulbs in conventional phototherapy units should be changed at least every 2,000 hours. Neonatal nurseries should be encouraged to get irradiance meters and measure irradiance of their phototherapy units periodically.[144] If bulbs are covered with a plastic shield, it should be clean and clear.[143] These plastic shields filter out ultraviolet light, not the wavelengths of visible light necessary for phototherapy.[145]

A phototherapy unit can be constructed using blue or white florescent bulbs. A blueprint for building homemade phototherapy devices is included in Box 20-5 and figures 20-13 through 20-16. These devices are intended for use in centers that do not have access to commercial phototherapy devices. As with all commercial units, irradiance should be checked; if it is not possible to check irradiance, bulbs should be changed as noted previously. Double phototherapy can be used by making lights that can be placed over the top of, and beside or under, the newborn's bed. Efficacy can be increased by using a white sling (cloth) over the lights or aluminum foil on either side of the baby.[145]

Box 20-5. Local Construction of Phototherapy Devices

Phototherapy devices can be constructed with locally available resources. The size of the device and orientation of the lamps are determined by the space in which the baby is to be treated. Incubators (isolettes) and cradles (40 x 80 cm) need 7 to 8 tubes oriented parallel to their length. Cribs (80 x 140 cm, not shown) need 8 or more tubes (depending on the number of babies to be treated simultaneously) oriented parallel to the crib width (figures 20-13 through 20-16).

A. **Supplies and Tools**
1. Frame lumber. Obtain soft wood from a lumberyard or sawmill; 7 cm wide x 3 cm high and up to 5 m long depending on the device to be constructed.
2. Cut 2 *device support bars* (Figure 20-13) to the width of the crib or bassinet *plus* 2 x 5 cm extensions.
3. Cut 2 *spacing bars* (Figure 20-13) to length of the lamp fixture *plus* 2 cm.
4. Obtain, from a lamp shop, a sufficient number of single or dual tube fixtures with 1 or 2 blue light fluorescent lamps each (20 W, 240 V alternating current [AC]), usually 59 cm long x 2.5 or 3.5 cm diameter. Do *not* use tubes that are painted blue. White tubes are not as effective as blue tubes, but if no blue lamps are available, white light is better than no light. Daylight tubes are more effective than cool white.
5. Wood saw.
6. Tape measure.
7. Marking pen(cil).
8. Screwdriver (Philips or blade).
9. Screws, 1 to 2 cm long, preferably sheet metal with approximately 8 mm in diameter Philips head, for mounting lamp fixtures (2 each per fixture).
10. Screws or nails, 4 cm long, to function as support bar stops (4 each per device frame).
11. Steel square.
12. Hammer.
13. Nails, thin, 1.0 to 1.5 mm, 4 cm long, 12 each per frame.
14. Wood glue.
15. Power cord, at least 200 cm long, with 240 V AC plug (Figure 20-14).
16. Vinyl electrician tape.
17. Power cord lock or restraint clamps (a strip of triple-folded aluminum cut with scissors from a soft drink can and bent as shown in Figure 20-14) will do).

B. **Frame Construction**
1. Mark 5-cm sections from each side of the center corresponding to the total number of lamp fixtures to be used (1–6, 1–7, or 1–8 or more tubes, for isolettes, cradles, or cribs, respectively).
2. Turn the device supporting bars over onto a flat surface, and align the spacing bars with the outer markings of the first and seventh (Figure 20-14).
3. Apply glue to the joints and connect the bars with one nail at each end of the spacing bar.
4. After making sure, using a steel square, that all the joints are square, apply a second and third nail to each joint, far enough from the edge to make sure that the wood does not split. The frame should now be square and sturdy.
5. When the glue has hardened, paint the frame with white latex or oil-based paint, making sure that you can still see the section markings. *Do not use lead-based paint.*

Box 20-5. Local Construction of Phototherapy Devices, continued

C. **Lamp Fixture Mounting and Wiring**

1. Mount each of the lamp fixtures with one screw at each end, in the center of the sections marked 1 to 8 or fewer; make sure that on one of the support bars a 2-cm space is left for mounting electrical wire connections. For the same reason, make sure that the power leads of the fixture exit toward this lamp support bar. A hole may need to be punched with a drill or hammer and nail 3 cm from each end of the fixture. The fixtures should be mounted with 0.5-cm spaces between them to allow for air circulation. In the case the device is to be used with a crib, it may be desirable to mount more than 8 tubes on the support bars.

2. It is recommended that a qualified electrician connect each of the lamp fixtures to the power cord. If such a person is not available, enlist the services of a person who understands how to make safe and effective electrical connections.

3. Start the process by making sure the lighting fixtures and lamps you obtained are in working condition. Test each lamp and fixture combination separately by connecting it to a power cord, insulating the junction, and making sure the lamp lights when the cord is plugged into a wall power socket.

4. There are 2 ways to make the electrical connections.
   (a) Using a so-called buzz wire connection or cord (Figure 20-14) is neater-looking but a more complicated and less reliable method.
   (b) The simpler and more reliable method (not shown) is to take one lead from each of the fixtures (same color, if the leads have different colors) and one of the power-carrying wires (not the ground wire) of the power cord and twist them firmly together. Then, preferably, fix them securely together with a so-called wire nut, if available. Do the same with the remaining fixture leads and power cord wires. Insulate each wire connection carefully with electrician tape. If the power cord has a ground wire, run separate wires to each of the light fixture frames.

5. For safety reasons, it is important that the power cord as well as the fixture leads be trimmed so that the wiring can be closely secured to the wood frame with one or more wire clamps (Figure 20-14).

6. The phototherapy device is now ready for testing on an empty bassinet or crib for fit and proper functioning of all lamps. The device is intended to be suspended upside down from the top rails of the cradle (Figure 20-15) or bassinet (Figure 20-16) with the lamps hanging down. The distance between the lamps and the baby should be minimized for maximum efficacy of the light but should be no less than 20 cm. You may need to limit or increase the number of mattresses beneath the baby or increase or decrease the height of the mattress support frame of a crib.

7. For use with a crib, the device support bars should be fitted with stops at each of the 4 extensions through installation of a screw or nail (approximately 0.5 cm) outside the crib's side rail so that the device remains solidly in place between the side rails of the crib and will not slide inside the crib when bumped.

8. Plug the power cord into an operating power socket and make sure all lamps are lit.

D. **Troubleshooting**

1. A lamp may not light up because it is defective, it is improperly placed into its sockets, or the fixture may have failed wiring. Test the lamp by placing it in a working fixture. If the lamp works, return it to its original socket. If it still does not light, try twisting the lamp gently in its sockets to make sure that the lamp pins connect with the socket connectors. If this does not light the lamp, you may have a faulty fixture or faulty wiring. To determine what is going on at this point, you may need to acquire a voltmeter or replace the fixture with a working one.

With permission of Hendrik J. Vreman, PhD.

Figure 20-13. Assembling a Locally Made Phototherapy Device

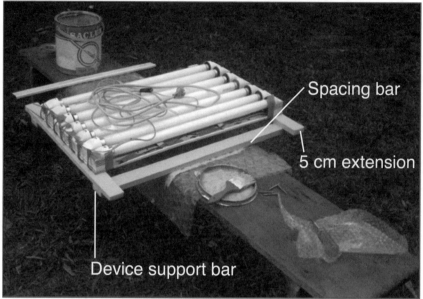

With permission of Hendrik J. Vreman, PhD.

Figure 20-14. Locally Made Phototherapy Device Inverted Over a Cradle to Display Fully Assembled Device

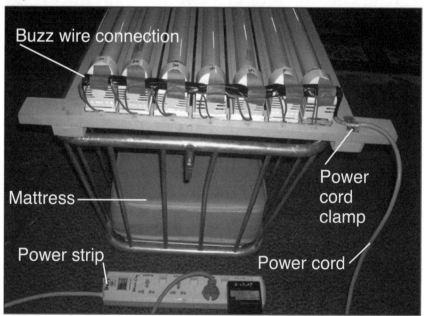

With permission of Hendrik J. Vreman, PhD.

Figure 20-15. Phototherapy Device in Use With a Cradle

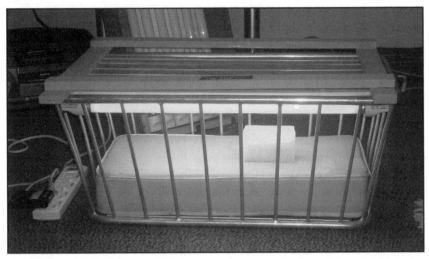

With permission of Hendrik J. Vreman, PhD.

Figure 20-16. Phototherapy Device Constructed for Use With a Bassinet (Note Extended Spacing Bars for Protection of Lamps)

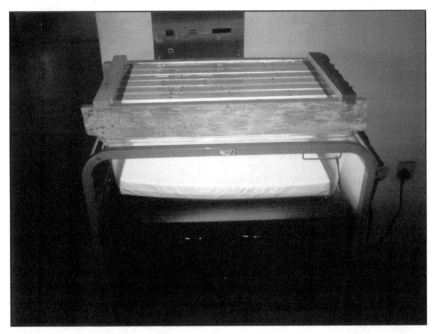

With permission of Hendrik J. Vreman, PhD.

White cloth is safer if there are any concerns about the electric wiring of the unit.

The newborn's eyes should be covered. Expose as much of the baby to the lights as possible, using only a small diaper, if needed.[131,144] Adequate hydration is important; however, routine supplementation is not advised in near-term and term newborns unless the breastfed baby is dehydrated.[131] Premature neonates on IVFs need an extra 0.5 to 1 mL/kg/hour while under phototherapy.[64]

Bilirubin should be checked at least every day in newborns receiving phototherapy. Bilirubin should be checked every 4 to 6 hours in newborns nearing exchange levels and less often (every 12 to 24 hours) in those whose bilirubin is stabilized or declining. Hematocrit or packed cell volume should be checked on a neonate admitted with jaundice and at least daily if the baby is hemolyzing or appears pale.

If a newborn's bilirubin rises to exchange blood transfusion (EBT) levels based on age and weight, or the newborn demonstrates signs of acute bilirubin encephalopathy, an exchange transfusion should be done as quickly as possible with fresh (less than 72 hours old) type O, Rh-specific, cross-matched blood.[64] A double volume exchange requires approximately 160 mL/kg plus blood for the tubing. Hold the exchange transfusion at 1 unit if the amount in the unit or blood bag is slightly less than that required for a double volume exchange; this decreases the potential increased infectious risk from using multiple units. Blood should be warmed before beginning the exchange. Because commercial blood warmers are rarely available in lower-income countries, other methods, such as water baths at 37°C, are most practical. Care should be taken not to overheat the blood because this can lead to hemolysis.

Most transfusions can be done through a single UVC. Sterile feeding tubes in size 5, 6, or 8 FR are generally used when umbilical catheters are not available. The exchange transfusion tubing should be set up so that blood is drawn from the newborn and discarded. Blood should then be drawn from the blood bag and infused into the newborn. The procedure should be repeated in a circular pattern without breaking the circuit. A 4-way stopcock is ideal but when not available, two 3-way stopcocks in tandem can be used. Ensure that all stopcocks and tubing are in the correct order before placing the catheter in the newborn; the cord is prepped and sterilely draped; and a tie is placed on the skin at the base of the cord, minimally tightened, and left in place to tighten further if needed to control bleeding. The cord is then cut, leaving about a 1-cm stump. The feeding tube or catheter is inserted until good blood flow is noted (usually 2 to 4 cm) and not advanced further; further insertion can lead to placement in the liver, which can lead to liver damage.

The EBT begins after the catheter is inserted. Use 5 to 10 mL aliquots in premature newborns and 15 to 20 mL aliquots in near-term and term newborns. Most EBTs are done over 90 minutes. Blood must be periodically agitated to prevent red cells from settling. Slowing the exchange leads to an increase in bilirubin withdrawal. Some clinicians give calcium gluconate 10% (1 mL)[64] after each 100 mL of blood exchanges via slow push to prevent bradycardia. Other clinicians suggest only giving calcium if the newborn develops signs or symptoms of hypocalcemia or serum calcium levels are low. However, because calcium levels are seldom checked in laboratories in lower-income countries, many clinicians favor giving calcium prophylactically. Check the bilirubin immediately before and after exchange transfusion and then every 4 to 6 hours depending on the bilirubin level. If hemolysis is ongoing, as it often is in newborns with G6PD deficiency or Rh incompatibility, a second or, rarely, third EBT may be needed.

Intravenous immunoglobulin (IVIG) (0.5–1 g/kg) decreases hemolysis and is indicated for treating hemolytic anemia, if available.[131] Older drugs, such as phenobarbital and phenobarbitone, are generally not beneficial in unconjugated (indirect) hyperbilirubinemia because it takes about 48 hours to induce liver enzymes that increase the rate of bilirubin excretion. However, one study suggested that phenobarbital use in low birth weight newborns may reduce the need for phototherapy and EBTs when given as prophylaxis.[146] Although maternal phenobarbital given prophylactically is controversial in hemolytic disease,[147] maternal phenobarbital administration can be considered in subsequent pregnancies of mothers whose prior babies had acute bilirubin encephalopathy, especially if appropriate and timely therapy for the newborn's jaundice is likely to be unavailable. Trevett et al recommends giving phenobarbital 30 mg per dose 3 times daily beginning at least 1 week before expected delivery.[148] It may be more practical to begin phenobarbital 2 to 3 weeks prior to the expected due date because ultrasounds are less common in lower-income countries and there is less accuracy in predicting due dates. Newer drug treatments may have a place in the future treatment of hyperbilirubinemia; some of the porphyrins currently being researched are especially promising.[131,149]

Figure 20-17 demonstrates the threshold for initiating phototherapy based on a newborn's age, serum bilirubin, and risk factors. Risk factors include jaundice in the first 24 hours, prematurity, previous sibling(s) with jaundice, cephalhematoma, bruising, breastfeeding, and racial groups known to have a high incidence of G6PD deficiency.[131]

Figure 20-17. Guidelines for Phototherapy in Newborns 35 Weeks' Gestation or Older

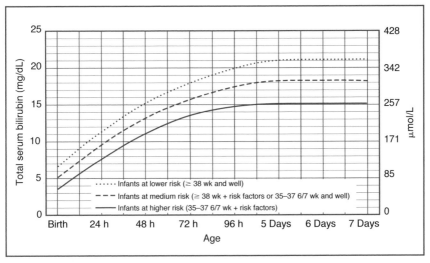

From American Academy of Pediatrics Subcommittee on Hyperbilirubinemia. Management of hyperbilirubinemia in the newborn infant 35 or more weeks of gestation. *Pediatrics.* 2004;114(1):297–316

Figure 20-18 demonstrates the threshold for performing an exchange transfusion based on a newborn's age, serum bilirubin, and risk factors.[139]

■ RESPIRATORY DISEASES

Respiratory distress is a common newborn problem worldwide. In India, a prospective study of more than 4,500 births was conducted to identify incidence of various causes of respiratory distress in a birth cohort. The overall incidence of respiratory distress was 6.7% in all births, with preterm births having the highest incidence at 30% of all premature births.[150]

The differential diagnosis of neonatal respiratory distress in term and preterm newborns is shown in Table 20-10. Although surfactant deficiency (respiratory distress syndrome [RDS]) is more common in the preterm newborn and transient tachypnea in the term newborn, there is considerable overlap in diagnoses. Other non-respiratory diagnoses to consider include neurologic injury, heart failure, choanal atresia, and tracheoesophageal fistula.

There are multiple signs of respiratory distress in the neonate, most commonly including tachypnea (respiratory rate greater than 60 BPM). Of note, it is important to count for a full 60 seconds, as newborns will normally vary their rate of breathing intermittently. Therefore, counting for less time may not accurately identify abnormalities. Other signs of

Figure 20-18. Guideline for Exchange Blood Transfusions in Newborns 35 Weeks' Gestation or Older

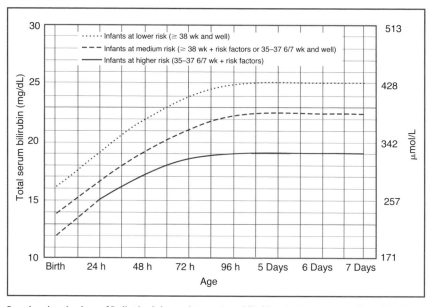

From American Academy of Pediatrics Subcommittee on Hyperbilirubinemia. Management of hyperbilirubinemia in the newborn infant 35 or more weeks of gestation. *Pediatrics.* 2004;114(1):297–316

Table 20-10. Differential Diagnosis of Neonatal Respiratory Distress in Preterm and Term Newborns

PRETERM	TERM
Respiratory distress syndrome Hyaline membrane disease Surfactant deficiency	Meconium aspiration (even more common in post-term newborns) or asphyxia
Infection (eg, sepsis, pneumonia, meningitis)	Infection (eg, sepsis, pneumonia, meningitis)
Transient tachypnea of the newborn	Congenital heart disease
Pneumothorax	Respiratory distress syndrome
Congenital diaphragmatic hernia	Pneumothorax
Persistent pulmonary hypertension	Congenital diaphragmatic hernia
Congenital heart disease	Persistent pulmonary hypertension

respiratory distress may include nasal flaring, grunting, tracheal tugging, retractions, and cyanosis. Grunting is an end-expiratory noise created when a newborn breathes against a partially closed glottis in an effort to create positive end-expiratory pressure (PEEP) to splint open airways. It may sound like the baby is saying, "EEEE."

Apnea, cessation of breathing effort for a minimum of 15 to 20 seconds, usually reflects brain stem immaturity in the preterm newborn but can also occur as a manifestation of respiratory distress or sepsis. It is important to distinguish prolonged apnea from normal respiratory patterns, such as periodic breathing. In the healthy term newborn, normal oxygen saturation in room air after 15 to 20 minutes of age is more than 95%. Cyanosis is not readily apparent to the eye until oxygen saturation is less than 70% due to characteristics of fetal hemoglobin. If possible, use an oximeter to determine the level of oxygen saturation.

Evaluating the Newborn With Respiratory Distress

Diagnosis and treatment of respiratory distress in the newborn are completely empirical in many lower-income countries with limited resources. The history and physical examination may be the only information available for diagnosis. The time course and response to treatment may be the only other information available to establish a diagnosis.

The evaluation should include

- *History.* Ask about maternal history, pregnancy complications, and delivery history, including prolonged labor, prolonged rupture of membranes, Apgar scores, presence of meconium, history of a difficult transition, or the need for resuscitation at birth.
- *Vitals.* Check heart and respiratory rates and temperature; include blood pressure and oxygen saturation if available.
- *Physical examination.* Look for increased work of breathing, including retractions, nasal flaring, grunting, tachypnea, and cyanosis.
- *Tests.*
  — Complete blood cell count with differential to look for anemia or evidence of infection. A blood culture or C-reactive protein (CRP) may be helpful if respiratory distress is not transient
  — Consider a chest radiograph if available. This is not routinely done for most newborns because of cost and availability. If the newborn is not responding to therapy as expected or has an atypical presentation, a chest radiograph should be obtained if possible.
  — Arterial or capillary blood gas, if available, may be indicated, especially if ventilator support is possible.
  — Oximeter, if available, to check or monitor oxygen saturation. Oximeters can also serve as cardiac monitors.

Specific Respiratory Conditions

Transient Tachypnea of the Newborn

Kumar and Bhat[150] noted that transient tachypnea of the newborn (TTN) was the most common cause of respiratory distress overall, occurring in approximately 43% of all newborns with respiratory distress. Although TTN is more common in term newborns, it occurs in preterm newborns as well. This generally benign condition, caused by delayed reabsorption of alveolar fluid, resolves without treatment within the first 48 to 72 hours after birth. Transient tachypnea of the newborn is more likely to occur with a cesarean delivery, especially in the absence of labor; after precipitous vaginal delivery; in newborns of diabetic mothers; and in males.

The physical examination should reveal a tachypneic baby in respiratory distress, which is typically mild but can be moderate. Lungs may be clear or sound wet with crackles. Chest radiograph, if available, may confirm but is not required for diagnosis. Typical chest radiograph patterns may include a starburst caused by increased vascular markings, fluid in the fissure, hyperinflation, and an overall wet appearance to the lungs.

Treatment of TTN is largely supportive; there is no known treatment to hasten the reabsorption of fluid into the lungs. Oxygen should be provided if saturation is less than 90%. Typically, patients with uncomplicated TTN will not require more than 40% oxygen.

Apnea of Prematurity

Apnea of prematurity, secondary to immature brain stem control of breathing, is very common in premature newborns, especially those who are younger than 34 weeks' gestation. These babies have intermittent periods of apnea that subsequently lead to bradycardia and desaturation when prolonged.

The definition of apnea of prematurity is cessation of airflow for a minimum of 20 seconds. These apneas are typically central in origin, although airway obstruction can lead to hypoxia and central apnea. Care must be taken to avoid obstructive apnea by carefully positioning the newborn's head and neck so the airway remains patent. Typically, apneic or bradycardic spells improve with tactile stimulation and usually resolve completely by term-adjusted age. Suspect infection as the cause of apnea when there is a sudden onset of apnea in a previously healthy premature newborn or if there is a marked increase in the severity or frequency of apnea in a preterm newborn with apnea of prematurity. Apnea in a term newborn is abnormal and the possibility of infection or neurologic injury should be investigated.

Theophylline, a methylxanthine that stimulates the respiratory drive, is used to treat apnea of prematurity. Caffeine, which is commercially available in the United States for this purpose, is expensive and may not be readily available. Dosing suggestions for theophylline and caffeine are included in Table 20-11. In addition to pharmacologic stimulant therapy, some newborns require intervention with a nasal cannula or nasal continuous positive airway pressure (CPAP), if available, to provide stimulation. Continuous positive airway pressure is indicated and often helpful in apnea of prematurity.

Respiratory Distress Syndrome

Respiratory distress syndrome, also referred to as hyaline membrane disease, occurs primarily in preterm newborns and is caused by surfactant deficiency. Surfactant reduces surface tension in the lungs. As the newborn takes his first breaths, surfactant is needed to help maintain alveolar expansion and lung volume during respiration. The incidence of RDS is inversely proportional to the gestational age. Risk factors for RDS include prematurity, maternal diabetes, asphyxia, and male gender.

On physical examination, newborns with RDS have tachypnea, increased work of breathing, nasal flaring, retractions, and expiratory grunting. There are no specific findings on physical examination that will confirm RDS; one must rely on history and risk factors. The onset of this condition is typically immediately after birth. The characteristic chest radiograph shows a diffuse ground glass opacity, air bronchograms, and hypoinflation.

A relatively simple and inexpensive gastric shake test (GST) can help identify newborns with surfactant deficiency. This qualitative test is done at the bedside by mixing an aliquot of early gastric aspirate with

Table 20-11. Drugs Used for Apnea of Prematurity

DRUG	THEOPHYLLINE	AMINOPHYLLINE[a]	CAFFEINE CITRATE
Loading Dose	Orally: 5 mg/kg	IV or orally: 5 to 6 mg/kg	IV or orally: 10 to 20 mg/kg
Maintenance Dose	Orally: 1 to 2 mg/kg/dose every 6 hours, up to 6 mg/kg/d	IV or orally: 1 to 2 mg/kg/dose every 6 to 8 h	IV or orally: 5 to 10 mg/kg once daily beginning 24° post-loading dose

Abbreviation: IV, intravenous.

[a] Typically, aminophylline is available in IV solution at a concentration of 250 mg in 10 mL. This can be diluted with sterile water or normal saline (1 mL aminophylline plus 9 mL sterile water), which will be a concentration of 2.5 mg/1 mL. This can be given orally or IV.

Adapted from Young TE, Magnum B. *Neofax 2010.* 23rd ed. New York, NY: Thomson Reuters; 2010

NSS and ethanol, then looking for the presence of bubbles. The GST can be done by aspirating a minimum of 0.5 mL of gastric fluid (before the newborn is 30 minutes old). Gastric fluid is then mixed with an equal volume of NSS for 10 seconds, followed by adding 1 mL of 95% ethanol. This mixture is then agitated for 10 seconds. The mixture rests for 15 minutes and is then examined for the presence of bubbles. The presence of bubbles is a positive test result indicating that surfactant is present.

In one small study by Chaudhari et al, the GST predicted the probability of RDS with reasonably good accuracy, with a positive predictive value of 100%.[151] The absence of bubbles (ie, a *negative* test) indicates the absence of surfactant and a high probability of developing RDS. There can be false negatives due to other substances in the gastric aspirate. On the other hand, a positive test does rule out RDS. The cost of surfactant and the attendant difficulties in storage (mainly refrigeration) and administration via intubation typically preclude the use of this medicine.

Two possibilities for giving surfactant in places where prolonged ventilation is not possible are administering surfactant via an ETT, which is then removed, or possibly administering surfactant via a laryngeal mask airway.[152] Newborns with RDS may benefit from the use of nasal CPAP (4 to 6 cm water) when possible. Oxygen should be administered by tent, nasal cannula, or nasal CPAP to maintain saturation between 88% and 94%. The natural history of RDS is clinical worsening over the first 48 to 72 hours, followed by gradual improvement, which is heralded by a spontaneous diuresis.

Persistent Pulmonary Hypertension of the Newborn

Persistent pulmonary hypertension is the pulmonary vasculature response to hypoxia, acidosis, asphyxia, and sepsis, as well as various causes of respiratory compromise, such as meconium aspiration, pneumonia, pneumothorax, and TTN. Sometimes an underlying cause cannot be found. Essentially this is persistence of the fetal pattern of circulation with continued right-to-left shunting through the patent ductus arteriosus (PDA) secondary to high pulmonary vascular resistance. These newborns present with tachypnea and cyanosis; they may not have increased work of breathing if there is no underlying lung disease. In developing countries, treatment is typically limited to oxygen administration, which is a pulmonary vasodilator via nasal cannula. If possible, saturation should be kept at 95% or more. Nasal CPAP is also helpful if there is underlying lung disease associated with persistent pulmonary hypertension. Magnesium sulfate infusion has also been used in developing countries with some success; however, hypotension is a risk and vasopressors or inotropic agents may be required.[153] A recent Cochrane review[154] did not recommend this treatment because of lack of evidence.

Meconium Aspiration

The incidence of meconium aspiration syndrome (MAS) in the developing world is likely substantially higher than in the developed world because of the much higher incidence of asphyxia and post-term delivery. A retrospective study in the West Indies found that 8% of admissions requiring ventilation were due to MAS.[155] In one study in India, 4.6% of all term neonates admitted to the neonatal intensive care unit had a diagnosis of meconium aspiration.[156] The newborn's history typically includes being term or postdates with fetal distress or difficult labor. Most meconium aspiration occurs before birth when the fetus reflexively gasps in response to intrapartum asphyxia and inhales amniotic fluid filled with meconium, which was passed in response to hypoxemia. If a neonate, born through meconium-stained fluid, is depressed at delivery and a skilled birth attendant is present, intubation may assist in suctioning out meconium from the proximal airway. Meconium aspiration syndrome often leads to pulmonary hypertension. These patients require support with face mask, hood, nasal cannula oxygen, or CPAP.

Pneumothorax

Pneumothorax may be spontaneous at birth, presumably because of the large negative intrathoracic pressures needed to initiate breathing; associated with underlying pulmonary disease (eg, RDS, pneumonia, TTN, MAS); or caused by overdistention of the lung by aggressive ventilation (including CPAP), especially in newborns with RDS or MAS. Symptoms include tachypnea, desaturation, and when very large, decreased breath sounds on the affected side. Small pneumothoraces resolve on their own. Symptomatic pneumothoraces can be aspirated by inserting a needle just over the rib at the second or third interspace at the midclavicular line. This may be done with a 20- or 22-gauge angiocatheter, a small-gauge needle, or a 23-gauge butterfly needle attached to a 3-way stopcock and syringe. The butterfly tubing can be placed in sterile water after aspirating air. This will serve as a water seal to see if the pneumothorax has resolved. Persistent bubbling indicates that the air leak is ongoing and insertion of a chest tube is probably necessary; however, chest tubes are often not available in low-resource settings.

Tracheoesophageal Fistula

Tracheoesophageal fistula (TEF) is another cause of respiratory distress in the neonate. In the most common type (85%),[64] the distal esophagus communicates with the posterior trachea. The esophagus ends blindly. It is often suspected in a newborn who is not handling his secretions well from birth. It can be diagnosed clinically by attempting to pass a nasogastric tube which fails to pass. An AP CXR demonstrates the nasogastric tube curled in the hypopharynx. The only treatment is surgical, which is often complicated or unavailable in low-resource settings.

Infection (Pneumonia/Sepsis)

Infection, such as pneumonia, sepsis, or meningitis, may present with respiratory distress. Typically, early onset pneumonia may be caused by gram-negative bacteria such as *Escherichia coli* or gram-positive bacteria such as group B *Streptococcus*. Later in infancy, the most common cause is gram-positive organisms, such as *Staphylococcus*. Other infections to consider are *Treponema pallidum*, HIV, *Chlamydia*, and *Listeria*. Pneumonia is impossible to distinguish clinically from noninfectious causes of respiratory distress; therefore, newborns with respiratory distress should be treated promptly with broad-spectrum antibiotics. Ampicillin and gentamicin are generally used as first-line agents for empiric treatment of neonatal infection. However, drug resistant organisms (eg, *E coli*, MRSA) are becoming more common. If at all possible, a blood culture should be obtained prior to beginning treatment and repeated if there is no clinical improvement within 48 hours to ensure the appropriate choice of antibiotic therapy.

Congenital Heart Disease

Congenital heart disease (CHD) may present with respiratory distress, cyanosis, or a heart murmur in the newborn period. The physical examination, chest radiograph, and electrocardiogram (ECG) can help determine the type of heart disease. Administering oxygen can help distinguish cyanotic heart disease from respiratory causes of cyanosis in the newborn. When 100% oxygen (hyperoxia test) is administered, the blue baby with a fixed right-to-left intracardiac shunt due to cyanotic CHD will remain cyanotic without any rise in oxygen saturation or improvement in color. Newborns with non-cyanotic heart disease or lung disease will usually have a rise in oxygen saturation and become pinker. Oxygen saturation greater than 95% to 100% generally rules out cyanotic CHD.

Echocardiography, which may be available in referral centers, is the most cost-effective way to diagnose CHD in low-resource settings. There is little treatment available in the developing world because of the complexity of the repairs required for most of these conditions. Depending on the condition, the life expectancy can be hours, weeks, months, or years.

Patent Ductus Arteriosus

Patent ductus arteriosus is a common problem in preterm newborns. A systolic murmur, hyperactive precordium, and bounding pulses (especially palmar or posterior tibial pulses) are typical signs. When a large left-to-right shunt occurs across the ductus, it may result in pulmonary over-circulation and congestion, increased oxygen requirements, tachypnea, increased work of breathing, and apnea; hepatomegaly may become evident. Treatment includes diuretics (furosemide, 1 mg/kg/dose every 12 to 24 hours), fluid restriction (less than or equal to 120 mL/kg/day), and administration of oxygen to maintain 90% to 95% saturation. If anemic, transfusion will help improve tissue oxygenation. If these measures are unsuccessful in closing the PDA, oral ibuprofen is a very effective treatment; this includes an initial dose of oral ibuprofen solution of 10 mg/kg nasogastric or orally followed by 5 mg/kg each at 24 and 48 hours after the initial dose. The regimen can be repeated once or twice if the PDA fails to close with the first 3-dose course.[157]

Congenital Diaphragmatic Hernia

Congenital diaphragmatic hernia should be considered in the term newborn with respiratory distress and a scaphoid abdomen, as the abdominal contents herniated into the chest. On examination there are diminished breath sounds on the side of the herniation and cardiac impulse is deviated to the right if, as is more often the case, the hernia is in the left chest. It is possible to make this diagnosis by prenatal ultrasound. Most newborns present at birth with respiratory distress and cyanosis. After birth, diagnosis can be confirmed with a lateral chest radiograph demonstrating bowel in the chest. Diaphragmatic hernias are very difficult to manage under the best of circumstances because of lung hypoplasia and severe pulmonary hypertension, often requiring inhaled nitric oxide, high-frequency ventilation, and extracorporeal membrane oxygenation in addition to surgical repair. The prognosis is extremely poor for these newborns in developing countries without access to sophisticated neonatal intensive care.

Oxygen

Oxygen should be considered a drug and used with caution. If available, a blender should always be used to minimize oxygen toxicity. Premature newborns can develop retinopathy of prematurity if administration of oxygen results in high oxygen levels in the blood. If saturation monitors are available, oxygen should be titrated to keep saturation between 88% to 95% in the absence of heart disease or other conditions that would require higher or lower oxygen saturation goals. Oxygen is most easily administered via nasal cannula. High oxygen concentrations can be administered to preterm newborns if the mouth is closed and the baby is not crying. As seen in Table 20-12, in contrast with the adult patient who gets about 24% oxygen from a nasal cannula running off 100% oxygen supply, a neonate can get around 66% from the same flow. Non–re-breather masks with a reservoir are needed if 100% oxygen is required for larger, term newborns. Regular face masks entrain room air and substantially reduce delivered oxygen concentration.

Continuous Positive Airway Pressure

Continuous positive airway pressure is indicated for mild to moderate respiratory distress and apnea of prematurity. It will not be effective for severe respiratory distress but can be lifesaving in less-severe disease. Continuous positive airway pressure has shown to decrease the need for mechanical ventilation in VLBW newborns with respiratory distress.[158] Continuous positive airway pressure can be delivered via nasal prongs, an ETT placed in the newborn's oropharynx, or an ETT placed in the trachea. Intubation is rarely done in low-resource settings because of the risk of the tube becoming dislodged or occluded.

Table 20-12. Nasal Cannula Conversion[a]				
	FIO$_2$			
FLOW RATE (L/MIN)	100%	80%	60%	40%
0.25	34%	31%	26%	22%
0.50	44%	37%	31%	24%
0.75	60%	42%	35%	25%
1.00	66%	49%	38%	27%

Abbreviation: FIO$_2$, fraction of inspired oxygen.

[a]Guideline only; numbers are not exact.

From Gomella TL, Cunningham MD, Eyal FG, et al. *Neonatology: Management, Procedures, On-Call Problems, Diseases, and Drugs.* New York, NY: McGraw-Hill; 2004. Reprinted with permission from The McGraw-Hill Companies.

Simple components needed for bubble CPAP include an oxygen source, an oxygen flowmeter, oxygen tubing, a container of sterile water, a humidifier device, and a device to deliver CPAP to the neonate. Most commonly, CPAP is administered through commercially available nasal prongs, which come in different sizes and should be snugly fitted in the newborn's nose with as little leaking as possible (Figure 20-19). If commercial prongs are not available, an ETT can be shortened to decrease the weight and likelihood of displacement and placed through the nose into the posterior oropharynx and the circuit attached to the ETT. Another option includes modifying a larger nasal cannula (Figure 20-20). An adult nasal cannula (for larger neonates) or pediatric nasal cannula (for small neonates) can be adapted for use if commercial prongs are not available (Figure 20-21).

Typically CPAP is started on 5 cm of water pressure, but this can be increased if the patient requires additional pressure. The range of pressure is generally between 5 and 8 cm of water. To administer the desired

Figure 20-19. Schematic of Bubble Continuous Positive Airway Pressure Using a Commercially Available Circuit

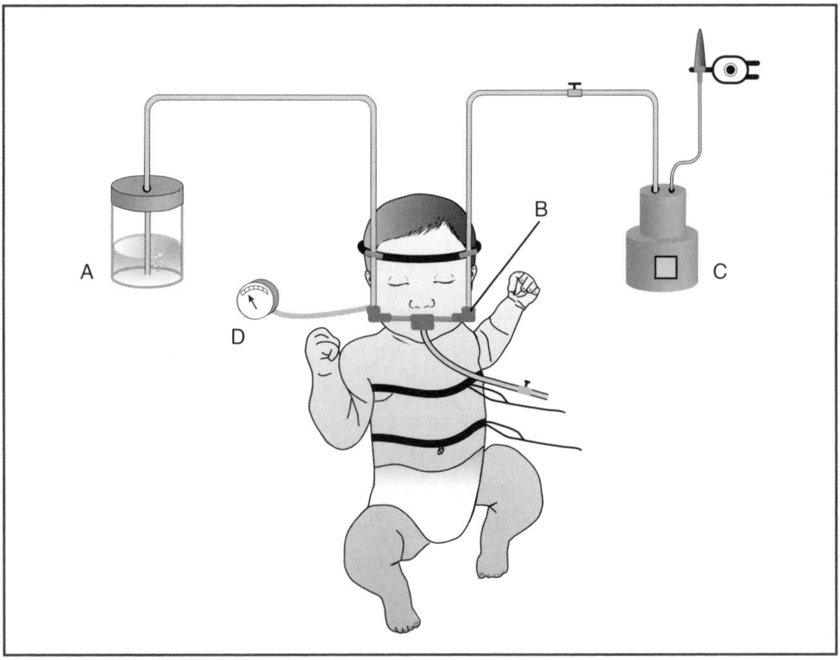

(A) Underwater bubble chamber; (B) Nasal CPAP prongs; (C) Heated humidifier attached to oxygen blender and flowmeter; (D) Manometer.

Modified from Liptsen E, Aghai ZH, Pyon KH, et al. Work of breathing during nasal continuous positive airway pressure in preterm infants: a comparison of bubble vs variable flow. *J Perinatol*. 2005;25:453–458, with permission from Nature Publishing Group.

Figure 20-20. Schematic of Bubble Continuous Positive Airway Pressure Using a Modified Nasal Cannula

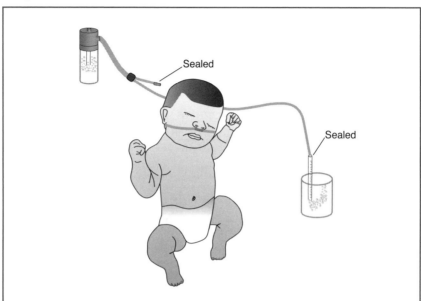

Adapted from Adrian Michael Slusher, BSME.

level of CPAP, the water container must be maintained securely in an upright position and the tube securely held in the desired position underwater. The level of CPAP can be titrated on the basis of oxygenation improvement, work of breathing improvement, or expansion of ribs on chest radiograph (goal of distending approximately 8 to 9 ribs) if available.

Continuous positive airway pressure can also be delivered with a pressure-limiting PEEP valve (Accu-Peep) that delivers a fixed (5 cm) amount of PEEP. This device is attached to the distal CPAP tubing and taped securely horizontally to the edge of the bassinet. While the amount of CPAP delivered cannot vary, 5 cm is high enough to be therapeutic in most circumstances and low enough to minimize the risk of air leak. Flow needs to be at 6 to 8 L or greater to use this device.

Continuous positive airway pressure can also be delivered by a high-flow nasal cannula with flows of 1 to 6 L per minute. However, the amount of CPAP delivered cannot be monitored and depends on variables baby size, cannula size, magnitude of air leak, and flow rate and is not consistent.[159] Depending on the circumstances, the CPAP actually delivered may be more or less than expected.

Figure 20-21. How to Make a Nasal Continuous Positive Airway Pressure Circuit From a Nasal Cannula

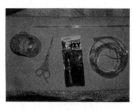

Equipment

A glass or bottle of water

Hard tube w/ numbers (ruler will work)

Nasal cannula

Scissors

Oxygen (preferably w/ humidifier)

Steps

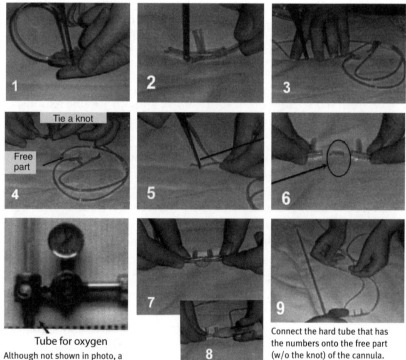

Tie a knot

Free part

Tube for oxygen

Although not shown in photo, a humidifier can be added here.

Connect the hard tube that has the numbers onto the free part (w/o the knot) of the cannula.

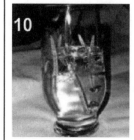

Insert the other side of the hard tube into the glass of water. If you put it under water up to 5 cm, there are 5 mm Hg of pressure for CPAP.

With permission from Janielle Nordell, MD; Ashely Baslam, MD; and Tina Slusher, MD.

Although CPAP is typically safe, too much distending pressure may cause pneumothorax, pneumomediastinum, or overdistension of the lung, which reduces venous return. Medical staff need to frequently monitor neonates on CPAP, as it is easy for the delivery device to dislodge, the apparatus to disconnect, or the prongs to become obstructed with secretions. In addition, the delivery device may cause trauma to the nares or oropharynx; patients must be examined frequently to ensure that there is no necrosis. Continuous positive airway pressure can also cause gaseous distension of the abdomen. Typically this is not harmful and an orogastric tube can be placed to decompress the abdomen. Gastric perforation has been described in synchronized noninvasive ventilation of the neonate but has not been described in those with CPAP only. One good source for training staff in the use of CPAP is a manual by Ammari et al.[160]

■ SEIZURES

Because neonatal seizures occur for treatable and untreatable reasons, determining the cause is of utmost importance. Seizure causes vary by the time of presentation. Brousseau and Sharieff developed a useful table that divides neonatal seizures into those most likely to occur on day 1 of life and those most likely to occur on the second day of life (Box 20-6). Generally, neonatal seizures can be classified as iatrogenic, or infectious; neurodevelopmental, which includes HIE; metabolic; traumatic or vascular; or toxicologic.[161]

Treatable causes of neonatal seizures include metabolic and electrolytic derangements, such as hypoglycemia, hypocalcemia or hypercalcemia, hyponatremia or hypernatremia, hypomagnesemia, and pyridoxine deficiency. Treating the underlying problem in these instances usually eliminates the seizure without the need for anticonvulsants. In addition, neonatal seizures secondary to herpes encephalitis, bacterial meningitis, and polycythemia require cause-specific treatment along with anticonvulsant therapy. Other causes of seizures, such as HIE, intracranial hemorrhage, cerebral infarction, congenital malformations of the brain, and developmental and non-herpetic TORCH infection, may require anticonvulsants, but care of these neonates is otherwise largely supportive.

Theophylline toxicity must be entertained as a cause in the neonate, especially if the possibility of incorrect dosing exists or if there are signs of theophylline toxicity, such as vomiting and tachycardia. Rarely, withdrawal from illicit drugs can cause seizures in the neonate. In these instances, although therapy is primarily supportive, the newborn may require anticonvulsant therapy until illicit drug levels fall.

Box 20-6. Causes of Seizures in Neonates

FIRST DAY OF LIFE

Anoxia/hypoxia
Drugs
Hypoglycemia/hyperglycemia
Infection
Intracranial hemorrhage
Pyridoxine deficiency
Trauma

SECOND DAY OF LIFE

Benign familial neonatal seizures
Congenital anomalies or developmental brain disorders
Drug withdrawal
Hyperphosphatemia
Hypertension
Hypocalcemia
Hypoglycemia
Hyponatremia/hypernatremia
Inborn errors of metabolism
Sepsis
Trauma

From Brousseau T, Sharieff GQ. Newborn emergencies: the first 30 days of life. *Pediatr Clin North Am.* 2006;53(1):69–84, with permission from Elsevier.

Clinical Manifestations

Diagnosis is usually based on close observation of the newborn and her movements. Although jitteriness and uncoordinated, random movements may be present in a normal neonate, the more premature the neonate, the more nonspecific the movements, which may suggest a diagnosis of seizures. The newborn brain is still in development; therefore, one does not see classic manifestations of seizures as in a more organized cortex. Seizures may present as

1. Tonic or clonic movements that cannot be interrupted by grasping the affected extremity
2. Stereotypic, slow rhythmic movements resembling bicycling or swimming, or posturing
3. Lateral or vertical deviation of the eyes
4. Autonomic instability, pupillary changes[64,162]

In contrast with older infants, focal deficits resulting from seizures in a neonate are not necessarily caused by focal lesions.

Diagnosis and Treatment

If a treatable cause of the seizure is identified, such as hypoglycemia, and the seizure resolves with that treatment, no further treatment is likely needed. The newborn will need to be observed closely for recurrence of the underlying cause (eg, hypoglycemia). Idiopathic seizures or seizures that persist despite specific treatment of underlying cause may require anticonvulsant therapy.

Hypocalcemia is best diagnosed using serum tests for ionized calcium. Because ionized calcium is not affected by the albumin level, it is preferable to total calcium. If serum calcium is not available but an ECG strip can be run immediately, probable hypocalcemia can be diagnosed by prolonged corrected QT (QTc) interval (see formula on page 501). If serum calcium or ECG strip are not available and hypocalcemia is clinically suspected, such as in post–exchange blood transfusion or SGA newborn, a trial of an IV calcium dose can be given. Ideally, hypocalcemic seizures are treated with IV calcium gluconate, 100 to 200 mg/kg/dose.[64] When administering calcium through a peripheral IV, it is crucial to verify that the IV is patent, preferably through a newly placed IV line. Intravenous calcium causes severe burns if it infiltrates. These burns may require skin grafting or an extended time to heal with marked scarring. Intravenous calcium should not be given through a scalp IV because these veins tend to be more fragile and prone to infiltration. The calcium dose should be diluted in 10 mL of sterile water or normal saline and given slowly over 10 minutes or longer with close observation for infiltration.

Rarely, severe hypercalcemia can cause seizures. Hypercalcemic seizures are treated with increasing fluids by about 25%, and the use of diuretics such as furosemide (1 mg/kg/dose every 12 hours) and phosphate, administered IV or enterically 30 to 40 mg/kg/day.[64]

Hypernatremia and hyponatremia can be associated with seizures. The diagnosis of sodium abnormalities requires confirmation by serum testing and the neonate may require anticonvulsants along with correction of electrolyte abnormalities. Hyponatremic seizures should be treated with 3% saline if available. To determine the proper amount of sodium, use the formula on page 435 (see "Fluids and Nutrition" on page 433 for prevention). Normal saline can be used when hypertonic saline is not available. Six mL/kg of 3% is approximately equal to 20 mL/kg of NSS. Normal saline contains 0.154 mEq/mL of sodium. Three-percent hypertonic saline contains 0.513 mEq/mL.

Hypernatremic seizures are often associated with dehydration and therefore should be treated with increased free water (water without added sodium, eg, D5W) and gradual reduction of serum sodium over 48 hours or more.[64]

Hypomagnesemia may be suspected clinically because testing serum levels for magnesium is largely unavailable in developing countries. Hypomagnesemia associated with seizures should be treated with magnesium sulfate (50 mg/kg/dose) given over at least 20 minutes IV[164] or 0.2 mEq/kg/dose every 6 hours[64] until symptoms resolve. Magnesium given orally is often associated with diarrhea and would not raise serum magnesium quickly enough to treat seizures.

Difficult to diagnose definitively in the developing world, presumptive herpes encephalitis in term and near-term newborns should be treated with IV acyclovir (20 mg/kg/dose) every 8 hours until herpes can be confirmed or ruled out.[162] Treat for at least 21 days if CNS infection is confirmed. If available, an EEG showing abnormalities in the temporal lobe may help support the diagnosis of herpetic encephalitis. Herpes encephalitis will require anticonvulsants in addition to acyclovir. These seizures may be difficult to control.

Bacterial meningitis requires high-dose antibiotic therapy in addition to anticonvulsant therapy. Seizures may occur at many different points in meningitis.

Seizures associated with polycythemia (central hematocrit greater than 65% if symptomatic) are treated with a partial exchange transfusion. Anticonvulsant therapy may be needed while waiting to perform a partial exchange transfusion. Normal saline is generally recommended for a partial exchange transfusion instead of blood products because of the lower infectious risks associated with its use. The procedure for doing a partial exchange for significant polycythemia is the same as described on page 481 for doing a double volume exchange; however, the volume of normal saline needed to reduce the hematocrit (HCT) appropriately is calculated using the following formula[64]:

$$\text{Volume exchanged} = \frac{(\text{weight [kg]} \times \text{blood volume*} \times [\text{patient's HCT} - \text{desired HCT}])}{\text{patient's HCT}}$$

*Blood volume = 80 mL/kg

Pyridoxine deficiency may be the cause in newborns who have difficult-to-control seizures. A trial 50 to 100 mg dose of pyridoxine, ideally with concurrent EEG monitoring, is reasonable in a neonate who continues to have seizures of undetermined etiology despite adequate anticonvulsant therapy. If the newborn is responsive to the test dose with resolution of seizures within 30 minutes, begin maintenance therapy with pyridoxine, 50 to 100 mg by mouth daily. If an EEG is not available, a trial of pyridoxine alone may clarify the underlying cause but should be reserved for a last resort in refractory seizures[162]; the newborn should be monitored because apnea and hypotension can occur.[162]

Seizures may be associated with an IVH. Intraventricular hemorrhage can be diagnosed with cranial ultrasonography. Other signs of clinical instability, such as hypotension, bulging fontanelle, posturing, and apnea, may point toward IVH, especially in the premature newborn. These seizures should be treated with anticonvulsants.

Anticonvulsants

(Note: Unless otherwise stated, all recommended loading doses for anticonvulsants are from the same source.[64])

First-line therapy for neonatal seizures without a specific treatment continues to be phenobarbital (also called phenobarbitone in many developing countries).[64,162,165] The loading dose for the neonate is 20 mg/kg IV followed by a maintenance dose of 5 mg/kg/day (1 or 2 doses per day depending on available dosing formulations). For many health care practitioners in low-resource settings, the only long-term option is 30-mg phenobarbital tablets, which can be divided in halves or quarters, limiting dosage options to 7.5 or 15 mg per day. In an actively seizing neonate, phenobarbital doses can be repeated in 5 mg/kg doses every 15 minutes up to a total dose of 40 mg/kg.[64,162]

If phenytoin or fosphenytoin are not available as a secondary treatment, sequential doses of phenobarbital can be tried. In one pediatric report, up to 80 mg/kg/day in sequential cumulative doses was used in children.[166] Cumulative doses above 40 mg/kg are associated with apnea requiring ventilatory support; availability of this support should be considered before giving excessively high doses. If levels are available, the therapeutic effect seems to plateau at 40 µg/mL.[167]

If seizures persist despite treating the cause and giving adequate phenobarbital, the next line of therapy is usually phenytoin[64,162] or fosphenytoin.[64] Both are given as a loading dose of 20 mg/kg IV and then in a maintenance dose of 5 to 8 mg/kg/day divided in 1 to 2 doses per day. In the neonate, phenytoin needs to be given IV because levels with oral dosing are totally unpredictable and variable without changes in dosage form or dosage. Phenytoin must be given slowly in non–glucose-containing fluids, such as NSS or sterile water (maximum of

1 mg/kg/minute) due to the risk of cardiac arrhythmia. Fosphenytoin may be given with glucose-containing fluids and is not as caustic to the vein as phenytoin; it is preferable over phenytoin in neonates, if available. Fosphenytoin should be refrigerated, which limits its use in some resource-poor settings.

Consider benzodiazepines if seizures still persist.[64,162] Their disadvantage is associated respiratory depression, which may be hard to manage in resource-poor settings without ventilator support. Diazepam is the most common available; it can be given in a dose of 0.3 to 0.75 mg/kg every 15 to 30 minutes up to a maximum of 2 to 5 mg.[163] Although rarely practical in resource-limited settings without ventilatory support, it can be used by continuous infusion in refractory seizures.

Oral carbamazepine[64] may be tried in seizures that fail to respond to other therapy. The starting dose is usually 5 mg/kg/day increased weekly, if needed, to a maximum of 20 mg/kg/day given in 3 to 4 divided doses with feedings.

Although rarely used, rectal paraldehyde has been used for seizures that are unresponsive to other therapies.[64,162] The dose is 0.3 mL/kg/dose every 4 to 6 hours if needed, mixed in mineral oil, and given rectally in a glass syringe. Opened containers should be discarded within 24 hours or sooner if they are discolored or smell like vinegar.

If seizures persist and are resistant to first-line and second-line therapies, refer the newborn, if possible, to a center at which a pediatric neurologist, special-care baby unit, EEG, cranial ultrasound, and computed tomography scans are available, or consult with a pediatric specialist or pediatric neurologist if available.

The recommended duration of seizure treatment depends on the cause, resources available, and recommendations of the neurologist or attending physician. However, most physicians recommend tapering the infant off anticonvulsants slowly somewhere between 3 and 6 months of age at the latest.[168] Observe closely for recurrent seizures.

Correction of Hyponatremia

(Desired sodium minus newborn's sodium) x weight (in kg) × 0.6. The desired sodium is usually around 130 mEq/L. Half the calculated correction is given over 12 to 24 hours.[64]

Measuring Corrected QT Interval

QTc = QT (seconds)/square root of the R-R interval (seconds).
0.44 seconds is the 97th percentile for a 3- to 4-day-old newborn.[163]

■ INFECTIONS

Neonatal sepsis is still one of the most common causes of morbidity and mortality in neonates in the developing world.[169] Untreated sepsis is rapidly fatal in the neonate. Sepsis can be very difficult to diagnose. Pending accurate cultures, sepsis must be suspected in almost any neonate who deviates from normal, with prompt evaluation and treatment. Signs of sepsis in the neonate are nonspecific and include almost any variation from normal in temperature, respiratory rate and effort, blood glucose level, feeding, activity, color, and mental status.[64,170] In a study by Weber et al looking at possible sepsis in more than 3,000 babies in lower-income countries, clinical signs alone could predict severe disease in neonates with a sensitivity of 87% and a specificity of 54%.[171] Investigators looked at signs of altered mental status and activity, feeding problems, respiratory distress, and signs of decreased perfusion. However, requiring more of these signs significantly lowered sensitivity.[171]

Although viral and fungal sepsis are important in the neonatal population, these are likely to be untreatable in most low-resource nurseries and therefore will not be covered in this chapter.

There are many risk factors for neonatal sepsis, including prematurity (less than 37 weeks); prolonged rupture of membranes; maternal fever or infection around the time of delivery; foul-smelling, purulent, or meconium-stained amniotic fluid; and the need for resuscitation at birth.[64,170] Early onset group B streptococcal infections in neonates are associated with more frequent maternal vaginal examinations during labor and maternal intrapartum fever.[172]

Per a recent review article by Zaidi et al, common bacterial causes of sepsis during the first week of life among home-born neonates in the developing world include gram-negative enteric organisms such as *Klebsiella* (25%) and *E coli* (15%), in addition to gram-positive organisms *Staphylococcus aureus* (14%) and group B *Streptococcus* (12%).[173] After the first week of life, 4 organisms caused most community-acquired neonatal infections, including *S aureus*, group B *Streptococcus*, *Streptococcus pneumonia*, and non-typhoidal *Salmonella*, each causing 12% to 14% of the disease.[171]

The best treatment of neonatal sepsis is always prevention. Clean deliveries, including good hand washing and clean instrumentation, are crucial in decreasing the incidence of neonatal sepsis. These principles should be incorporated into safe motherhood training throughout the world.[69,174,175] It is important to identify mothers at risk of delivering an infected newborn and to consider treatment with appropriate intrapartum antibiotics to the mother and postpartum antibiotics to the neonate.

Early recognition and treatment are important because septic neonates often die very quickly and have such nonspecific signs of infection. Equally important is minimizing the duration of treatment in newborns who are not infected. This can be especially challenging in situations in which diagnostics are very limited and cultures are unavailable, unreliable, or expensive.

Diagnosis

Reliable cultures are the gold standard for diagnosing sepsis.[170,176] Ideally, more than 1 blood culture should be obtained because a single blood culture may miss 10% to 15% of positive blood cultures.[170,176] This is generally not recommended because difficulty in obtaining multiple specimens from neonates may delay treatment. However, in much of the developing world, even a single blood culture is unavailable[177] or unreliable, necessitating reliance on other methods to diagnosis and treat presumed sepsis. Ancillary tests are especially helpful where there are no reliable cultures available. No single laboratory evaluation, including total leukocyte counts, differential leukocytes counts, absolute neutrophil count, ratio of immature to total neutrophil (I:T ratio), leukocyte morphology, platelet counts, or acute phase reactants such as CRP, can be relied on to confirm or exclude sepsis in the newborn. These tests are particularly insensitive indicators of infection during the first hours of early onset (within 48 hours of birth) neonatal sepsis. However, a total or absolute neutrophil count outside normal range for gestational age (high or low) will point toward or away from sepsis in the symptomatic neonate. Neutropenia with respiratory distress is particularly associated with early onset (less than 48 hours) sepsis from group B *Streptococcus*[178] as well as other bacterial pathogens such as pneumococci[179,180] and gram-negative organisms.[181] A CBC with indices (Table 20-13) is more helpful if followed over time. A combination of abnormalities is useful (Table 20-14 and Figure 20-22). Like most other screening tools, it is better at predicting the absence of sepsis versus the presence of sepsis. Per Rodwell et al, a score of 2 or less predicted the absence of sepsis 99% of the time.[182]

Another adjunct is a CRP. C-reactive protein is a marker of acute tissue inflammation and injury and plays a role in classic complement pathway activation and regulation of leukocyte function and phagocytosis. Many studies of neonatal sepsis have shown elevations of CRP at the time of neonatal symptom onset, with sensitivity between 35% and

Table 20-13. Neonatal Neutrophil Indices Reference Ranges (Per mm)

VARIABLE	BIRTH	12 H	24 H	48 H	72 H	>120 H
Absolute neutrophil count	1,800–5,400	7,800–14,400	7,200–12,600	4,200–9,000	1,800–7,000	1,800–5,400
Immature neutrophil count	<1,120	<1,440	<1,280	<800	<500	<500
Ratio	<0.16	<0.16	<0.13	<0.13	<0.13	<0.12

From Gomella TL, Cunningham MD, Eyal FG, et al. *Neonatology: Management, Procedures, On-Call Problems, Diseases, and Drugs.* New York, NY: McGraw-Hill; 2004

Table 20-14. Rodwell Hematologic Abnormality Scoring System

HEMATOLOGIC ABNORMALITY	SCORE
Immature to total neutrophil ratio ↑	1
Total PMN/neutrophil count ↑ or ↓	1
Immature to mature neutrophil count >0.3	1
Immature PMN/neutrophil count ↑ (if no mature PMNs seen, score 2 rather than 1 for abnormal total PMN count)	1
Total white blood count abnormal	1
Degenerative changes in neutrophils (>3 + vacuolization, toxic granulations, or Döhle bodies [graded 0–4+])	1
Platelet count ≤150,000/mm^3	1

Abbreviation: PMN, abnormal total neutrophil.

From Rodwell RL, Leslie AL, Tudehope DI. Early diagnosis of neonatal sepsis using a hematologic scoring system. *J Pediatr.* 1988;112:761–767, with permission from Elsevier.

94%.[183–186] Unfortunately, its elevation is not always indicative of bacterial infection, and CRP levels may be elevated in viral infections and noninfectious conditions of the newborn, including fetal distress, birth asphyxia, meconium aspiration, and intracranial hemorrhage.[184,185]

Because it is difficult to tell these conditions apart from serious bacterial infections, elevated CRP values are limited in their specificity and positive predictive value for infection. Thus, similar to absolute neutrophil count values, CRP determinations are most helpful in ruling out sepsis (negative predictive value) and should be followed over time whenever possible. Two CRPs less than 1 mg/dL obtained 24 hours apart and 8 to 48 hours after presentation indicate that bacterial infection is unlikely.[184,185]

Figure 20-22. Portion of Immature to Total Neutrophils in the First 60 Hours of Life

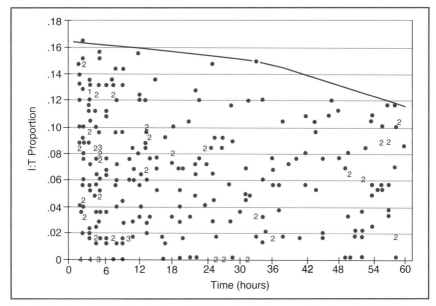

Adapted from Manroe BL, Weinberg AG, Rosenfeld CR, Browne R. The neonatal blood count in health and disease. I. Reference values for neutrophilic cells. *J Pediatr.* 1979;95(1):89–98, with permission from Elsevier.

A small study in Pakistan looked at 28 babies with culture-proven sepsis and found that combining CRP values with absolute neutrophil count led to 100% sensitivity and 86% specificity in culture-proven sepsis.[187] Combining a positive gastric acid cytology (GAC) with an elevated CRP led to 100% sensitivity and 92% specificity. A positive GAC is defined as greater than 5 polymorphonuclear cells (PMNs) per high-power field.[187] In an older study by Chandna et al,[188] the combination of CRP plus GAC was also considered the best combination among the tests they studied for differentiating between septic and non-septic babies. Studies by Yeung[189] and Vasan[190] also suggest that a GAC is helpful. The cost of CRP has come down to the point that it may be affordable in low-resource settings and easier to perform with a faster turnaround than blood cultures.

Using clinical presentation, clinical course, and a combination of tests available to determine the workup and duration of treatment is the most practical approach in situations in which blood cultures are unreliable or unavailable. Table 20-15 contains the uses and limitations of screening tests often done to screen for or rule out neonatal sepsis, including those mentioned previously. When no laboratory studies are available, the diagnosis of sepsis must be empiric, based only on the newborn's clinical

Table 20-15. Screening Tests for Septicemia: Uses and Limitations

TEST FINDING	FINDING SUPPORTING POSSIBLE INFECTION	COMMENT(S)
Total white blood cell count (cells/mm³)	<5000 or >20 000	<50% of those with finding have proved infection
Total neutrophil (polymorphonuclear: PMN count (cells/mm³)	<4000	Particularly useful in first hours of life
Total immature PMN count (cells/mm³)	>1100 (cord blood) >1500 (12 h) >600 (>60 h)	Relatively insensitive; finding unusual in uninfected infants
Ratio of immature PMNs to total PMNs	>0.2	Sensitivity 30–90%; good negative predictive value
Platelet count (cells/mm³)	<100 000	Insensitive, nonspecific, and late finding
C-reactive protein (mg/dL)	>1.0	Sensitivity 50%–90% at onset
Interleukin-6 (pg/mL)	>15	Sensitivity >80%; cutoff points vary; serial determinations may be required
Procalcitonin (ng/mL)	>0.5	Promising for early- and late-onset infection
Erythrocyte sedimentation rate (mm/h)	>5 (1st 24 h) >Infant's age in days +3 (through age 14 d) >20 (>2 wk of age)	Individual laboratories must establish normal values; normal value varies inversely with hematocrit
Fibronectin (g/mL)	<120–145	Sensitivity 30%–70%
Haptoglobin (mg/dL)	>10 (cord blood) >50 (after delivery)	Unreliable due to poor sensitivity
Granulocyte colony-stimulating factor (pg/mL)	>200	Good sensitivity but low specificity

From Long SS, Pickering LK, Prober CG. *Principles and Practice of Pediatric Infectious Diseases.* 3rd ed. Philadelphia, PA: WB Saunders; 2009, with permission from Elsevier.

presentation and course. Treatment should be directed against the most likely organisms depending on clinical setting and specific country. Initial treatment is broad spectrum and parenteral. In many low-resource settings the course of antibiotics may be completed using oral antibiotics. The efficacy of this approach is unknown but presents a significant risk for newborns in whom sepsis is likely.

The duration of treatment depends on the infection being treated and the newborn's response to treatment. In general, pneumonia is treated for 7 days, sepsis for 10 days, and meningitis for 14 to 21 days. It is equally important to discontinue treatment promptly in newborns who are not likely to be infected. This may be a difficult decision, especially if laboratory tests are not available; however, it is important to decrease development of resistant organisms, limit unnecessary drug toxicity, and contain costs.[170,174,177]

Meningitis should always be considered in a newborn with possible sepsis. Clinical examination alone cannot differentiate a neonate with bacteremia from one with bacteremia with meningitis. Up to 15% of all neonates with bacterial sepsis will have meningitis. A lumbar puncture is indicated in newborns with possible sepsis unless there is a contraindication. Blood cultures may be negative in newborns with meningitis.[64,191] Wiswell and colleagues found that up to 28% of newborns with meningitis had sterile blood cultures.[191] In a neonate, a normal cerebrospinal fluid (CSF) white blood cell count may be up to 32, normal protein may be up to 170 mg/dL, and glucose is half to two thirds of serum glucose.[64] Bacterial microorganisms are detected on a Gram stain of CSF in approximately 80% of newborns with group B streptococcal and gram-negative meningitis.[192] In contexts in which CSF cultures are not easily obtained, there may be still be value in obtaining CSF for evaluation of cell count and Gram stain examination.

Urinary tract infections should be considered in suspected late-onset sepsis. Urine cultures are not needed in early onset sepsis.[170] However, a sepsis workup after the first 48 hours should include a urine culture obtained by suprapubic tap or bladder catheterization whenever possible.[170,193]

Treatment Considerations and Options

Antibiotic doses and timing are based on gestational and postnatal age (Table 20-16).

The combination of ampicillin and gentamicin is still inexpensive and considered the appropriate first line to treat suspected neonatal sepsis. However, gentamicin does not penetrate well into the CSF and should not be used if meningitis is suspected. In addition, many recent studies, including studies from Tanzania, Nigeria, and India, show an alarming rate of resistance of gram-negative organisms to gentamicin (23%–68%) as well as high resistance rates to other commonly used antibiotics including cephalosporins.[194–196]

Table 20-16. Antibiotic Dosage for Neonates (mg/kg/d)

ANTIBIOTICS	ROUTE	< 2,000 G (0–7 D)	< 2,000 G (8–28 D)	> 2,000 G (0–7 D)	> 2,000 G (8–28 D)	> 28 D
Ampicillin	IV, IM	100 ÷ every 12 h	150 ÷ every 8 h	150 ÷ every 8 h	200 ÷ every 6 h	200 ÷ every 6 h
Cefotaxime	IV, IM	100 ÷ every 12 h	150 ÷ every 8 h	100 ÷ every 12 h	150 ÷ every 8 h	200 ÷ every 6 h
Ceftazidime	IV, IM	100 ÷ every 12 h	150 ÷ every 8 h	100 ÷ every 12 h	150 ÷ every 8 h	150 ÷ every 8 h
Ceftriaxone	IV, IM	50 every day	50 every day	50 every day	75 every day	100 every day
Erythromycin	IV, PO	20 ÷ every 12 h	30 ÷ every 8 h	20 ÷ every 12 h	40 ÷ every 8 h	40 ÷ every 6 h
Metronidazole	IV, PO	7.5 ÷ every 24 h	15 ÷ every 12 h	7.5 ÷ every 12 h	15 ÷ every 12 h	30 ÷ every 8 h
Penicillin G	IV	300,000 U ÷ every 12 h	450,000 U ÷ every 8 h	300,000 U ÷ every 8 h	450,000 U ÷ every 6 h	450,000 U ÷ every 6 h
Cloxacillin[a]	IV	50 mg ÷ every 12 h	75 mg ÷ every 8 h	75 ÷ every 8 h	150 ÷ every 6 h	150 ÷ every 6 h
Gentamicin	IV, IM	≤29 wk and ≤7 d 5 mg/kg/48 h; >34 wk 4 mg/kg every 24 h	≤29 wk and 8–28 d 4 mg/kg every 36 h	30–34 wk and ≤7 d 4.5 mg every 36 h; >34 wk 4 mg/kg every 24 h	≥30 and >8 d 4 mg/ kg every 24 h	≤29 wk and >28 d 4 mg/kg every 24 h
OR						
Gentamicin	IV, IM	≤26 wk 2.5 every 24 h	27–34 wk 2.5 every 18 h	35–42 wk 4 every 24 h	≥43 wk 4 every 24 h	

Abbreviations: IM, intramuscular; IV, intravenous.

[a] Recommendations for cloxacillin based on nafcillin/oxacillin dosing as recommended doses found in the literature vary around these doses. Cloxacillin IV is no longer available in the United States, and therefore doses are not in US drug books.

Modified from Bradley JS, Nelson JD. 2010–2011 Nelson's Pocket Book of Pediatric Antimicrobial Therapy. 18th ed. Elk Grove Village, IL: American Academy of Pediatrics; 2010

If staphylococcal infection is common in the nursery, cloxacillin can be substituted for ampicillin, sacrificing coverage for *Listeria,* which is rare.

If the newborn has meningitis, cefotaxime is more appropriate than gentamicin. If the newborn is not responding to ampicillin and gentamicin, or if sensitivities indicated resistance, substitute cefotaxime or other antibiotics to which the organism is sensitive.

Ceftriaxone should be avoided whenever possible in jaundiced neonates as the drug reduces the protein-binding sites available for bilirubin and may increase the risk of bilirubin toxicity. The level of jaundice at which protein binding is significantly affected is unknown. Caution should be exercised in using ceftriaxone in newborns receiving calcium supplementation because of death in a small number of neonates requiring calcium after receiving ceftriaxone.

Syphilis should be treated with IV penicillin. Remember to treat the mother and her partner as well.

Gonorrheal conjunctivitis should be treated with single-dose ceftriaxone. It is also helpful to irrigate the eyes frequently. Neonates with gonococcal ophthalmia should be evaluated for disseminated infection and hospitalized if sepsis, meningitis, or arthritis is present.

All IM injections, including antibiotics, should be given in the upper outer thigh, not the buttock, to avoid sciatic nerve damage.

Please note: Gentamicin is stated *per dose based on gestational age* in Table 20-16, while the dosage of other antibiotics is stated *per day based on weight* and needs to be divided to arrive at the individual dose.

Tetanus

Neonatal tetanus is still one of the leading causes of neonatal mortality worldwide, accounting for about 5% to 7% of neonatal deaths.[197] Tetanus is caused by the toxin produced by *Clostridium tetani.* The bacteria itself is noninvasive and nontoxic.[197]

The portal of entry is usually the umbilical stump, although circumcision, tattooing, and scarification can also be portals of entry. Susceptible babies are those whose cords were cut or dressed with an instrument or substance contaminated with *C tetani* and whose mothers were not adequately immunized before birth. Administering 2 to 3 tetanus immunizations to the mother before giving birth is effective in preventing neonatal tetanus.[96] Cutting or dressing the cord (or circumcising or tattooing) with a clean instrument can also eliminate neonatal tetanus.[96]

The incubation period is generally 3 to 31 days, with most cases occurring between 3 and 14 days after birth.[197] The shorter the incubation period, the worse the prognosis.[170]

Symptoms and Treatment

Tetanus symptoms are initially nonspecific, such as difficulty feeding, fever, and irritability, but rapidly progress to provoked and unprovoked tetanic spasms with trismus or sardonic smile and generalized stiffness.[170,197] The goals of treating tetanus include

1. Controlling spasms
2. Supporting respirations
3. Providing nutrition
4. Neutralizing toxin
5. Eradicating *C tetani*
6. Educating the mother, family, and community or village on the prevention of tetanus

Tetanus must be treated until presynaptic nerve endings are regenerated, which usually takes about 2 to 3 weeks. This prolonged hospitalization can be challenging to family resources that are already stretched.

Controlling spasms is usually done with a combination of drugs, including diazepam, phenobarbital, and chlorpromazine. In one study in Turkey, this drug combination led to the lowest mortality of their babies.[198] Diazepam is usually started at 2.5 mg every 4 hours per nasogastric tube and escalated to a much as 7.5 to 10 mg every 4 hours. Breakthrough spasms are treated with diazepam at doses of 2.5 mg IV as needed. Chlorpromazine is usually given in a dose of 6.25 mg (quarter of 25-mg tablet) every 4 hours and is alternated with diazepam. Phenobarbital is given at a dose of 5 mg/kg/day divided twice a day. Consider adding magnesium to this regimen, as it may decrease the need for massive doses of diazepam. Although not yet reported in neonates, case studies have found magnesium to be safe and useful in older children.[199,200] If magnesium is used, it can be given as a bolus dose of 25 to 50 mg/kg every 6 hours slowly over 30 minutes, or ideally as a drip of 25 mg/kg/hour titrated to have an effect as long as reflexes (ie, knee jerks) remain present. Magnesium levels should not be toxic if knee jerks remain present and, therefore, can be followed to assess for magnesium toxicity even in facilities where magnesium levels cannot be checked.

Supporting respirations is often necessary for survival. In hospitals where conventional ventilation is not an option, place the neonate on a continuous pulse oximeter with appropriate set pulse oximeter limits. Instruct nursing staff to check on the patient and provide positive-pressure ventilation when the patient is apneic. With close monitoring and quick response, mortality rates for neonatal tetanus can be lowered to below the present accepted mortality of 70% to 95%.[201]

Providing nutrition is essential for a good outcome secondary to the prolonged nature of this illness. In neonates this is usually achieved by nasogastric tube feeding with expressed human milk.

Recommended doses of tetanus immunoglobulin (TIG) and tetanus antitoxin (TAT) vary drastically from study to study and center to center. In a meta-analysis by Kabura et al,[202] the range of dosing for TIG was 250 to 40,000 units IM and for TAT was 250 to 10,000 units IM. Per that same meta-analysis, intrathecal of TIG or TAT was felt to be more beneficial than dosing them IM. The dosing range in this meta-analysis for intrathecal administration ranged from 50 to 1,500 units.[202]

Eradication of *C tetani* is done by thoroughly cleaning the wound and giving the newborn metronidazole or penicillin G. See Table 20-17 for antibiotic doses. Metronidazole is now considered by some to be the drug of choice,[170] but extensive studies comparing the 2 antibiotics have not been done. At least 1 study in patients older than 12 years compared benzathine penicillin, metronidazole, and benzyl penicillin and found equal efficacy among the drugs.[203]

Table 20-17. Antibiotics for Treatment of Neonatal Tetanus		
Metronidazole Oral or IV Doses	< 2,000 g 0–7 d	7.5 mg/kg/d divided every 24 h for 10–14 d
	< 2,000 g > 7 d	15 mg/kg/d divided every 12 h for 10–14 d
	> 2,000 g 0–7 d	7.5 mg/kg/d divided every 24 h for 10–14 d
	> 2,000 g > 7 d	15 mg/kg/d divided every 12 h for 10–14 d
Penicillin G IV	< 2,000 g 0–7 d	50,000 units/kg/d divided every 12 h for 10–14 d
	< 2,000 g > 7 d	75,000 units/kg/d divided every 8 h for 10–14 d
	> 2,000 g 0–7 d	50,000 units/kg/d divided every 8 h for 10–14 d
	> 2,000 g > 7 d	100,000 units/kg/d divided every 6 h for 10–14 d

Abbreviations: IV, intravenous.

Modified from Bradley JS, Nelson JD. *2010–2011 Nelson's Pocket Book of Pediatric Antimicrobial Therapy.* 18th ed. Elk Grove Village, IL: American Academy of Pediatrics; 2010

Prevention

Take this opportunity to educate the parent, extended family, and community about prevention of tetanus. Immunize as many as patients as possible while they are in the hospital. Stress the need to complete the series of immunizations. Five immunizations are considered a completed series for an adult. See Table 20-18 for the current WHO-recommended tetanus immunization, which provides immunity at least through the childbearing years. Although maternal immunization rates have been steadily increasing with concomitant decreases in neonatal tetanus, unfortunately the disease is still not eradicated (Figure 20-23). Most immunization programs in the developing world do not have booster programs beyond childbearing years and unfortunately most do not include men and boys. Suggest that men and boys also get immunized. Patients need to be immunized because tetanus does not provide lasting immunity and patients can have repeated tetanus if reexposed without immunizations.

■ EDUCATION

Educating others in newborn care is essential and effective in improving the health of mother and newborn.[204] The majority of women in the developing world go through pregnancy, delivery, and early neonatal care without seeing a physician or other trained health care practitioner; this alone contributes to a staggering number of deaths.[46] Structured training for advanced health care practitioners needs to begin in the training institutions.[5] Teaching the basics of maternal and newborn care can potentially have a significant effect on the health of mother and newborn. Teaching simple things such as clean delivery, including hand washing and clean instruments and supplies to clean and cut the cord;

Table 20-18. Tetanus Toxoid Schedule and Period of Protection for Women of Childbearing Age		
DOSE	**WHEN GIVEN**	**PERIOD OF PROTECTION**
TT1	At first contact with woman of childbearing age, or as early as possible in pregnancy	No protection
TT2	At least 4 weeks after TT1	3 years
TT3	At least 6 months after TT2	5 years
TT4	At least 1 year after TT3	10 years
TT5	At least 1 year after TT4	All childbearing years

From World Health Organization. Core information for the development of immunization policy. Geneva, Switzerland: World Health Organization; 2002: 130. http://www.who.int/immunization_delivery/policy_programmes/globalgoals/en/CorePolicy.pdf. Accessed June 23, 2011

Figure 20-23. Neonatal Tetanus Global Annual Reported Incidence and 2-Dose Tetanus Toxoid Coverage, 1980–2007

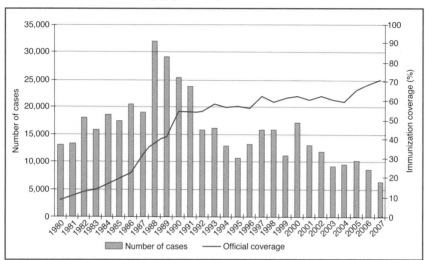

From World Health Organization. WHO vaccine-preventable diseases: monitoring system. 2010 global summary. http://whqlibdoc.who.int/hq/2010/WHO_IVB_2010_eng.pdf. Accessed June 29, 2011

basic neonatal resuscitation; thoroughly wiping the baby's eyes after delivery; preventive measures, such as vitamin A for the mother; keeping the newborn warm; exclusive breastfeeding, using colostrum; recognizing danger signs in the newborn; and referring appropriately is possible even in resource-poor settings.[96,205,206]

Trained health care workers must first be aware of the need for training all health care practitioners, including those at the community level. Recognizing the need to train community health workers, traditional birth attendants, and other health care practitioners at the village level is the second step to realizing this goal. Although having advanced health care professionals at every delivery is a worthy goal, it is simply not realistic for most women and babies in lower-income countries. Traditional birth attendants must be included in the training to maximally decrease birth asphyxia,[46] decrease infection, detect significant jaundice, and treat early or provide lifesaving care to the premature newborn.

It is important to ensure that basic supplies are available and to use locally available materials whenever possible.[7] When appropriate, items such as positive-pressure bags will need to be purchased. Providing a culturally appropriate approach to training with reinforcement and ongoing instruction during the learning period is essential and possible.[206] Finally, retraining every 1 to 2 years will most likely be necessary if results are to be sustainable.

■ KEY POINTS

Neonatal Resuscitation

- Neonatal resuscitation is one of most important tools in preventing neonatal death and asphyxia.
- Equipment and supplies needed for neonatal resuscitation in low-resource settings include 2 clean cloths, suction, and positive-pressure bag and mask.
- Initial steps of newborn resuscitation are warm, position, suction (if needed), dry, and stimulate.
- Positive-pressure ventilation should begin by 1 minute for any newborn who is not breathing or not breathing well.
- Oxygen is not essential in most newborn resuscitations and, in fact, may actually be harmful when not indicated.
- Epinephrine and volume are the only medications needed in the delivery room.
- Epinephrine should be diluted to 1:10,000 and given in a dose of 0.01 to 0.03 mg/kg (0.1 to 0.3 mL) IV if heart rate persists at less than 60 BPM after effective positive-pressure ventilation.
- Intubation may be indicated to provide more effective positive-pressure ventilation and to suction the trachea in depressed newborns with meconium.
- Resuscitation may be discontinued when the newborn's heart rate is above 100 BPM and the newborn is breathing well.
- Resuscitation may also generally be discontinued after 10 to 20 minutes of resuscitation without signs of life. Judgment must be used to determine when to stop resuscitation in other scenarios.

Fluids and Nutrition

- Fluid requirements in terms of content and amount change based on gestational age and weight of a neonate.
- When possible, IV fluids should be given with an IV pump or micro-drip set.
- Weight should be monitored, followed, and plotted regularly in all sick and premature newborns.
- Ideal nutrition is provided by human milk.
- Calories per kg to gain weight vary with each individual neonate, as well as gestational and chronologic age.
- Feeding in premature newborns should be systematically increased as tolerated to full feeds.

- Lacto-engineering with use of a creamatocrit and hindmilk often allows the use of high-calorie human milk without the risks of artificial feeds.
- Counseling, encouragement, breast pumps, and medications can all be used to increase milk production for a newborn who is not gaining weight or not gaining weight well.
- Breastfeeding only rarely needs to be discontinued for medications or other reasons.
- Iron and vitamin supplements are needed in most premature newborns.
- The newest recommendations addressing the use of human milk in babies of mothers who are HIV positive include the fact that unless human milk substitutes are "acceptable, feasible, affordable, sustainable and safe," human milk is best, but decisions about the type of feeding should always be made in accordance with the mother's desires.
- Two options to drastically decrease maternal-to-child transmission of HIV include daily nevirapine to the baby for the entire duration of breastfeeding or antiretroviral therapy to the mother for the entire time the baby is breastfeeding.
- Blood transfusions should only be given when needed, following hematocrit routinely.

Thermal Regulation
- Keeping premature neonates warm is essential to life.
- A warm, dry environment coupled with a hat helps prevent hypothermia.
- Skin-to-skin care helps prevent hypothermia as well as provides other benefits to the neonate.
- Low-cost incubators can be built.
- If available, functioning commercial isolettes and overhead warmers may be used if the newborn is monitored closely.

Preventive Care
- The umbilical cord should be cut with a clean instrument.
- Other cord care depends on circumstances, but dangerous practices such as applying cow dung should be avoided and a more benign substitute found.
- Delayed cord clamping raises hematocrit.
- Several options exist for eye prophylaxis, including tetracycline, erythromycin, sliver nitrate, and povidone iodine, which can be made locally and inexpensively.

- Vitamin K$_1$ can prevent hemorrhagic disease of the newborn.
- Hepatitis B vaccine should be incorporated into all newborn immunization programs.
- HIV prophylaxis is important and locally available protocols should be implemented.

Neonatal Dermatology

- Skin care is important and often overlooked.
- Delayed bathing is recommended for temperature control and because vernix is antibacterial and an excellent skin cleanser.
- Harmful practices such as applying mustard oil and mentholated compounds need to be avoided.
- Some oils or emollients may be beneficial.
- Several benign rashes are common in the neonate, including erythema toxicum, transient pustular melanosis, milia, sebaceous gland hyperplasia, Epstein pearls, neonatal acne, miliaria, and seborrheic dermatitis.
- Other rashes that are not benign and may require treatment are herpes simplex, petechiae, and syphilis.

Birth Asphyxia

- Birth asphyxia is a leading cause of neonatal morbidity and mortality worldwide.
- A simple definition of birth asphyxia is failure to breathe at birth.
- Preventing and recognizing intrapartum hypoxia is key to reducing the incidence of birth asphyxia.
- Having at least 1 person trained in positive-pressure ventilation is also key to reducing the incidence of birth asphyxia.
- Hypoxic-ischemic encephalopathy is the neurologic sequelae of birth asphyxia and the usual cause of death and disability.
- Severity of HIE can be graded and is predictive of outcome.
- Maternal fever and neonatal hyperthermia exacerbate asphyxia birth injury.
- Asphyxia is the most common cause of neonatal seizures.
- Spastic cerebral palsy, mental retardation, ongoing seizures, microcephaly, and hearing deficits are some of the neurodevelopmental sequelae of HIE.
- Anticonvulsants such as phenobarbital are often required for treating seizures related to HIE.

Hypoglycemia

- Hypoglycemia is common in the neonatal period, especially in developing countries.
- Newborns who are premature, SGA, and IDM are more likely to develop hypoglycemia.
- Screening asymptomatic term newborns for hypoglycemia is not recommended.
- Newborns with symptomatic hypoglycemia should be treated immediately with breastfeeding or formula-feeding. If breastfeeding or formula-feeding is not available, glucose water can be used orally.
- Very low glucose levels in symptomatic newborns should be treated with IV glucose infusion of D10W.
- Concentrated glucose solutions such as D25W or D50W should not be used in neonates.

Jaundice

- Neonatal jaundice is common, affecting the majority of newborns.
- Although most neonatal jaundice is benign, severe neonatal jaundice is a significant cause of morbidity and mortality.
- Bilirubin encephalopathy occurs acutely and chronically (kernicterus) and can lead to tone abnormalities, abnormal cry, and abnormal facies acutely, and choreoathetoid cerebral palsy, deafness, and dental enamel dysplasia chronically.
- Screening programs using transcutaneous bilirubin measurements or micromethod serum bilirubin levels should be instituted.
- An etiologic diagnosis should be established whenever possible.
- Common causes, such as hemolysis (G6PD deficiency, Rh incompatibility, ABO incompatibility) and infection, should be identified.
- Phototherapy should begin at or below the guidelines suggested by the AAP for newborns at least 35 weeks' gestational age.
- Other guidelines are recommended for premature and sick newborns.
- Phototherapy is generally the first line of treatment.
- Phototherapy should be optimized whenever possible by using effective phototherapy, changing bulbs often, measuring irradiance level, and using special blue bulbs.
- Support, including eye protection and adequate hydration, should be provided.
- Exchange blood transfusions should be performed when a newborn meets EBT criteria based on risk, gestational age, or age, or at any time the newborn demonstrates evidence of acute bilirubin encephalopathy.

- Exchange blood transfusions are generally performed through a UVC; sterile feeding tubes are appropriate substitutes for commercial catheters when these are not available.
- Guidelines for performing EBTs using fresh whole blood are straightforward and can be adapted to low-resource settings.
- Other treatments such as IVIG or phenobarbital prophylactically to mother or newborn can be considered in high-risk situations.

Respiratory Diseases

- Respiratory illness is a common cause of neonatal morbidity and mortality worldwide.
- Differential diagnosis of respiratory distress or cyanosis is large and includes etiologies such as prematurity, surfactant deficiency, infection, congenital heart and lung disease, meconium aspiration, transient tachypnea, TEF, and persistent pulmonary hypertension.
- Transient tachypnea of the newborn is common and generally benign, and requires only minimal oxygen support.
- Apnea of prematurity can be treated with theophylline, aminophylline, or caffeine, prophylactically or symptomatically.
- Respiratory distress syndrome or hyaline membrane disease is common in the premature neonate and can be treated with surfactant.
- Continuous positive airway pressure is used to treat mild to moderate respiratory distress and apnea. A CPAP device can be made from locally available supplies and used in setting with minimal monitoring available.
- Persistent pulmonary hypertension occurs primarily in late preterm and term newborns and the only treatment available in low-resource settings is usually oxygen. High fraction of inspired oxygen is usually required.
- Meconium aspiration often causes severe respiratory distress. Treatment is generally limited to oxygen therapy. Endotracheal intubation and suctioning at birth is indicated if health care practitioners capable of intubating are available.
- Pneumothoraces can cause respiratory distress and can often be treated with simple aspiration of the air without the need for a chest tube.
- Infection should always be considered in respiratory distress, and newborns with respiratory distress should be treated promptly for infection until this is ruled out.
- Congenital heart disease should be considered in cyanosis not responding to oxygen therapy.

- Patent ductus arteriosus is common, especially in preterm newborns. Patent ductus arteriosus can sometimes be closed using an oral agent such as ibuprofen.
- Oxygen should be considered a drug and used conservatively when indicated.
- Blended oxygen is preferable.
- Low-flow nasal cannulas are one mechanism of providing lower fraction of inspired oxygen to newborns.
- Continuous positive airway pressure is indicated for mild to moderate respiratory distress and can be provided using several devices in low-resource settings, including homemade CPAP devices.
- Continuous positive airway pressure is generally safe when used in the 3 to 10 cm range; however, it can be associated with pneumothorax, over-distention of the lungs, and gastric distention.

Seizures

- Seizures in the neonate occur from treatable and untreatable causes.
- Easily treatable causes may include metabolic and electrolyte abnormalities. Treating these abnormalities, such as hypoglycemia, may obviate the need for anticonvulsants in these newborns.
- Other illnesses, such as meningitis and polycythemia, require treatment of the underlying cause and anticonvulsants as well.
- Diagnosis is generally made by observing the newborn's movements carefully, excluding jitteriness, startles, and nonspecific movements.
- Treat the underlying cause of the seizure when possible.
- For seizures that are not caused by specific treatable etiology or when seizures persist despite treatment of cause and correction of metabolic or electrolyte abnormalities, anticonvulsants are indicated.
- Phenobarbital is the anticonvulsant of choice in neonates.

Infections

- Neonatal sepsis remains a leading cause of neonatal morbidity and mortality.
- Untreated neonatal sepsis is rapidly fatal.
- Diagnosis of sepsis in the absence of reliable cultures is challenging, but adjuncts like CRP, CBC with differential, and platelet count can be helpful, especially when followed over time.
- Ampicillin and gentamicin remain the recommended intial, inexpensive choices for most neonatal sepsis in low-resource settings.

- For sepsis not responding to ampicillin and gentamicin and for meningitis, cefotaxime is the cephalosporin of choice. If staphylococcal sepsis is suspected, an anti-staphylococcal agent such as cloxacillin should be added. Increasing resistance to these common antibiotics will necessitate changes in these recommendations over time.
- Antibiotics should be dosed according to weight and postnatal age.
- Despite immunizations, tetanus is still a significant cause of neonatal death.
- Immunizations to the mother prior to delivery (minimum of 2) or cutting and caring for the cord in a clean manner will prevent neonatal tetanus.
- Controlling spasms, supporting respirations, providing nutrition, and educating and immunizing family members are the most important elements in caring for a neonate with tetanus.
- Controlling spasms is usually done with a combination of high-dose diazepam, chlorpromazine, and possibly magnesium.
- Tetanus immunoglobulin or tetanus antitoxin or immune antiserum, along with antibiotics (penicillin or metronidazole), are also given.

Education

- Educating others, including the mother herself, extended family, traditional birth attendants, and other health care practitioners, is essential to the ultimate health of the newborn.
- Teaching the basics, such as clean delivery, hand washing, preventive measures, breastfeeding, danger signs, and when to refer, is important, especially in resource-limited settings.
- Positive-pressure bags and training in their use should be promoted for all birth attendants, including the community level.

■ REFERENCES

1. World Health Organization. *Make Every Mother and Child Count*. Geneva, Switzerland: World Health Organization; 2005. http://www.who.int/whr/2005/whr2005_en.pdf. Accessed June 9, 2011

2. American Academy of Pediatrics, American Heart Association. *Textbook of Neonatal Resuscitation*. Kattwinkel J, ed. 6th ed. Elk Grove Village, IL: American Academy of Pediatrics; 2011

3. Zhu XY, Fang HQ, Zeng SP, Li YM, Lin HL, Shi SZ. The impact of the neonatal resuscitation program guidelines (NRPG) on the neonatal mortality in a hospital in Zhuhai, China. *Singapore Med J*. 1997;38(11):485–487

4. O'Hare BA, Nakakeeto M, Southall DP. A pilot study to determine if nurses trained in basic neonatal resuscitation would impact the outcome of neonates delivered in Kampala, Uganda. *J Trop Pediatr*. 2006;52:376–379

5. Deorari AK, Paul VK, Singh M, Vidyasagar D. Impact of education and training on neonatal resuscitation practices in 14 teaching hospitals in India. *Ann Trop Paediatr.* 2001;21(1):29–33

6. Choudhury P. Neonatal Resuscitation Program: first golden minute. *Indian Pediatr.* 2009;46(1):7–9

7. Carlo WA, Wright LL, Chomba E, et al. Educational impact of the neonatal resuscitation program in low-risk delivery centers in a developing country. *J Pediatr.* 2009;154(4):504–508

8. Opiyo N, Were F, Govedi F, Fegan G, Wasunna A, English M. Effect of newborn resuscitation training on health worker practices in Pumwani Hospital, Kenya. *PLoS ONE.* 2008;3(2):e1599

9. Senarath U, Fernando DN, Rodrigo I. Effect of training for care providers on practice of essential newborn care in hospitals in Sri Lanka. *J Obstet Gynecol Neonatal Nurs.* 2007;36(6):531–541

10. Daga SR, Daga AS, Dighole RV, Patil RP, Dhinde HL. Rural neonatal care: Dahanu experience. *Indian Pediatr.* 1992;29(2):189–193

11. Singhal N, Bhutta ZA. Newborn resuscitation in resource-limited settings. *Semin Fetal Neonatal Med.* 2008;13(6):432–439

12. American Academy of Pediatrics, American Heart Association. Simply NRP. Laerdal's Neonatal Resuscitation Simulation Solution. 2009. http://www.laerdal.com/binaries/ AAGLAHYI/4971_SimplyNRP_SS.pdf

13. American Academy of Pediatrics. Helping Babies Breathe. The First Golden Minute. http://www.helpingbabiesbreathe.org

14. Kattwinkel J, et al. Part 15: neonatal resuscitation: 2010 American Heart Association Guidelines for Cardiopulmonary Resuscitation and Emergency Cardiovascular Care. *Circulation.* 2010;122(18 Suppl 3):S909–S919

15. International Liaison Committee on Resuscitation. http://www.ilcor.org/en/news/ news-archive/new-guidelines-2010-now-available

16. Saugstad OD. New guidelines for newborn resuscitation. *Acta Paediatr.* 2007;96(3): 333–337

17. Saugstad OD, Ramji S, Soll RF, Vento M. Resuscitation of newborn infants with 21% or 100% oxygen: an updated systematic review and meta-analysis. *Neonatology.* 2008;94(3):176–182

18. Richmond S, Goldsmith JP. Refining the role of oxygen administration during delivery room resuscitation: what are the future goals? *Semin Fetal Neonatal Med.* 2008;13(6):368–374

19. Wyllie J, Niermeyer S. The role of resuscitation drugs and placental transfusion in the delivery room management of newborn infants. *Semin Fetal Neonatal Med.* 2008;13(6):416–423

20. Eglash A, Montgomery A, Wood J. Breastfeeding. *Dis Mon.* 2008;54(6):343–411

21. Uhing MR, Das UG. Optimizing growth in the preterm infant. *Clin Perinatol.* 2009;36(1):165–176

22. Young TE, Magnum B. *Neofax 2010.* New York, NY: Thomson Reuters; 2010

23. Exclusive breastfeeding for six months best for babies everywhere. http://www. who.int/mediacentre/news/statements/2011/breastfeeding_20110115/en

24. Stuebe A. The risks of not breastfeeding for mothers and infants. *Rev Obstet Gynecol.* 2009;2(4):222–231

25. Venneman MM, Bajanowski T, Brinkman B, et al. Does breastfeeding reduce the risk of sudden infant death syndrome? *Pediatrics.* 2009;123(3):e406–e410

26. World Health Organization. Effect of breastfeeding on infant and child mortality due to infectious diseases in less developed countries: a pooled analysis. *Lancet.* 2000;355:451–455

27. Sisk PM, Lovelady CA, Dillard RG, et al. Early human milk feeding is associated with a lower risk of necrotizing enterocolitis in very low birth weight infants. *J Perionatol.* 2007;27(7):428–433

28. Loland BF, Baerug AB, Nylander G. Human milk immune responses and health effects. *Tidsskr Nor Laegeforen.* 2007;127(18):2395–2398

29. Kramer MS. "Breast is best": the evidence. *Early Hum Dev.* 86(11):729–732

30. Vohr BR, Poindexter BB, Dusick AM, et al. NICHD Neonatal Research Network. Beneficial effects of breast milk in the neonatal intensive care unit on the developmental outcome of extremely low birth weight infants at 18 months of age. *Pediatrics.* 2006;118(1):e115–1e23.

31. Schanler RJ. The use of human milk for premature infants. *Pediatr Clin North Am.* 2001;48(1):207–219

32. Baby-Friendly Hospital Initiative. Revised, updated and expanded for integrated care. World Health Organization, UNICEF; 2009. http://www.who.int/nutrition/publications/infantfeeding/9789241594950/en

33. Mathur NB, Dwarkadas AM, Sharma VK, et al. Anti-infective factors in preterm human colostrum. *Acta Paediatr Scand.* 1990;79:1039

34. Breastfeeding the infant with a problem. In: Lawrence RA, Lawrence RM. *Breastfeeding: A Guide for the Medical Professional.* 5th ed. St. Louis, MO: Mosby; 1999

35. Meier PP, Engstrom JL, Murtaugh MA, et al. Mothers' milk feedings in the neonatal intensive care unit: accuracy of the creamatocrit technique. *J Perinatol.* 2002;22(8):646–649

36. Lemmons JA, Moye L, Hall D, et al. Differences in the composition of preterm and term human milk during early lactation. *Pediatr Res.* 1982;16:113–117

37. Slusher TM, Slusher IL, Keating EM, et al. Comparison of maternal milk (breast milk) expression methods in an African Nursery. *Breastfeed Med.* Accepted for publication

38. Griffin TL, Meier PP, Bradford LP, et al. Mothers' performing creamatocrit measures in the NICU: accuracy, reactions, and cost. *J Obstet Gynecol Neonatal Nurs.* 2000;29(3):249–257

39. Morton J, Hall JY, Wong RJ, et al. Combining hand techniques with electric pumping increases milk production in mother of preterm infants. *J Perinatol.* 2009;29(11):757–764

40. Betzold C. Galactagogues. *J Midwifery Women Health.* 2004;49(2):151–154

41. Hale TW. *Medications and Mothers' Milk.* 13th ed. Amarillo, TX: Hale Publishing; 2008

42. Anderson PO, Valdés V. A critical review of pharmaceutical galactagogues. Breastfeed Med. 2007;2(4):229–242

43. Newman J. Domperidone. http://www.breastfeedingonline.com/Dom19abcombinedpdf.pdf. Accessed July 5, 2009

44. Kuhn L, Aldrovandi G. Survival and health benefits of breastfeeding versus artificial feeding in infants of HIV-infected women: developing versus developed world. *Clin Perinatol.* 2010;37(4):843–862

45. Bland RM, Rollins NC, Coovadia HM, Coutsoudis A, Newell ML. Infant feeding counselling for HIV-infected and uninfected women: appropriateness of choice and practice. *Bull WHO.* 2007;85(4):289–296

46. United Nations Children's Fund. *Monitoring the Situation of Children and Women.* UNICEF; 2009

47. Coovadia HM, Coutsoudis A. HIV, infant feeding, and survival: old wine in new bottles, but brimming with promise. *AIDS*. 2007;21(14):1837–1840

48. Iliff PJ, Piwoz EG, Tavengwa NV, et al. Early exclusive breastfeeding reduces the risk of postnatal HIV-1 transmission and increases HIV-free survival. *AIDS*. 2005;19(7):699–708

49. World Health Organization. HIV and Infant Feeding 2010. http://www.who.int/hiv/topics/mtct

50. Kesho Boro Study. http://www.who.int/reproductivehealth/publications/rtis/keshobora/en/index.html

51. World Health Organization. *Rapid Advice: Use of Antiviral Drugs for Treating Pregnant Women and Preventing HIV Infection in Infants*. 2010 rev ed. Geneva, Switzerland: World Health Organization; 2010

52. Piwoz, Ellen G. *What Are the Options? Using Formative Research to Adapt Global Recommendations on HIV and Infant Feeding to the Local Context*. World Health Organization; 2004

53. Savage F, Lhotska L. Recommendations on feeding infants of HIV positive mothers. In: Berthold Koletzko et al, eds. *Short and Long Term Effects of Breast Feeding on Child Health*. Kluwer Academic/Plemum Publishers; 2000:225–230

54. Marinelli K, Hamelin K. Breastfeeding and the use of human milk in the neonatal intensive care unit. In: MacDonald MG, Mullett MD, Seshia MMK, eds. *Avery's Neonatology Pathophysiology & Management of the Newborn*. Lippincott Williams & Wilkins; 2005:435

55. Hurst NM, Valentine CJ, Renfro L, Burns P, Ferlic L. Skin-to-skin holding in the neonatal intensive care unit influences maternal milk volume. *J Perinatol*. 1997;17(3):213–217

56. Charpak N, Ruiz JG, Zupan J, et al. Kangaroo mother care: 25 years after. *Acta Paediatr*. 2005;94(5):514–522

57. American Academy of Pediatrics. Transfer of drugs and other chemicals into human milk. *Pediatrics*. 2001;108(3):776–789

58. Ronai C, Taylor JS, Dugan E, Feller E. The identifying and counseling of breastfeeding women by pharmacists. *Breastfeed Med*. 2009;4(2):91–95

59. American Academy of Pediatrics. *Red Book: 2009 Report of the Committee on Infectious Diseases*. 28th ed. Pickering LK, ed. Elk Grove Village, IL: American Academy of Pediatrics; 2009

60. Kumar V, Shearer JC, Kumar A, Darmstadt GL. Neonatal hypothermia in low resource settings: a review. *J Perinatol*. 2009;29(6):401–412

61. Soll RF. Heat loss prevention in neonates. *J Perinatol*. 2008;28(Suppl 1):S57–S59

62. World Health Organization. *Thermal Protection of the Newborn: A Practical Guide*. Geneva, Switzerland: World Health Organization; 1997

63. Dragovich D, Tamburlini G, Alisjahbana A, et al. Thermal control of the newborn: knowledge and practice of health professional in seven countries. *Acta Paediatr*. 1997;86(6):645–650

64. Gomella TL, Cunningham MD, Eyal FG, et al. *Neonatology: Management, Procedures, On-Call Problems, Diseases, and Drugs*. McGraw-Hill; 2004

65. Goldsmith JR, Arbeli Y, Stone D. Preventability of neonatal cold injury and its contribution to neonatal mortality. *Environ Health Perspect*. 1991;94:55–59

66. da Mota Silveira SM, Goncalves de Mello MJ, de Arruda Vidal S, et al. Hypothermia on admission: a risk factor for death in newborns referred to the Pernambuco Institute of Mother and Child Health. *J Trop Pediatr*. 2003;49(2):115–120

67. Sodemann M, Nielsen J, Veirum J, et al. Hypothermia of newborns is associated with excess mortality in the first 2 months of life in Guinea-Bissau, West Africa. *Trop Med Int Health.* 2008;13(8):980–986

68. Ogunlesi TA, Ogunfowora OB, Ogundeyi MM. Prevalence and risk factors for hypothermia on admission in Nigerian babies <72 h of age. *J Perinat Med.* 2009;37(2):180–184

69. World Health Organization. *Essential Newborn Care—Report of a Technical Working Group.* In: Chapter 1; 1996

70. Speer M, Perlman JM. Modest hypothermia as a neuroprotective strategy in high-risk term infants. *Clin Perinatol.* 2006;33(1):169–182

71. Azzopardi D, Strohm B, Edwards AD, et al. Treatment of asphyxiated newborns with moderate hypothermia in routine clinical practice: how cooling is managed in the UK outside a clinical trial. *Arch Dis Child Fetal Neonatal Ed.* 2008

72. Ogunlesi TA, Ogunfowora OB, Adekanmbi FA, et al. Point-of-admission hypothermia among high-risk Nigerian newborns. *BMC Pediatr.* 2008;8:40

73. Basu S, Rathore P, Bhatia BD. Predictors of mortality in very low birth weight neonates in India. *Singapore Med J.* 2008;49(7):556–560

74. Kumar R, Aggarwal AK. Accuracy of maternal perception of neonatal temperature. *Indian Pediatr.* 1996;33(7):583–585

75. Marchini G, Lindow S, Brismar H, et al The newborn infant is protected by an innate antimicrobial barrier: peptide antibiotics are present in the skin and vernixcaseosa. *Br J Dermatol.* 2002;147:1127–1134

76. Ibrahim CPH, Yoxall CW. Use of plastic bags to prevent hypothermia at birth in preterm infants—do they work at lower gestations? *Acta Paediatr.* 2009;98:256–260

77. Bergman NJ, Linley LL, Fawcus SR. Randomized controlled trial of skin-to-skin contact from birth versus conventional incubator for physiological stabilization in 1200- to 2199-gram newborns. *Acta Paediatr.* 1993;93:779–785

78. Bogale Worku Assaye Kassie. Kangaroo mother care: a randomized controlled trial on effectiveness of early kangaroo mother care for the low birthweight infants in Addis Ababa, Ethiopia. *J Trop Pediatr.* 2005;51(2):93–97

79. Ludington-Hoe SM, Nguyen N, Swinth JY, Satyshur RD. Kangaroo care compared to incubators in maintaining body warmth in preterm infants. *Biol Res Nurs.* 2000;2(1):60–73

80. Conde-Agudelo A, Diaz-Rossello JL, Belizan JM. Kangaroo mother care to reduce morbidity and mortality in low birthweight infants (review). *Cochrane Database Syst Rev.* 2003;(2):1–38

81. World Health Organization. *Care of the Umbilical Cord: A Review of the Evidence.* Geneva, Switzerland: World Health Organization; 1998

82. Zupan J, Garner P, Omari AA. Topical umbilical cord care at birth. *Cochrane Database Syst Rev.* 2004;(3):CD001057

83. Fraser N, Davies BW, Cusack J. Neonatal omphalitis: a review of its serious complications. *Acta Paediatr.* 2006;95(5):519–522

84. Ononeze AB, Hutchon DJ. Attitude of obstetricians towards delayed cord clamping: a questionnaire-based study. *J Obstet Gynaecol.* 2009;29(3):223–224

85. van Rheenen PF, Gruschke S, Brabin BJ. Delayed umbilical cord clamping for reducing anaemia in low birthweight infants: implications for developing countries. *Ann Trop Paediatr.* 2006;26(3):157–167

86. Rabe H, Reynolds G, Diaz-Rossell J. A systematic review and meta-analysis of a brief delay in clamping the umbilical cord of preterm infants. *Neonatology.* 2008;93(2):138–144

87. Rabe H, Jewison A, Alvarez RF, et al. Milking compared with delayed cord clmaping to increase placental transfusion in preterm neonates: a randomized controlled trial. *Obstest Gynecol*. 2011;117(2 Pt 1):203–204

88. Hosono S, Mugishima H, Fujita H, et al. Umbilical cord milking reduces the need for red cell transfusions and improves neonatal adaptation in infants born at less than 29 weeks' gestation: a randomized controlled trial. *Arch Dis Child Fetal Neonatal Ed*. 2008;93(1):F14–F19

89. Grajeda R, Perez-Escamilla R, Dewey KG. Delayed clamping of the umbilical cord improves hematologic status of Guatemalan infants at 2 mo of age. *Am J Clin Nutr*. 1997;65(2):425–431

90. Foster A, Klauss V. Ophthalmia neonatorum in developing countries. *N Engl J Med*. 1995;332(9):600–601

91. Schaller UC, Klauss V. Is Crede's prophylaxis for ophthalmia neonatorum still valid? *Bull WHO*. 2001;79(3):262–263

92. Isenberg SJ, Apt L, Wood M. A controlled trial of povidone-iodine as prophylaxis against ophthalmia neonatorum. *N Engl J Med*. 1995;332(9):562–566

93. Puckett RM, Offringa M. Prophylactic vitamin K for vitamin K deficiency bleeding in neonates. *Cochrane Database Syst Rev*. 2000;(4):CD002776

94. Wynn RM. The obstetric significance of factors affecting the metabolism of bilirubin, with particular reference to the role of vitamin K. *Obstet Gynecol Surv*. 1963;18:333–354

95. Finkel MJ. Vitamin K1 and the vitamin K analogues. *Clin Pharmacol Ther*. 1961;2:794–814

96. World Health Organization. *Introduction of Hepatitis B Vaccine Into Childhood Immunization Services*. Geneva, Switzerland: World Health Organization; 2001

97. Bhutta ZA, Darmstadt GL, Hasan BS, et al. Community-based interventions for improving perinatal and neonatal health outcomes in developing countries: a review of the evidence. *Pediatrics*. 2005;115(2 Suppl):519–617

98. Darlow BA, Graham PJ. Vitamin A supplementation to prevent mortality and short and long-term morbidity in very low birthweight infants. *Cochrane Database Syst Rev*. 2007;(4):CD000501

99. Gogia S, Sachdev HS. Neonatal vitamin A supplementation for prevention of mortality and morbidity in infancy: systematic review of randomised controlled trials. *BMJ*. 2009;338:b919

100. Fernandez A, Patkar S, Chawla C, et al. Oil application in preterm babies—a source of warmth and nutrition. *Indian Pediatr*. 1987;24(12):1111–1116

101. Darmstadt GL, Mao-Qiang M, Chi E, et al. Impact of topical oils on the skin barrier: possible implications for neonatal health in developing countries. *Acta Paediatr*. 2002;91(5):546–554

102. Moraille R, Pickens WL, Visscher MO, Hoath SB. A novel role for vernix caseosa as a skin cleanser. *Biol Neonate*. 2005;87(1):8–14

103. Akinbi HT, Narendran V, Pass AK, Markart P, Hoath SB. Host defense proteins in vernix caseosa and amniotic fluid. *Am J Obstet Gynecol*. 2004;191(6):2090–2096

104. World Health Organization. Pregnancy, childbirth, postpartum and newborn care: a guide for essential practice. In: *Integrated Management of Pregnancy and Childbirth*. 2nd ed. Geneva, Switzerland: World Health Organization; 2006

105. Owa JA. Relationship between exposure to icterogenic agents, glucose-6-phosphate dehydrogenase deficiency and neonatal jaundice in Nigeria. *Acta Paediatr Scand*. 1989;78(6):848–852

106. Tielsch JM, Darmstadt GL, Mullany LC, et al. Impact of newborn skin-cleansing with chlorhexidine on neonatal mortality in southern Nepal: a community-based, cluster-randomized trial. *Pediatrics.* 2007;119(2):e330–e340

107. Parish JL. Treponemal infections in the pediatric population. *Clin Dermatol.* 2000;18(6):687–700

108. Stanton C, Lawn JE, Rahman H, Wilczynska-Ketende K, Hill K. Stillbirth rates: delivering estimates in 190 countries. *Lancet.* 2006;367(9521):1487–1494

109. Lawn JE, Cousens S, Zupan J. 4 million neonatal deaths: when? Where? Why? *Lancet.* 2005;365(9462):891–900

110. Bryce J, Boschi-Pinto C, Shibuya K, Black RE. WHO estimates of the causes of death in children. *Lancet.* 2005;365(9465):1147–1152

111. Lawn J, Shibuya K, Stein C. No cry at birth: global estimates of intrapartum stillbirths and intrapartum-related neonatal deaths. *Bull WHO.* 2005;83(6):409–417

112. Lawn JE, Osrin D, Adler A, Cousens S. Four million neonatal deaths: counting and attribution of cause of death. *Paediatr Perinat Epidemiol.* 2008;22(5):410–416

113. Keyes LE, Armaza JF, Niermeyer S, Vargas E, Young DA, Moore LG. Intrauterine growth restriction, preeclampsia, and intrauterine mortality at high altitude in Bolivia. *Pediatr Res.* 2003;54(1):20–25

114. Murphy SC, Breman JG. Gaps in the childhood malaria burden in Africa: cerebral malaria, neurological sequelae, anemia, respiratory distress, hypoglycemia, and complications of pregnancy. *Am J Trop Med Hygiene.* 2001;64(1-2 Suppl):57–67

115. Siza JE. Risk factors associated with low birth weight of neonates among pregnant women attending a referral hospital in northern Tanzania. *Tanzan J Health Res.* 2008;10(1):1–8

116. Davis PG, Tan A, O'Donnell CP, Schulze A. Resuscitation of newborn infants with 100% oxygen or air: a systematic review and meta-analysis. *Lancet.* 2004;364(9442):1329–1333

117. Tan A, Schulze A, O'Donnell CP, Davis PG. Air versus oxygen for resuscitation of infants at birth. *Cochrane Database Syst Rev.* 2005;(2):CD002273

118. Jacobs S, Hunt R, Tarnow-Mordi W, Inder T, Davis P. Cooling for newborns with hypoxic ischaemic encephalopathy. *Cochrane Database Syst Rev.* 2007;(4):CD003311

119. Robertson NJ, Nakakeeto M, Hagmann C, et al. Therapeutic hypothermia for birth asphyxia in low-resource settings: a pilot randomised controlled trial. *Lancet.* 2008;372(9641):801–803

120. Levene MI, de Vries L. Hypoxic-ischemic encephalopathy. In: Martin RJ, Fanaroff AA, Walsh MC, eds. *Fanaroff and Martin's Neonatal-Perinatal Medicine. Diseases of the Fetus and Infant.* 8th ed. Philadelphia, PA: Mosby Elsevier; 2006:938–1033

121. Odd DE, Lewis G, Whitelaw A, Gunnell D. Resuscitation at birth and cognition at 8 years of age: a cohort study. *Lancet.* 2009;373(9675):1615–1622

122. van Handel M, Swaab H, de Vries LS, Jongmans MJ. Long-term cognitive and behavioral consequences of neonatal encephalopathy following perinatal asphyxia: a review. *Eur J Paediatr.* 2007;166(7):645–654

123. Anderson S, Shakya KN, Shrestha LN, Costello AM. Hypoglycaemia: a common problem among uncomplicated newborn infants in Nepal. *J Trop Pediatr.* 1993;39(5):273–277

124. Bhat MA, Kumar P, Bhansali A, Majumdar S, Narang A. Hypoglycemia in small for gestational age babies. *Indian J Pediatr.* 2000;67(6):423–427

125. Kalhan S, Parimi P. Disorders of carbohydrate metabolism. In: Martin RJ, Fanaroff AA, Walsh MC, eds. *Fanaroff and Martin's Neonatal-Perinatal Medicine. Diseases of the Fetus and Infant.* 8th ed. Philadelphia, PA: Mosby Elsevier; 2006:138–144

126. Marx JA, Hockenberger RS, Walls RM. *Rosen's Emergency Medicine Concepts in Clinical Practice.* 7th ed. Philadelphia, PA: Mosby Elsevier; 2010

127. Owa JA, Ogunlesi TA. Why we are still doing so many exchange blood transfusion for neonatal jaundice in Nigeria. *World J Pediatr.* 2009;5(1):51–55

128. Owa JA, Osinaike AI. Neonatal morbidity and mortality in Nigeria. *Indian J Pediatr.* 1998;65(3):441–449

129. English M, Ngama M, Musumba C, et al. Causes and outcome of young infant admissions to a Kenyan district hospital. *Arch Dis Child.* 2003;88(5):438–443

130. Salas AA, Mazzi E. Exchange transfusion in infants with extreme hyperbilirubinemia: an experience from a developing country. *Acta Paediatr.* 2008;97(6):754–758

131. American Academy of Pediatrics. Management of hyperbilirubinemia in the newborn infant 35 or more weeks of gestation. Pediatrics. 2004;114(1):297–316

132. Nair PA, Al Khusaiby SM. Kernicterus and G6PD deficiency—a case series from Oman. *J Trop Pediatr.* 2003;49(2):74–77

133. Tiker F, Gulcan H, Kilicdag H, Tarcan A, Gurakan B. Extreme hyperbilirubinemia in newborn infants. *Clin Pediatr (Phila).* 2006;45(3):257–261

134. Ogunlesi TA, Dedeke IO, Adekanmbi AF, Fetuga MB, Ogunfowora OB. The incidence and outcome of bilirubin encephalopathy in Nigeria: a bi-centre study. *Niger J Med.* 2007;16(4):354–359

135. Bhutani VK, Johnson LH, Keren R. Diagnosis and management of hyperbilirubinemia in the term neonate: for a safer first week. *Pediatr Clin North Am.* 2004;51(4):843–861

136. Webster J, Blyth R, Nugent F. An appraisal of the use of the Kramer's scale in predicting hyperbilirubinaemia in healthy full term infants. *Birth Issues.* 2005;14(3):83–89

137. Bilgen H, Ince Z, Ozek E, et al. Transcutaneous measurement of hyperbilirubinaemia: comparison of the Minolta jaundice meter and the Ingram icterometer. *Ann Trop Paediatr.* 1998;18(4):325–328

138. Madlon-Kay DJ. Recognition of the presence and severity of newborn jaundice by parents, nurses, physicians, and icterometer. Pediatrics. 1997;100(3):E3

139. Manzar S. Cephalo-caudal progression of jaundice: a reliable, non-invasive clinical method to assess the degree of neonatal hyperbilirubineaemia. *J Trop Pediatr.* 1999; 45(5):312–313

140. Moyer VA, Ahn C, Sneed S. Accuracy of clinical judgment in neonatal jaundice. *Arch Pediatr Adolesc Med.* 2000;154(4):391–394

141. Volpe JJ. Bilirubin and brain injury. In: *Neurology of the Newborn.* 5th ed. Philadelphia, PA: Saunders Elsevier; 2008:635–637

142. Slusher TM, Owa JA, Painter MJ, Shapiro SM. The Kernicteric Facies: facial features of acute bilirubin encephalopathy. *Pediatr Neurol.* 2011;44(2):153–154

143. Jirapaet K. Thai healthy newborns have a higher risk. *J Med Assoc Thai.* 2005;88(9):1314–1318

144. Wentworth S. Neonatal phototherapy—today's lamps, lights and devices. *Infant.* 2005;1(1):14–19

145. Maisels MJ, McDonagh AF. Phototherapy for neonatal jaundice. *N Engl J Med.* 2008;358(9):920–928

146. Chawla D, Parmar V. Phenobarbitone for prevention and treatment of unconjugated hyperbilirubinemia in preterm neonates: a systematic review and meta-analysis. *Indian Pediatr.* 2010;47(5):401–407

147. Thomas JT, Muller P, Wilkinson C. Antenatal phenobarbital for reducing neonatal jaundice after red cell isoimmunization. *Cochrane Database Syst Rev*. 2007;(2):CD005541

148. Trevett TN Jr, Dorman K, Lamvu G, Moise KJ Jr. Antenatal maternal administration of phenobarbital for the prevention of exchange transfusion in neonates with hemolytic disease of the fetus and newborn. *Am J Obstet Gynecol*. 2005;192(2):478–482

149. Morioka I, Wong RJ, Abate A, Vreman HJ, Contag CH, Stevenson DK. Systemic effects of orally-administered zinc and tin (IV) metalloporphyrins on hemeoxygenase expression in mice. *Pediatr Res*. 2006;59(5):667–672

150. Kumar A, Bhat BV. Respiratory distress in newborn. *Indian J Matern Child Health*. 1996;7(1):8–10

151. Chaudhari R, Deodhar J, Kadam S, Bavdekar A, Pandit A. Gastric aspirate shake test for diagnosis of surfactant deficiency in neonates with respiratory distress. *Ann Trop Paediatr*. 2005;25(3):205–209

152. Trevisanuto D, Grazzina N, Ferrarese P, Micaglio M, Verghese C, Zanardo V. Laryngeal mask airway used as a delivery conduit for the administration of surfactant to preterm infants with respiratory distress syndrome. *Biol Neonate*. 2005;87(4):217–220

153. Chandran S, Haqueb ME, Wickramasinghe HT, et al. Use of magnesium sulphate in severe persistent pulmonary hypertension of the newborn. *J Trop Pediatr*. 2004; 50(4):219–223

154. Ho JJ, Rasa G. Magnesium sulfate for persistent pulmonary hypertension of the newborn. *Cochrane Database Syst Rev*. 2007;(3):CD005588

155. Trotman H. The neonatal intensive care unit at the University Hospital of the West Indies: the first few years' experience. *West Indian Med J*. 2006;55(2):75–79

156. Singh BS, Clark RH, Powers RJ, et al. Meconium aspiration syndrome remains a significant problem in the NICU: outcomes and treatment patterns in term neonates admitted for intensive care during a ten year period. *J Perinatol*. 2009;29(7):497–503

157. Cherif A, Khrouf N, Jabnoun S, et al. Randomized pilot study comparing oral ibuprofen with intravenous ibuprofen in very low birth weight infants with patent ductusarteriosus. *Pediatrics*. 2008;122(6):e1256–e1261

158. Nowadzky T, Pantoja A, Britton JR. Bubble continuous positive airway pressure, a potentially better practice, reduces the use of mechanical ventilation among very low birth weight infants with respiratory distress syndrome. *Pediatrics*. 2009;123(6):1534–1540

159. Lampland AL, Plumm B, Meyers PA, Worwa CT, Mammel MC. Observational study of humidified high-flow nasal cannula compared with nasal continuous positive airway pressure. *J Pediatr*. 2009;154(2):177–182

160. Ammari A, Kashlan F, Exxedeen F, et al. Bubble nasal CPAP manual. http://earlybubblecpap.com/.../CPAP%20Educational%20Files/CPAP_Manual.pdf

161. Blumstein MD, Friedman MJ. Childhood seizures. *Emerg Med Clin North Am*. 2007;25(4):1061–1086

162. Sankar MJ, Agarwal R, Aggarwal R, Deorari AK, Paul VK. Seizures in the newborn. *Indian J Pediatr*. 2008;75(2):149–155

163. Custer JW, Rau RE. *The Harriet Lane Handbook: A Manual for Pediatric House Officers*. 18th ed. Philadelphia, PA: Mosby/Elsevier; 2009

164. Bradley JS, Nelson JD, eds, *2009 Nelson's Pocket Book of Pediatric Antimicrobial Therapy*. 17th ed. Elk Grove Village, IL: American Academy of Pediatrics; 2009

165. Bartha AI, Shen J, Katz KH, et al. Neonatal seizures: multicenter variability in current treatment practices. *Pediatr Neurol*. 2007;37(2):85–90

166. Lee WK, Liu KT, Young BW. Very-high-dose phenobarbital for childhood refractory status epilepticus. *Pediatr Neurol.* 2006;34(1):63–65

167. Gilman JT, Gal P, Duchowny MS, et al. Rapid sequential phenobarbital treatment of neonatal seizures. *Pediatrics.* 1989;83(5):674–678

168. Clancy RR. Summary proceedings from the neurology group on neonatal seizures. *Pediatrics.* 2006;117(3 Pt 2):S23–S27

169. World Health Organization. The newborn deaths that went unnoticed. In: *The World Health Report 2005.* Geneva, Switzerland: World Health Organization; 2005

170. Long SS, Pickering LK, Prober CG, eds. *Principles and Practice of Pediatric Infectious Diseases.* 3rd ed. Philadelphia, PA: Churchill Livingstone/Elsevier; 2008

171. Weber MW, Carlin JB, Gatchalian S, et al. Predictors of neonatal sepsis in developing countries. *Pediatr Infect Dis J.* 2003;22(8):711–717

172. Schuchat A, Zywicki SS, Dinsmoor MJ, et al. Risk factors and opportunities for prevention of early-onset neonatal sepsis: a multicenter case-control study. *Pediatrics.* 2000;105(1 Pt 1):21–26

173. Zaidi AK, Thaver D, Ali SA, et al. Pathogens associated with sepsis in newborns and young infants in developing countries. *Pediatr Infect Dis J.* 2009;28(1 Suppl):S10–S18

174. Costello A, Manandhar D. *Improving Newborn Infant Health in Developing Countries.* London, England: Imperial College Press; 2000

175. Gardner SL. Sepsis in the neonate. *Crit Care Nurs Clin North Am.* 2009;21(1):121–141

176. Krugman S, Gershon AA, Hotez PJ, eds. *Krugman's Infectious Diseases of Children.* 11th ed. Philadelphia, PA: Mosby; 2004

177. Sharma A, Kutty CV, Sabharwal U, et al. Evaluation of sepsis screen for diagnosis of neonatal septicemia. *Indian J Pediatr.* 1993;60(4):559–563

178. Menke JA, Giacoia GP, Jockin H. Group B beta hemolytic streptococcal sepsis and the idiopathic respiratory distress syndrome: a comparison. *J Pediatr.* 1979;94(3):467–471

179. Bortolussi R, Thompson TR, Ferrieri P. Early-onset pneumococcal sepsis in newborn infants. *Pediatrics.* 1977;60(3):352–355

180. McAdams RM, Garza-Cox S, Yoder BA. Early-onset neonatal pneumococcal sepsis syndrome. *Pediatr Crit Care Med.* 2005;6(5):595–597

181. Christensen RD, Rothstein G, Anstall HB, Bybee B. Granulocyte transfusions in neonates with bacterial infection, neutropenia, and depletion of mature marrow neutrophils. *Pediatrics.* 1982;70(1):1–6

182. Rodwell RL, Leslie AL, Tudehope DI. Early diagnosis of neonatal sepsis using a hematologic scoring system. *J Pediatr.* 1988;112(5):761–767

183. Mannan MA, Shahidullah M, Noor MK, et al. Utility of C-reactive protein and hematological parameters in the detection of neonatal sepsis. *Mymensingh Med J.* 2010;19(2):259–263

184. Benitz WE, Han MY, Madan A, et al. Serial serum C-reactive protein levels in the diagnosis of neonatal infection. *Pediatrics.* 1998;102(4):E41

185. Nuntnarumit P, Pinkaew O, Kitiwanwanich S. Predictive values of serial C-reactive protein in neonatal sepsis. *J Med Assoc Thai.* 2002;85(Suppl 4):S1151–S1158

186. McWilliam S, Riordan A. How to use C reactive protein: postscript. *Arch Dis Child Educ Pract Ed.* 2010;95(6):194–195

187. Ahmed Z, Ghafoor T, Waqar T, et al. Diagnostic value of C- reactive protein and haematological parameters in neonatal sepsis. *J Coll Physicians Surg Pak.* 2005;15(3):152–156

188. Chandna A, Rao MN, Srinivas M, et al. Rapid diagnostic tests in neonatal septicemia. *Indian J Pediatr.* 1988:55(6):947–953

189. Yeung CY, Tam ASY. Gastric aspirate findings in neonatal pneumonia. *Arch Dis Child.* 1972;47:735–740

190. Vasan U, Lim DM, Greenstein RM, et al. Origin of gastric aspirate polymorpho-nuclear leukocytes in infants born after prolonged rupture of membranes. *J Pediatr.* 1977;91(1):69–72

191. Wiswell TE, Baumgart S, Gannon CM, et al. No lumbar puncture in the evaluation for early neonatal sepsis: will meningitis be missed? *Pediatrics.* 1995;95(6):803–806

192. Sarff LD, Platt LH, McCracken GH Jr. Cerebrospinal fluid evaluation in neonates: com-parison of high-risk infants with and without meningitis. *J Pediatr.* 1976;88(3):473–477

193. Visser VE, Hall RT. Urine culture in the evaluation of suspected neonatal sepsis. *J Pediatr.* 1979;94(4):635–638

194. Kayange N, Kamugisha E, Mwizamholya DL, et al. Predictors of positive blood cultures and deaths among neonates with suspected neonatal sepsis in a tertiary hospital, Mwanza-Tanzania. *BMC Pediatrics.* 2010;10:39

195. Ogunlesi TA, Ogunfowora OB, Osinupebi O, et al. Changing trends in newborn sepsis in Sagamu, Nigeria: Bacterial aetiology, risk factors and antibiotic susceptibility. *J Paediatrics and Child Health.* 2011;47:5–11

196. Joshi SG, Ghole VS, Niphadkar KB. Neonatal gram-negative bacteremia. *Indian J Pediatr.* 2000;67(1):27–32

197. Roper MH, Vandelaer JH, Gasse FL. Maternal and neonatal tetanus. *Lancet.* 2007; 370(9603):1947–1959

198. Kurtoglu S, Caksen H, Ozturk A, et al. A review of 207 newborn with tetanus. *J Pak Med Assoc.* 1998;48(4):93–98

199. Puliyel MM, Pillai R, Korula S. Intravenous magnesium sulphate infusion in the management of very severe tetanus in a child: a descriptive case report. *J Trop Pediatr.* 2009;55(1):58–59

200. Ceneviva GD, Thomas NJ, Kees-Folts D. Magnesium sulfate for control of muscle rigid-ity and spasms and avoidance of mechanical ventilation in pediatric tetanus. *Pediatr Crit Care Med.* 2003;4(4):480–484

201. Ertem M, Cakmak A, Saka G, Ceylan A. Neonatal tetanus in the South-Eastern region of Turkey: changes in prognostic aspects by better health care. *J Trop Pediatr.* 2004;50(5):297–300

202. Kubura L, Ilibagiza D, Menten J, et al. Intrathecal vs. intramuscular administration of human antitetanusimmunoglobin or equine tetanus antitoxin int the treatment of tetanus: a meta-analysis. *Trop Med Int Health.* 2006;11(7):1075–1081

203. Ganesh Kumar AV, Kothari VM, Krishnan A, Karnad DR. Benzathine penicillin, metro-nidazole and benzyl penicillin in the treatment of tetanus: a randomized, controlled trial. *Ann Trop Med Parasitol.* 2004;98(1):59–63

204. Chomba E, McClure EM, Wright LL, et al. Effect of WHO newborn care training on neonatal mortality by education. *Ambul Pediatr.* 2008;8(5):300–304

205. Greenwood AM, Bradley AK, Byass P, et al. Evaluation of a primary health care pro-gramme in The Gambia. I. The impact of trained traditional birth attendants on the outcome of pregnancy. *J Trop Med Hyg.* 1990;93(1):58–66

206. Kumar V, Mohanty S, Kumar A, et al. Effect of community-based behaviour change management on neonatal mortality in Shivgarh, Uttar Pradesh, India: a cluster-ran-domised controlled trial. *Lancet.* 2008;372(9644):1151–1162

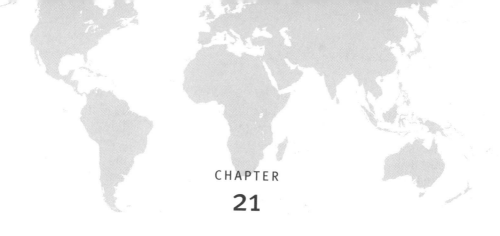

CHAPTER

21

Promoting Early Child Development

Aisha K. Yousafzai, PhD
Zulfiqar A. Bhutta, MD, PhD, FAAP

◼ INTRODUCTION

Early child development (ECD) strategies are now widely regarded as key
components to improving child health and nutrition programs in developing countries. In 2007, Grantham-McGregor and colleagues reported
that globally at least 219 million children younger than 5 years did
not meet their development potential. This substantial loss of human
capital affects subsequent educational achievement and future economic
productivity. The global challenge to avoid the loss of development
potential in the early years must be addressed by the international child
health community.

◼ GLOBAL CONTEXT OF CHILD SURVIVAL

In 2003, the Bellagio Study Group on Child Survival reported that 10.8
million children die before their fifth birthday, with one third of these
deaths occurring in the neonatal period.[1] The leading causes of early
childhood mortality include pneumonia and diarrheal disease.[1] More
than two thirds of these deaths are preventable.[2,3] While improvements
in child survival rates have been observed since 1990 with an estimated
27% decline in younger-than-5 mortality,[4] there remains significant
disparities across and within populations. Developing more effective
strategies to reach the most vulnerable children to achieve Millennium
Development Goal (MDG) 4 (reduce younger-than-5 mortality by two
thirds) resulted in strengthening understanding about the circumstances
in which children survive. Exposure to risk factors such as malnutrition,

HIV/AIDS, malaria, conflict, and lack of access to safe water and adequate sanitation not only increase the likelihood of childhood mortality and morbidity but also have long-term detrimental implications on motor, cognitive, language, social, and emotional development.[5] The global data on child health is discussed more extensively in Chapter 1, The Reality of Child Mortality.

The number of young children worldwide surviving and not fulfilling their development potential far exceeds 200 million—a figure reached by looking at worldwide prevalence of people living in absolute poverty and early childhood stunting.[6] Stunting and poverty are indicators closely associated with poor cognitive outcome and educational performance. Understanding the common pathways that lead to poor development, health, and nutrition status can facilitate the identification of a host of interventions that will enhance early childhood outcomes. Integrated early child survival and development strategies will therefore not only help achieve MDG 4 but also contribute to the achievement of MDG 2 (universal primary education).

■ RATIONALE FOR INTEGRATING EARLY CHILD DEVELOPMENT INTERVENTIONS IN EXISTING CHILD HEALTH SERVICES

Understanding the Early Child Development Period

Understanding the factors influencing early development can help identify interventions that can complement existing child survival, health, and nutrition programs. Child development is shaped by continuous interactions among biology, experience, and the environment. There are several interdependent domains of development, including motor, cognitive, language, social, and emotional development. The ECD period generally includes children from birth to 8 years of age; however, the critical period of early development is usually defined as the first 3 years of life. During this early period there is rapid development of pathways in the brain that influence health, learning, and behavior throughout the life cycle.[7]

Brain development is an interaction among genetics, experience, and the quality of the environment. Evidence from animal experiments demonstrates that deprivation of nutrition, exposure to environmental toxins, maltreatment, and poor quality of social interaction affect brain structure and function, thereby influencing learning ability and behavioral responses throughout the life cycle.[7,8] In humans exposure to violence, maltreatment, and inadequate caregiving practices in early life are shown to have long-lasting negative implications on subsequent behavior patterns observed in longitudinal studies and studies of brain structure and function.[9-13]

The basic premise that early development is shaped by nature (biology) and nurture (quality of the environment and maternal care) has helped to elucidate the pathways that operate through poor cognitive and social development, leading to educational failure and subsequent low economic productivity. This loss of developmental potential is in part caused by poor health and undernutrition, but it is also the result of non-stimulating environments and inadequate care practices. While many of the risk factors associated with poor health and undernutrition are well recognized and often addressed in child survival, health, and nutrition programs (eg, iodine deficiency, iron deficiency, stunting), stimulation and care is less well understood.

There are many theories about how children learn. Developmental psychologists generally agree that children learn through a process of observation, exploration, imitation, and practice of any given task at developmentally appropriate stages. Social interaction is an important aspect of development; skills are acquired with the guidance of an adult, where the child is encouraged to observe, imitate, explore, and practice a particular task (a *scaffolding* process). Many studies show that young children who receive psychosocial stimulation support (ie, learning and language development opportunities through interaction with caregivers) can improve their cognitive functioning; thus, young children acquire the skills needed for future school readiness.[14-17]

The term *care* within the household can extend the provision of appropriate health, hygiene, and feeding practices to also include psychosocial stimulation. Maternal emotional availability is an important factor that can determine the quality of care provided by the mother (or other significant caregiver). The mother's level of sensitivity and responsiveness to her child's needs influences the child's cognitive, social, and emotional development. *Sensitivity* is the mother's capacity to be aware of the infant and his acts and vocalizations that communicate his needs and wants. *Responsiveness* is the caregiver's capacity to contingently and appropriately respond to the infant's signals. The way a child expresses these needs will change as he develops and the mother must be able understand the changing signals. Therefore, the caregiver must be sensitive to be responsive.

Parenting programs are interventions designed to enhance caregiving capacity. In addition to providing health, nutrition, and development information, support to enhance caregiving capacity (in particular sensitivity and responsiveness) must be an integral component of a parenting program. These caregiving behaviors will also support the child's physical well-being through timely observation and judgment of her health and nutritional needs.[18]

Emotional availability is a determinant of the quality of early attachment and bonding with the child. Studies on children growing up in low-quality institutional care, where they may lack supportive and stable caregiving relationships, show increased risks for failure to thrive, as well as compromised social and emotional development. While the association of maternal physical health and nutritional status with early child outcomes on growth, health, and development are well known, there is now growing recognition to address factors that can impede the mother's ability to provide appropriate emotional care for her child (eg, maternal depression).[18–20] Helping mothers, particularly those who are vulnerable, to be more responsive caregivers through guidance and provision of adequate support, including health, nutrition, and economic resources as well as social-emotional support, is essential for their children's survival, well-being, and development.

Development is shaped by risk and protective factors throughout the life cycle. The timing of early experience is important and the course of development can be most effectively modified in the early childhood period by strategically timed interventions that strengthen resilience and reduce vulnerability. For the health sector, this window of opportunity is in the first 3 years of a child's life when vital stages of brain development are occurring. This period is also a time when a child and family may see health care professionals more regularly for newborn care, immunizations, and other early childhood services.

Existing health services provide a range of interventions that will benefit child development outcome; however, stimulation, caregiving support, and maternal mental health remain as gaps that, if filled, could strengthen overall outcomes for development, growth, and health (Table 21-1).

Critical Links to Support Vulnerable Groups

The case for integrated child health services is strengthened further when one considers that many children growing up in developing countries face multiple and co-occurring risks leading to poor development, health, and nutrition status. In a systematic review of risk factors for adverse child development outcomes in lower-income countries, Walker and colleagues identified 4 important factors: stunting, inadequate cognitive stimulation, iodine deficiency, and iron deficiency anemia, which affect 20% to 25% of all children in developing countries.[5] In addition, there was considered to be sufficient evidence to warrant intervention

Table 21-1. Framework for Early Child Development Programming Across the Early Years

ECD PERIOD (AGE, Y)	0	1	2	3	4	5	6	7	8
GOAL	PROMOTE OPTIMAL DEVELOPMENT, ENABLING CHILDREN TO THRIVE AND ACQUIRE CONTEXTUALLY RELEVANT SKILLS AND BEHAVIORS.								
POSSIBLE INDICATORS			STUNTING IMPAIRMENT			SCHOOL READINESS		ACADEMIC ACHIEVEMENT, ENROLLMENT/DROP OUT	
Interventions[a]	Antenatal Care Services								
		Key Newborn and Young Child Health and Nutrition Services							
		Parenting Programs: Education for Health, Nutrition, Development, and Enhancement of Caregiving Capacity							
		Early Stimulation							
		Maternal Support: Mental Health Services							
		Growth and Development Monitoring and Intervention							
					Early Child Education: Preschool Programs				
							Primary Early Child Education: Primary School		
						School Health and Life Skills Programs			

Table 21-1. Framework for Early Child Development Programming Across the Early Years, continued

GOAL	PROMOTE OPTIMAL DEVELOPMENT, ENABLING CHILDREN TO THRIVE AND ACQUIRE CONTEXTUALLY RELEVANT SKILLS AND BEHAVIORS.								
ECD PERIOD (AGE, Y)	0	1	2	3	4	5	6	7	8
POSSIBLE INDICATORS			STUNTING IMPAIRMENT			SCHOOL READINESS	ACADEMIC ACHIEVEMENT, ENROLLMENT/DROP OUT		
Main Sector Involvement	Health Services Educational Services → Social Protection and Welfare →								
Policy Considerations	National plan of action, leadership, coordination, and financing								

Abbreviation: ECD, early child development.

a Interventions represent areas where ECD can be strengthened by the health sector.

to address exposure to malaria, maternal depression, violence, low birth weight with intrauterine growth restriction, and exposure to heavy metals for improved child development outcomes in the domains of cognitive, social-emotional, and motor-sensory development.

It is noteworthy to observe that nutrition-related factors accounted for 4 of the 9 identified risk factors for poor development. The delivery of effective evidence-based nutrition services for pregnant women, infants, and young children will have benefits for the development of the child; however, the benefits will be greater if these interventions are combined with psychosocial stimulation and improved caregiving strategies.

There is substantial evidence linking stunting with poor cognitive development and academic achievement.[21–24] Prevention of early stunting through improved early feeding strategies is a priority intervention; however, the delivery of such strategies can be combined with the delivery of psychosocial stimulation and responsive care for the development of greater benefits. This was demonstrated in studies of Jamaican infants with and without stunting who received nutritional supplementation, psychosocial stimulation, or combined interventions. It was identified that supplementation and stimulation had independent effects, and that the effects were additive. Follow-up of these children into adolescence showed that over time, only the benefits from the stimulation intervention were sustained.[21–23]

Psychosocial stimulation can be used to universally promote healthy child development. This intervention can also be used as part of the management or rehabilitation strategy for children especially at risk, such as those with moderate-severe malnutrition.[15,25] Benefits of psychosocial stimulation as a component of the overall management strategy were also observed for other at-risk children and families such as those affected by HIV/AIDS, although more research is required to support program development.[25] A few studies also show that engaging mothers in psychosocial care for their child may reduce symptoms associated with maternal depression; again, the evidence base can be strengthened through research by ensuring a range of outcome measures affecting child and family are assessed in ongoing and future studies.[26]

Children growing up in poor and disadvantaged communities are often exposed to more than one risk factor that will affect development, health, and nutrition status. Disentangling specific risk factors from the complexity of poverty, and determining which combination of interventions should be provided in any given approach to yield optimal benefits for young children and their families, are important decisions that are likely to be context and program specific. Such decisions must be guided by evidence for effectiveness.

■ OPPORTUNITIES FOR INTERVENTION IN EXISTING HEALTH SERVICES

In Western contexts, ECD services are delivered through health sectors. Over the last 20 years, evidence from developing countries has been emerging and a number of ECD intervention studies conducted in developing countries, including Jamaica, Turkey, Bangladesh, Vietnam, and India, have been reported in peer-reviewed literature. The interventions range from parenting education programs to early childhood education preschool programs, psychosocial stimulation, and nutrition supplementation. Program delivery ranges from home visits to center-based sessions with individual counseling or group sessions and center-based activities for children. Overall, a number of key lessons can be ascertained about what works in ECD.[27] The characteristics of successful ECD programs are shown in Table 21-2.

Despite the knowledge gained from a number of efficacy studies on what interventions work, the coverage of ECD programs remains low. The opportunity to improve coverage of ECD programs through integrating services in existing health systems is another benefit to the integrated approach. Integration into existing health services requires review of the local health care scenario and identification of points of integration for action to promote ECD, prevent developmental loss, and implement rehabilitation strategies (Table 21-3). However, few studies evaluate the feasibility and effect of integrating ECD interventions in existing health systems. While most ECD intervention studies recruited community workers specifically to deliver ECD interventions, Powell and colleagues demonstrated that it was feasible to integrate a psychosocial stimulation program into the primary health care system in an urban setting in Jamaica.[17]

While the authors report significant improvements in the development quotient for the intervention group, several issues were raised for consideration when incorporating such interventions within a government system. First, while it is recognized that the intensity of the intervention is an important parameter of how much children will benefit, health workers were unable to make the recommended weekly visits as a result of the workload. It was determined that if such a program was to be sustained in the health care system, each worker could only support 3 to 5 families in addition to other responsibilities. Second,

Table 21-2. Characteristics of Successful Early Child Development Programs	
CHARACTERISTIC	
Targeted toward disadvantaged children (eg, poverty, malnourished)	**Core features of services**
Initiate services for younger children (younger than 3 years) with strategies to continue throughout early childhood.	
High quality, defined by structure (child-staff ratio, staff training, intensity) and processes (responsive interactions, variety of activities)	
Provide direct services to children and parents (provide families with skills for providing quality psychosocial support to their children) and whether individually or in groups ensure parents can practice with their child.	
Enable children to initiate their own learning through opportunity for exploration of their environment through developmentally appropriate activities. Encourage use of low-cost/no-cost items for exploration.	
Support caregivers (especially mothers).	
Integrated into existing health, nutrition, or education systems	**Important issues for sustainability of services**
Value traditional beliefs and practices combined with evidence-based strategies.	
Developed with and for communities	
Adopt rights-based approaches that value all children.	
Cost-effectiveness and sustainability	

cost of integrating ECD in the health care system was not studied. Costs would include training and intervention materials in addition to a full-time coordinator to support this component of primary health care for children.[17]

Opportunities for integrating new interventions to strengthen ECD outcome in existing health services must first review what is feasible in terms of delivery approach, frequency of intervention delivery, existing personnel, training requirements, resource input requirements, and monitoring processes. The evidence base for the effectiveness of integrating ECD interventions into existing health services in developing countries requires further strengthening.

Table 21-3. Opportunities for Early Child Development Interventions

COVERAGE	EXISTING SERVICES	NEW INTERVENTION TO INTEGRATE
Universal to promote health development and prevent developmental loss	Family Planning Services	Parenting Program and Key Messages for Newborn Development Care
Community-based and primary health care	Antenatal Care	Psychosocial Stimulation
	EPI Program	
	IMCI Program	
	Growth Monitoring Program	Key Developmental Milestones
Selected to support those children at high risk for developmental loss	Nutritional Supplementation	Psychosocial Stimulation and Parenting Programs
Community-based and primary health care	HIV/AIDS Programs	Maternal/Family Support: Mental Health Services
	Community-based/Outreach Programs for vulnerable communities: slums, remote rural/ tribal areas	
	Cash Transfers	Conditions linked to ECD services
Indicated to support those with disability for prevention of secondary conditions	Existing services for children with disabilities	Inclusion in ECD Programs and Outreach/Community-based rehabilitation, including the training of multiskilled development therapists
Community-based and primary health care		

Abbreviations: ECD, early child development; EPI, expanded program on immunization; IMCI, integrated management of childhood illness.

■ CHALLENGES IN SCALING UP EARLY CHILD DEVELOPMENT STRATEGIES

In a review of strategies to avoid the loss of developmental potential, Engle and colleagues noted that awareness of child development is increasing in many countries.[28] Governments, multilateral and bilateral agencies, and civil society have invested in a range of ECD programs. For example, by 2005 the World Bank Group financed loans to 52 lower-income countries for child development programs. Available evaluations of these programs are few but necessary to help meet the challenge of ensuring that ECD strategies will reach the most vulnerable populations. In this review, the integration of ECD programs in existing systems (eg, health care services) was considered a crucial future direction.[28] While many opportunities can be identified for points of integrating ECD interventions in existing health systems, more information is needed to ensure that coverage, quality, and effectiveness are achieved.

Program Sustainability

Program sustainability necessitates investigating feasibility within existing health services. Additional costs may limit the service to selected populations (those identified most at risk) rather than universal coverage. The constraints on going to scale in health-related interventions are well described, and particular attention needs to be paid to such constraints that may occur at many levels of the system. Focus must be paid to the quality of the program as well as the constraints that may prevent scaling up, eg, the level of family and community acceptance, competing priorities within the health program, cost and cost benefit of scaling up, and general environmental and contextual issues that exist. Attention to these issues is required if effective ECD scale-up is to be demonstrated.

Compliance

Compliance at the program or community level within ECD studies has not been extensively reported. It is essential to capture information relating to facilitators and barriers for participation in the program and compliance with activities to understand processes of information flow and behavioral change across the population. For example, families are often highly motivated by seeing their child's improved development, which may encourage them to more regularly visit health services. While at the health service level, the extent to which health personnel comply with the delivery of the additional interventions may need to be identified. This will help identify factors that can be strengthened in a new integrated program design.

Monitoring and Evaluation

Currently, there is no internationally agreed-on set of indicators to monitor child development. Existing programs may have a set of indicators already collected (eg, prevalence of stunting) that might be helpful for evaluating child development status in the population. There may also be value in reviewing whether the addition of ECD interventions benefits other parameters of child health and nutrition status in a given population (eg, reduced morbidity because of improved responsive care strategies). In addition to reanalyzing existing indicators, a simple-to-collect but effective set of population level indicators needs to be agreed on to directly assess child development outcomes.

Policy

The United Nations Convention on the Rights of the Child values the child's right to survival and development. A coordinated ECD policy is important to ensure that children's holistic needs are met by all sectors. A common policy situation is when the education sector has a policy or action plan to improve ECD through effective preschool programming and early childhood education strategies, while the health sector has no specific action plan. Health policy makers need to be convinced of the importance of ECD and the benefits to integrated survival and development services.

Inclusion of Children With Disabilities

While this chapter primarily focuses on ECD promotion for healthy development and reduction of risk for loss of developmental potential, it can also be argued that the rationale for integrated services can be expanded to include children with a disability. International estimates suggest 4.5% prevalence of moderate to severe impairment leading to disability in a developing country. However, it is acknowledged that the accurate estimate of people living with a physical, visual, hearing, communication, or intellectual impairment poses many challenges, not the least of which are the difficulties in identifying impairment in settings where there are limited screening and rehabilitation services.[29,30]

In a recent study on neurodevelopmental outcomes of preterm infants in Bangladesh, the authors comment that while the overall prevalence of disability remained constant over the last decade, there was a shift from more severe disabilities to milder problems related to cognitive impairment, behavioral problems, hearing impairments, and communication impairments. It may be argued that these children will also benefit from the types of interventions suggested.[31] An expanded rationale to include treating physical conditions, reducing the effect of impairments and preventing secondary conditions, and supporting families with additional caregiving demands brings another dimension to the existing services that have yet to be discussed extensively in the ECD literature with respect to developing countries.[32]

Therefore, when integrating new interventions to strengthen overall ECD in health care services, program planners need to review local health scenarios to identify gaps and opportunities. Planning must evaluate the most effective combination of interventions, feasible delivery mode, additional time and cost taken for delivery, and training and materials, as well as monitor the benefits to the development, health, and nutrition status of the target population.

■ FUTURE ACTION

Several important actions must be prioritized to address the challenges mentioned herein, to improve coverage of ECD strategies, and to ensure quality and effectiveness if new interventions are integrated into existing systems.

1. Rigorous research is required to look at the effectiveness of integrating what is known to work from ECD intervention studies in existing health programs.
2. International experts must agree to a minimal set of standard indicators that countries can collect at the national level for ECD across the early year age range. For the health sector, particular focus should be on a set of standards for the first 3 years of life.
3. There must be capacity development of personnel that can plan, educate, and train in ECD in the health services.
4. Health policy makers must be convinced of the case for integrating survival and development services. They must also be persuaded that they have a critical role in improving the development status of children so they will act on it.

■ KEY POINTS

- The loss of developmental potential in more than 200 million young children worldwide and its implications for future human development cannot be ignored.
- The health sector has a critical role in helping to avoid early developmental loss in the first 3 years of life when children are in regular contact with health services. The goal of ECD programs is to promote optimal development by enabling children to thrive and to acquire contextually relevant skills and behaviors.
- Evidence suggests that children with higher risk factors for developmental loss, such as malnourishment or living in poverty, will benefit most from participating in ECD programs.
- Integrated interventions (ie, survival, health, nutrition, stimulation, and maternal support) together with responsive care practices are likely to result in successful child development, health, and nutrition outcomes.

- Research is needed to understand the nature and composition of integration according to local context and feasibility, and to support quality and effectiveness in integrated models for advocacy and capacity development.

■ REFERENCES

1. Black RE, Morris SS & Bryce J (2003) Where and why are 10 million children dying every year? Lancet 361; 2226–2234
2. Jones G, Steketee RW, Black RE et al (2003) How many child deaths can we prevent this year? Lancet 362; 65–71
3. Bryce J, Black RE, Walker N et al (2005) Can the world afford to save the lives of 6million children each year? Lancet 365; 2193–2200
4. UNICEF (2008) State of the World's Child Report. UN: New York
5. Walker S, Wachs T, Gardner J et al. (2007) Child development: risk factors for adverse outcomes in developing countries. Lancet 369; 145–157.
6. Grantham-McGregor S, Cheung YB, Cueto P et al (2007) Developmental potential in the first five years for children in developing countries. Lancet 369; 60–70
7. Shonkoff JP, Phillips DA (Eds) (2004). From Neurones to Neighbourhoods- The Science of Early Child Development National Academy Press: Washington DC.
8. Mustard JF (2006) Early child development and experience based brain development- the scientific underpinnings of the importance of early child development in a globalised world. World Bank International Symposium on Early Child Development- A Priority for Sustained Growth and Equity. 27–29 September 2005.
9. Teicher MH (2003) The neurobiological consequences of early childhood stress and maltreatment. Neuroscience and Biobehavioural Reviews 27; 33–44
10. Teicher MH (2002) Scars that won't heal- The neurobiology of child abuse. Scientific American. March 2003; 68–75.
11. Tremblay RE, Hartup WW, Archer J (Eds) (2005) Developmental Origins of Aggression. The Guilford Press: New York
12. Trembely RE (2004) Physical aggression in early childhood: Trajectories and Predictors. Paediatrics 4; (e) 43–50.
13. Trembley RE (1999) When Social Development Fails in Developmental Health and the Wealth of Nations. Keating DP, Hertzman C (Eds). The Guilford Press: New York
14. Kagitcibasi C, Sunar D, Bekman S (2001). Long-term effects of early intervention: Turkish low-income mothers and children J Appl Dev Psychol 22; 333–61.
15. Hamadani J, Huda S, Khatun F & Grantham-McGregor S (2006) Psychosocial stimulation improves the development of undernourished children in rural Bangladesh. Journal of Nutrition 136; 2645–2652.
16. Ertem IO, Atay G, Bingoler E et al (2006). Promoting child development at sick-child visits: A controlled trial J Amr Acad Paed 118; 124–131
17. Powell C, Baker-Henningham H, Walker S, Gernay J & Grantham-McGregor S (2004). Feasibility of integrating early stimulation into primary care for undernourished Jamaican children: cluster randomised control trial. British Medical Journal 329; 89–92.

18. Richter L (2004). The importance of caregiver-child interactions for the survival and healthy development of young children World Health Organisation: Geneva.
19. Patel V, Rahman A, Jacob KS & Huges M (2004). Effect of maternal mental health on infant growth in low income countries: new evidence from South Asia. British Medical Journal 328; 820–823.
20. Poobalan AS, Aucott LS, Ross L et al. (2007) Effects of treating postnatal depression on mother-infant interaction and child development. British Journal of Psychiatry 191; 378–386.
21. Grantham McGregor S, Powell C, Walker S et al (1994). The long-term follow-up of severely malnourished children who participated in an intervention program. Child Dev 65: 428–39.
22. Grantham McGregor SM, Powell CA, Walker SP, Himes JH (1991). Nutritional supplementation, psychosocial stimulation, and mental development of stunted children: the Jamaican Study. Lancet 338(8758): 1–5
23. Walker SP, Chang SM, Powell CA, Grantham-McGregor SM (2005). Effects of early childhood psychosocial stimulation and nutritional supplementation on cognition and education in growth-stunted Jamaican children: prospective cohort study. Lancet 366:1804–7.
24. Super CM, Herrera MG, Mora JO (1990). Long-term effects of food supplementation and psychosocial intervention on the physical growth of Colombian infants at risk of malnutrition. Child Dev 61; 29–49.
25. WHO (1999). A Critical Link- Interventions for physical growth and psychological development. World Health Organisation: Geneva.
26. King E, De Silva M, Stein A & Patel V (2009) Interventions for Improving the psychosocial well being of children affected by HIV and AIDS. Cochrane Review. The Cochrane Library 2009, Issue 2.
27. Baker-Henningham H, Powell C, Walker S, Grantham-McGregor S (2005). The effect of early stimulation on maternal depression: cluster randomised control trial. Archives of Diseases in Childhood 90; 1230–1234.
28. Engle P, Black M, Behrman J et al. (2007). Strategies to avoid the loss of developmental potential in more than 200 million children in the developing world. Lancet 369; 229–242.
29. Helander E (1992). Prejudice and Dignity: An Introduction to Community-Based Rehabilitation. UNDP: New York.
30. Maulik PK & Darmstadt GL (2007) Childhood disability in low and middle income countries: Overview of screening, prevention, services, legislation, and epidemiology. Pediatrics 120; S1–S55.
31. Khan NZ, Muslima H, Parveen M et al (2006). Neurodevelopmental outcomes of preterm infants in Bangladesh. Pediatrics 118; 280–289.
32. Simeonsson RJ. (1991). Early prevention of childhood disability in developing countries. Int J Rehabil Res 14(1); 1-12

CHAPTER

22

Malnutrition

Karin Karlsson, RD
David Fox II, MD
Philip R. Fischer, MD, FAAP

■ INTRODUCTION

Even in our current affluent high-technology era, more than 1 billion people do not have enough to eat.[1] Malnutrition kills approximately 2 million children per year and contributes to the deaths of approximately 4 million other children. One out of 4 children in developing countries are underweight.[2] Specific micronutrient deficiencies (eg, vitamin A, iron, iodine, zinc) affect more than half the children in developing countries and contribute heavily to additional morbidity and mortality.[3] While nearly two thirds of the world's hungry individuals are in just 7 African and Asian countries,[4] malnutrition is indeed a global problem—global in its distribution as well as the effect it has on the lives of children, families, communities, and entire countries. While overweight and obesity are major problems in developed countries and growing problems in resource-limited countries, this chapter focuses on undernutrition. Indeed, the first of the United Nations Millennium Development Goals is to "end extreme poverty and hunger."[5,6]

■ PEDIATRIC MALNUTRITION

To identify malnutrition it is necessary to know what is meant by being well nourished and where one crosses the line from being nourished to being malnourished.[7] Simply stated, with pediatric malnutrition there is a discrepancy between a child's dietary needs (ie, protein, energy/calories, and micronutrients) and what is actually consumed.[8] Conditions such as wasting, stunting, kwashiorkor, and marasmus are all types of generalized malnutrition and unfortunately are common in many of the world's lower-income countries.[8,9]

Wasting refers to a weight for height more than 2 standard deviations (SD) below a reference population mean. *Stunting* is the state of having a height for age more than 2 SD below a reference population mean. *Underweight* is defined as a weight for age more than 2 SD below the mean of a reference population.

Severe malnutrition can present as kwashiorkor (with edema) or marasmus (without edema). In addition to generalized malnutrition resulting from macronutrient deficiencies, specific micronutrient deficiencies also plague many children in the developing world. In whatever form, insufficient nutrient intake at a young age affects the child's physical stature and neurodevelopmental progress with adverse effects on subsequent mental and cognitive abilities.[10,11] To effectively combat the problem of pediatric malnutrition, it is important to define measurable features of malnutrition so as to accurately identify those who truly are at risk and need nutritional aid while excluding those who do not. The criteria by which the condition is screened will determine who is identified to be at nutritional risk and who receives treatment.[7]

■ GLOBAL SIGNIFICANCE AND CONSEQUENCES

Pediatric malnutrition occurs worldwide, making a global perspective necessary for strategic interventions to reduce mortality rates. Understanding the various etiologies of malnutrition is crucial for successfully combating the problem on a global level. Solutions should be specific for each targeted population, identifying needs, parameters, and goals tailored for that population. Practical, strategic nutrition interventions are necessary to understand and meet specific nutritional needs and deficits in high-risk areas.[11,12]

Collaboration of skills to reduce pediatric malnutrition and the consequent risks of mortality is of great importance. By joining academic, health, economic, and political knowledge and putting policies into place, one might actively combat malnutrition, adequately train staff, and provide the necessary resources.[7] Due to their practical experience and knowledge, health professionals have the opportunity to play a valuable role in initiating action to combat the problem of malnutrition.[12] To help ensure that programs are sustainable and adequate for culturally specific needs, whole communities should be involved, engaging them in the education process. Fighting malnutrition can then be done on a larger scale when knowledge is passed on by those who possess the skills and knowledge needed to help those who are in need.[7,12] Encouraging education and awareness of available resources, and examining proven methodology and current research, are important components in empowering health professionals, communities, families, and individuals.[12]

In addition to malnutrition's direct adverse effects, there are also secondary health, societal, and economic effects. These economic challenges represent a large burden, particularly affecting areas in Asia, Africa, and South America.[7] Adverse effects of widespread malnutrition include

1. *Increased mortality.* Ending avoidable deaths is not merely a financial issue but an ethical challenge in which access to necessary resources tends to predict the chance of survival.[12]

2. *Additive decreases in health.* Individuals with inadequate nutrient stores become more susceptible to illness and have greater difficulty fighting illness. The cycle of illness becomes inevitable in which it is progressively harder for the child to recover.[12]

3. *Loss of educational potential.* Inadequate nutrient intake is shown to affect cognition, the child's ability to learn, and the degree of education achieved, thus affecting the child's ability to succeed in school and potential opportunities that may follow.[11] Severe malnutrition tends to delay the age at which schooling is initiated. Furthermore, children affected by malnutrition are often sick more frequently than other children, causing them to be absent from school more often.[13] Impairment in cognitive development has long-term economic consequences for individuals, families, and nations.

4. *Loss of labor earnings.* A common trend is if malnutrition is not resolved but continues through childhood, individuals' poor health may affect labor forces' earnings throughout that person's lifetime.[12,13]

Addressing such issues is vital in ensuring the future development of affected individuals, communities, and countries.[11]

■ EPIDEMIOLOGY

Incidence, Distribution, and Control of Malnutrition

Current and Historical Trends

Malnutrition continues to be a worldwide problem.[14] In the developing world it is estimated that there are more than 800 million individuals who suffer from various degrees of malnutrition. This currently represents approximately 20% of the developing world's population.[14,15] Pediatric malnutrition is particularly a problem in Asia (ie, Bangladesh, Pakistan, India, China, and Indonesia) and Africa (ie, Democratic Republic of the Congo, Ethiopia, and Somalia).[4] Deficiencies of macronutrients (ie, protein, carbohydrates, and fat) often lead to protein-energy malnutrition (PEM), which is currently the most common type of malnutrition among children in India.[11,15] Current trends in hunger and malnourishment around the world are often associated with the increase of migration to urban settings, as families settle in slums where there is a high prevalence of poverty and hunger.[11] In contrast with the very poorest countries, many others are now seeing trends of children consuming a high intake of fat, which is contributing to a different type of malnutrition, often referred to as *overnutrition*. Despite the high caloric consumption, a balance of sufficient nutrients is often not achieved, which causes other problems such as diet-related chronic diseases.[12]

Africa

Some African countries (ie, Nigeria, Niger, Angola, Malawi, Madagascar, Ghana, Tanzania, and some northern Africa nations) are seeing a decline in malnutrition. In contrast, Africa's eastern countries now have the most rapidly increasing rates of underweight children.[12] Despite progress, malnutrition continues to increase in sub-Saharan Africa. A high incidence of preschool malnutrition is associated with the devastating effect of the HIV/AIDS epidemic.[12] Current predictions suggest that between 2000 and 2020, the overall prevalence of malnutrition in Africa will drop from 34% to 31%. However, because of an increasing population, the number of malnourished children will actually increase from 44 million to 48 million in that same period.[16] The prevalence of malnutrition in sub-Saharan Africa is increasing rapidly, such that it will soon surpass malnutrition in Asia. Projections show that there will soon be an increase in wasted (low weight for height) preschoolers in every region in Africa. East Africa is currently experiencing the highest increase in prevalence and numbers of underweight children.[12]

Asia

The majority (70%) of malnourished children live in Asia. South-central Asia has the world's highest prevalence of wasted children. With substantial increases in dietary fat and sugar intake, the Chinese population reported a significant reduction in the number of undernourished children. Unfortunately, this is contributing to other unhealthy trends in mortality related to chronic diseases, such as coronary vascular disease and type 2 diabetes, in areas that already have high mortality rates.[12,16]

The current and predicted trend toward urban migration of children in rural India is of great concern because of the high prevalence of malnutrition in urban slums. Strategic plans should be initiated to reverse malnutrition among children living in urban slums; these children are a reasonable target population for pro-nutrition activities.[11]

South America, Latin America, and the Caribbean

In South America, malnutrition commonly manifests as stunting and micronutrient deficiency, which are significant public health concerns. A large hurdle in the fight against malnutrition in Latin American countries is the lack of malnutrition-related curricula in health professional training programs.[7] It is predicted that the number of stunted children in Latin America and the Caribbean will decrease between 2000 and 2020.[16] There has been significant progress in the fight against malnutrition in South America, in contrast with Central America, where there has been little progress and acute malnutrition has a high fatality rate. Ending avoidable deaths of malnutrition remains a major health challenge and represents an ethical imperative.[7]

Developed Countries

To a certain degree, malnutrition even affects developed countries; underweight can be seen. But developed countries especially see the other extreme of malnutrition, caused by overnutrition, in which nutrients are eaten in excess, causing an increase in obesity among children. Reasons for this trend have been associated with the increased availability and convenience of calorically dense foods high in sugar and fat, as well as reduced physical activity in children.[16,17]

Pediatric Mortality Related to Malnutrition

Young children bear the greatest brunt of malnutrition.[14] Currently, malnutrition contributes directly or indirectly to more than 50% of all infant deaths.[7,14] Nearly 10 million preschool-aged children die each year; most of these deaths occur in developing countries where malnutrition is a strong factor. Table 22-1 outlines (by region) the prevalence of the various types of PEM in children younger than 5 years. Adequate nutrition would likely prevent many of these tragic deaths.[12]

In developing countries, 31% of preschoolers are underweight, 38% have stunted growth, and 9% show signs of wasting.[15] Figure 22-1 shows that the acute causes of death in malnourished children are often diarrhea, pneumonia, malaria, measles, AIDS, and perinatal conditions. Micronutrient deficiencies, such as inadequate zinc or vitamin A, further

Table 22-1. Prevalence of Protein-Energy Malnutrition Among Children Younger Than 5 Years in Developing Countries

REGION	STUNTING %	UNDERWEIGHT %	WASTING %
Africa	39	28	8
Asia	41	35	10
Latin America and Caribbean	18	10	3
Oceania	31	23	5

From Müller O, Krawinkel M. Malnutrition and health in developing countries. *CMAJ.* 2005;173(3):279–286. © Access Copyright. Reprinted with permission. No further reproductions are permitted.

Figure 22-1. Causes of Death Among Children Younger Than 5 Years Between 2000 and 2003 Worldwide

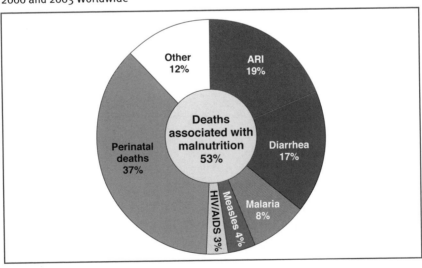

Abbreviation: ARI, acute respiratory infection.

From Müller O, Krawinkel M. Malnutrition and health in developing countries. *CMAJ.* 2005;173(3):279–286. © Access Copyright. Reprinted with permission. No further reproductions are permitted.

contribute by increasing the severity and length of infectious illnesses. With nutrition affecting immunity, malnutrition frequently contributes to infection-related deaths. Continuing a vicious cycle, malnutrition leads to prolonged infectious illnesses, which then lead to increased caloric needs during a time of anorexia, thus further worsening nutritional status. Similarly, gastrointestinal diseases and malnutrition combine to further decrease intestinal absorption of nutrients, leaving the child even more vulnerable to subsequent illnesses.[12]

Low birth weight is often linked to poor maternal nutrition and can, in part, be prevented by improved prenatal nutrition. Intrauterine growth retardation leads to low birth weight (less than 2,500 g) in children. Children who are born with low birth weight are at high risk for stunting, continued underweight, increased infant mortality, and more chronic diseases during childhood.[12]

■ ETIOLOGY

Environmental Factors

The etiology of malnutrition is multifaceted and best described when the many factors contributing to its cause are examined.[11] On a population level, the problem goes deeper than a simple lack of food being available in the home. Despite etiologic complexity and regional variance, factors contributing to global pediatric malnutrition in developing countries include

1. Food production, intake, and availability[15]
2. Political and economic situation, and overall poverty[10,15]
3. Prevalence of sickness, infectious diseases, and access to and quality of health services[15]
4. Seasonal natural disasters and climate conditions[15]
5. Maternal nutritional status and breastfeeding habits[15]
6. Education level, sanitation practices, and access to uncontaminated water[15]
7. Availability and effectiveness of nutrition programs for the population[15]
8. Cultural and religious food customs and practices[15]
9. Most immediate and detrimental causes—inadequate dietary intake with severe and repeated infectious diseases[15]

Poverty

Poverty is often seen as an underlying theme in malnutrition and food insecurity. However, reducing the prevalence of malnutrition has the potential of simultaneously contributing to reducing poverty. Good nutritional status not only contributes to lessening the risk of diet-related disease; slowing the progression of some diseases, such as AIDS; and increasing the survival rate of malaria, but is also a significant factor in improving learning and educational capabilities. Better educational outcomes can be expected if good nutrition is provided in childhood. Improved nutrition directly reduces poverty by contributing to increased productivity, thus creating a healthier workforce. Another way in which nutrition directly affects poverty is by its relationship to health care costs. Individuals who have a good nutritional base tend to need fewer days to recover from sickness, are less likely to suffer from diet-related chronic diseases, have an increased likelihood of surviving malaria, and have a slower onset of AIDS, thus reducing costs otherwise needed for health care. There is also a positive correlation between improved nutritional status and the empowerment of women.[12,18]

Inadequate Food Intake, Availability, and Security

Food security is often seen in the context of a nation's ability to produce adequate food for the entire population. However, food security for an individual depends on the national situation as well as the personal availability of and access to that food.[19,20] Food insecurity "exists whenever the availability of nutritionally adequate and safe foods or the ability to acquire acceptable foods in socially acceptable ways is limited or uncertain."[21] Viewed from the positive side, "Food security exists when all people, at all times, have physical and economic access to sufficient, safe nutrition food to meet their dietary needs and food preference for an active and healthy life."[20]

Discrepancies in food security occur within family units in which adequate food may be available but not distributed in accordance to varying needs of family members. This in turn may cause malnutrition in some family members while sparing others.[19] According to the Food and Agriculture Organization of the United Nations, 18% of the population in the developing world was undernourished in the mid-1990s, presumably related to insecure food sources. The situation improved slightly to "just" 17% between 1990 and 2001.[12]

There are varying degrees of food insecurity. Some people experience insecurity but do not necessarily have hunger or malnourishment. Others have micronutrient deficiency diseases or are food deprived and severely malnourished. Identifying at-risk populations is a helpful step in developing effective preventive interventions to obviate detrimental physical and economic outcomes.[20] Table 22-2 shows different levels of food insecurity and examples of what they may look like.

Table 22-2. Levels of Household Food Insecurity Experienced Across Cultures

LEVEL	DESCRIPTION	ILLUSTRATION
Core domains	The deepest structure, the universal food insecurity experience	Inadequate quality of food
Sub-domains	Elements of core domains that are likely to be of concern in many but possibly not all cultures	Lack of dietary diversity
Items	Expression of sub-domains using culturally relevant examples and language	Limited food variety offered to child; eg, just rice and vegetable curry

From Coates J, Frongillo EA, Rogers BL, Webb P, Wilde PE, Houser R. Commonalities in the experiences of household food insecurity across cultures: what are measures missing? *J Nutr.* 2006;136(5):1438S–1448S, with permission from American Society for Nutrition.

Reasons for Food Insecurity

Although there are instances in which children are malnourished because of a community-wide lack of adequate intake due to limited food access, there are some areas where children are not meeting adequate food requirements even though there is not a food shortage.[19] One reason (of many) is lack of knowledge of sufficient intake of the various food groups needed for health during different stages of life. In fact, nutritional education and adequate provision of nutritional intake have the potential to prevent low birth weight deliveries and malnutrition in poor urban households for women of childbearing age. Malnutrition becomes especially high risk in situations in which there is not a responsible caregiver to look after and care for a child. A child is at particular risk for malnutrition between the ages of 6 months and 2 years because she cannot provide her own food and is particularly dependent on someone else to do so.[19]

Solutions to Food Insecurity

One approach to resolving food insecurity is by educating women about the specific needs for them and their infants to avoid deficits and prevent nutrition-related complications.[12] There are various approaches that may be used to reach this population; even the use of mass media, such as television and radio, may have the potential to educate through relevant nutrition messages.[12]

Sickness and Disease

The majority of pediatric morbidity and mortality in the developing world is the consequence of

1. Acute respiratory infection
2. Diarrheal disease
3. Malaria
4. Measles
5. HIV/AIDS
6. Anemia
7. Maternal factors

Malnutrition aggravates and is aggravated by each of these conditions.

Acute Respiratory Infection

Pneumonia is one of the leading causes of pediatric mortality and morbidity, causing approximately 20% (3 million per year) of all deaths occurring in children younger than 5 years; most take place in developing countries and are amenable to health and nutritional interventions.[22] There are many nutrition-related factors that positively correlate to the risk of contracting pneumonia, including low birth weight, anemia, acute malnutrition, rickets, and lack of breastfeeding.[22]

Children in developing countries are commonly deficient in zinc, which is an important micronutrient specifically involved in cell growth and differentiation. Severe deficiency can lead to stunting of growth, an impaired immune system, anorexia, and impaired cognitive ability.[23] In addition, a child suffering from zinc deficiency is at increased risk of contracting pneumonia. Insufficient zinc stores contribute to a higher risk of mortality and morbidity, as well as pneumonia severity.[12]

Zinc supplementation prevents and reduces the severity of respiratory illness primarily in children who have severely depleted zinc stores. Healthy children who preventively receive zinc supplementation have fewer incidences of lower respiratory illness. Carefully monitored zinc supplementation programs in areas where zinc deficiency is common would likely improve child health. Children with marginal or very poor nutritional status are especially likely to benefit from supplementation.[22]

Vitamin D deficiency and rickets are associated with increased risks of acute respiratory infection and death from pneumonia,[24,25] which is likely related to hypovitaminosis D causing reductions in B cells and natural killer cell numbers.[26]

Promotion of breastfeeding and maternal lactation education enhances a child's immune system and gives the child the advantage of protection against contracting pneumonia at an early age. While the protective mechanisms of breastfeeding are not completely understood, current research indicates that exclusive breastfeeding in the first 6 months of life protects the infant's immune system by maturational, anti-inflammatory, immunomodulatory, and antimicrobial actions. On average, children who are not breastfed spend longer periods in the hospital with acute respiratory infection, are more likely to contract pneumonia, and often need multiple antibiotic regimens for successful treatment, all of which contribute to an overall increased mortality rate. By initiating and implementing effective community programs, targeting specific risk factors, the incidence of pneumonia may be reduced and its complications prevented.[22]

Diarrhea

There has been great progress in reducing diarrhea-related mortality over the past 20 years, which is largely related to an increased use of oral rehydration solution (ORS). Approximately 4.6 million children died each year from diarrhea in the early 1980s. Currently, about 1.5 million die of diarrheal disease each year.[27] Notwithstanding this improvement, diarrhea remains a leading reason for morbidity and mortality in much of the developing world. Up to 30% of hospital admissions and a fourth of pediatric deaths in developing countries are associated with diarrheal infections.[28,29] In many cases, diarrhea can lead to undernutrition in children, contributing to compromised immune function, increased incidence of hospitalization, and even increased mortality rates.[30] Box 22-1 outlines the most common reasons for hospitalization in children with diarrhea in lower-income countries.[29] In the case of acute diarrhea, overall survival rates have improved; however, incidence remains relatively unchanged.[28] Clearly, diarrhea and malnutrition interact in devastating ways, with each aggravating the other.

Box 22-1. Contributing Factors Increasing Risk of Hospitalization Due to Diarrhea

- Malnutrition
- Diarrheal episode lasting longer than 7 days
- Low socioeconomic status
- Poor sanitation at home
- Presence of *Escherichia coli* in stool
- Parents with poor education and high multiparity
- Unawareness of benefits of using oral rehydrating solutions in dehydrated children

From Khalili B, et al. Risk factors for hospitalization of children with diarrhea in Shahrekord, Iran. *Iran J Clin Infect Dis.* 2006;1:131–136

Intervention and Prevention

Much success in the decrease in mortality rate associated with acute diarrhea is because of successful implementation of use of oral rehydration therapy. Breastfeeding education is another factor that has minimized incidence and severity in the pediatric population.[27] Basic nutritionally sound interventions to prevent and manage diarrhea and thus prevent subsequent fatality include

• Breastfeeding promotion
• Appropriate complementary feeding (eg, use of nutritional weaning foods when transitioning beyond exclusive breastfeeding)
• Hygiene and sanitation
• Zinc and vitamin A supplementation
• Oral rehydration therapy
• Education of these practices

Breastfeeding

Breastfeeding has a protective effect against the incidence of diarrhea. Breastfed infants tend to have lower incidence and duration of general illnesses compared with non-breastfed infants. Lactoferrin and lysozyme, which are present in breast milk, may play a protective role. Lactoferrin has bacteriostatic and bactericidal activity, protecting against a large range of harmful pathogens even when the infant's iron stores are low. Lysozyme kills gram-positive bacteria.

Encouraging mothers to exclusively breastfeed for the initial 6 months not only reduces the risk of diarrhea related to unsanitary formula-feeding practices but also provides biologic protection against diarrhea and other illnesses by enhancing the infant's immune system.[30]

Sanitation

The etiology of some diarrhea is of bacterial and viral origin associated with a lack of sanitation, hygiene, and clean water. Vaccinations for rotavirus, the primary source of viral diarrhea, are commonly used and shown to be effective in Latin America, the United States, and Europe. It is estimated that approximately 30% of diarrheal illness could be eradicated by simply following sanitary hand-washing guidelines.[27]

Zinc Supplementation

The use of zinc in treating diarrhea in children older than 6 months is shown to be safe and beneficial. Studies indicate that giving ORS together with zinc reduces the risk of morbidity caused by diarrhea, as well as hospitalization. Zinc supplements given for 10 to 14 days following an episode of acute diarrhea can prevent subsequent episodes over ensuing months. Providing this supplement may also be financially beneficial because it reduces the overall cost of antidiarrheal drugs and can prevent or reduce hospital stay duration.[27,31]

Hydration and Electrolytes

Optimal care is vital to prevent possible adverse outcomes from high fluid losses and electrolyte imbalances present in diarrheal episodes. A standardized ORS was first created in 1978 by the World Health Organization (WHO) and United Nations Children's Fund (UNICEF) to prevent and treat diarrhea. Since then, millions of childhood deaths have been avoided secondary to the successful treatment of diarrhea with ORS. Initially, the formula replaced needed nutrients and fluid but did not reduce the volume of stool or duration of the diarrheal episode. When used to treat children and infants, the formula tended to be some-what hyperosmolar compared with their bodies' plasma, which caused hypernatremia and created an osmotic-related diarrhea. In response to this problem, modified solutions were made with a lower sodium con-tent, creating a more favorable, lower osmolarity that proved to be effec-tive. Table 22-3 outlines the composition of the original ORS formula and the modified glucose ORS formula.[30,32]

Oral, instead of intravenous (IV), rehydration is safer and more effec-tive in treating malnourished children with diarrhea even when they are moderately dehydrated. In fact, IV fluids given to severely malnour-ished children can precipitate or exacerbate existing heart failure, which may be fatal. For this reason, IV fluids should never be used in severely malnourished children unless the child is in shock. Osmotic diarrhea is likely the case if diarrhea increases when a hyperosmolar starter formula (eg, F-75) is used in malnourished children with diarrhea but decreases when the glucose load is reduced. In such cases, switching to a formula

Table 22-3. Composition of Oral Rehydration Solution		
CONTENT	**G-ORS**	**ORS**
Sodium	75 mmol/L	90 mEq/L
Potassium	20 mmol/L	20 mEq/L
Chloride	80 mmol/L	98 mEq/L
Citrate	10 mmol/L	290 mg/dL
Glucose	20.0 g/L	20 g/L (111 mmol/L)
Osmolarity	224 mOsm/L	311 mOsm/L

Abbreviations: G-ORS, glucose oral rehydration solution; ORS, oral rehydration solution.

Adapted from Zavaleta N, Figueroa D, Rivera J, Sánchez J, Alfaro S, Lönnerdal B. Efficacy of rice-based oral rehydration solution containing recombinant human lactoferrin and lysozyme in Peruvian children with acute diarrhea. *J Pediatr Gastroenterol Nutr.* 2007;44(2):258–264; and Alam NH, Yunus M, Faruque AS, et al. Symptomatic hyponatremia during treatment of dehydrating diarrheal disease with reduced osmolarity oral rehydration solution. *JAMA.* 2006;296(5):567–573

with a lower osmotic load is recommended.[33] Alternatively, Rehydration Solution for Malnutrition (ReSoMal) (detailed later in this chapter) should be used for malnourished children with diarrhea. While the initial phases of malnutrition management in children with diarrhea focus on fluids, subsequent phases move toward stepwise nutritional support.[35]

Malaria

It is estimated that malaria causes 1 million childhood deaths each year, mostly in Africa. Most of the casualties (90%) are children younger than 5 years.[27] Despite substantial progress in the prevention and management of malaria, it is still considered to be "out of control" in sub-Saharan Africa and has a devastating effect on the child mortality rate.[9] Countries with a high prevalence of malaria often have high incidences of malnutrition. Factors contributing to an increased risk of contracting malaria include poor nutritional status, underweight, and the rainy season.[9] Severity, longevity, and mortality are affected by micronutrient deficiencies, such as vitamin A and zinc, as well as general malnutrition and being underweight. Poor nutritional status creates an additional burden on public health (ie, financially, resources, and staff) in such areas. Research also suggests that socioeconomic factors may contribute to malarial morbidity in situations in which poverty is the major contributor to poor nutritional status.[9,12]

Signs and Symptoms

Malaria is sometimes defined as "any parasitemia plus fever." Anemia almost always accompanies severe malaria and is considered one of the main features. Contrary to the previous belief that chronic malnutrition is a protective factor against malaria morbidity, current research reveals that children who are malnourished are more susceptible to malaria and have a harder time fighting it because of a compromised immune response to the pathogens involved.[9]

Interventions

Interventions for malaria include insecticide-treated bed nets, complementary feeding, and prompt antimalarial use.[27] Because nutritional status strongly correlates with susceptibility to and recovery from malaria, providing appropriate dietary needs has the potential to positively affect morbidity and mortality. Currently, early diagnosis and treatment are the primary methods by which malaria control is attempted in sub-Saharan Africa; bed nets and residual insecticides are used in communities and intermittent preventive treatment is being explored. Because anemia is considered an independent risk factor for contracting malaria, it is reasonable to assume that by identifying and preventing factors contributing to the prevalence of anemia, a decrease in the susceptibility to and severity of malaria may occur as well. Studies suggest that by including nutritional counseling and education for the malnourished population as part of malaria-control programs, one might directly target one of the main contributing factors of malaria.

Health professionals of various disciplines should be able to identify children with poor nutritional status that would benefit from such education. Education should be provided for mothers, families, and the susceptible population. These programs should include recommendations for feeding programs that focus on improving nutritional health to decrease overall morbidity caused by malaria.[9]

Measles

The incidence of death associated with measles is significantly higher in lower-income countries when compared with higher-income countries; there were approximately 770,000 deaths in 2000 and 164,000 in 2008.[35,36] The severity of existing malnutrition contributes proportionally to the risk of death from infections such as measles, and prolonged measles illness often leads to subsequent malnutrition. Approximately 45% of all measles-related pediatric deaths are directly attributable to malnutrition.[7,9,13] Preschool-aged children are at particular risk of serious morbidity and mortality from measles.[35] There is also some correlation between childhood mortality from measles and maternal education level, presumably because maternal education leads to improved nutritional activities and health-seeking behaviors.[37] Other reasons for increased mortality rates associated with measles in developing countries include young age at which the infection occurs, lack of previous vaccination, malnutrition, vitamin A deficiency, and compromised immune system due to other underlying conditions. Environmental factors, such as crowding, lack of access to medical care, poor hygiene, and the presence of famine and warfare, also contribute to its prevalence, complications, and severity.[19,35] Infants are often initially protected by antibodies received maternally and during breastfeeding. However, in cases in which children are born to mothers with compromised immune systems, such as mothers who are HIV-infected, susceptibility and severity to measles tend to be heightened.[35]

Signs and Symptoms

There are many complications commonly seen during and after contracting measles, which affect practically every organ system in the body. Pneumonia tends to be the most common severe complication and contributes to the risk of mortality. Nutrition-related complications seen with measles include

- Hypocalcemia
- Renal failure
- Malnutrition
- Diarrhea
- Croup
- Stomatitis
- Death

Common complications occurring after measles include

- Mouth sores, including cancrum oris
- Decreased food intake
- Protracted diarrhea
- Weight loss
- Severe protein calorie malnutrition
- Disruption of epithelial surfaces

Having an underlying vitamin A deficiency increases the risk of fatality in children with measles in developing countries. Vitamin A deficiency also makes the child more susceptible to severe keratitis, corneal scarring, and blindness. This is one of the most common causes of acquired childhood blindness in developing countries. The risk of death associated with pneumonia caused by measles is also increased when lacking adequate stores of vitamin A.

Children who are already suffering from malnutrition and are infected with measles tend to have more severe complications and a higher risk of death due to a weak immune system and prolonged excretion of the immune system. On the other hand, having measles also makes the child more susceptible to malnutrition because of decreased intake while having higher metabolic needs, often causing significant protein loss. Anthropometric measures, such as weight for age, also tend to be significantly reduced in cases in which measles were developed early on in life.[35]

Interventions

Provision of adequate nutrition, including vitamin A micronutrient supplementation, has proven to be effective and necessary in treating measles. Along with antibiotics for bacterial superinfections, these interventions reduce the risk of mortality.

Because measles often leads to a deficiency in vitamin A and vitamin A treatment of children with measles is known to reduce morbidity and mortality, the WHO recommends including vitamin A as part of the treatment plan for all children who have measles. This treatment has shown to reduce the rate of mortality by approximately 50% in countries where the incidence of mortality tends to be high. The suggested regimen for hospitalized patients is vitamin A treatments once daily for 2 days.

- Twelve months and older: 200,000 IU
- Six to 12 months: 100,000 IU[35]
- Younger than 6 months: 50,000 IU

According to the WHO recommendation, to reduce the risk of further infections and improve general health, it is beneficial to regularly continue vitamin A supplementation every 4 to 6 months in children between 6 and 59 months of age.[38] Studies also show that in cases in which pneumonia is developed secondary to measles, large doses of vitamin A supplementation have a favorable effect on the incidence and severity of secondary pneumonia. The current recommendation is a total of 400,000 IU on the first 24 hours of admission.[39]

Prevention

Vaccination is the most effective way to reduce the incidence of measles; it protects more than 90% of those inoculated. Before vaccine use, between 95% and 98% of children were infected by the measles virus by the age of 18 years. While becoming one of the most economically beneficial health interventions, the measles vaccine also saves the lives of approximately 5 million children yearly who would likely have been a casualty to measles without it.[35]

HIV/AIDS

Despite progress in the fight against malnutrition, the rapid spread of HIV/AIDS presents a significant hurdle to eradicating malnutrition and risks reversing previous progress.[12] HIV currently affects approximately 2.5 million children younger than 15 years worldwide, causes premature death, and devastates the family structure, leaving many children orphaned with limited resources and access to food.[27] The majority of new cases involving children younger than 10 years are caused by the transmission occurring between mother and child.[12] Infant mortality rates are directly associated with the prevalence of malnutrition and its complications in those who have contracted HIV/AIDS.[28] Thus, nutritional intervention to prevent and halt the progress of malnutrition in children with HIV/AIDS plays an important role in reducing overall mortality rates. Dietary education plays a vital role in the solution, equipping mothers and other care providers with adequate and accurate knowledge of safe feeding practices for their infants to minimize risk and complications.[12]

Nutrition Intervention

The body's nutritional demands increase prior to the symptomatic phase of HIV. Weight loss and malnutrition are strongly associated with increased risks of mortality. Providing adequate nutrition has shown to slow the progression of HIV to AIDS. The primary nutritional concern is to optimize daily dietary intake to meet increased estimated needs and maintain a good nutritional status. By doing so, good nutritional health can contribute to quality of life by providing nutrients necessary to function in daily activities. Medical treatment also tends to be more effective and symptoms reduced when an adequate diet is maintained. Dietary needs increase and malnutrition becomes more prevalent as infection progresses.

Strategies for nutritional intervention include multiple components. Because HIV/AIDS often devastates the family structure, communities play a central role in nutrition care. Awareness of adequate nutritional intake, meal planning, and nutritional counseling are needed to provide for nutritional needs. It is important to be aware that certain antiviral drugs often used to slow the progression of HIV/AIDS alter the metabolism of energy, fat, and bone. These drugs may also alter the way various nutrients are used in the body, the amount eaten, and overall nutritional status.[12] It is common to use replacement feeding as part of the intervention.[27]

Prevention

Replacement Feeding

It is imperative that mothers are correctly informed about the risks and benefits of available feeding options for their newborns to minimize the spread of HIV and to reduce infant mortality risks associated with malnutrition. The following recommendations are based on those proposed by the UNFPA/UNICEF/WHO/UNAIDS Inter-Agency Task Team on Mother-to-Child Transmission of HIV.[12] To reduce transmission of HIV, replacement feeding is recommended over breastfeeding only when it is "acceptable, feasible, affordable, sustainable and safe."[12] Possible clinical risks associated with unsafe replacement feeding practices include infections, diarrhea, and malnutrition.[28] Therefore, optimal feeding practices must be evaluated on an individual basis to determine the risks associated with the woman's situation; the evaluation should also include the social environment and circumstances where the feeding will take place.[12]

- Breastfeeding is recommended early in life if any of these requirements are not met. There is an absolute risk of HIV transmission (10% to 20%) for breastfed infants.[12]
- A study showed lower HIV transmission when infants were exclusively breastfed for the first 3 months rather than using replacement feeding and breastfeeding.[12]

Multiple studies confirm the likely relationship between nutritional status and HIV transmission. Implementing vitamin supplementation decreases mother-to-child infection transmission when nutritionally compromised mothers receive a multivitamin supplement while breastfeeding.[12]

Multifactorial Anemia

Anemia is commonly seen in infants and children in developing countries and is often prevalent in more than 50% of the pediatric population. Iron deficiency affects more than a billion people worldwide; thus, it is the most common nutrient deficiency. However, many additional factors contribute to the etiology of widely prevalent anemia, which contributes to the difficulty of reducing its prevalence. If hemoglobin levels are the sole test available, the etiologic diagnosis of anemia will often be missed.[40-42]

Many illnesses and diseases are more difficult to treat if simultaneously battling anemia due to poor treatment response, resulting in an increased risk of morbidity. Pediatric anemia is also known to have a negative effect on learning, language, and development, often resulting in poor scholastic results. It can cause poor coordination, motor, and behavioral skills.[43,44]

Pathophysiology

The etiology of anemia is multifactorial. Figure 22-2 outlines the major factors influencing an infant's total iron stores.[45]

Factors leading to anemia include
- Poor dietary intake and choices
  —Inadequate intake of food containing heme iron
  —Presence of nutritional deficiencies
  —Poor intake and practices when weaning infant from breast milk
- Inappropriate intake of cow's milk
  —High intake of calcium inhibiting iron absorption
  —Milk protein intolerance provoking intestinal blood loss

Figure 22-2. Factors Contributing to Infant Iron Status

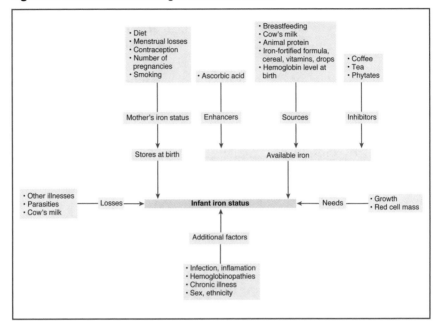

From Lozoff B, Kaciroti N, Walter T. Iron deficiency in infancy: applying a physiologic framework for prediction. *Am J Clin Nutr.* 2006;84(6):1412–1421, with permission from American Society for Nutrition.

- Lack of breastfeeding in the first 4 months of infancy
- Excessive blood loss
- Parasitic infections
  — Presence of malaria or hookworm contributing to poor anemia
- Cellular micronutrient deficiencies
  — Iron
  — Retinol (vitamin A)
  — Folate (vitamin B₉)
    ▪ Associated with macrocytic anemia (elevated mean corpuscular volume)
  — Cobalamin (vitamin B₁₂)
    ▪ Associated with macrocytic anemia (elevated mean corpuscular volume)
- Presence of infections and diseases
  — Presence of malaria, HIV/AIDS, and chronic or repeated infections
- Premature birth
  — Smaller amounts of absolute iron in the body, predisposing the infant to postnatal iron deficiency

- Genetic blood disorders
  - Genetic variations
  - Common within particular ethnic groups
  - Affecting hemoglobin production[19,40–42,45,46]

Malarial episodes are often associated with anemia; sometimes anemia preceded the acute malarial infection. There is a complex relationship among malnutrition, anemia, and malaria, with each affecting the other. Typically, severe anemia is a symptom of severe malaria. It is important to ensure that treatment and prevention strategies include antimalarial agents, as well as address the nutritional issues present to provide optimal treatment and ultimately reduce the incidence of childhood deaths.[9] Helminth infection should be investigated or presumptively treated in anemic, malnourished children in areas where helminthiasis is common.

Anemia is often present in hospitalized HIV-infected children. Studies show that the presence of HIV infection tends to increase the risk of anemia up to 6 times that of a child who does not have HIV. In many cases, a poor hemoglobin value is indicative of the progression of HIV to AIDS. Specific factors making HIV-infected infants more prone to anemia include

- Repeated illness
- Early age of HIV infection
- Low maternal CD4+ lymphocyte count[40]

Because vitamin A plays a role in the creation of new blood cells, a retinol deficiency also contributes to anemia. Infants are born with very poor stores of this vitamin and rely heavily on dietary intake to supply needs. In most cases, the mother's breast milk contains an easily absorbed and adequate source. However, if the mother is deficient (approximately 20% of cases in developing countries), breast milk will not supply adequate needs and the infant is likely to become anemic.[40]

Intervention

Because the presence of anemia in an infant is strongly related to the mother's nutrient intake, a key intervention is to encourage expecting mothers to consume adequate amounts of iron, as well as other prenatal vitamins, to optimize their nutritional status. In some cases, providing iron supplementation to children may be necessary to treat anemia. Options for such supplementation include formulas fortified with bioavailable iron or, in some cases, medical supplementation. However, it is important to verify the etiology to ensure that the right treatment is provided because lack of iron may not be the root cause of anemia. Providing additional iron may in fact worsen the problem instead of curing the anemia, especially in cases of infection and certain other micronutrient deficiencies. The safety of iron supplementation in the case of HIV-related anemia is unknown. However, there is currently not sufficient documentation of adverse effects that outweigh potential benefits to discourage implementation of iron.[38,40]

Prevention

To prevent and treat anemia, great care should be given to provide infant and mother with optimal nutrition and health. Initially exclusive breast-feeding in infancy has shown a positive effect in preventing anemia, and exclusive breastfeeding for 6 months typically provides adequate iron for the infant.[40] Recommendations for additional preventive measures during pregnancy, according to the WHO guidelines, include daily iron-folate supplementation of 60 mg of iron and 400 mg of folate during the final 6 months of pregnancy. Twice this daily dose should be used if the mother is severely anemic. It is also beneficial to use a multivitamin supplement that includes vitamin B complex, vitamin C, and vitamin E to reduce the risk of adverse pregnancy outcomes and encourage healthy birth weight. It is recommended that mothers continue taking a multi-vitamin while breastfeeding to reduce infant mortality and morbidity, as well as increase the infant's CD4+ cell counts. Multivitamins are also recommended for HIV-positive women during pregnancy and lactation.[38] In remote locations where there are insufficient resources to determine underlying causes of anemia, once malaria and serious infection is ruled out, many physicians treat empirically with iron, folate, and anti-helminths (in areas where helminthiasis is common).

Breastfeeding/Maternal Advantage

The nutritional status of the mother giving birth has a large effect on the future nutritional well-being of the infant and later on as the child develops. Malnutrition may be replicated from generation to generation. When a malnourished pregnant woman gives birth, the baby is often malnourished as well; this cycle of malnutrition is likely to continue if there is not an intervention.[12]

Reducing malnutrition, especially in women, may be a key to reducing many cases of infant malnutrition and thus preventing the continuation of intergenerational malnutrition and poverty. Children who are already malnourished in the womb are unable to fully catch up to the nutritional status of infants who were not malnourished in the womb. Children born with a low birth weight are at a greater risk of

• Increased morbidity and mortality
• Poor neurodevelopment outcomes

- Reduced strength and work capacity
- Chronic disease in adulthood
- Shorter and lighter than normal birth weight infants on average[12]

The first 2 years of life are deemed critical to the effect of nutrition on health, as these years represent a child's most rapid growth and most critical period of brain development. Sadly, the devastating consequences of poor nutrition are only partially reversible at best, which underscores the need for preventive measures, as well as early recognition and treatment of nutrition-related disorders.

■ DIAGNOSIS AND MANAGEMENT OF MALNUTRITION

More than 50% of all childhood mortality is directly or indirectly related to undernutrition.[46] Of the 556 million children living in lower-income countries, 112 million are underweight and 55 million are wasted. Of these 55 million, 36 million, or 65% of these children, are found to be moderately malnourished.[47] Severely and moderately malnourished children are at increased risk for short- and long-term mortality and morbidity, including cognitive deficiencies that may feed the cycle of poverty in many of these countries. Clearly, diagnostic screening tools are needed that will accurately identify those children at risk for mortality and morbidities associated with undernutrition early in the course of their disease. It is important that these tools identify not only those at immediate risk of mortality from malnutrition (ie, those with severe malnutrition) but also those who display warning signs of impending severe malnutrition and its sequelae (ie, those with signs of moderate malnutrition or growth faltering).

Many approaches have been developed over the years in an attempt to identify and categorize undernutrition disorders. In 1956, Gomez introduced the concept of measuring anthropometric data to identify malnutrition by using weight for age as a clinical indication for PEM.[7,48] To determine the parameters of normal nutritional status, Gomez used a comparative reference population with the mean reference value serving as the standard against which subjects were compared (using *percent of the mean*, not percentiles, as on routine American growth curves).[7] Table 22-4 outlines the criteria for mild to severe weight-for-age loss according to Gomez's criteria.

In 1970, Wellcome proposed a method of distinguishing among different clinical forms of malnutrition by using weight for age as well as the absence or presence of edema. Through his definition a differentiation was made among various types of PEM, such as kwashiorkor and marasmus, as outlined in Table 22-5.

Table 22-4. Gomez's Criteria of Malnutrition (Weight-for-Age Loss)

Mild	10% to 25% deficit of the reference
Moderate	26% to 40% deficit of the reference
Severe	More than 40% deficit of the reference

Based on Gómez F. Desnutrición. *Bol Med Hosp Infant Mex.* 1946;3:543–551

Table 22-5. Wellcome's Classification of Protein-Energy Malnutrition

WEIGHT FOR AGE	EDEMA PRESENT	EDEMA ABSENT
80% to 60%	Kwashiorkor	Underweight
Less than 60%	Marasmic kwashiorkor	Marasmus

From Gernaat HB, Voorhoeve HW. A new classification of acute protein-energy malnutrition. *J Trop Pediatr.* 2000;46(2):97–106, with permission from Oxford University Press.

Despite promising progress, both definitions have a few limitations. One of the problems in using these diagnostic tools is that exact age is not always available or known, making comparison to a certain standard difficult. Furthermore, when evaluating normal weight for age, factors such as stunting and wasting should also be considered in the equation.[48] For example, a stunted child who is chronically malnourished may have only modestly reduced weight for age. In this instance, the child's degree of malnutrition may be underestimated if only weight for length is compared. The true extent of his nutritional deficiency would best be exhibited with height-for-age comparison. This demonstrates an important point in the diagnosis of malnutrition disorders—the best way to diagnose malnutrition is not through the evaluation of a single anthropometric measurement. Rather, malnutrition is best diagnosed and defined by evaluating numerous anthropometric measurements (as defined in the following section) in combination with a developmental screening and clinical evaluation for evidence of macronutrient and micronutrient deficiencies.

■ ANTHROPOMETRY

Numerous anthropometric measurements may be used in evaluating the nutritional status of a child. As already mentioned, weight for age may be used to determine if the child is underweight or overweight. Height for age may be used to determine if the child is stunted. Weight for height is used to determine if the child is wasted or obese; this particular measurement is useful when the exact age of the child is unknown. When combined with the presence or absence of edema, weight for height may be the most useful measurement in assessing those who are severely malnourished. For this reason among others, this measurement is the preferred method of diagnosing severe malnutrition based on a one-time measurement only. Furthermore, other measurements, such as mid-upper arm circumference (MUAC) and tri-fold skin thickness, can be used to determine the degree of wasting of lean body mass or loss of subcutaneous fat, respectively. Many of these measurements are most useful when measured in series over time. In this way, loss of growth velocity can be identified early, with subsequent intervention also initiated early. Unfortunately, this most desirable strategy is often not possible in the developing world. Many children are seen only once and often in an emergency situation. As a result, the WHO and UNICEF developed a new strategy for identifying those children most at risk for mortality and morbidity from undernutrition. Box 22-2 provides a summary of the new elements included in the WHO child growth standards. These criteria have been clinically shown to identify those children most likely to benefit from nutritional intervention, making this diagnostic tool perhaps the most clinically useful.[49]

The aims of this new set of references are to represent normal early childhood growth and be applicable for the pediatric population across ethnic, socioeconomic status, and feeding types. Therefore, the new guidelines were developed through evaluating children from numerous countries around the world who were faced with conditions such as poor diets and infections likely to affect growth patterns and development. These children were born to mothers who practiced healthy breastfeeding habits and did not smoke during or after pregnancy. The new guidelines recognize that despite different environmental factors, children throughout the world grow and develop similarly when their nutritional and health care needs are met.[50] Because these new reference anthropometric values were developed from children around the developing world, they can truly be used as the new standards of pediatric growth in lower-income countries.

Box 22-2. New Elements Included in the World Health Organization Child Growth Standards

- Prescriptive approach; focusing on a standard for growth and development in contrast to a growth reference.
- Population reference is based on a global pediatric population and can therefore be used worldwide.
- Links between physical growth and motor development.

From World Health Organization. *WHO Child Growth Standards: Methods and Development.* Geneva, Switzerland: World Health Organization; 2006. http://www.who.int/childgrowth/standards/technical_report/en/index.html. Accessed June 20, 2011

The WHO criteria are based on *z* scores, which represent individuals in relation to SDs from the population mean. A *z* score of 0 would represent a child whose measurement is the same as the mean of her comparison group. A *z* score of +1 represents a measurement equal to 1 SD *above* the mean in the comparison group, while a *z* score of -2 represents a measurement equal to 2 SD *below* the mean in the comparison group. As seen in Figure 22-3, only about 2% of a population will have a *z* score below -2 and only 0.1% of a population will have a *z* score below -3.

Table 22-6 demonstrates appropriate diagnoses, including severity for various anthropometric measurements relative to their *z* score.[51]

For clinical utility in the developing world it is useful to consider children with weight-for-height *z* scores between -2 and -3 as having moderate malnutrition and those with weight-for-height *z* scores less than

Figure 22-3. Prevalence of Normal Population *Z* Scores

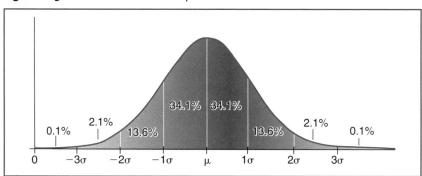

Table 22-6. Classification of Nutritional Status by *Z* Scores

Z SCORE	WEIGHT FOR AGE	HEIGHT FOR AGE	WEIGHT FOR HEIGHT
Above 3	Possibly overweight[a]	Very tall	Obese
Above 2	Possibly overweight[a]	Normal	Overweight
Above 1	Possibly overweight[a]	Normal	Possible risk of overweight
0	Median	Median	Median
Below -1	Normal	Normal	Normal
Below -2	Underweight	Stunted	Wasted
Below -3	Severely underweight	Severely stunted	Severely wasted

[a]A child whose weight for age falls in this range may have a growth problem, but this is better assessed from weight for length/height or body mass index for age.

World Health Organization. Training course on child growth assessment. Geneva, Switzerland: World Health Organization; 2010. http://www.who.int/childgrowth/training/module_C_interpreting_indicators.pdf. Accessed July 7, 2011

-3 as having severe malnutrition. Height for age below -2 is also likely to have at least moderate malnutrition. These definitions of moderate versus severe malnutrition can be useful in therapeutic decision-making. Children with severe malnutrition will likely need to be hospitalized and require intensive treatment. However, outpatient or community-based treatment may be appropriate in children with severe malnutrition who maintain a healthy appetite and have no medical complications. On the other hand, children who fall into the moderate malnutrition category often do not need hospitalization and can be managed at home with appropriate dietary and other counseling with regular follow-up. Fortified milks and ready-to-use therapeutic food (RUTF) are not usually needed for these children but rather an appropriate diet based on locally available foods.

Recently, the WHO changed the cutoff for malnutrition based on MUAC for children between the ages of 6 and 60 months. Previously, the cutoff was placed at 110 mm. However, the same study used to develop z score criteria also revealed that lowering the MUAC criteria to 115 mm increased sensitivity to nearly 99% while still maintaining high specificity for severe acute malnutrition (SAM).[47] The MUAC is easily measured in children with a standard tape measure; however, many prefer color-coded tapes made specifically for identifying these cutoffs. This makes MUAC measurements a useful tool in community screening programs in which height and weight measuring tools may be unavailable or burdensome. The main MUAC disadvantage for diagnosing SAM is the often-observed inconsistency in technique. For this reason, many malnutrition programs use weight for height as the primary measurement. Table 22-7 describes the diagnostic criteria used for diagnosing SAM in children between the ages of 6 and 60 months.

Table 22-7. Diagnostic Criteria for Diagnosing Severe Acute Malnutrition in Children Aged 6 to 60 Months		
INDICATOR	MEASURE	CUTOFF
Severe wasting[a]	Weight for height[b]	Less than -3
Severe wasting[a]	MUAC	Less than 115 mm
Bilateral pedal edema[a]	Clinical sign	

Abbreviation: MUAC, mid-upper arm circumference.

[a]Independent indicators of severe acute malnutrition that require urgent action.
[b]Based on World Health Organization standards (www.who.int/childgrowth/standards).

Adapted from World Health Organization, United Nation Children's Fund. *WHO Child Growth Standards and the Identification of Severe Acute Malnutrition in Infants and Children.* Geneva, Switzerland; World Health Organization; 2009. http://www.who.int/nutrition/publications/severemalnutrition/9789241598163_eng.pdf. Accessed June 20, 2011

■ DEVELOPMENTAL MILESTONES

As mentioned previously, the diagnosis of malnutrition is best made with a holistic approach to the child rather than on the basis of anthropometric measurements alone. The child's developmental status is often useful when making the diagnosis of malnutrition, as many children with true SAM will demonstrate developmental delay or regression. There are numerous developmental screening tools available; however, many are time consuming and may present difficulties in training others in their proper use. The WHO recommends a simplified approach to developmental screening that focuses on 6 major developmental milestones from ages 3 to 24 months. These milestones are easy to remember and train staff to recognize.[52]

- Sitting without support
- Standing with assistance
- Hands-and-knees crawling
- Walking with assistance
- Standing alone
- Walking alone

Charts demonstrating appropriate age ranges for these milestones are available for download from the WHO Web site and are useful in gathering further information in those children at risk for malnutrition.

■ CLINICAL MANIFESTATIONS OF MACRONUTRIENT DEFICIENCY

A full history and physical examination are indispensable in determining evidence of macronutrient or micronutrient deficiencies leading to the diagnosis of malnutrition. Micronutrient deficiencies are covered starting on page 600, limiting the focus of this discussion to clinical manifestations of macronutrient deficiency, namely PEM. Protein-energy malnutrition develops from deficiencies of caloric intake and protein quantity and quality. The child who is not receiving appropriate calories (energy) is likely to have a diet deficient in protein as well. Furthermore, if the diet contains insufficient calories, even what little protein is consumed will be used as an energy source instead of building lean body mass. Protein-energy malnutrition is most prevalent in children 6 months to 2 years of age.[15] Because of children's complete dependency on their caregiver for intake, children in this age range are at a particularly high risk for multiple nutritional problems associated with inappropriate feeding practices. Educational gaps, certain cultural traditions, and taboos are a few reasons leading to this deficit. This particular population is at high risk due to potential errors in the many feeding transitions during this time of life, such as

- Early weaning
- Late introduction of complementary foods
- Inadequate protein intake
- Frequent or severe infections and illness

Deficiency of energy and protein largely manifests as 2 different clinical pictures, marasmus and kwashiorkor. Traditionally, the differences between these 2 clinical manifestations of PEM have been explained with reference to the amount of protein deficiency relative to energy deficiency. However, both conditions result from deficiencies in protein and caloric intake and cannot be explained simply on the basis of protein content in diets. Furthermore, some children will have manifestations of both clinical pictures, so-called marasmic kwashiorkor (see Wellcome criteria in Table 22-5). Although some controversy remains as to the mechanisms leading to the differences seen in these 2 clinical pictures, one of the best explanations comes from the "adaptation hypothesis."[53] According to this hypothesis, children with predominantly marasmic clinical features are well adapted. In response to energy and protein deficiency, these children break down fat and lean muscle stores to produce the needed energy to survive. In a way, their bodies act appropriately in response to the deprivation.

On the other hand, children who manifest kwashiorkor seem to have a maladaptive response to deprivation—they retain some subcutaneous fat while continuing to break down lean muscle in addition to developing edema, which further complicates their ability to adapt. This maladaptive process is likely a combination of genetic as well as environmental factors, such as infections and aflatoxin exposure. Marasmus tends to be easier to treat and has fewer clinical complications. This may be because the marasmic reaction to malnutrition is the "correct" response to nutrient deprivation, whereas the maladaptation displayed in kwashiorkor places the child at a metabolic disadvantage. Thus, recovery rates in marasmus tend to be higher than those in kwashiorkor.[54]

Several factors influence the clinical manifestations of PEM, including the magnitude and duration of deprivation, the relative deficiency of different nutrients, accompanying infections or chronic disease, and exposure to environmental toxins (ie, aflatoxins). It is useful to think of PEM as a metabolic disorder resulting from a "reductive adaptation."[46] To preserve energy, reductions occur in physical activity, growth, and basal metabolic rate. These metabolic derangements form the basis of many of the treatments initiated in the WHO-recommended 10 steps for successfully treating severe malnutrition (detailed on page 586).

Water, Electrolytes, and Minerals

Total body water is increased in marasmus and kwashiorkor, with more severely malnourished children having higher total body water. Thirst is paradoxically increased because of a defective thirst mechanism despite the increase in total body water. In addition, total body potassium is reduced while total body sodium is increased.[46] For this reason, fluid resuscitation in severely malnourished children should be accomplished using a solution that is low in sodium and high in potassium, such as ReSoMal. Numerous other minerals are also deficient in many children with severe malnutrition, including calcium, iron, magnesium, zinc, copper, phosphorus, and chromium.

Protein and Amino Acids

As expected, total serum protein is reduced with hypoalbuminemia, leading to pitting edema, which is a hallmark of kwashiorkor.

Lipids

Chronic malnutrition often leads to atrophy of the gastric as well as intestinal mucosa. This in turn leads to reduction of fat absorption from the gut. As a result, there is often increased fecal fat that may present as chronic diarrhea. There is also abnormal lipid metabolism, which results in fatty infiltration of the liver in kwashiorkor. Fatty liver may be observed as an increase in liver transaminases or as hepatomegaly, which contributes to the characteristic abdominal distension seen in kwashiorkor.

Carbohydrates and Metabolism

Multiple abnormalities may exist in carbohydrate metabolism and endocrine function in the malnourished child. Among these abnormalities are impaired glucose absorption, transient disaccharide intolerance, and a low basal metabolic rate. These changes, in turn, may lead to bradycardia, hypothermia, and hypoglycemia, which can be fatal. Circulating thyroglobulins are often reduced in PEM, although the thyroid stimulating hormone may remain normal.[55]

Immunity

Severely malnourished children are relatively immunocompromised and are therefore subject to numerous infectious diseases. Often, lymphopenia with reduced T-helper cells is present along with impaired cell-mediated immunity. There may also be a reduced response to antigens with reduction in cytokine production and antibodies.[56] These changes place the child at increased risk for common, as well as uncommon, childhood infections, which forms the basis for the WHO recommendation to give broad-spectrum antibiotics to all children treated for severe malnutrition. These children will also often benefit from anti-parasitic and anti-helminth treatment.

Cardiac

The effects of malnutrition on cardiac size and function must not be overlooked, as heart failure often leads to death in these children, especially if unrecognized. Weight and heart size, and thereby cardiac function, are often reduced in proportion with the severity of wasting elsewhere in the body.[57] Bradycardia and reduced blood flow are common findings that further contribute to the common finding of hypothermia, which can be fatal. High vigilance must be kept when rehydrating the malnourished child to prevent the onset or exacerbation of heart failure. Intravenous fluids should never be used for rehydration unless the child shows clear signs of shock. Furthermore, as previously mentioned, a low-sodium (high-potassium) oral solution is preferred.

Renal

As elsewhere in the body, malnutrition affects the renal system. The glomerular filtration rate is reduced and there is inefficient acid excretion due to tubular damage.[58] However, despite this inefficiency, urine remains acidic secondary to excretion of hydrogen ions in the body's attempt to preserve potassium through the hydrogen/potassium pump.

Gastrointestinal

Lastly, diarrhea is commonly associated with malnutrition, although it is often difficult to determine if it is a contributor to the malnutrition or part of the sequelae; often it is both. In fact, the prevalence and duration of diarrhea are increased in malnourished children.[59] Diarrhea may result from a combination of bacterial, parasitic, or candidal causes in addition to common viral causes. Furthermore, there is often intestinal and gastric mucosal damage from prolonged malnutrition, which leads to malabsorption, particularly in marasmic patients; this in turn may cause further diarrhea. Of course, chronic or recurrent diarrhea itself is also a risk factor for developing malnutrition.

These metabolic and functional changes resulting from PEM are the basis for many of the treatments for malnutrition discussed as follows.

■ CLINICAL FEATURES OF PROTEIN-ENERGY MALNUTRITION

Marasmus

There may be numerous clinical findings in a child with marasmus, but the principle signs include severe wasting manifested by weight for age less than 60% of expected and the absence of edema (Table 22-5). The child will often have a wizened appearance or the so-called "old man facies." There will also be visible wasting with loss of subcutaneous fat and lean muscle mass (Figure 22-4). These losses could also be measured with MUAC and tri-fold thickness, but the wasting in marasmus should be apparent on simple inspection of the child, who is often withdrawn and apathetic (figures 22-5 and 22-6). Table 22-8 classifies the degree of wasting based on anatomic location of subcutaneous fat loss.

Kwashiorkor

Kwashiorkor may also present with numerous clinical manifestations. However, the following 4 major signs are most agreed on:

• Body weight that is 60% to 80% of predicted for age.
• There is retention of at least some subcutaneous fat even though muscle wasting may be present.
• Psychomotor changes (apathy).
• Pitting edema (Figure 22-7).
   —Often seen in the feet bilaterally
   —May be present only in the periorbital region

However, some diagnostic tools, such as the Wellcome criteria, focus only on the percentage of the mean weight for age and the presence of pitting edema. In fact, the presence of edema alone in a young child is cause for concern for severe malnutrition in many malnutrition programs, including those advocated by the WHO.[46] In addition to these major findings, evidences of macronutrient and micronutrient deficiency may be seen in various systems throughout the body in the child with kwashiorkor. There are frequently skin and hair changes including hypopigmented or hyperpigmented areas of skin, areas of desquamation especially in the groin and axilla, peeling skin (so-called "flaky paint" rash [figures 22-8 through 22-10]), sparse or patchy hair, and darkening or whitening of the hair.[14] These children will also often have striking abdominal distention. At first glance, when combined with edema, these children may be incorrectly diagnosed as overnourished. The abdominal distension is not the result of ascites, as some may presume, but is often the result of hepatomegaly from fatty infiltration of the liver and weakened abdominal muscles from loss of muscle mass. Table 22-9 provides a summary of critical laboratory values to consider in assessing

Figure 22-4. Clinical Features of Marasmus

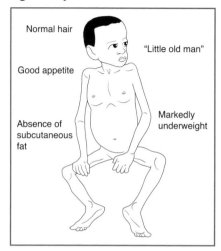

From Fischer PR. Tropical pediatrics. *Pediatr Rev.* 1993;14(3):95–99

Figure 22-6. Improvement in Marasmus

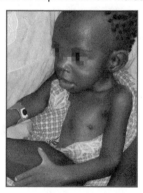

Substantial improvement was observed following only 2 weeks of treatment at an inpatient therapeutic feeding center.

From Spector JM, Gibson TE. *Atlas of Pediatrics in the Tropics and Resource-Limited Settings.* Elk Grove Village, IL: American Academy of Pediatrics; 2009

Figure 22-5. Marasmus

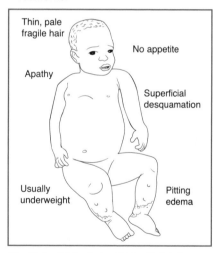

Marasmus in a young child whose family had been displaced as a result of civil conflict in Angola.

From Spector JM, Gibson TE. *Atlas of Pediatrics in the Tropics and Resource-Limited Settings.* Elk Grove Village, IL: American Academy of Pediatrics; 2009

Figure 22-7. Clinical Features of Kwashiorkor

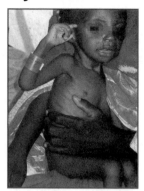

From Fischer PR. Tropical pediatrics. *Pediatr Rev.* 1993;14(3):95–99

Table 22-8. Grading of Nutritional Marasmus

1	Loss of fat from axilla/groin
2	Loss of fat from abdominal wall and gluteal region
3	Loss of fat from chest and back
4	Loss of buccal fat (composed of fatty acid and the last area to be affected)

Figure 22-8. Kwashiorkor Showing Edema

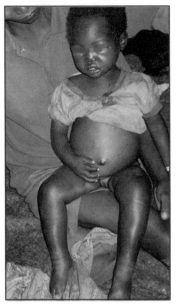

From Spector JM, Gibson TE. *Atlas of Pediatrics in the Tropics and Resource-Limited Settings.* Elk Grove Village, IL: American Academy of Pediatrics; 2009

Figure 22-9. Kwashiorkor Showing Peeling Skin ("Flaky Paint")

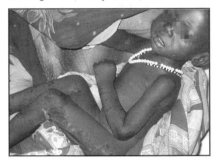

From Spector JM, Gibson TE. *Atlas of Pediatrics in the Tropics and Resource-Limited Settings.* Elk Grove Village, IL: American Academy of Pediatrics; 2009

Figure 22-10. Kwashiorkor Showing Abdominal Distention and Peeling Skin ("Flaky Paint")

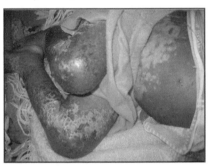

Courtesy of David Fox II, MD.

severe malnutrition. It is clinically important to distinguish between marasmus and kwashiorkor, as some aspects of the treatment, prognosis, and follow-up may differ. The easiest way to identify the presence of kwashiorkor is with the observation of lower extremity pitting edema or periorbital edema in an underweight child.

Prevention of PEM should be an integral part of any comprehensive plan to manage malnutrition. Preventive measures to reduce the incidence of kwashiorkor and marasmus include increasing nutritional education to people of various incomes, ages, and education levels. Mothers, children, and communities at particularly high risk may also benefit from supplemental food programs, subsidiaries, and maternal-infant support programs. Encouraging immunization use, early treatment of infectious diseases, and good sanitary practices are vital in

Table 22-9. Laboratory Features of Severe Malnutrition

BLOOD OR PLASMA VARIABLES	INFORMATION DERIVED
Hemoglobin, hematocrit, erythrocyte count, mean corpuscular volume	• Degree of dehydration and anemia; type of anemia (iron/folate and vitamin B_{12} deficiency, hemolysis, malaria)
Glucose	• Hypoglycemia
Electrolytes and alkalinity Sodium Potassium Chloride, pH bicarbonate	• Hyponatremia, type of dehydration (despite increased total body sodium content) • Hypokalemia • Metabolic alkalosis or acidosis
Total protein, transferring, (pre-) albumin	• Degree of protein deficiency
Creatinine	• Renal function
C-reactive protein, lymphocyte count, serology, thick and thin blood films	• Presence of bacterial or viral infection or malaria
Stool examination	• Presence of parasites

From Müller O, Krawinkel M. Malnutrition and health in developing countries. *CMAJ*. 2005;173(3):279–286. © Access Copyright. Reprinted with permission. No further reproductions are permitted.

preventing illnesses that are likely to put a child at high risk of PEM and prevent growth and development.[15]

■ TREATMENT OF MALNUTRITION

Moderate Malnutrition

Moderate malnutrition includes all children with *moderate wasting,* which is defined as weight for height between -3 and -2 z scores, and all those with *moderate stunting,* which is defined by height for age between -3 and -2 z scores, both from the WHO child growth standards. Most of these children will be *moderately underweight* (weight for age between -3 and -2)[60]; research concerning morbidity and mortality in moderate malnutrition clearly reveals that both are increased. Death from diarrhea, pneumonia, malaria, and measles are all significantly increased in moderately malnourished children. Furthermore, many of these children will progress to severe malnutrition on their way to fatality.[60] Unfortunately, moderate malnutrition has not received the same intensity of research or intervention as severe malnutrition. As previously mentioned, nearly two thirds of undernourished children are in the moderately malnourished category. It is clear that moderate malnutrition requires the most serious attention.

Unfortunately, the optimum strategy for treating moderate malnutrition has yet to be definitively described. What is clear is that more specific strategies and counseling are needed for treatment to be effective. Previous attempts at generic nutritional advice have proven ineffective. In many resource-poor areas, it is likely that treating moderate malnutrition with the same supplements as severe malnutrition, while likely to be effective, is cost or resource prohibitive.[61] While recognizing that further research is needed, recent research and consensus panels reached some conclusions concerning the most appropriate diet for moderately malnourished children. These dietary recommendations include the following components[62]:

High Energy Density

Malnourished children should receive a diet with a high energy density. This can be accomplished by reducing the meal's bulk by reducing water content. Foods that contain large amounts of water may cause the child early satiety before she consumes enough calories. The child should be offered clean water between meals to ensure adequate hydration. Additionally, adding oil or sugar to meals, when appropriate (ie, porridge), can increase the food's energy content.

Adequate Protein Quantity, Quality, and Bioavailability

Clearly, children suffering from PEM need to consume adequate amounts of protein if they are to recover. However, there is also concern that too much protein may adversely affect appetite as well as provide undue financial burden on caregivers. Therefore, it has been suggested that protein should account for 12% of daily energy consumption in moderately malnourished children. In addition, protein quality and bioavailability are important. Protein consumed from meat sources is of higher quality and greater bioavailability than protein consumed from vegetable sources. These advantages must be balanced with the higher cost of meat-based proteins. So, for instance, reasonable plant-based protein can be feasibly provided in many low-resource settings.

Fat Quantity and Quality

Fat has more than twice the energy of protein or carbohydrates. Therefore, it is a key component to the diet of malnourished children as a source of high energy density. It is recommended that 35% to 50% of daily calories come from fat. Furthermore, fat quality is also important; in fact, it is likely that deficiency of essential fatty acids is responsible for many of the cutaneous manifestations of malnutrition. Therefore, malnourished children should receive appropriate amounts of polyunsaturated fatty acids with an appropriate n-3/n-6 ratio.

Animal Source Foods

As previously mentioned, meat is an excellent source of high-quality and highly bioavailable proteins. Meat products are also high in micronutrients and low in anti-nutrients. In addition, the so-called meat factor allows for greater absorption of iron from nonheme (plant-based) sources. Animal products, especially milk protein, are shown to increase linear growth as well as lean muscle mass. Although meat products are often the most expensive ingredients in meals, they are indispensable in the diets of malnourished children. Every effort should be made to introduce at least some meat product into the diet of these children.

Micronutrients

Typically, diets for malnourished children focus on energy and protein content. However, it is now clear that foods high in micronutrients should be added to meals. Micronutrients are often only needed in small quantities and can be obtained from a variety of animal, fruit, and vegetable sources.

Anti-nutrients

The term *anti-nutrients* refers to compounds largely found in plant-based foods that bind nutrients found in other foods consumed simultaneously. Phytates and tannins are important anti-nutrients that bind to numerous positively charged minerals, such as calcium, magnesium, and iron, preventing their absorption. Phytates are found in numerous legumes and vegetables while tannins are found in black tea and dark sorghum. Although it is impossible to avoid these foods altogether, methods such as roasting, malting, and fermenting can reduce the content of phytates before consumption. Black tea should be avoided in all malnourished children.

In addition to these recommendations, any dietary advice should include meals containing a low risk of contamination. For example, if lack of clean water is a concern, powdered milk is not the best option because it is likely to be contaminated while being mixed with the water. Also, the foods must have an appropriate taste and texture, be culturally appropriate, be easy to prepare, be made with locally available products, and be affordable. Tension is constant between choosing the best foods (usually animal products), which are typically the most expensive, and choosing the cheapest foods (usually roots or cereals). Research is making it clear that not only the cheapest foods should be recommended but rather the proper balance of those foods that provide the best nutrients and are the most affordable.[62]

Severe Malnutrition

Guidelines for treating severe malnutrition are much more clearly defined subsequent to more extensive research and testing. Although many children with severe malnutrition will need intensive inpatient treatment, there is a subset of patients who will do well with outpatient, community-based treatment. Treatment in hospitals mainly occurs when PEM is severe, appetite is poor, and infections complicate the case.[5] When considering the most appropriate location for SAM treatment, factors that should be considered include coexisting medical complications, access to a treatment center, availability of a supportive caregiver, sanitary conditions, prevalence of severe malnutrition in the area, and availability of a complementary feeding program.[7]

The WHO growth standards are designed as indicators to identify the need for nutritional intervention. Treatment methods are largely based on the presence of medical complications (Table 22-10). According to the WHO child growth standards (Table 22-6), a child between the ages of 6 and 60 months with signs of bilateral edema or severe wasting, with a weight for height of less than -3 SD or MUAC less than 115 mm, is considered to have SAM and should be treated. Table 22-10 outlines factors that should be considered when discerning approaches to treatment. A medical facility is recommended when symptoms are severe, appetite is lacking, and there are medical complications. On the other hand, an outpatient, community-based management approach may be more appropriate if no medical complications are evident and the child has an appetite.[49]

The importance of community and family involvement leading to empowerment in successful malnutrition prevention and treatment is well known. Treatment options in which cultural settings are taken into consideration have been implemented with good results. For example, the National Health Service in Chile provides an alternative to hospital treatment with psychomotor stimulation in addition to nutritional care. Additionally, the child's caregiver participates in the recovery process. Because this approach was used among some of the poorest in Chile, there was also an emphasis on improving the socioeconomic situation of the families involved. Not only did these centers show results in treating the malnutrition, but they also demonstrated reductions in mortality rates related to malnutrition through simultaneous education. The main problems with this approach are the financial costs of the program

Table 22-10. General Management of Severe Acute Malnutrition

TREATMENT LOCATION	FACILITY-BASED	OUTPATIENT COMMUNITY-BASED
Symptoms	• Lack of appetite • Medical complications	• Appetite preserved • No medical complications
Interventions	• F-75 (starter formula)[a] • Progress to F-100 (catch-up formula)[b] or RUTF • 24-hour medical care	• RUTF • Basic medical care
Discharge criteria	• Reduced edema • Good appetite • Z score greater than -1 • Acceptable intake of RUTF (at least 75% of estimated RUTF daily ration) • Discharged to community-based care	• 15% to 20% weight gain

Abbreviation: RUTF, ready-to-use therapeutic food.

[a]World Health Organization (WHO)- and United Nation Children's Fund (UNICEF)-provided starter milk-based formula, commonly available in developing countries.
[b]WHO- and UNICEF-provided catch-up milk-based formula, commonly available in developing countries.

Adapted from World Health Organization, United Nation Children's Fund. *WHO Child Growth Standards and the Identification of Severe Acute Malnutrition in Infants and Children.* Geneva, Switzerland; World Health Organization; 2009. http://www.who.int/nutrition/publications/severemalnutrition/9789241598163_eng.pdf. Accessed June 20, 2011

as well as the potential disruption to a family's daily dynamics. Today, alternative programs are implemented, including treatments based in child care centers as well as staff monitoring children in their home. These programs appear to be more cost-effective while providing care that does not disrupt the family's normal life.[7]

When considering inpatient management for SAM, the format outlined in the WHO guidelines[33] provides a tested method to treat signs and symptoms associated with severe protein-energy deficiency. This proven approach can be divided into 2 phases, initial stabilization and rehabilitation. Table 22-11 describes the approximate timeline of when various interventions take place in the treatment process.[33] Key treatment elements include[13]

• Initial phase of emergency
  — Provide cautious low-lactose, low-protein feeding and hydrate with a low-sodium solution to reduce the risk of hypoglycemia, hypothermia, and dehydration.
  — Closely monitor volume loads (oral, enteral, and parenteral intake) to avoid heart failure.
  — Modify a standard ORS (eg, by using ReSoMal) to reduce sodium concentrations and increase potassium, magnesium, copper, selenium, and zinc concentrations.

Table 22-11. Elements in the Management of Severe Protein-Energy Malnutrition (According to the World Health Organization)

STEP	MANAGEMENT	STABILIZATION DAYS 1–2	STABILIZATION DAYS 3–7	REHABILITATION WEEKS 2–6
1. Prevent and treat hypoglycemia.	Monitor blood glucose; provide oral (or intravenous) glucose as indicated; initiate early cautious feeding every 2 hours.	⟶		
2. Prevent and treat hypothermia.	Warm patient and keep dry; maintain and monitor body temperature; initiate early cautious feeding every 2 hours; administer broad-spectrum antibiotics.	⟶		
3. Dehydration	Rehydrate carefully with oral solution containing less sodium and more potassium than standard mix (ReSoMal).	⟶		
4. Electrolytes	Supply plenty of potassium and magnesium.	⟶		⟶
5. Infections	Administer broad-spectrum antibiotics; consider antihelminth, antiparasitic, and antimalarial therapy (if indicated); begin/continue immunizations (especially measles).	⟶	No iron	With iron
6. Micronutrients	Provide copper, zinc, iron, folate, and multivitamins.	⟶		⟶
7. Starter nutrition	Keep protein and volume load low (F-75 if available).	⟶		
8. Tissue-building nutrition, catch-up growth	Furnish a rich diet dense in energy, protein, and all essential nutrients that are easy to swallow and digest (F-100 if available or RUTF such as Plumpy'nut).		⟶	

Table 22-11. Elements in the Management of Severe Protein-Energy Malnutrition (According to the World Health Organization), continued

| | | PHASE | | |
| | | STABILIZATION | | REHABILITATION |
STEP	MANAGEMENT	DAYS 1–2	DAYS 3–7	WEEKS 2–6
9. Sensory stimulation and emotional support	Prevent permanent psycho-social effects of starvation with psychomotor stimulation and tender, loving care.		→	
10. Prevention of relapse; prepare for follow-up.	Start early to identify causes of protein-energy malnutrition in each case; involve family and community in prevention.			→

Abbreviation: RUTF, ready-to-use therapeutic food.

Modified from Müller O, Krawinkel M. Malnutrition and health in developing countries. *CMAJ*. 2005;173:279–286. © Access Copyright. Reprinted with permission. No further reproductions are permitted; and Ashworth A, Jackson A, Khanum S, Schofield C. Ten steps to recovery. *Child Health Dialogue*. 1996;(3-4):10–12

— Treat concomitant infections with broad-spectrum antibiotics (bacteremia, especially with gram-negative bacteria, is not uncommon).
- Early phase of rehabilitation
  — Limit protein intake to less than 1 g/kg to avoid ammonia buildup due to
    - Impaired liver function with breakdown of the urea cycle
    - Reduced urine excretion with dehydration

Phases of Management of Malnourished Children

For treatment purposes, SAM management is divided into 3 phases: acute, nutritional rehabilitation, and follow-up. Table 22-12 provides a summary describing the focus and management of each phase.

Acute

In the acute phase, treatment is focused on the most critical and urgent problems at hand, which commonly include dehydration, infection, hypoglycemia, hypothermia, and water/electrolyte imbalance. The first 48 hours of hospitalization are usually the most critical and when mortality rates tend to be highest. The focus of treatment in this phase includes preventing hypoglycemia and hypothermia, treating dehy-

Table 22-12. Phases of Management of Diarrhea in Malnourished Children

PHASE	FOCUS	MANAGEMENT
Acute	• Dehydration • Infection • Hypoglycemia • Hypothermia • Water/electrolyte imbalance	• Correction of micronutrient imbalances with supplementation. • Broad-spectrum antibiotics. • Initiate feeding immediately after admission or 2 h after rehydration started. • Scheduled frequent, small feedings. • Rehydration.
Nutritional rehabilitation	• Regaining weight lost • Maintaining weight	• Intensive feeding • Involvement/instruction of caregiver • Child given emotional and physical stimuli
Follow-up	• Minimize relapse. • Ensure optimal physical and mental growth and development.	• Follow-up instruction and education to meet needs and prevent recurrence of diarrhea

dration, discovering electrolyte imbalances and infection, correcting micronutrient imbalances, and cautiously initiating feeding.

For successful treatment it is important to adhere to a specific feeding schedule. Feeding should be initiated immediately after admission or 2 hours after rehydration is started. The purpose of these early feedings is not weight gain but rather to prevent hypothermia and hypoglycemia while preparing the child's lethargic metabolism for more intensive feeding in the rehabilitation phase. Micronutrient supplementation is often needed to replenish and normalize serum values. Rational use of rehydration is a key component of this phase, which should be slow, gradual, and preferably oral. ReSoMal is the oral solution of choice when rehydrating malnourished children because of its lower sodium and higher potassium content. Every effort should be made to use this oral solution over IV rehydration unless the malnourished child shows signs of shock. Using a broad-spectrum antibiotic to prevent and treat concurrent infection is also recommended. For the seriously ill child, IV broad-spectrum antibiotics are recommended, while an oral regimen may be considered for those children who do not appear septic or otherwise distressed. During the acute phase one should be aware of the potential risk for various complications and thus start treatment in a timely manner.[34]

Nutritional Rehabilitation

At this phase focus is put on the patient regaining weight with high-calorie and high-protein intensive feedings to compensate for weight previously lost. It is important to have the child's caregiver involved in this stage to learn how to best care for the child's needs once he is well enough to be discharged. The child should also be stimulated emotionally and physically to help in the recovery process.[34]

Follow-up

Follow-up should be part of the management plan to reduce the chance of relapse and to ensure optimal physical and mental growth and development of the child.[34]

Despite advances in the understanding and treatment of SAM, fatality rates remained about the same in children who were hospitalized with malnutrition from 1950 through 1990. However, mortality rates in treatment centers range from 50% to less than 5%. Accordingly, it is clear that mortality rates can be dramatically reduced if tested strategies are implemented. Those severely malnourished children who die in the hospital typically die from 4 main causes: hypoglycemia, hypothermia, heart failure, and infection.[46] In response, the WHO developed a strategic treatment plan to address the common elements present in severe malnutrition[33] as outlined and detailed in the following charts and tables. Currently, the widespread availability of special feedings designed for malnourished children (ReSoMal, F-75, F-100, Plumpy'nut) in developing countries has been very beneficial in improving clinical management.

Treating and Preventing Hypoglycemia and Hypothermia

1. Hypoglycemia often occurs in combination with hypothermia, indicating infection.
2. Monitor temperature regularly and check for hypoglycemia whenever the child is hypothermic.
3. Provide small, frequent feedings (eg, F-75 every 2 hours) to control hypoglycemia and hypothermia.
4. Severely malnourished children should be treated as though they are hypoglycemic if it is not possible to measure blood glucose levels.
5. Refer to tables 22-13 and 22-14 for detailed treatment plans.

Table 22-13. Treatment and Prevention of Hypoglycemia

	SYMPTOMS: CONSCIOUS WITH BLOOD GLUCOSE BELOW 54 MG/DL	SYMPTOMS: UNCONSCIOUS, LETHARGIC, OR CONVULSING
Treatment	1. 50 mL bolus of 10% glucose or 10% sucrose solution (1 rounded teaspoon of sugar in 3.5 table-spoons water), orally or by naso-gastric tube	1. IV sterile 10% glucose (5 mL/kg), followed by 50 mL of 10% glucose or sucrose by nasogastric tube
	2. Feed starter F-75 every 30 minutes for 2 hours (giving one quarter of the 2 hourly feedings each time).	
	3. Provide antibiotics.	
	4. Provide 2 hourly feeds, day and night.	
Monitor	• Glucose level: monitor after 2 hours (most children stabilize within 30 minutes after treatment). • Blood glucose less than 54 mg/dL — Additional 50 mL bolus 10% glucose or sucrose solution. — Feed continuously every 30 minutes until stabilized. • Retest blood sugar if — Rectal temperature is below 35.5°C or axillary temperature below 35°C. — Level of consciousness deteriorates.	
Prevention	• Initiate 2 hourly feedings immediately or after rehydration if needed. • Provide feedings day and night.	

Abbreviation: IV, intravenous.

Adapted from Ashworth A, Khanum S, Jackson A, Schofield C. *Guidelines for the Inpatient Treatment of Severely Malnourished Children.* Geneva, Switzerland: World Health Organization; 2003. http://www.who.int/nutrition/publications/guide_inpatient_text.pdf. Accessed June 21, 2011

Treating and Preventing Dehydration

1. The degree of dehydration in severely malnourished children is often difficult to assess when only using clinical signs. Signs, such as sunken eyes, reduced skin turgor, and lethargy, may be caused by the malnutrition or dehydration. Even children with edema may be dehydrated.
2. All children with watery stools should be assumed to have dehydration and be treated.
3. Oral rehydration is preferred and should be used whenever possible.
4. ReSoMal
   - Solution formulated especially for severely malnourished children with reduced sodium and increased potassium.
   - Standard solutions often are too high in sodium and too low in potassium for severely malnourished children.
5. Refer to Table 22-15 for detailed treatment plans and tables 22-16 and 22-17 for ReSoMal and electrolyte solution recipes.

Table 22-14. Treatment and Prevention of Hypothermia	
	SYMPTOMS: RECTAL TEMPERATURE BELOW 35.5°C (95.9°F), AXILLARY BELOW 35°C
Treatment	1. Initiate feeding immediately, or after rehydration if needed.
	2. Rewarm child.
	3. Provide antibiotics.
Monitor	• Rectal temperature: Monitor every 2 hours until above 36.5°C (every half hour if heater is used). • Cover child at all times. • Feel for warmth. • If hypothermic: check for hypoglycemia.
Prevention	• Initiate 2 hourly feedings. • Provide feedings day and night. • Cover child and keep away from drafts (kangaroo care is best). • Keep child dry (eg, change wet diapers, clothes, bedding). • Avoid exposure (eg, bathing, prolonged medical examinations). • Let child sleep with mother or caregiver at night for warmth.

Adapted from Ashworth A, Khanum S, Jackson A, Schofield C. *Guidelines for the Inpatient Treatment of Severely Malnourished Children*. Geneva, Switzerland: World Health Organization; 2003. http://www.who.int/nutrition/publications/guide_inpatient_text.pdf. Accessed June 21, 2011

6. Intravenous rehydration
   • *Only* used in cases of shock.
   • Careful, slow infusion of 15 mL/kg over 1 hour to avoid excess fluid flooding the circulation and overloading the heart.
   • Give isotonic saline or Ringer lactate solution with 5% dextrose.

Correcting Electrolyte Imbalance

1. Sodium
   • High in all severely malnourished children even when plasma sodium may be normal or low.
   • Providing high concentrations of sodium is often fatal.
2. Potassium and magnesium
   • Deficient in severely malnourished children.
   • Takes at least 2 weeks for levels to normalize.
   • Additional potassium and magnesium can be added to feeds when indicated (see Table 22-18 for recipe).
3. Edema
   • May be partly caused by electrolyte imbalances.
   • Do not use diuretics to treat edema in severely malnourished children.

Table 22-15. Treatment and Prevention of Dehydration

Treatment	**SYMPTOMS: WATERY STOOLS**

	1. ReSoMal
	  • 5 mL/kg every 30 minutes for 2 hours.
	  • Orally or by nasogastric tube.
	  • 5 to 10 mL/kg/h for the next 4 to 10 hours as clinically indicated.
	  • Target volume replacement is around 5% body weight.
	  • Determine the exact amount by taking into consideration
	    — How much the child wants
	    — Stool and vomiting losses

	2. Replace the ReSoMal doses at 4, 6, 8, and 10 hours with F-75 if rehydration is continuing at these times.
	3. Continue feeding starter F-75.
	4. During treatment, rapid respiration and pulse rates should slow down and the child should begin to pass urine.

Monitor	• Monitor every half hour for the first 2 hours.
	• Monitor hourly for the next 6 to 12 hours, recording
	  — Pulse rate
	  — Respiratory rate
	  — Urine frequency
	  — Stool/vomit frequency
	• Signs of rehydration (will not appear in children who are severely malnourished until fully rehydrated)
	  — Return of tears
	  — Moist mouth
	  — Eyes and fontanels appearing less sunken
	  — Improved skin turgor
	• Signs of excess fluid (overhydration) or infection
	  — Increasing respiratory rate (greater than 5 bpm)
	  — Increasing pulse rate (greater than 25 bpm)
	  — Increasing edema
	  — Puffy eyelids
	• Stop fluids immediately and reassess needs after an hour if overhydration occurs. Do not routinely give diuretics.

Prevention	When diarrhea is present • Continue starter F-75 feedings. • Replace stool volume losses with ReSoMal. • Provide 50 to 100 mL after each watery stool. • If the child is breastfed, encourage continuation.

Adapted from Ashworth A, Khanum S, Jackson A, Schofield C. *Guidelines for the Inpatient Treatment of Severely Malnourished Children.* Geneva, Switzerland: World Health Organization; 2003. http://www.who.int/nutrition/publications/guide_inpatient_text.pdf. Accessed June 21, 2011

Table 22-16. Recipe for ReSoMal Oral Rehydration Solution

INGREDIENTS	AMOUNT
Water (boiled and cooled)	2 L
WHO oral rehydration solution	One 1-L packet (includes 3.5-g sodium chloride, 2.9-g trisodium citrate dihydrate, 1.5-g potassium chloride, 20-g glucose)
Sugar	50 g
Electrolyte/mineral solution	40 mL

Abbreviation: WHO, World Health Organization

Adapted from Ashworth A, Khanum S, Jackson A, Schofield C. *Guidelines for the Inpatient Treatment of Severely Malnourished Children.* Geneva, Switzerland: World Health Organization; 2003. http://www.who.int/nutrition/publications/guide_inpatient_text.pdf. Accessed June 21, 2011

Table 22-17. Recipe for Electrolyte/Mineral Solution (Used in Preparation of ReSoMal and Milk Feeds)

- Weigh the following ingredients and make up to 2,500 mL.
- Add 20 mL of electrolyte/mineral solution to 1,000 mL of milk feed.

INGREDIENTS	QUANTITY (G)	MOLAR CONTENT OF 20 ML
Potassium chloride	224	24 mmol
Tripotassium citrate	81	2 mmol
Magnesium chloride	76	3 mmol
Zinc acetate	8.2	300 μmol
Copper sulphate	1.4	45 μmol
Water	2,500 mL	

Note: Add selenium if available (sodium selenate 0.028 g) and iodine (potassium iodine 0.012 g) per 2,500 mL.

PREPARATION

- Dissolve the ingredients in cooled boiled water.
- Store the solution in sterilized bottles in the refrigerator to slow deterioration.
- Discard solution if it turns cloudy.
- Make fresh solution each month.

Adapted from Ashworth A, Khanum S, Jackson A, Schofield C. *Guidelines for the Inpatient Treatment of Severely Malnourished Children.* Geneva, Switzerland: World Health Organization; 2003. http://www.who.int/nutrition/publications/guide_inpatient_text.pdf. Accessed June 21, 2011

<table>

| **Table 22-18. Potassium and Magnesium Solution** |
</table>

- Provide 20 mL of liquid potassium and magnesium solution to 1 L of feeds or ReSoMal.

INGREDIENTS

| Additional potassium | 3–4 mmol/kg/d |
| Additional magnesium | 0.4–0.6 mmol/kg/d |

- When rehydrating, provide a low-sodium rehydration solution (eg, ReSoMal).
- Food prepared should be without salt.

Adapted from Ashworth A, Khanum S, Jackson A, Schofield C. *Guidelines for the Inpatient Treatment of Severely Malnourished Children.* Geneva, Switzerland: World Health Organization; 2003. http://www.who.int/nutrition/publications/guide_inpatient_text.pdf. Accessed June 21, 2011

Treating and Preventing Infections

1. Normal signs and symptoms of infection (eg, fever) are usually not present in the severely malnourished due to a weakened immune system.
2. Providing a broad-spectrum antibiotic as well as measles vaccine (if child is older than 6 months and not vaccinated; delay if child is in shock) is therefore recommended on admission.
   - Intravenous antibiotic choices
     — Ampicillin and gentamicin
     — Chloramphenicol
     — Third-generation cephalosporin (ie, ceftriaxone)
   - Oral antibiotic choices (if child is stable with no obvious complications)
     — Amoxicillin with or without gentamicin intramuscularly
     — Co-trimoxazole
     — Augmentin
3. Anorexia
   - If anorexia persists after 5 days of antibiotic treatment
     — Continue a full 10 days of antibiotic treatment.
   - If anorexia persists after 10 days of antibiotic treatment
     — Reassess child, checking
       ■ Infection sites
       ■ Potentially resistant organisms
       ■ Micronutrient supplements provided correctly
4. Consider anti-helminth therapy for all children with SAM.
5. Consider metronidazole to help with healing damaged intestinal mucosa as well as possible concurrent parasitic infections.
6. Consider antimalarial treatment if in an endemic area or if otherwise indicated.

Correcting Micronutrient Deficiencies

1. Providing a micronutrient solution to feedings is beneficial because all severely malnourished children have vitamin and mineral deficiencies (Table 22-19).
2. Anemia
   - Common in malnutrition.
   - Iron may be provided once appetite is regained and signs of weight gain are evident (often in the second week of treatment).
     — Providing iron too early may suppress appetite and can be fatal.

Starting Cautious Feedings

1. The stabilization phase
   - The initial days of treatment, usually lasting 3 to 7 days.
   - Return of appetite is the primary sign of recovery, signaling the need for transition to catch-up feedings.
   - Hospitalization is crucial because of the critical and complicated condition during this state.[63]
   - In this phase, cautious feedings are initiated as soon as possible after admission to maintain basic physiologic functions and needs, and provide adequate energy and protein (Table 22-20).
     — The goal is not to begin weight gain but only to provide enough nutrients for proper physiologic functioning.
     — Diarrhea usually starts to resolve.
     — Weight loss is seen in children with edema.[33]

Table 22-19. Treating Micronutrient Deficiencies

Day 1, provide
- Vitamin A orally
  — Older than 12 months: 200,000 IU
  — Six to 12 months: 100, 000 IU
  — Birth to 5 months: give 50,000 IU

Unless there is definite evidence that a dose has been given in the last month.

Provide daily, starting on day 1, for at least 2 weeks.
1. Multivitamin supplement
2. Folic acid, 1 mg/d (5 mg on day 1)
3. Zinc, 2 mg/kg/d
4. Copper, 0.3 mg/kg/d
5. Iron, 3 mg/kg/d (but only when gaining weight)

Adapted from Ashworth A, Khanum S, Jackson A, Schofield C. *Guidelines for the Inpatient Treatment of Severely Malnourished Children.* Geneva, Switzerland: World Health Organization; 2003. http://www.who.int/nutrition/publications/guide_inpatient_text.pdf. Accessed June 21, 2011

Table 22-20. Treatment During Stabilization Phase

Treatment	Feeding route	• Oral or nasogastric feeds (never parenteral preparations). • Feed from a cup; very weak children may be fed by spoon, dropper, or syringe. • Breastfeeding — Encourage mother to continue breastfeeding. — Provide the prescribed amounts of starter formula to make sure the child's needs are met. • Indication for nasogastric feeds — Provide remaining feed by nasogastric tube if, after allowing for any vomiting, intake does not reach 80 kcal/kg/d (105 mL starter formula/kg) despite frequent feedings and encouraging. — Do not exceed 100 kcal/kg/d in this phase.
	Composition	• Small, frequent feeds of low osmolarity and low lactose. • In most cases, milk-based starter F-75 is adequate for most children. • Starter F-75 provides — 75 kcal/100 mL — 0.9 g protein/100 mL
	Needs	• 100 kcal/kg/d • 1–1.5 g protein/kg/d • 130 mL/kg/d of fluid (100 mL/kg/d if the child has severe edema
	Intake	**Recommended Feeding Schedule** See table below.

Recommended Feeding Schedule

DAYS	FREQUENCY	VOL/KG/FEED	VOL/KG/D
1–2	2 hourly	11 mL	130 mL
3–5	3 hourly	16 mL	130 mL
6–7+	4 hourly	22 mL	130 mL

• With good appetite and no edema, this schedule can be completed in 2 to 3 days (eg, 24 hours at each level).

Monitor and Record	• Intake amounts offered and left over • Vomiting • Frequency of watery stool • Daily body weight

Adapted from Ashworth A, Khanum S, Jackson A, Schofield C. *Guidelines for the Inpatient Treatment of Severely Malnourished Children*. Geneva, Switzerland: World Health Organization; 2003. http://www.who.int/nutrition/publications/guide_inpatient_text.pdf. Accessed June 21, 2011

Achieving Catch-up Growth/Rehabilitation Phase

1. The rehabilitation phase
   - Typically starts at around week 2 after the return of the child's appetite and lasts until week 6 of treatment.
   - Aims to replenish lost nutrient stores to attain healthy weight gain.[33] This is accomplished by changing to a milk (ie, F-100) or RUTF (ie, Plumpy'nut) that contains higher protein and energy content (Table 22-21).

Providing Sensory Stimulation and Emotional Support

1. Malnutrition can lead to delays in mental and behavioral development.
2. To avoid such delays it is important to provide emotional care and sensory stimulation as part of the treatment process, involving the child's caregiver as much as possible.

Preparing for Follow-up and Recovery

1. Recovery criteria
   - Ninety-percent weight for length (equivalent to -1 *z* score).
     — Weight for age tends to be low secondary to stunting in children recovering from severe malnutrition.
   - Close follow-up as outpatient or with home visits are crucial for long-term recovery.
   - To reduce relapse risk it is very important that the caregiver is aware of diet goals and is instructed on how to continue to provide necessary care. Needs
     — Macronutrients
       - At least 150 kcal/kg/d.
       - At least 4 g protein/kg/d.
       - Consider discharging the caregiver with RUTFs to cover these demands if available.
     — Micronutrients
       - Provide 20 mL (4 teaspoon) electrolyte/mineral solution daily in feeds to mask flavor (1 teaspoon/200 mL fluid).
       - Provide vitamin A every 6 months.
   - Meals
     — At least 5 meals per day.
     — High energy and protein content.
       - Approximately 100 kcal and 2 to 3 g protein per 100 g
     — Encourage child to finish entire meal.

Table 22-21. Treatment During the Rehabilitation Phase

	TREATMENT DURING TRANSITION	MONITOR DURING TRANSITION
Initiate	• Approximately 1 week after admission. • Signaled by return of appetite. • Gradually transition to avoid risk of heart failure, which can occur if a child suddenly consumes huge amounts.	• Respiratory rate • Pulse rate If respirations increase by 5 or more breaths per min and pulse by 25 or more beats per minute for 2 successive 4 hourly readings, reduce the volume per feed (give 4 hourly F-100 at 16 mL/kg/feed for 24 hours, then 19 mL/kg/feed for 24 hours, then 22 mL/kg/feed for 48 hours, then increase each feed by 10 mL as above).
Goal	• Vigorous feeding to achieve very high intake and rapid weight gain of more than 10 g gain/kg/d	
Intake	• F-100 — Milk based — Containing 100 kcal and 2.9 g protein/100 mL • RUTFs such as Plumpy'nut • Modified porridges — If with comparable energy and protein concentrations to F-100 • Modified family foods — If with comparable energy and protein concentrations	
Method	• Transition between starter and catch-up formula — Replace starter F-75 with the same amount of catch-up formula F-100 for 48 hours. — Thereafter, increase each successive feed by 10 mL until some feed remains uneaten. — The point when some remains unconsumed is likely to occur when intake reaches about 30 mL/kg/4-h feed (200 mL/kg/d).	

Table 22-21. Treatment During the Rehabilitation Phase, continued

TREATMENT AFTER TRANSITION		MONITOR AFTER TRANSITION
Intake	1. Frequent feeds (at least 4 hourly) of unlimited amounts of a catch-up formula. 2. 150 to 220 kcal/kg/d. 3. 4 to 6 g protein/kg/d. 4. If the child is breastfed, encourage to continue (*note*: breast milk does not have sufficient energy and protein to support rapid catch-up growth).	• Weigh child each morning before feeding. • Plot weight. • Each week calculate and record weight gain as g/kg/d. **To calculate weight gain** (example for a 7-day period) • Subtract from today's weight (in g) the child's weight 7 days earlier. • Divide by 7 to determine the average daily weight gain (g/d). • Divide by the child's average weight in kg to calculate the weight gain as g/kg/d. • Weight gain — Poor (less than 5 g/kg/d): requires full reassessment. — Moderate (5–10 g/kg/d): check if intake targets are met or for presence of infection. — Good (greater than 10 g/kg/g): continue to praise staff and mothers.

Adapted from Ashworth A, Khanum S, Jackson A, Schofield C. *Guidelines for the Inpatient Treatment of Severely Malnourished Children*. Geneva, Switzerland: World Health Organization; 2003. http://www.who.int/nutrition/publications/guide_inpatient_text.pdf. Accessed June 21, 2011

- Snacks
  - —Provided between meals with high energy content.
  - —Often continuation of RUTF supplements can be helpful during this transition period.
2. Encourage follow-up and booster immunizations to minimize chance of relapse.

Special Circumstances: Malnutrition in Infants Younger Than 6 Months

Traditionally, little has been know about the prevalence of malnutrition in infants younger than 6 months, and the hallmark of prevention is exclusive breastfeeding for the first 6 months of life. Recent research, however, has shown that the prevalence of malnutrition in the younger-than-6-months age group is quite prevalent, reaching levels of greater than 30% in some countries, with a mean prevalence of 15% in many lower-income countries. Furthermore, using the new WHO standards nearly doubles the prevalence.[64] The goals of treatment for severe malnutrition are generally the same in this age group, with a couple of differences. First of all, because most of these children have not been exclusively breastfed, the goal is to return the child to exclusive breastfeeding whenever possible. Often there is a transitional period when supplemental formula is used until the mother is able to give adequate breast milk feedings and the child is gaining weight well. The WHO recommends using diluted F-100 (1:1.5 ratio of formula to water) instead of F-75 to reduce solute load on the young infant's kidneys. If the child has been adequately and exclusively breastfed from birth, an organic cause should be sought for the malnutrition. Often, these young infants will require a higher caloric intake than older children to gain appropriate weight.

■ MICRONUTRIENT DEFICIENCIES

For centuries, generalized malnutrition has plagued many people, especially those who are economically disadvantaged and those who are displaced by political and social problems. During the second half of the 20th century, the Green Revolution involved using new agricultural technologies and procedures to boost overall production. As a result, generalized malnutrition became less common. At the same time, however, dietary intake became less varied in many regions, and micronutrient deficiencies again emerged as causes of specific pathologic clinical conditions in children.

Today, millions of children around the world suffer from specific micronutrient deficiencies. Rather than relegating conditions (eg, scurvy, beriberi, rickets) to history books, clinicians must be prepared to recognize and manage micronutrient deficiencies when caring for children in lower-income countries.

Table 22-22 summarizes key features of important micronutrients. Figure 22-11 identifies common symptoms and signs of micronutrient deficiencies.

■ SPECIFIC MICRONUTRIENT DEFICIENCIES

Vitamin A[65,66]

Importance

Vitamin A deficiency is the major cause of preventable blindness in the world. Hypovitaminosis A is also linked to increased infection-related morbidity and mortality, especially following diarrhea and measles. Of course, vitamin A deficiency is also seen anywhere in the world where a child has a problem with fat malabsorption, such as celiac disease, cystic fibrosis, and hepatic insufficiency.

Physiology

Vitamin A refers to retinol and related compounds that share a beta-ionone ring; eg, retinal and retinoic acid. Dietary vitamin A consists of retinyl esters from animal sources (ie, liver, dairy, kidney, and eggs) and from plants (ie, carotenoids, such as beta-carotene in green and yellow vegetables). Vitamin A is absorbed through the intestines and stored in the liver. Retinol is important in the growth and integrity of epithelial cells; the retina uses retinal to promote normal vision; and retinoic acid promotes glycoprotein synthesis.

Epidemiology

Approximately 28 million preschool-aged children suffer from clinical vitamin A deficiency (xerophthalmia with serum vitamin A level less than 0.35 mmol/dL), and 251 million have subclinical deficiency (no xerophthalmia but deficient levels).[67,68] Two thirds of Asian children are thought to have vitamin A deficiency, while about half of African children are affected; deficiency is less common in other areas. Vitamin A deficiency is very common in children with generalized malnutrition, and vitamin A levels fall during the course of infections, such as measles.

Table 22-22. Causes, Manifestations, Management, and Prevention of Major Micronutrient Deficiencies

NUTRIENT	ESSENTIAL FOR THE PRODUCTION OR FUNCTION OF	CAUSES OF DEFICIENCY	MANIFESTATION OF ISOLATED DEFICIENCY	MANAGEMENT AND PREVENTION
Iron	• Hemoglobin • Various enzymes • Myoglobin	• Poor diet • Elevated needs (eg, while pregnant, in early childhood) • Chronic loss from parasite infections (eg, hookworms, schistosomiasis, whipworm)	• Anemia and fatigue • Impaired cognitive development • Reduced growth and physical strength	• Foods richer in iron and with fewer absorption inhibitors • Iron-fortified weaning foods • Low-dose supplements in childhood and pregnancy • Cooking in iron pots
Iodine	• Thyroid hormone	• Except where seafood or salt fortified with iodine is readily available, most diets worldwide are deficient.	• Goiter, hypothyroidism, constipation • Growth retardation • Endemic cretinism	• Iodine supplement • Fortified salt • Seafood
Vitamin A	• Eyes • Immune system	• Diets poor in vegetables and animal products	• Night blindness • Xerophthalmia • Immune deficiency • Increased childhood illness • Early death • Contributes to development of anemia	• More dark-green leafy vegetables, animal products • Fortification of oils and fats • Regular supplementation
Zinc	• Many enzymes • Immune system • Wound healing	• Diets poor in animal products • Diets based on refined cereals (eg, white bread, pasta, polished rice)	• Immune deficiency • Poor wound healing • Acrodermatitis • Increased childhood illness, early death • Complications in pregnancy and childbirth	• Zinc treatment for diarrhea and severe malnutrition • Improved diet

Table 22-22. Causes, Manifestations, Management, and Prevention of Major Micronutrient Deficiencies, continued

NUTRIENT	ESSENTIAL FOR THE PRODUCTION OR FUNCTION OF	CAUSES OF DEFICIENCY	MANIFESTATION OF ISOLATED DEFICIENCY	MANAGEMENT AND PREVENTION
Thiamine (B_1)	• Coenzyme for various metabolic pathways	• Diets poor in meat, eggs, legumes • Poor dietary diversity	• Beriberi (causing heart failure and peripheral neuropathy) • Wernicke encephalopathy (ophthalmoplegia with nystagmus and ataxia)	• Maternal intake during pregnancy and lactations • Supplementation
Riboflavin (B_2)	• Metabolism of protein, fat, and carbohydrate • Metabolism of other B vitamins	• Diets poor in animal protein and green vegetables • Restrictive diets	• Oral and ocular problems • Other vitamin B deficiencies • Stomatitis, glossitis, keratitis, dry skin	• Consuming a broad diet • Multivitamin supplementation • Supplementation
Niacin (B_3)	• Component of enzyme used in glycolysis	• Poor intake of meat, milk, and eggs • High intake of corn without animal protein intake	• Pellagra (with diarrhea, dementia, and dermatitis)	• Consuming a well-balanced diet • Adequate intake of animal protein • Multivitamin supplementation if on a restrictive diet • Supplementation
Folate (B_9)	• Cell growth • DNA synthesis • Red blood cell maturation	• Diets poor in fresh green vegetables and fruit • Malabsorption due to celiac disease • Short gut syndrome with bacterial overgrowth • Chronic diarrhea • Sickle cell disease	• Anemia • Neural tube defects in children born of mothers with deficiencies • Failure to thrive	• Adequate intake of fruits and vegetables • Supplementation

Table 22-22. Causes, Manifestations, Management, and Prevention of Major Micronutrient Deficiencies, continued

NUTRIENT	ESSENTIAL FOR THE PRODUCTION OR FUNCTION OF	CAUSES OF DEFICIENCY	MANIFESTATION OF ISOLATED DEFICIENCY	MANAGEMENT AND PREVENTION
Cobalamin (B_{12})	• Contributes to DNA synthesis	• Diet restricting animal products • Absent or diseased ileum	• Macrocytic anemia	• Adequate intake of animal products • Supplementation
Vitamin C (ascorbic acid)	• Hydroxylation of collagen • Capillary epithelium and osteoid tissue integrity • Antioxidant • Wound healing	• Diets poor in fruit and vegetable intake	• Scurvy (often with symptoms of severe fatigue, joint pain, excessive bruising, and bleeding gums) • Poor wound healing	• Adequate dietary intake of vitamin C • Supplementation
Vitamin D and calcium	• Vitamin D stimulates the absorption of calcium. • Calcium is for bone health.	• Poor dietary intake (fortified milk or liver). • Lack of exposure to ultraviolet sunlight. • Darkly pigmented skinned people are at higher risk for deficiency.	• Rickets • Osteomalacia • Stunting • Infantile heart failure and muscle weakness • Negatively affects risk and severity of other diseases and conditions	• Adequate sun exposure. • Vitamin D supplementation. • Adequate calcium intake. • Breastfed infants should be supplemented with vitamin D daily.
Selenium	• Several enzymes • Metabolism of free radicals	• Soil depletion of selenium causing inadequate amounts in food sources	• Myxedematous cretinism (in combination with iodine deficiency) • Keshan disease (a form of cardiomyopathy) • Kashin-Bek osteoarthropathy • Poor pregnancy outcomes • Poor longitudinal growth	• Selenium supplementation; preventively if in an area of high risk or as treatment if deficiency is identified

Figure 22-11. Affects of Micronutrient Deficiencies

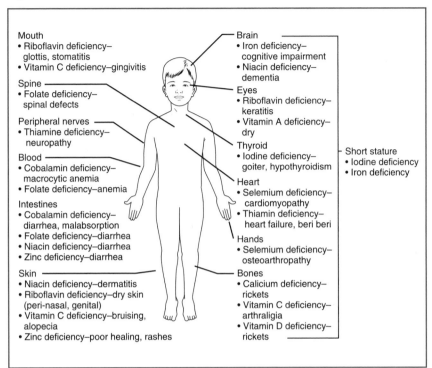

Mouth
- Riboflavin deficiency–
  glottis, stomatitis
- Vitamin C deficiency–gingivitis

Spine
- Folate deficiency–
  spinal defects

Peripheral nerves
- Thiamine deficiency–
  neuropathy

Blood
- Cobalamin deficiency–
  macrocytic anemia
- Folate deficiency–anemia

Intestines
- Cobalamin deficiency–
  diarrhea, malabsorption
- Folate deficiency–diarrhea
- Niacin deficiency–diarrhea
- Zinc deficiency–diarrhea

Skin
- Niacin deficiency–dermatitis
- Riboflavin deficiency–dry skin
  (peri-nasal, genital)
- Vitamin C deficiency–bruising,
  alopecia
- Zinc deficiency–poor healing, rashes

Brain
- Iron deficiency–
  cognitive impairment
- Niacin deficiency–
  dementia

Eyes
- Riboflavin deficiency–
  keratitis
- Vitamin A deficiency–
  dry

Thyroid
- Iodine deficiency–
  goiter, hypothyroidism

Heart
- Selemium deficiency–
  cardiomyopathy
- Thiamin deficiency–
  heart failure, beri beri

Hands
- Selemium deficiency–
  osteoarthropathy

Bones
- Calicium deficiency–
  rickets
- Vitamin C deficiency–
  arthraligia
- Vitamin D deficiency–
  rickets

Short stature
- Iodine deficiency
- Iron deficiency

Clinical Presentations

Inadequate tissue integrity, poor healing, and complications of infections, such as diarrhea and measles, occur with low levels of vitamin A, even before seeing the pathognomonic feature of hypovitaminosis A— xerophthalmia (dry eyes). Skin over extensor surfaces is dry and scaly, and similar keratinization of the conjunctiva and lacrimal glands leads to dry eyes with follicular conjunctivitis (xerophthalmia). Night blindness results from delays in rhodopsin synthesis and is considered the earliest eye manifestation of vitamin A deficiency. Bitot spots can be seen as small, silvery, triangle-shaped patches on the conjunctiva where keratinization occurred. Inflammatory changes in the eyes lead to keratomalacia, corneal ulceration, and blindness.[65] Symptoms can be reversed with treatment as long as scarring has not already occurred. Therefore, it is imperative to recognize the symptoms of vitamin A deficiency early before keratomalacia and corneal ulcerations develop.

Prevention

Unless mothers are vitamin A deficient, breast milk contains adequate levels of this vitamin to support a growing child. Supplementation (single doses of 200,000 to 400,000 IU) to postpartum women can increase vitamin A content in breast milk.[69] When maternal hypovitaminosis A is common, supplementation is recommended during the first postpartum visit; high-dose supplementation during pregnancy might carry a risk for teratogenesis and is usually avoided. Vitamin A supplementation is suggested in areas where childhood vitamin A deficiency is common. Many countries require vitamin A to be added to frequently ingested foods, such as milk, oils, and margarines, which may be recommended. Direct supplementation with vitamin A may be preventive if such fortified foods are unavailable. Since 1987, the WHO has recommended oral supplementation with 100,000 IU vitamin A at 6 to 9 months of age (the time of routine measles vaccination).[70] Additional booster doses of 200,000 IU can be given every 4 to 6 months until age 4 years. In fact, in many areas in the developing world the WHO immunization campaigns now include routinely giving vitamin A supplementation. While smaller daily doses could be considered, care providers in developing countries usually find that intermittent large doses are more feasibly delivered.

Treatment

Children with documented low levels of vitamin A (in the rare situations where testing is done in developing countries) or with clinical findings of xerophthalmia or night blindness should be treated for vitamin A deficiency. Daily doses of 200,000 IU (100,000 IU if younger than 1 year) for 2 days are effective. Similarly, children younger than 2 years in lower-income countries should be given 2 days of treatment at the onset of measles.[71]

Thiamine (B$_1$)[65,66]

Importance

Thiamine deficiency, which causes beriberi, is widespread in Southeast Asia. Affected infants are at risk of death because of heart failure, while older children are at risk of peripheral neuropathy complications.

Physiology

Thiamine is a water-soluble vitamin that serves as a coenzyme in various metabolic pathways, including acetylcholine synthesis. It is readily available in meat, eggs, legumes, and rice but is inactivated during the cooking process. Natural rice is a good source of thiamine; however, the thiamine remains with the husks. Therefore, it is lost during the de-husking or polishing process.

Epidemiology

As previously mentioned, thiamine deficiency is common in Southeast Asia[72,73] and is a significant cause of infantile death. Wet beriberi is associated with populations who discard the washings produced during rice preparation, have low socioeconomic status, and have minimal dietary diversity. Beriberi is common in some refugee populations.

Clinical Presentations

Infants 1 to 6 months of age manifest thiamine deficiency as wet beriberi with heart failure. They often are irritable with a hoarse or absent cry. They sleep poorly, often vomit, and can sweat excessively. They appear critically ill (septic) and can die of heart failure within hours to days on development of symptoms.

Older children with dry beriberi have peripheral neuropathy that progresses to increasing muscle weakness, gait abnormalities, ataxia, and dysesthesias; areflexia is noted on examination. Ophthalmoplegia with nystagmus and ataxia (Wernicke encephalopathy) has been reported with thiamine deficiency.

Prevention

Infantile beriberi is prevented by ensuring adequate maternal thiamine intake during pregnancy and lactation. Mothers may be supplemented orally with 50 mg thiamine daily.

Treatment

The diagnosis of infantile beriberi should prompt treatment of mother and child. Infants are treated once with 50 mg of thiamine intramuscularly; a repeat dose can be given if symptoms are not resolving over several hours (while also evaluating and treating for sepsis and other potential confounding conditions). Less acute cases of beriberi in older children and mothers can be treated with 10 (young child) to 50 (adult) mg of oral thiamine daily for 1 month (assuming that adequate subsequent thiamine intake is assured).

Riboflavin (B$_2$)[63,64]

Importance

Riboflavin deficiency is an occasional cause of oral and ocular problems in poorly nourished children.

Physiology

Riboflavin is a precursor of enzyme cofactors important to oxidation-reduction reactions related to protein, carbohydrate, and fat metabolism. It is found in animal protein and green vegetables. Riboflavin plays a role in the metabolism of other B vitamins; other B-vitamin deficiencies are often identified concurrently with riboflavin deficiency.

Epidemiology

Riboflavin deficiency is found in malnourished children with extremely restricted diets.

Clinical Presentations

Angular stomatitis, glossitis, keratitis, and dry skin around the nose and genital area are physical signs suggesting riboflavin deficiency.

Prevention

Riboflavin deficiency is fully preventable by using a broad diet particularly consisting of at least some meat products or multivitamin preparations.

Treatment

Riboflavin deficiency is treated with 1 mg riboflavin orally 3 times daily until signs of deficiency are resolved.

Niacin (B$_3$)[65,66]

Importance

Niacin deficiency, commonly known as pellagra (Italian for "rough skin"), is still seen in some developing countries where malnutrition is widespread.

Physiology

Niacin is the end product of tryptophan metabolism and is a building block for enzymes that are required for protein transport and glycolysis. Niacin is found in milk, meat, and eggs.

Epidemiology

Pellagra is most often seen in individuals who primarily eat maize (corn) without animal protein. Other signs of generalized malnutrition and other micronutrient deficiencies often coexist with pellagra. Individuals on isoniazid can develop isolated niacin deficiency.

Clinical Presentations

Pellagra is characterized by 3 Ds: diarrhea, dermatitis, and dementia. Glossitis and angular stomatitis accompany the diarrhea (perhaps in part because of concurrent riboflavin deficiency). Sun-exposed skin becomes painful and erythematous (or hyperpigmented in dark-skinned individuals); repeat sun exposure can lead to blistering and bullae formation. Eventually, sun-exposed skin becomes rough and scaly; hair, nails, and sun-unexposed areas are spared. Individuals may have insomnia, fatigue, irritability, and mental dullness, which progress to frank dementia.

Prevention

Regular ingestion of animal protein can prevent pellagra, as can multivitamin preparations in individuals with severely restricted diets. Maize contains some niacin but only in a poorly absorbed bound form.

Treatment

Niacin deficiency is treated orally with 50 to 100 mg of nicotinamide 3 times daily. A varied diet should be instituted and other potentially co-occurring vitamin deficiencies should be treated at the same time. Pharmacologic supplementation can be discontinued when signs and symptoms of deficiency resolve.

Folate (B_9)[65,66]

Importance

Folate deficiency contributes to anemia in many parts of the world. However, the greatest effect of this deficiency is associated with neural tube defects in children because of a deficiency in women of childbearing potential.

Physiology

Dietary folate, as contained in fresh green vegetables and some fruit, is absorbed through the small intestines. It affects cell growth by providing purine and thymine, and thus, DNA synthesis. Its effects are most obvious as they relate to red cell maturation and, with deficiency, a risk of anemia.

Epidemiology

Inadequate folate intakes are common around the world, but frank deficiency is most common in children with intestinal malabsorption caused by celiac disease, short gut with bacterial overgrowth, and chronic diarrhea. Deficiency does not seem specific to any particular geographic region or population group.[74] Children with chronic hemolysis caused by sickle cell disease have an increased need for folate and frequently become deficient.

Clinical Presentations

Folate deficiency presents with anemia, irritability, and failure to thrive. Chronic diarrhea is often present, frequently because diarrhea predisposed the child to becoming folate deficient.

Prevention

Eating multiple daily servings of fruits and vegetables is effective in preventing folate deficiency. Folate supplements (1 to 5 mg per day, given orally) are actually better absorbed than folate in food. Preemptive or preventive folate supplementation should be considered for children with chronic diarrhea, sickle cell disease, and other chronic hemolytic anemias (ie, thalassemias, glucose-6-phosphate dehydrogenase deficiency) and for women of childbearing age.

Treatment

When suspected or diagnosed, folate deficiency may be treated orally (or parenterally, if required) with 1 (young infants) to 5 (adolescents) mg daily. Treatment should be continued until the symptoms resolve and adequate dietary intake is established.

Cobalamin (B$_{12}$)[65,66]

Importance

Vitamin B$_{12}$ (cobalamin) deficiency occurs around the world but usually in individuals with no intake of animal products or with absent or diseased ilea.

Physiology

Vitamin B$_{12}$ is produced by microorganisms living in animals; however, humans are not capable of producing it. Ingested B$_{12}$ combines with intrinsic factor in the stomach and is eventually absorbed in the ileum. It is stored in the liver and contributes to DNA synthesis.

Epidemiology

Vitamin B$_{12}$ deficiency is seen around the world but is not specifically associated with any particular geographic area or population subgroup.[74] Deficiency is most common in strict vegetarians who do not eat animal products and in patients who had surgical resection involving the stomach or terminal ileum.

Clinical Presentations

Vitamin B_{12} deficiency manifests itself as macrocytic anemia, often with diarrhea and, in young infants, failure to thrive. Hypersegmented neutrophils are noted on peripheral blood smears of deficient individuals.

Prevention

Vitamin B_{12} deficiency is avoided by eating animal products or taking supplements.

Treatment

Vitamin B_{12} deficiency is readily treated with parenteral (or oral if absorption is adequate) administration of 1 mg of vitamin B_{12}. Hematologic improvement occurs within a few days. Subsequent assurance of adequate B_{12} intake is necessary (monthly doses of 0.1 mg if dietary intake is not possible).

Vitamin C[65,66,75,76]

Importance

Scurvy, the vitamin C deficiency bane of 18th-century citrus-deprived sailors, is uncommon. Nonetheless, it is still seen from time to time in children who do not eat fruits and vegetables.

Physiology

Some animals are able to synthesize vitamin C, but humans depend on exogenous sources. Vitamin C, otherwise known as ascorbic acid, is contained in citrus fruits, papaya, tomatoes, potatoes, spinach, and cabbage. About 90% of a human's intake of vitamin C comes from fruit and vegetable sources. Cooking reduces active vitamin C content by about a third. Vitamin C is active in the hydroxylation of collagen and is therefore important in the formation and integrity of capillary epithelium and osteoid tissue. Ascorbic acid is an antioxidant and, thus, is relevant to several disease states. It reduces dietary iron from the ferric to the ferrous form to facilitate iron absorption.

Epidemiology

Scurvy is uncommon but does present in individuals with restricted diets (because of poverty, presumed food intolerances, or misconceptions about dietary needs). A review of 28 children with scurvy in Thailand[77] identified associations not only with an absence of dietary fruit and vegetable but also with ultra–high-temperature milk processing; the role of heat-treated milk in altering vitamin C is not well understood. Preschoolers are more affected by scurvy than older children.

Clinical Presentations

Children with scurvy often have severe fatigue and weakness, as well as a limp because of joint pain. They may demonstrate a frog-leg posture (pseudoparalysis) because of the severe joint pain. Pseudoparalysis should be distinguished from true paralysis by lifting the child from under her axilla and allowing the legs to hang freely. The child with pseudoparalysis will flex her hips from the pain caused by the sudden extension of her legs, while the child with true paralysis will be unable to flex her hips. Capillary fragility is seen as unusual skin bruising and swollen bleeding gums; splinter hemorrhages of the nail beds and subconjunctival hemorrhage may be seen. Hyperkeratotic papules and corkscrew hairs and alopecia can develop. Subperiosteal hemorrhages lead to severe bone pain and radiographic evidence of separated epiphyses. Arthralgia and myalgia are common, and hemarthrosis is possible. Wound healing is delayed. Normochromic normocytic anemia is common. Some may present with a scorbutic rosary in the costochondral regions, which can be distinguished from the rachitic rosary of vitamin D deficiency by its more angular nature and its exquisite tenderness. A serum vitamin C level below 11 mmol/L confirms vitamin C deficiency as the cause of clinical findings. Symptoms and signs of scurvy resolve rapidly with treatment.

Prevention

A daily intake of 50 mg of ascorbic acid (the amount in 1 orange) is recommended; however, 10 mg per day should be adequate to prevent childhood scurvy. Children should be encouraged to eat a wide variety of uncooked fruits, including guava (which contains nearly 3 times the vitamin C as oranges) and other citrus fruits.

Treatment

Children with scurvy should receive 25 mg of vitamin C 4 times a day for 1 week. Symptoms resolve within hours to days. Subsequently, adequate vitamin C intake should be ensured.

Vitamin D and Calcium[65,66,78,79]

Importance

Rickets, a consequence of calcium or vitamin D deficiency, affects up to 10% of the population in some parts of the developing world. More subtly, osteomalacia and stunting result from combined or isolated calcium and vitamin D deficiencies. In addition, hypovitaminosis D likely affects the risk and severity of diabetes, cancer, multiple sclerosis, chronic pain, and infections, including tuberculosis, leprosy, and HIV. Rickets increases the risk of mortality with acute respiratory infection.[24]

Physiology

Vitamin D is produced in ultraviolet light-exposed skin or ingested in fortified dairy products or liver. Following hepatic and renal hydroxylation, biologically active 1,25-dihydroxyvitamin D stimulates calcium absorption from the intestines, calcium deposition into bones, and a variety of other metabolic actions through interactions with parathyroid hormones. In addition, there are potential metabolic, infectious, and neoplastic actions that seem to result from the influence of vitamin D receptors scattered throughout the body. Rickets results when a child's isolated calcium or vitamin D deficiency leads to an inadequate delivery of minerals to developing bones. Calcium deficiency also leads to an increased metabolic need for vitamin D, and many children get rickets with a combined insufficiency of calcium and vitamin D. Less commonly, rickets occurs because of renal disease with inadequate bioactivation of 25-hydroxyvitamin D.

Epidemiology

For centuries, rickets has been reported in northern climates of industrialized countries where young children are minimally exposed to sunlight because of weather and cultural conditions. Rickets has reemerged as a clinical problem in North America, especially in breastfed babies with darkly pigmented skin. In developing countries, rickets occurs in infants, young children, and adolescents who are shielded from the sun (sometimes because of cultural practices, such as the Muslim purdah, or from living in crowded slum dwellings), as well as in older infants and young children with calcium-insufficient diets. Rickets has been reported in most countries of the world in recent decades. Calcium-deficiency rickets seems especially common in Nigeria, South Africa, India, and Bangladesh.

Clinical Presentations

Vitamin D–deficiency rickets traditionally presents late in the first year of life with hypocalcemic tetany, or during the toddler years with curving deformities of lower limbs. Calcium-deficiency rickets usually presents with limb deformities during the toddler and childhood years. Bowed legs, knock-knees, and anterior curvature of the tibiae are all possible. Widened wrists and ankles, beaded ribs which are typically non-tender, large fontanelles, chest wall deformities, and dental hypoplasia are seen with either form of rickets. Bone pain and increased fractures result from calcium or vitamin D deficiency. Infantile heart failure and muscle weakness are possible with vitamin D deficiency. When available, laboratory testing can show hypovitaminosis D (levels less than 10 nmol/L associated with rickets, levels 10 to 25 nmol/L subnormal but unlikely to cause rickets without concurrent calcium deficiency). Serum levels of 1,25-dihydroxyvitamin D are low in vitamin D–deficiency rickets but elevated in children with calcium-deficiency rickets. Alkaline phosphatase levels are elevated due to rapid bone turnover in rachitic children. Radiographs show osteopenia along with cupping, fraying, and epiphyses widening. An x-ray scoring system for the severity of rickets was developed[80] and is useful in following the adequacy of a child's response to treatment.

Prevention

Rickets is avoidable by fostering adequate sun exposure, taking vitamin D supplements, or ensuring adequate calcium intake. Infants should get at least 60 minutes per week of sunshine exposure to the head, and older children should get at least 60 minutes of head and extremity sun exposure. Breast milk does not contain adequate vitamin D for children who do not have another source, but fortified formulas and processed milk often do contain adequate vitamin D. As needed, all infants and children can be supplemented with additional vitamin D to ensure at least 400 IU of daily intake.

Nigerian and South African children with calcium-deficiency rickets take in less than 25% of the recommended 800 mg elemental calcium daily allotment. Calcium intake can be encouraged by the use of dairy products, eating small fish with the bones included (ground, as in many parts of Africa, or whole, as in parts of Asia), or taking calcium supplements. Adolescents should take at least 1,200 mg of elemental calcium per day; ultimate adult bone strength likely depends on the peak bone mass achieved during adolescence.

Treatment

Children with tetany require aggressive calcium supplementation and intensive care monitoring. Children with rickets, especially when vitamin D levels are not available, should receive adequate vitamin D; this can be done by giving 2,000 to 5,000 IU vitamin D orally per day for 3 to 6 months or by giving 300,000 to 600,000 IU vitamin D intramuscularly every 3 to 6 months. After acute treatment of rickets over 6 months (and normalization of the serum alkaline phosphatase level and resolution of radiographic abnormalities, if such tests were indeed available), ongoing adequacy of sun exposure or vitamin D intake should be ensured.

Concurrently, in areas where calcium-deficiency rickets is common and in a child who presents with rickets after 12 months of age, with a history of seemingly adequate sun exposure, daily oral calcium supplements should be given to provide 1,000 mg of elemental calcium (as found in 2.5 g of calcium carbonate).

Ongoing adequacy of calcium intake should be ensured after 6 months of treatment and resolution of laboratory and radiographic abnormalities. Even striking leg deformities can straighten over time with ongoing growth. Beading of ribs can persist for years. Surgery (whether scraping or stapling growth plates or actual osteotomies) should be considered when deformities limit function years after actual bone mineralization defects are resolved. Children with rickets caused by renal disease need full treatment for the underlying kidney condition.

Iodine[66,67,81]

Importance

Iodine deficiency is the world's leading cause of preventable brain damage. Primarily through its affects on thyroid function, iodine deficiency plagues about half of children in Asia and a third of children in Africa.

Physiology

Iodine is an essential component of thyroid hormone. Deficiency in pregnant women can lead to endemic cretinism (severe irreversible mental retardation along with hypothyroidism). Acquired iodine deficiency in children causes goiter, hypothyroidism, and subclinical learning difficulties. Humans eat iodine when they ingest plants grown in iodine-rich soil or iodine-fortified products (eg, salt in North America). Natural products contain inadequate iodine in most parts of the world, and people must depend on iodine-fortified foods for their intake. The metabolism of iodine depends on selenium and iron to some degree, and iodine-deficient children do not respond completely to iodine treatment until their selenium and iron statuses are normal.

Epidemiology

Most people in the world are at risk of iodine deficiency, but the widespread use of iodized salt obviates this risk in industrialized areas. Iodine deficiency remains common in developing countries where salt is not routinely fortified or where there is not a central (fortifiable) source of salt. Nonetheless, 35% of the world's children have inadequate iodine intakes. Approximately 90% of salt is iodized in the Americas and Caribbean and approximately only two thirds of salt is iodized in Asia and Africa—children in these areas remain at significant risk. Consequences of iodine deficiency are most severe during pregnancy and childhood.

Clinical Presentations

Infants born to severely iodine-deficient mothers may be heavy, sluggish, and mentally retarded. Mental deficits persist even after hypothyroidism is corrected. Cretins vary from myxedematous (large and slow) to spastic (hypertonic with trouble ambulating) with deafness depending on whether selenium deficiency concurrently affected the children. Acquired iodine deficiency usually presents as goiter and is reversible with iodine replacement. Iodine-deficient children have a lower IQ by 30 points and more fine-motor control problems than do iodine-replete children. Chronically iodine-deficient children have short stature.

Prevention

Preventing iodine deficiency depends on adequate iodine intake and is best approached at community, regional, and national levels. In areas where salt fortification is not yet feasible, supplementing individual children with iodized oil leads to decreased goiter rates and decreased hypothyroidism. Some studies also reported significant improvement in cognitive function, psychomotor ability, and growth with iodized oil.[81]

Treatment

Successfully treating iodine deficiency depends on adequate selenium and iron status; iodine therapy will be incompletely effective if other deficiencies are not corrected concurrently. Iodine may be given safely as potassium iodide orally (usually 150 µg per day; 200 µg per day if pregnant) or, if treatment compliance is uncertain, an intramuscular iodized oil injection (200 mg) is adequate for 1 year of coverage.

Iron[66,82]

Importance

Iron deficiency is the most common form of malnutrition in the world; by current estimates, 42% of young children on this planet are iron deficient. More than one third of iron-deficient children are anemic, but even without anemia, iron deficiency causes neurodevelopmental compromise and altered activity tolerance.

Physiology

Iron is available in dairy products, vegetables, and meat. However, absorption varies with the iron source. Iron from vegetable sources (non-heme iron) is less well-absorbed than iron from dairy or meat sources (heme iron). Iron from human milk is best absorbed (50%), while only 4% to 10% is absorbed from (bioavailable in) infant formulas and cow's milk. Iron absorption is facilitated by vitamin C and inhibited by antacids, phytic acid (legumes, rice, and grains), polyphenol (eg, tea), and other divalent cations (ie, calcium and zinc). Pathologic iron loss occurs with gastritis, infantile cow's milk protein intolerance, and hookworm infection; excessive blood or iron loss can occur with menstruation. Iron deficiency results when iron absorption is inadequate to balance iron loss and iron needs (which increase during times of growth). Iron is directly required for red cell synthesis. Even without anemia, iron deficiency has been associated with neurodevelopmental compromise, poor academic performance, activity intolerance, and sleep disorders (specifically restless leg syndrome).

Epidemiology

In developing countries, dietary limitations (eg, minimal meat intake) combine with excessive iron losses (from cow's milk protein intolerance in some young infants and hookworm in many older infants and children) to produce a high prevalence of iron deficiency. Normal hemoglobin levels vary with age, and anemia is defined as a hemoglobin concentration less than 10 g/dL at 4 to 6 months of age, less than 10.5 g/dL at 9 months of age, and less than 11 g/dL after a baby's first birthday.

Iron deficiency is assumed to be the cause of the anemia when it is associated with hypochromia and microcytosis or a low serum ferritin level. However, iron deficiency is 2.5 times more common than iron deficiency anemia in developing countries. Low serum ferritin levels suggest iron deficiency in the absence of an acute inflammatory condition; similarly, a low iron binding saturation suggests iron deficiency. Iron deficiency is common by whatever diagnostic criteria are used.

Three fourths of infants in sub-Saharan Africa are anemic. About half of Asians and South Americans and one third of North Africans are similarly affected; half of these anemic children are thought to be iron deficient. Iron deficiency is more common in resource-limited areas and former premature babies. The prevalence of iron deficiency is higher in infants and young children than in older children and adolescents. Overall, nearly half of the young children on this planet are thought to be iron deficient.

Clinical Presentations

A majority of young children in developing countries are iron deficient, but they rarely present for medical care due to their nutritional deficiency. Thus, screening (often by simply determining hemoglobin levels or hematocrits) is important and public health measures should be instituted in addition to managing individually diagnosed children.

Prevention

Prevention of iron deficiency should start before a child is born. Pregnant women should eat iron-rich foods and, in areas of risk, receive iron supplementation. Testing (or presumptive treatment) for hookworm is indicated in areas of high prevalence. At the time of birth, delayed cord clamping (approximately 2 minutes, until pulsations cease) allows for greater maternal-infant transfer of blood and iron.

Breastfeeding should be encouraged and supported for the first year of the infant's life. Premature and low birth weight babies should have iron supplementation (2 to 3 mg elemental iron per kg per day). Iron-rich foods should be added to the routine infant diet at about 6 months of age. Iron supplements should be considered for at-risk infants. Stool testing for helminths (or presumptive deworming) every 6 months during childhood is advisable in lower-income countries. Widespread professional and lay education can help mobilize efforts to implement these interventions at community levels.

Treatment

Children found to be iron deficient should be treated with iron supplements to provide 4 to 6 mg elemental iron per kg per day for at least 3 months, and subsequent adequacy of dietary intake should be assured. Anemic children can be presumptively treated with iron in areas with limited laboratory testing—an increase of 1 g/dL or more in hemoglobin concentration after 1 month confirms an iron-deficiency diagnosis. A lack of response to treatment (with known adherence to therapeutic regimen) could prompt a search for other causes of anemia. Blood transfusions are given when there are signs of cardiovascular decompensation due to the anemia, realizing that children with chronic anemia often become tolerant to hemoglobin levels in the 5 to 8 g/dL range.

Selenium

Importance

Rarely, selenium deficiency is seen in children with inadequate parenteral nutrition. Selenium deficiency is also seen as 3 clinical situations in distinct geographic areas of the world: central Africa in combination with iodine deficiency causing myxedematous cretinism; southwest China as a unique form of cardiomyopathy, Keshan disease; and southwest China as Kashin-Bek osteoarthropathy. These conditions are increasingly rare thanks to improved selenium nutrition.

Physiology

Selenium deficiency is uncommon except in a few areas of the world. Dietary selenium intake depends on local soil content, which determines how much selenium is in water, plants, animals, and milk. Selenium is necessary for the functioning of several enzymes and the metabolism of free radicals through glutathione peroxidase.

It is likely that selenium deficiency serves as a cofactor with other agents or conditions to produce unique clinical problems. It seems that coxsackievirus infection might interact with selenium deficiency to cause a unique cardiomyopathy in and around the Keshan province of China; the clinical presentation is similar to mitochondrial cardiomyopathies.[83] Combined selenium and iodine deficiencies affect cartilage integrity and longitudinal growth, but the exact mechanism by which selenium deficiency contributes to Kashin-Bek osteoarthropathy is unknown; in fact, even the relevance of low selenium levels to this condition has been debated.[84]

Epidemiology

A belt running through several provinces of southwest China is associated with low selenium levels in soil, animals, and humans. Up to 100% of children show some signs of disease in some areas of China. Selenium levels are lower in parts of Scandinavia than in most other parts of the world. Northern regions of the Democratic Republic of the Congo are also relatively selenium deficient. Children are more affected than adults, and poor pregnancy outcomes (miscarriages) are also seen with selenium deficiency during pregnancy.

Clinical Presentations

Selenium deficiency in Central Africa manifests itself by combining with prevalent iodine deficiency to produce myxedematous cretinism (rather than the more common spastic cretinism seen in other areas). Kashin-Bek osteoarthropathy presents as painful destruction of joint cartilage at about 5 years of age and progresses to multiple joints. Progressive joint deformity and stunting are common. Keshan cardiomyopathy occurs in children and presents with heart failure and dysrhythmia; it is often fatal and myocardial necrosis is seen on autopsy.

Prevention

To prevent selenium deficiency in recipients of parenteral nutrition, the IV solution should include 2 µg of selenium per kg per day. In endemic areas, prevention of selenium deficiency is effective with supplementation (usually 1 mg orally each week if younger than 10 years; 2 mg orally each week if older than 10 years). Supplementation leads to significant reductions in overt disease and mortality in high-risk areas.

Treatment

Keshan cardiomyopathy is reversible with early treatment (100 µg per day IV has been used).[85] Outcome studies are limited, but a diagnosis of selenium deficiency in a patient who is not critically ill should prompt supplementation as dosed for prevention.

Zinc[66]

Importance

Zinc deficiency contributes directly to morbidity and mortality due to infectious illnesses in impoverished communities around the world. It is estimated that zinc deficiency accounts for 4% of childhood deaths and 1% of childhood disease in Africa, Asia, and Latin America.[86] Specifically, zinc deficiency was identified as an exacerbating factor in 2 of the most common killers of children, diarrhea and pneumonia.

Physiology

Zinc is an essential cofactor in a variety of metabolic pathways that greatly affect protein and energy metabolism. Zinc is readily available in meats, cheese, legumes, and grains. Deficiency affects transcription pathways and cellular synthetic functions, which result in problems with growth and resistance to infections.

Epidemiology

Zinc deficiency is widespread, especially in developing countries where generalized malnutrition is common. A majority of children in slums in some parts of Asia are zinc deficient.[87] It is estimated that one fourth of the world's population is at risk of zinc deficiency.[86]

Clinical Presentations

Isolated severe zinc deficiency is rare and presents as perioral and perianal dermatitis, diarrhea, increased susceptibility to infection, and poor growth. Less severe zinc deficiency is not characterized by the dermatologic findings but aggravates gastrointestinal and respiratory diseases in children who grow poorly.

Prevention

Adequate general dietary intake prevents zinc deficiency. Daily (20 mg) or weekly (70 mg) supplements are effective for children in deprived areas of the world. In areas where zinc deficiency is common, children with diarrhea recover better if they are concurrently treated with zinc (10 mg daily for 2 weeks if younger than 6 months; 20 mg per dose for older infants and children).[86,88] Pre-illness zinc supplementation decreases the incidence of childhood pneumonia but likely does not alter the course of established respiratory infection.[89]

Treatment

Severe zinc deficiency responds within days to daily zinc supplements of 20 to 30 mg orally. Daily (1 mg/kg/d) and weekly (70 mg) supplements for mildly deficient young children have similar favorable effects.

■ MALNUTRITION: THE FUTURE

What We Know

It is said that Isaac Newton claimed he could only extend scientific knowledge "by standing on the shoulders of giants"; that is, by building on the foundation others laid for him. Like Newton, we are poised to extend the scientific and clinical conquest of malnutrition to greater levels of success. We do so, however, not by standing on the shoulders of giants but by rising above the collective experience of the starving, shriveled masses who have gone before us. We learn from their tragic sacrifices and we implement better strategies to avoid the intolerable burden of childhood malnutrition.

Malnutrition is often an economic problem directly related to living in poverty. Meanwhile, much of the planet's population lives in luxury. We know that more than 1 billion people on the planet are hungry.[1] We know that 2 million children, mostly in the resource-limited countries of Asia and Africa, die each year from malnutrition.[2,3,90] We know that up to half of children in developing countries suffer from subtle (and not-so-subtle) effects of generalized malnutrition or specific micronutrient deficiencies.[3] These children are sometimes crippled or blinded by their malnutrition. Other times, they are weakened and diseased. And sometimes, they look OK but fail to reach their developmental, academic, social, and economic potential because of their nutritional deficiencies. We know that families, communities, and countries are suffering from inadequate nutrition.

We know that poverty is a problem, yet we realize that much of the planet's population lives in luxury. We know that there are significant disparities in the allocation of resources, with 20% of the world's population garnering 76% of the planet's resources.[90] We know that more than half of the world's people live on less than the equivalent of $2.50 per day.[91] Yet we also know that there are ways to combat poverty—top-down,[92] community-up,[93] and social mobilization.[94]

However, we also know that malnutrition is complex. It is often a matter of poverty, but it is also often a matter of other social and political issues. It is affected by war. Armed conflict, for instance, diverts agricultural workers to soldiering, decreases security of gardens and food, and displaces families, all with resulting increases in malnutrition. Overall, nearly a fifth of children in the developing world lack secure sources of daily food.[11]

We know that malnutrition is a health problem and that malnutrition aggravates and is aggravated by other health problems. We know that major child killers such as diarrhea, pneumonia, malaria, and birth asphyxia are tangled up with malnutrition.[95]

We know how to define and diagnose various forms of malnutrition. We know how to assess and alter the course of malnutrition. We know how to use individual supplements and integrated systems to combat malnutrition.

And we know that we care. We are involved with this chapter and this book precisely because we want to get involved in solutions. To us, malnutrition is not merely an academic exercise but rather, an active experience. We know that we must personally and collectively engage in the battle to improve individual and societal outcomes for people currently suffering from malnutrition, and we know that we must support ongoing efforts to prevent malnutrition in the next generation.

What We Need to Do

Aware of large issues and societal approaches to malnutrition, we must now work to help children who are suffering from generalized malnutrition or micronutrient deficiency. Affected children must be identified and monitored. Appropriate care for concurrent illnesses must be instituted. A holistic approach, as identified by the WHO,[11] must be followed to help those most severely affected. We must consider the possibility of micronutrient deficiency while caring for asymptomatic and ill children in developing countries, and we must treat those deficiencies appropriately. Treating malnutrition is not glamorous or easy, but it is necessary. While working clinically with malnourished individuals, we must also work to improve systems that foster malnutrition. We must advocate for food, security, protection of children from the effects of armed conflict, equitable distribution of vaccines, development of improved water sources and better sanitation, and child-appropriate health policies. At the same time, we should partner with multinational organizations to improve distribution of resources. We should support research about micronutrients and cognition, food fortification and supplementation, and population-based implementation of nutritional programs.

The Next Generation

Science has advanced enough to adequately inform our prescriptions of care for malnourished children. We know what needs to be done for individuals and groups, but we must continually use evidence-based research to improve our care.[96] What mostly remains, however, is to learn to implement systems better to ensure that appropriate care reaches the most needy children. We must continue to work toward systems that rectify existing disparities in the availability of adequate nutritional care and health interventions. Mostly, though, we must avoid paralysis of analysis. The children of our current and next generations need action—action that we are now able to undertake.

■ KEY POINTS

- Childhood malnutrition is a serious global health issue resulting from a multiplicity of complex and interrelated factors, including financial, geographic, political, cultural, and educational causes.
- Though Asia has typically been the area of highest prevalence of malnutrition, East Africa is currently experiencing the greatest increase in malnutrition disorders.

- Malnutrition increases morbidity and mortality associated with the most common causes of childhood illness including diarrheal, acute respiratory, malaria, measles, and HIV/AIDS.
- Proper nutrition, often including supplementation of important micronutrients such as zinc and vitamin A, can reduce mortality from these common illnesses.
- Anemia in children living in underdeveloped countries is often multifactorial. Malaria should be considered in addition to dietary and helminth causes.
- Exclusive breastfeeding for the first 6 months of life reduces malnutrition in infants and reduces frequency and severity of numerous common childhood illnesses; as such, it is an important strategy for reducing the devastating effects of malnutrition.
- Malnutrition is arguably the most critical health issue facing children in the developing world, contributing to more than 50% of the mortality in children younger than 5 years.
- Malnutrition results in numerous metabolic abnormalities that form the basis for proven treatment strategies.
- Malnourished children should be identified and treated early in the course of their disease to prevent sequelae and mortality.
- Diagnosis of malnutrition should be based on multiple anthropometric measurements when available, developmental survey, and clinical signs of macronutrient and micronutrient deficiencies.
- Once identified, malnourished children should be placed in a community- or hospital-based treatment plan as appropriately determined by appetite and presence of comorbidities.
- The WHO 10 steps are a proven beneficial strategy for treatment of SAM and should be strictly adhered to for inpatient treatment of malnutrition.
- Despite reductions in generalized malnutrition rates, micronutrient deficiencies continue to plague much of the developing world because of lack of diversity in diets, cultural issues, and lack of education concerning pediatric nutritive needs.
- Many of these nutritional deficiencies can be prevented simply by providing a balanced meal plan, including fresh fruits and vegetables and some animal products. In fact, children receiving adequate animal products in their diets rarely develop generalized malnutrition or micronutrient deficiencies.
- Adequate maternal micronutrient supplementation is important for preventing micronutrient deficiencies in newborns and breastfed infants.

- Treatment of micronutrient disorders requires acute replacement of the deficient nutrient as well as continued adequate dietary intake throughout childhood.

■ REFERENCES

1. Food and Agriculture Organization of the United Nations. 1.02 billion people hungry. June 2009. http://www.fao.org/news/story/en/item/20568/icode. Accessed April 20, 2010

2. United Nations Children's Fund. *The State of the World's Children 2007*. Geneva, Switzerland: United Nations Children's Fund; 2007. http://www.unicef.org/sowc07/docs/sowc07.pdf. Accessed June 17, 2011

3. World Food Programme. Hunger Stats. http://www.wfp.org/hunger/stats. Accessed April 20, 2010

4. Ghanem H. *The State of Food Insecurity in the World 2008*. Rome, Italy: Food and Agriculture Organization of the United Nations; 2008. http://www.fao.org/docrep/011/i0291e/i0291e00.htm. Accessed June 17, 2011

5. United Nations Millenium Development Goals. http://www.un.org/milleniumgoals.poverty.shtml

6. Keating EM, Chock M, Fischer PR. Big hopes for the children of the world: a review of the Millenium Development Goals. *Ann Trop Paediatr*. In press

7. Weisstaub G, Araya M. Acute malnutrition in Latin America: the challenge of ending avoidable deaths. *J Pediatr Gastroenterol Nutr*. 2008;47(Suppl 1):S10–S14

8. Alp H, Orbak Z, Kermen T, Uslu H. Bone mineral density in malnourished children without rachitic manifestations. *Pediatr Int*. 2006;48:128–131

9. Ehrdardt S, Burchard GD, Mantel C, et al. Malaria, anemia and malnutrition in African children—defining intervention priorities. *J Infect Dis*. 2006;194:108–114

10. Cole CR, Lifshitz F. Zinc nutrition and growth retardation. *Pediatr Endocrinol Rev*. 2008;5:889–896

11. Mehra S, Agrawal D. Indian pediatrics—environmental health project. *Indian Pediatr*. 2004;41:137–145

12. United Nations Systems Standing Committee on Nutrition. *5th Report on the World Nutrition Situation*. Geneva, Switzerland: United Nations; 2004. http://www.unscn.org/layout/modules/resources/files/rwns5.pdf. Accessed April 20, 2010

13. McLachlan M. Tackling the child malnutrition problem: from what and why to how much and how. *J Pediatr Gastroenterol Nutr*. 2006;43(Suppl 3):S38–S46

14. Heath ML, Sidbury R. Cutaneous manifestations of nutritional deficiency. *Curr Opin Pediatr*. 2006;18:417–422

15. Müller O, Krawinkel M. Malnutrition and health in developing countries. *CMAJ*. 2005;173:279–286

16. De Onis M, Blössner M. The World Health Organization global database on child growth and malnutrition: methodology and applications. *Int J Epidemiol*. 2003;32:518–526

17. Albala C, et al. Effects of replacing the habitual consumption of sugar-sweetened beverages with milk in Chilean children. *Am J Clin Nutr*. 2008;88:605–611

18. World Health Organization. *The World Health Report 2008: Primary Health Care Now More Than Ever*. http://www.who.int/whr/2008/whr08_en.pdf. Accessed August 19, 2009

19. Ghosh S, Shah D. Nutrition problems in urban slum children. *Indian Pediatr.* 2004;41:682–696

20. Webb P, et al. Measuring household food insecurity: why it's so important and yet so difficult to do. *J Nutr.* 2006;136(Suppl):S1404–S1408

21. Coates J, et al. Commonalities in the experiences of household food insecurity across cultures: what are measures missing? *J Nutr.* 2006;136(Suppl):S1438–S1448

22. Tiewsoh K, et al. Factors determining the outcome of children hospitalized with severe pneumonia. *BMC Pediatr.* 2009;9

23. Aggarwal R, Sentz J, Miller MA. Role of zinc administration in prevention of childhood diarrhea and respiratory illnesses: a meta-analysis. *Pediatrics.* 2007;119:1120–1130

24. Muhe L, Lulseged S, Mason KE, Simoes EA. Case-control study of the role of nutritional rickets in the risk of developing pneumonia in Ethiopia children. *Lancet.* 1997;349:1801–1804

25. Banajeh SM. Nutritional rickets and vitamin D deficiency—association with the outcomes of childhood very severe pneumonia: a prospective cohort study. *Pediatr Pulmonol.* 2009;44:1207–1215

26. Dogan M, Erol M, Cesur Y, Yuca SA, Dogan Z. The effect of 25-hydroxyvitamin D_3 on the immune system. *J Pediatr Endocr Metab.* 2009;22:929–935

27. Oettgen B. Every child counts: the global reality of child survival. *Pediatr Ann.* 2008;37:799–805

28. Amadi B. Role of food antigen elimination in treating children with persistent diarrhea and malnutrition in Zambia. *J Pediatr Gastroenterol Nutr.* 2002;34(Suppl 1):S54–S56

29. Khalili B, et al. Risk factors for hospitalization of children with diarrhea in Shahrekord, Iran. *Iran J Clin Infect Dis.* 2006;1:131–136

30. Zavaleta N, et al. Efficacy of rice-based oral rehydration solution containing recombinant human lactoferrin and lysozyme in Peruvian children with acute diarrhea. *J Pediatr Gastroenterol Nutr.* 2007;44:258–264

31. Bhandari N, et al. Effectiveness of zinc supplementation plus oral rehydration salts compared with oral rehydration salts alone as a treatment for acute diarrhea in a primary care setting: a cluster of randomized trial. *Pediatrics.* 2008;121:1279–1285

32. Alam NH, et al. Symptomatic hyponatremia during treatment dehydrating diarrheal disease with reduced osmolarity oral rehydration solution. *JAMA.* 2006;296:567–573

33. Ashworth A, Khanum S, Jackson A, Schofield C. *Guidelines for the Inpatient Treatment of Severely Malnourished Children.* Geneva, Switzerland; World Health Organization; 2003. http://www.who.int/nutrition/publications/guide_inpatient_text.pdf. Accessed October 24, 2009

34. Ahmed T, Begum B, Badiuzzam Ali M, et al. Management of severe malnutrition and diarrhea. *Indian J Pediatr.* 2001;68:45–51

35. Perry R, Halsey NA. The clinical significance of measles: a review. *J Infect Dis.* 2004;189(Suppl 1):S4–S16

36. World Health Organization. Measles. http://www.who.int/mediacentre/factsheets/fs286/en. Accessed January 29, 2011

37. Moss WJ, et al. HIV type 1 infection is a risk factor for mortality in hospitalized Zambian children with measles. *Clin Infect Dis.* 2008;46:523–527

38. Fawzi W, Msmanga G, Spiegelman D, Hunter DJ. Studies of vitamins and minerals and HIV transmission and disease progression. *J Nutr.* 2005;135:938–944

39. Rodriguez A, et al. Effects of moderate doses of vitamin A as an adjunct to the treatment of pneumonia in underweight and normal-weight children: a randomized, double-blind, placebo-controlled trial. *Am J Clin Nutr.* 2005;82:1090–1096
40. Miller M, et al. Effect of maternal and neonatal vitamin A supplementation and other postnatal factors on anemia in Zimbabwean infants: a prospective, randomized study. *Am J Clin Nutr.* 2006;84:212–222
41. Thurlow R, et al. Only a small portion of anemia in northeast Thai schoolchildren is associated with iron deficiency. *Am J Clin Nutr.* 2005;82:380–387
42. Zimmermann MB, et al. Serum transferring receptor and zinc protoporphyrin as indicators of iron status in African children. *Am J Clin Nutr.* 2005;81:615–623
43. Kordas K. Iron, lead, and children's behavior and cognition. *Annu Rev Nutr.* 2010. In press
44. Shafir T, Angulo-Barroso R, Jing Y, Angelilli ML, Jacobson SW, Lozoff B. Iron deficiency and infant motor development. *Early Hum Dev.* 2008;84:479–485
45. Lozoff B, Kaciroti N, Walter T. Iron deficiency in infancy: applying a physiologic framework for prediction. *Am J Clin Nutr.* 2006;84:1412–1421
46. World Health Organization. *Serious Childhood Problems in Countries With Limited Resources.* Geneva, Switzerland: World Health Organization; 2004. http://whqlibdoc.who.int/publications/2004/9241562692.pdf. Accessed June 17, 2011
47. Black RE, Allen LH, Bhutta ZA, et al. Maternal and child undernutrition: global and regional exposures and health consequences. *Lancet.* 2008;371:243–260
48. Gernaat HBPE, Voorhoeve HWA. A new classification of acute protein-energy malnutrition. *J Trop Pediatr.* 2000;46:97–106
49. World Health Organization, United Nations Children's Fund. *WHO Child Growth Standards and the Identification of Severe Acute Malnutrition in Infants and Children.* Geneva, Switzerland: World Health Organization, United Nations Children's Fund; 2009. http://www.who.int/nutrition/publications/severemalnutrition/9789241598163_eng.pdf. Accessed June 17, 2011
50. World Health Organization. WHO child growth standards. http://www.who.int/childgrowth/standards/technical_report/en/index.html. Accessed July 13, 2009
51. World Health Organization. *Training Course on Child Growth Assessment: WHO Child Growth Standards.* Geneva, Switzerland: World Health Organizaiton; 2008. http://www.who.int/childgrowth/training/module_h_directors_guide.pdf. Accessed June 17, 2011
52. WHO Multicentre Growth Reference Study Group. WHO Motor Development Study: windows of achievement for six gross motor development milestones. *Acta Paediatr.* 2006;450(Suppl):86–95
53. Badaloo AV, Forrester T, Reid M, Jahoor F. Lipid kinetic differences between children with kwashiorkor and those with marasmus. *Am J Clin Nutr.* 2006;83:1283–1288
54. Jahoor F, Badaloo A, Reid M, Forrester T. Protein kinetic differences between children with edematous and nonedematous severe childhood undernutrition in the fed and postabsorptive states. *Am J Clin Nutr.* 2005;82:792–800
55. Abrol P, Verma A, Hooda HS, et al. Thyroid hormone status in protein energy malnutrition in Indian children. *Indian J Clin Biochem.* 2001;16:221–223
56. Beisel, WR. Nutrition and immune function: overview. *J Nutr.* 1996;126:2611S–2615S
57. Phornphatkul C, Pongprot Y, Suskind R, et al. Cardiac function in malnourished children. *Clin Pediatr.* 1994;33:147–154
58. Benabe JE, Martinez-Maldonado M, et al. The impact of malnutrition on kidney function. *Miner Electrolyte Metab.* 1998;24:20–26

59. Guerrant RL, Schorling JB, McAuliffe JF, de Souza MA. Diarrhea as a cause and an effect of malnutrition: diarrhea prevents catch-up growth and malnutrition increases diarrhea frequency and duration. *Am J Trop Med Hyg.* 1992;47(Suppl 1):28–35

60. Ashworth A, Ferguson E. Dietary counseling in the management of moderately malnourishment in children. *Food Nutr Bull.* 2009;30(3 Suppl):S405–S433

61. Briend A, Prinzo ZW, et al. Dietary management of malnutrition: time for a change. *Food Nutr Bull.* 2009;30(3 Suppl):S265–S266

62. Michaelsen, et al. Choice of foods and ingredients for moderately malnourished children aged 6 months to 5 years of age. *Food Nutr Bull.* 2009;30(3Suppl):S343–S404

63. Bernal C, Velasquez C, Alcaraz G, et al. Treatment of severe malnutrition in children: experience in implementing the World Health Organization guidelines in Turbo, Colombia. *J Pediatr Gastroenerol Nutr.* 2008;46:322–328

64. Kerac M, Blencowe H, Grijalva-Eternod C, et al. Prevalence of wasting among under 6-month-old infants in developing countries and implications of new case defi nitions using WHO growth standards:a secondary data analysis. *Arch Dis Child.* 2011

65. Sethuraman U. Vitamins. *Pediatr Rev.* 2006;27:44–55

66. Kleinman RE, ed. *Pediatric Nutrition Handbook.* 6th ed. Elk Grove Village, IL: American Academy of Pediatrics; 2009

67. Ramakrishnan U, Darnton-Hill I. Assessment and control of vitamin A deficiency disorders. *J Nutr.* 2002;132(Suppl):2947S–2953S

68. Ramakrishnan U. Prevalence of micronutrient malnutrition worldwide. *Nutr Rev.* 2002;60:S46–S52

69. Caminiha MF, Batista Filho M, Fernandes TF, Arruda IK, Diniz Ada S. Vitamin A supplementation during puerperium: systematic review. *Rev Saude Publica.* 2009;43:699–706

70. World Health Organization. *Vitamin A Supplementation.* Geneva, Switzerland: World Health Organization. http://www.who.int/vaccines/en/vitamina.shtml. Accessed June 17, 2011

71. Huiming Y, Chaomin W, Meng M. Vitamin A for treating measles in children. *Cochrane Database Syst Rev.* 2005;4:CD001479

72. McGready R, Simpson JA, Cho T, et al. Postpartum thiamine deficiency in a Karen displaced population. *Am J Clin Nutr.* 2001;74:808–813

73. Soukaloun D, Kounnavong S, Pengdy B, et al. Dietary and socio-economic factors associated with beriberi in breastfed Lao infants. 2003;23:181–186

74. McLean E, de Benoist B, Allen LH. Review of the magnitude of folate and vitamin D_{12} deficiencies worldwide. *Food Nutr Bull.* 2008;29(2 Suppl):S38–S51

75. Heymann WR. Scurvy in children. *J Am Acad Dermatol.* 2007;57:358–359

76. Olmedo JM, Yiannias JA, Windgassen EB, Gornet MK. Scurvy: a disease almost forgotten. *Int J Dermatol.* 2006;45:909–913

77. Ratanachu-Ek S, Sukswai P, Jeerathanyasakun Y, Wongtapradit L. Scurvy in pediatric patients: a review of 28 cases. *J Med Assoc Thai.* 2003;86(Suppl 3):S734–S740

78. Fischer PR, Thacher TD, Pettifor JM. Pediatric vitamin D and calcium nutrition in developing countries. *Rev Endocr Metab Disord.* 2008;9:181–192

79. Thacher TD, Fischer PR, Strand MA, Pettifor JM. Nutritional rickets around the world: causes and future directions. *Ann Trop Paediatr.* 2006;26:1–16

80. Thacher TD, Fischer PR, Pettifor JM, Lawson JO, Manaster BJ, Reading JC. Radiographic scoring method for the assessment of the severity of nutritional rickets. *J Trop Pediatr.* 2000;46:132–139

81. Angermayr L, Clar C. Iodine supplementation for preventing iodine deficiency disorders in children. *Cochrane Database Syst Rev.* 2004;2:CD003819

82. Lutter CK. Iron deficiency in young children in low-income countries and new approaches to its prevention. *J Nutr.* 2008;138:2523–2528

83. Fuyu Y. Keshan disease and mitochondrial cardiomyopathy. *Sci China C Life Sci.* 2006;49:513–518

84. Zou K, Liu G, Wu T, Du L. Selenium for preventing Kashin-Beck osteoarthropathy in children: a meta-analysis. *Osteoarthritis Cartilage.* 2009;17:144–151

85. Saliba W, El Fakih R, Shaheen W. Heart failure secondary to selenium deficiency, reversible after supplementation. *Int J Cardiol.* 2008. In press

86. Scrimgeour AG, Lukaski HC. Zinc and diarrheal disease: current status and future perspectives. *Curr Opin Clin Nutr Metab Care.* 2008;11:711–717

87. Dhingra U, Hiremath G, Menon VP, Dhingra P, Sarkar A, Sazawal S. Zinc deficiency: descrptive epidemiology and morbidity among preschool children in peri-urban population in Delhi, India. *J Health Popul Nutr.* 2009;27:632–639

88. Patro B, Golicki D, Szajewska H. Meta-analysis: zinc supplementation for acute gastroenteritis in children. *Aliment Pharmacol Ther.* 2008;28:713–723

89. Natchu UCM, Fataki MR, Fawzi WW. Zinc as an adjunct for childhood pneumonia—interpreting early results. *Nutr Rev.* 2008;66:398–405

90. World Bank Development Indicators 2008. http://www.globalissues.org/article/26/poverty-facts-and-stats. Accessed April 22, 2010

91. Shah A. Poverty facts and stats. http://www.globalissues.org/article/26/poverty-facts-and-stats. Accessed April 22, 2010

92. Sachs J. *The End of Poverty: Economic Possibilities for Our Time.* New York, NY: Penguin Press; 2005

93. Easterly W. *The White Man's Burden: Why the West's Efforts to Aid the Rest Have Done So Much Ill and So Little Good.* New York, NY: Oxford University Press; 2006

94. One. http://www.one.org/us. Accessed April 22, 2010

95. United Nations Children's Fund. *The State of the World's Children 2008.* Geneva, Switzerland: United Nations Children's Fund; 2008. http://www.unicef.org/sowc08/docs/sowc08_execsummary.pdf

96. Brewster Dr. Inpatient management of severe malnutrition: time for a change in protocol and practice. *Ann Trop Paediatr.* 2011;31:97–107

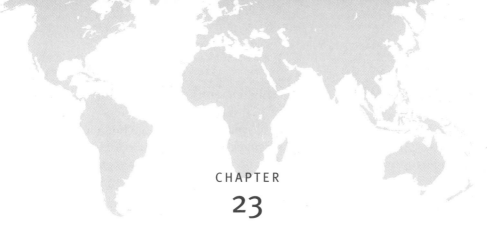

CHAPTER

23

Fever

John C. Christenson, MD, FAAP

■ INTRODUCTION

Fever is a frequent manifestation of disease in children. In most cases, it is indicative of an infectious process. Fortunately, most are mild and self-limiting and require no medical intervention. However, in endemic regions, fever may be the initial presentation of a serious infection such as malaria, dengue, or enteric fever. In most countries, respiratory infections caused by viruses or bacteria are responsible for a significant degree of morbidity and mortality in children. Measles still remains an important cause. Of the estimated 8.795 million deaths in children younger than 5 years reported worldwide in 2008, 68% were caused by infectious diseases. While pneumonia was the most common cause of death, diarrhea was responsible for approximately 1.336 million deaths and malaria was responsible for approximately 732,000.[1]

On a daily basis clinicians are faced with determining the cause of fever in their pediatric-aged patients and the most appropriate treatment. This chapter provides a framework for care providers to assist with care of patients. Special emphasis is given to the approach to the febrile child, especially those that reside in developing countries and who traveled back into non-endemic regions. Malaria, enteric fever, and dengue will receive specific attention.

Stanfield provided one of the first comprehensive reviews detailing the diverse spectrum of etiologies for fever in children living in the tropics.[2] Bacteremia, malaria, meningitis, otitis media, pneumonia, diarrheal infections, and acute rheumatic fever were among the most common.[2] Among hospitalized children returning from the tropics with febrile illnesses, diarrhea and malaria were the most common. A treatable cause for the febrile illness was identified in 46% of children.[3] In parts of Asia and Latin America, dengue is a frequent cause of fever. In parts of Africa, rickettsial infections are a major cause. Eight percent of ill children returning from international travel were found to have malaria; 69% of these children required hospitalization. Most cases were caused by *Plasmodium falciparum* following travel to sub-Saharan Africa. Only 1% to 2% had dengue and enteric fever.[4]

■ APPROACH TO THE CHILD WITH FEVER

Because morbidity and mortality associated with infections acquired in developing countries in the tropics is significant, recognition and early treatment is imperative. Clinicians must differentiate between minor, self-limiting illnesses and diseases such as malaria, enteric fever, shigellosis, and meningococcal meningitis. In most instances, fever will not be the only manifestation of disease. Chills, sweats, headaches, fatigue, neck pain, malaise, vomiting, diarrhea, and abdominal pain may be present and help with the clinical diagnosis. However, challenges remain. Malnourished and immunocompromised children with serious infections may not mount a febrile reaction or may have atypical clinical features.

At times, clinical presentations in children will differ from those observed in adults. The well-described classical fever patterns associated with malaria in adults were rarely observed in children, in which patterns are more erratic. It is important to remember that not all febrile illnesses represent an infection. Fever is frequently part of systemic juvenile idiopathic arthropathies, acute rheumatic fever, Kawasaki disease, and certain malignancies.

Integrated Management of Childhood Illness guidelines were developed by the World Health Organization (WHO) and United Nations Children's Fund to assist clinicians in the management of children with febrile illnesses. Their goal is to help identify those patients most likely to have malaria and other serious bacterial infections and provide prompt and appropriate therapy. They were mostly developed for regions of the world with limited access to care and therapies.

A history of fever, "feels hot," or an axillary temperature of 37.5°C or above was used as the definition for fever. A classification into a high or low malaria risk category determines if the child receives empiric antimalarial or antibiotic therapy. A runny nose or an exanthem diminishes the likelihood of malaria. Febrile children who are likely to have malaria would receive antimalarial therapy, and those with suspected bacterial infections would receive antibiotics. The ultimate goal is to diminish morbidity and mortality and use resources efficiently.[5]

A test of the guidelines in a region of low malaria prevalence revealed that 78% of those with bacterial infections received antibacterial therapy; 100% with meningitis; 95% with pneumonia; and 95% of children with otitis media. Children with bacteremia, dysentery, or skin infections received therapy, but at a lower percentage—less than 50%.[6] Guideline improvements are still merited.

Using WHO guidelines can lead to undertreating of children with bacterial infections. In an area of high malaria transmission, use of guidelines failed to identify close to one third of children with invasive bacterial disease.[7]

The etiologic diagnosis of a febrile illness is easier when the person traveled to an endemic area and returned to a non-endemic area. Specific incubation periods are helpful in determining a possible etiology. A too-short or too-long incubation period could eliminate consideration of some conditions. However, this may not be possible for children living in endemic regions. Box 23-1 lists diseases according to incubation period. Incubation periods of less than 14 days would support the diagnosis of malaria, dengue, rickettsial infection, leptospirosis, and typhoid fever. Incubation periods greater than 14 days would rule out dengue. Known exposures to individuals with an infectious condition, such as measles or chickenpox, may help the clinician by providing a precise incubation period.

It is important to remember that more than 30% of febrile illnesses are caused by more cosmopolitan-type infections, such as acute otitis media, pharyngitis, infectious mononucleosis, soft tissue, and urinary tract.

Physical findings on examination may lead to a diagnosis. Purpura may suggest meningococcal disease; eschars and chagomas may support the diagnosis of rickettsioses or Chagas disease, respectively. The presence of lymphadenopathy, tonsillitis, and hepatosplenomegaly would suggest infectious mononucleosis, possibly by Epstein-Barr virus. A person with fever and polyarthropathy in northern Australia may represent Ross River fever, but it may represent Chikungunya viral infection on islands of the Indian Ocean. Vesicular and vesiculopustular exanthems can be observed with a multiplicity of different conditions, such as rickettsialpox, disseminated herpes simplex virus in a young infant, or chickenpox. Vesicular lesions were observed in patients with monkeypox. Endemic mycoses, such as coccidioidomycosis and histoplasmosis, can present with erythema nodosum. Persons with tuberculosis may

Box 23-1. Incubation Periods for Common Infections That Cause Fever

INCUBATION PERIOD LESS THAN 14 DAYS
- Malaria
- Dengue
- Rickettsial infections (eg, *Rickettsia africae, Ehrlichia)*
- Acute HIV retroviral syndrome
- Leptospirosis
- Enteric fever (ie, typhoid, paratyphoid fever)
- Diarrheal illnesses (eg, shigellosis, salmonellosis, campylobacteriosis)
- Brucellosis
- Viral respiratory infections (eg, influenza, hantavirus, respiratory syncytial virus)
- Endemic mycoses (eg, histoplasmosis, coccidioidomycosis, blastomycosis)
- Acute toxoplasmosis
- Relapsing fever
- Trichinellosis
- Trypanosomiasis
- Viral hemorrhagic fevers
- Yellow fever
- Meningococcal sepsis and meningitis
- Pneumococcal sepsis and meningitis
- Enteroviral infections (including poliomyelitis)

INCUBATION PERIOD 2 TO 6 WEEKS
- Malaria
- Enteric fever (ie, typhoid, paratyphoid)
- Hepatitis A and E
- Acute schistosomiasis (eg, Katayama fever)
- Leptospirosis
- Amebic liver abscess
- Q fever
- Acute HIV retroviral syndrome
- Tuberculosis
- Brucellosis
- Infectious mononucleosis
- Toxoplasmosis

INCUBATION PERIOD GREATER THAN 6 WEEKS
- Malaria
- Tuberculosis
- Hepatitis B
- Visceral leishmaniasis
- Schistosomiasis
- Amebic liver abscess
- Brucellosis
- Visceral larva migrans
- Bartonellosis
- Histoplasmosis
- Coccidioidomycosis
- Paracoccidioidomycosis
- Filariasis
- Fascioliasis

have a similar exanthem. Regional lymphadenopathy with an eschar may suggest tularemia. Unfortunately, fever may be the only manifestation early in the illness; physical examination may still be of limited benefit. Box 23-2 provides differential diagnoses according to syndromic features. Signs and symptoms, such as meningismus, headache, vomiting, and photophobia, all suggest a central nervous system infection such as meningitis. A diagnostic flow chart based on clinical manifestations is provided in Table 23-1 as a tool to assist clinicians in the management of febrile children.

Clinicians must be familiar with the epidemiology of infectious pathogens frequently observed in regions of interest. There are also epidemiologic variations within countries. For example, most of South Africa is malaria free, with the exception of the northeast regions around Kruger National Park.

Approximately 10% of people who travel to a developing country experience a febrile illness during or after travel, which frequently requires medical consultation. Stays in sub-Saharan Africa and Southeast Asia-Pacific regions are most often associated with febrile illnesses. Tropical diseases account for close to 40% of febrile illness cases. A cause cannot be determined for one fourth of patients.

The type of disease is greatly influenced by the country visited. Malaria (mostly by *P falciparum)* and rickettsial infections are the leading diagnoses associated with travel to Africa, while dengue and enteric fever lead with travel to Asia, and dengue and malaria lead with travel to Latin America. *P falciparum* malaria is the most frequent cause of hospitalization.[8] In Thailand, dengue and leptospirosis were common causes of febrile illnesses.[9] In the Ecuadorian Amazon basin, leptospirosis, malaria, rickettsioses, and dengue were the most common causes of acute undifferentiated febrile illnesses.[10]

Access to medical facilities with diagnostic and therapeutic capabilities could influence observed outcomes. In addition, parental responses to fever, especially in regions endemic with malaria, also influence how promptly effective therapy is initiated. While urban and rural mothers in Nigeria are aware that malaria causes fevers in children, urban mothers tend to respond better. However, rural mothers recognize childhood fever and danger signs better than urban mothers. Rural mothers frequently use leftover medicines from prior episodes.[11]

Many factors influence the likelihood of a febrile child receiving effective therapy. Access can be impeded by lack and cost of transportation, cost of medications, and the need to care for other children, prepare food for others, and work. Access to medicines at home or

(continued on page 640)

Box 23-2. Febrile Syndromes

FEVER AND HEPATITIS
- Hepatitis A, B, and E
- Leptospirosis
- Infectious mononucleosis
- Amebiasis (eg, liver abscess)

FEVER AND EOSINOPHILIA
- Schistosomiasis (eg, Katayama fever)
- Ascariasis
- Strongyloidiasis

FEVER AND LYMPHADENOPATHIES
- Toxoplasmosis (mononucleosis-like)
- Epstein-Barr virus (mononucleosis-like)
- Cytomegalovirus
- Tularemia
- HIV (eg, acute retroviral syndrome)
- Brucellosis

FEVER AND ARTHROPATHIES
- Ross River virus
- Chikungunya virus
- Dengue
- Lyme borreliosis
- Pyogenic septic arthritis
- Acute rheumatic fever
- Human parvovirus B19

FEVER AND DIARRHEA
- Shigellosis
- Salmonellosis
- Amebiasis
- Campylobacteriosis
- *Clostridium difficile* enteritis
- Diarrheagenic *Escherichia coli* (eg, enterotoxigenic, enterohemorrhagic, enteroadherent)
- Rotavirus

FEVER—CHRONIC, RELAPSING, RECURRENT
- Malaria
- Relapsing fever (eg, louse-borne, tick-borne)
- Enteric fever
- Brucellosis
- Q fever
- Leptospirosis
- Familial Mediterranean fever

FEVER AND HEMORRHAGIC MANIFESTATIONS
- Dengue
- Yellow fever
- Lassa fever
- Rift Valley fever
- Viral hemorrhagic fevers (eg, Machupo, Marburg, Ebola)
- Meningococcal

Box 23-2. Febrile Syndromes, continued

FEVER AND EXANTHEM (TYPE)
- Dengue (maculopapular)
- Chikungunya (maculopapular)
- Measles (maculopapular)
- Rubella (maculopapular)
- Rickettsial (maculopapular, eschar, petechial, vesiculopustular)
- *Neisseria meningitidis* (petechial, purpura)
- Enterovirus (maculopapular)
- Drug reactions (erythema multiforme)
- Varicella-zoster virus (vesicular)
- Histoplasmosis, coccidioidomycosis, blastomycosis (erythema nodosum)
- Tuberculosis (erythema nodosum, papulonecrotic tuberculids)
- Monkeypox (vesicular)
- Syphilis (maculopapular)
- Yellow fever (maculopapular)

FEVER AND CENTRAL NERVOUS SYSTEM DISEASE
- *Neisseria meningitidis* meningitis
- *Streptococcus pneumoniae* meningitis
- Enterovirus
- Coccidioidomycosis
- Malaria
- Arboviral meningoencephalitis
- Rabies
- Japanese encephalitis virus
- West Nile virus
- Tuberculosis
- *Angiostrongylus* (eg, eosinophilic meningitis)

FEVER AND ABDOMINAL PAIN
- Enteric fever (eg, typhoid, paratyphoid)
- Yersiniosis
- Adenovirus
- Liver abscess

FEVER, RESPIRATORY SYMPTOMS, AND PNEUMONIA
- Pneumococcal
- Influenza
- Respiratory syncytial virus
- Tuberculosis
- Histoplasmosis
- Coccidioidomycosis
- Adenovirus
- Legionellosis
- Q fever
- Plague
- Tularemia
- Diphtheria
- Anthrax
- Hantavirus

Table 23-1. Approach to the Febrile Child Living in the Tropics

Step 1: Is the child febrile? *Fever* is defined as axillary temperature ≥37.5°C, history of fever, or "feels hot."

Step 2: Decide management of the febrile child based on signs and symptoms.

Rule: **Before considering etiologies, clinicians must be familiar with specific conditions that may present with fever that are endemic to the region where they practice or at-risk activities that may lead to exposure and disease; eg, malaria, dengue, rickettsial infections, leptospirosis.**

I. RESPIRATORY SYMPTOMS OR FINDINGS

A. Nasal congestion, rhinorrhea, watery eyes, sore throat, +/- coughing: **Upper respiratory tract infection, most likely viral**

> Supportive care only. No antibacterial therapy needed.

B. Sore throat, no coughing, no congestion, foul-smelling breathe, pharyngitis/tonsillitis with exudates: **Streptococcal pharyngitis—tonsillitis likely**

> Oral antibacterial therapy indicated—penicillin, amoxicillin

C. Coughing, tachypnea; may be accompanied by congestion, sore throat, +/- wheezing; crackles on examination: **Pneumonia likely. Nasal congestion with wheezing: likely viral.**

> Antibacterial therapy indicated—amoxicillin, amoxicillin-clavulanic acid, cephalosporin, macrolide

II. SKIN OR MUCOSAL FINDINGS

A. Nasal, congestion, coughing, maculopapular exanthem, +/- Koplik spots: **Measles, highly probable**

> Supportive care

B. Purpura, petechial exanthem; poor perfusion: **Meningococcal sepsis**

> Intravenous fluids, intravenous antibacterial therapy—third-generation cephalosporin such as ceftriaxone

C. Eschars, +/- regional adenopathy; +/- petechial exanthem: **Rickettsial infection**

> Antibacterial therapy, all ages—doxycycline

D. Jaundice, +/- hepatosplenomegaly, +/- adenopathy: **Hepatitis A and E likely. Hepatitis B and C possible. Acquired toxoplasmosis may have similar presentation.**

> Supportive care

Table 23-1. Approach to the Febrile Child Living in the Tropics, continued

II. SKIN OR MUCOSAL FINDINGS, CONTINUED

E. Jaundice, hepatosplenomegaly, adenopathy, exudative tonsillitis: **Infectious mononucleosis due to Epstein-Barr virus or cytomegalovirus**

Supportive care. Prednisone for marked tonsillar hypertrophy.

F. Jaundice, hepatosplenomegaly, conjunctival suffusion, renal dysfunction, +/- mental status changes: **Leptospirosis**

Antibacterial therapy—penicillin is agent of choice. Alternatives—erythromycin or doxycycline.

III. CENTRAL NERVOUS SYSTEM FINDINGS

A. Headaches, neck pain, vomiting, altered mental status, nuchal rigidity, +/- seizures: **Acute bacterial meningitis likely**

Intravenous antibacterial therapy—third-generation cephalosporin such as ceftriaxone. Supportive care.

B. Chills, myalgias, sweats, absence of respiratory symptoms, altered mental status, seizures; malaria-endemic regions: **Cerebral malaria**

Antimalarial therapy, +/- intravenous antibacterial therapy

IV. NONSPECIFIC FEBRILE SYNDROMES

A. Chills, myalgias, sweats, absence of respiratory symptoms; malaria-endemic regions: **Malaria**

Antimalarial therapy

B. Chills, myalgias, sweats, absence of respiratory symptoms; non–malaria-endemic regions: **Dengue**

Supportive care. Watch for hemorrhagic/shock changes.

C. Chills, myalgias, sweats, exposure to freshwater, floods: **Leptospirosis possible**

Antibacterial therapy—penicillin is agent of choice. Alternatives—erythromycin or doxycycline.

D. Poor perfusion, signs of sepsis, no exanthems, no meningismus, +/- altered mental status: **Bacterial sepsis possible**

Intravenous antibacterial therapy, regimen based on local resistance patterns; supportive care

V. GASTROINTESTINAL SYMPTOMS AND FINDINGS

A. Abdominal pain, diarrhea with mucus or blood: **Bacterial enteritis possible. Shigellosis, salmonellosis (including enteric fever) or campylobacteriosis.**

Antibacterial therapy—azithromycin is preferred empiric agent. Ciprofloxacin could be used in regions with low resistance (eg, Africa).

from neighborhood shops or vendors may improve access to effective therapy.[12] Birthplace, feeding type, parental education, maternal visits to antenatal clinics, household economic status, and place of residence influence the incidence of fevers and resulting mortality. Children living in urban areas have a lower risk of fever than those living in rural regions.[13] Urban areas in developing countries may have a lower risk of malaria. Stays at higher elevations (higher than 2,500 m) are associated with a lower risk as well. Sleeping accommodations protected from mosquitoes by using bed nets reduced the incidence of malaria.

Vaccinations diminish the risk of yellow fever and Japanese encephalitis virus infection. When resources are available, an initial workup may consist of a complete blood cell count and differential, liver function tests, blood cultures for bacteria, stool culture, urinalysis, and thick and thin smears for malaria. Serologic testing may be needed to confirm dengue. Patients with a cough may require a chest film, and evidence of pneumonic infiltrates may require respiratory viral testing or sputum for Gram stain and culture or gastric aspirates for acid-fast bacilli cultures. A stool culture may be useful in patients with diarrhea, as determined by the duration and type of symptoms; some may require testing for *Clostridium difficile* toxin. Examination for ova and parasites may be useful in persons with chronic diarrhea. Antigen assays for *Cryptosporidium* and *Giardia* are particularly sensitive. Individuals with complaints of pharyngitis and evidence of exudative disease would benefit from rapid streptococcal antigen assay with a backup throat culture if necessary. Patients with symptoms suggestive of meningitis require a lumbar puncture. Some individuals may require diagnostic imaging with a computed tomography scan or magnetic resonance imaging. Aspiration of joints is required for patients with suspected pyogenic septic arthritis. Tuberculin skin testing or interferon-gamma release assays may be needed as a way of confirming the diagnosis of tuberculosis in a young child with an atypical or complex disease.

■ SPECIFIC INFECTIOUS CAUSES OF FEVER

Malaria

Malaria is a mosquito-borne protozoan infection that involves erythrocytes. The most important species infecting humans are *P falciparum*, *P vivax*, *P ovale*, *P malariae*, and *P knowlesi*, a simian species, which was most recently recognized as an important human pathogen. The major vector is the *Anopheles* mosquito, which is endemic in many regions of the world, including the United States. Regions of the world with the most malarial transmission are sub-Saharan Africa, Southeast Asia-Pacific,

Amazonian South America, and parts of Central America. *P knowlesi* is widely distributed in Malaysian Borneo, Peninsular Malaysia, and the Philippines. The spectrum of disease is variable, with many recovering without sequelae; however, mortality is estimated at 10%.[14,15]

More than 40% of the world's population is exposed to malaria. According to WHO estimates, 1.5 to 2.7 million people are infected each year, resulting in approximately 900,000 deaths. Most deaths (80%) are in children younger than 5 years, and most deaths occur in Africa.[16]

Most deaths are caused by *P falciparum* resulting from cerebral involvement, bacterial superinfection, and multi-organ failure. In addition, severe anemia is responsible for delayed growth and development. Unfortunately, regions affected by malaria are also plagued by HIV, tuberculosis, and typhoid fever.

Resistance to antimalarial agents in *P falciparum* contributed to its uncontrolled prevalence in Africa. Most *P falciparum* strains are resistant to chloroquine outside Central America. *P falciparum* is resistant to mefloquine in some Asian countries (ie, regions bordering Thailand, Myanmar, Laos, and Cambodia). *Plasmodium vivax* is the most prominent species outside Africa, especially in Asia where better diagnosis and antimalarial treatments are available, resulting in less *P falciparum*. However, resistance does not escape *P vivax*. Chloroquine resistance is reported in areas of Indonesia and Malaysia. *Plasmodium ovale* is rarely observed outside Africa. Recently, *P ovale* was detected in southeastern Bangladesh.[17]

In a study from The Gambia, the incidence of non-typhoidal *Salmonella* infections decreased along with a decrease in the prevalence of malaria parasitemia, which suggests an association between the infections.[18]

Nonspecific clinical features are usually observed in children with malaria. Fever, vomiting, headaches, chills, myalgias, and anorexia are common. Gastrointestinal symptoms, such as diarrhea, abdominal pain, and distension, are also observed. In one study, the absence of thrombocytopenia had a negative predictive value of 97% for malaria.[3] Other conditions, such as influenza, typhoid fever, and dengue, may have similar complaints.

Severe malaria may result from cerebral involvement, acute respiratory distress syndrome, and multi-organ involvement. Most of these children will die unless they are hospitalized and promptly treated with effective support and antimalarial medications. Coma, seizures, metabolic acidosis, profound hypoglycemia, and shock are associated with high mortality.[19] While most of the serious complications are observed with *P falciparum,* severe malarial anemia in young infants is seen more often with *P vivax.* Severe thrombocytopenia is also seen more often with *P vivax.*[20] Children with severe malaria have a lower mortality than individuals older than 50 years—6.1% versus 36.5%, respectively. The incidence of anemia and convulsions decreases with age, but the degree of hyperparasitemia, jaundice, and renal insufficiency increases with age.[21]

While it is known that the sickle cell trait (hemoglobin genotype AS) protects against malaria, it is assumed that children with sickle cell disease are at increased risk of malaria when compared with children who do not have sickle cell disease. Evidence from a study in a rural area on the coast of Kenya could not support such a notion. However, children with sickle cell disease are more likely to die from malaria.[22,23]

Visualization of the parasite on blood smears has been the method of choice for malaria diagnosis for decades. Unfortunately, there is great variability of practitioners' ability to perform proper microscopy. In addition, a functioning microscope may be unavailable in some areas. Because many febrile illnesses share clinical features, overuse of antimalarial agents is a problem. Of interest, even when malaria was excluded, individuals with acute undifferentiated fever still frequently received antimalarial therapy.[24] Diagnostic tests have to be sensitive and accurate.

Driven by this problem, the use of rapid diagnostic tests (RDTs) is becoming more widespread. In clinical settings where access to microscopy is not available, RDT results in less overuse of antimalarial agents and improved focused use of antibiotics. However, in the same study from Ghana, the use of RDT at 4 peripheral clinics added very little if microscopy was available.[25] In a laboratory-based study, RDT performed better than the Giemsa-stained blood smears (GS). Rapid antigen capture assay (BinaxNOW Malaria test) had a sensitivity of 97% compared with 85% of GS with a negative predictive value of 99.6% versus 98.2% with GS for all malaria. The sensitivity was 100% for *P falciparum.*[26] In regions of high endemicity, performing RDT on all patients with suspected malaria was not cost-effective when compared with presumptive treatment of all febrile children.[27] In a low-transmission area, RDT use decreased drug costs and improved management of patients and compliance with test results.[28]

Other diagnostic methodologies may eventually replace GS in laboratory settings. Polymerase chain reaction (PCR) has become the gold standard for diagnosis. However, its availability is still limited in most financial-strained countries. In a study from Thailand, Pöschl and coworkers[29] compared loop-mediated isothermal amplification (LAMP) to nested PCR and microscopy. Loop-mediated isothermal amplification is a molecular method that compares favorably with PCR but is cheaper, simpler, and faster. Using PCR as a gold standard, LAMP detected 100% of blood specimens with *P falciparum* with 100% specificity. Microscopy demonstrated 92% sensitivity and 93% specificity. Loop-mediated isothermal amplification performed just as well with specimens containing *P vivax,* while microscopy detected only 68% of positive specimens. The use of LAMP may eliminate the need for a subjective interpretation of microscopic findings. However, its use as a field tool needs further study.[29] The new fluorescent assay Partec Rapid Malaria Test may be easier to perform and provides quicker results compared with GS.[30]

Recently, the WHO updated its guidelines for malaria treatment.[31] Artemisinin-based combinations are the recommended treatment for uncomplicated *P falciparum* malaria. Artemether-lumefantrine, artesunate plus amodiaquine, artesunate plus mefloquine, and artesunate plus sulfadoxine-pyrimethamine are being used throughout the world. Of these, only artemether-lumefantrine (Coartem) is licensed in the United States. Artemisinin derivatives should never be used as monotherapy. Artemisinin-based therapy is given for 3 days.

When compared with mefloquine alone, artesunate-mefloquine cleared parasitemia and reduced gametocyte carriage more rapidly in Nigerian children, and there was a lesser fall in hematocrit.[32] Of interest, individuals coinfected with *Plasmodium* and *Schistosoma* who received treatment with the combination artesunate-mefloquine for malaria had clearance of their malaria parasitemia and a reduction in schistosomiasis-related morbidity; artesunate-mefloquine, therefore, appeared to be more effective than praziquantel.[33] In a trial in Bangladesh, an artesunate-azithromycin combination was found to be just as effective as an artemether-lumefantrine regimen. The combination was also well tolerated.[34]

Second-line antimalarial treatments may consist of artesunate plus tetracycline or doxycycline or clindamycin, or quinine plus tetracycline or doxycycline or clindamycin. These combination therapies are to be administered for at least 7 days. Atovaquone-proguanil, artemether-lumefantrine, or quinine plus doxycycline or clindamycin are recommended for travelers returning to non-endemic countries where they develop malaria.

Severe malaria is always a medical emergency. Parenteral antimalarial treatment should be started immediately. Not all agents may be available for use in developing countries. Therapy should be started with whichever effective antimalarial is first available. For children living in endemic regions, especially Africa, the following antimalarial agents are recommended: intravenous (IV) or intramuscular (IM) artesunate, quinine (IV infusion or divided IM injection), or IM artemether. Parenteral antimalarials are usually IV administered for a minimum of 24 hours and then switched to an oral regimen consisting of an artemisinin-based combination therapy, artesunate plus clindamycin or doxycycline, or quinine plus clindamycin or doxycycline, to complete the therapy. Quinidine can be used when parenteral quinine is not available. Artemisinin derivatives were found to be equivalent to quinine in the treatment of cerebral malaria in children.[35,36]

Chloroquine combined with primaquine is the treatment of choice for chloroquine-susceptible *P vivax* infections. An artemisinin-based combination regimen is recommended for infections suspected to be caused by chloroquine-resistant *P vivax*. Primaquine is recommended for 14 days to eliminate the hepatic hypnozoite stage and prevent relapses. Severe *P vivax* or *P knowlesi* infections should be treated with artemisinin-combination regimens. To avoid medication-induced hemolysis, testing to rule out glucose-6-phosphate dehydrogenase deficiency is advised before treating with primaquine.

Children with severe malaria presenting with respiratory distress and metabolic acidosis benefit from blood transfusions. Close monitoring for hypoglycemia is imperative. Seizures can be a complication of cerebral malaria or profound hypoglycemia.

Vector control, intermittent preventive treatments, and insecticide-treated bed nets are strategies used to reduce transmission and the effect of malaria on children. In Sierra Leone, the presence of splenomegaly is highly suggestive of malaria. However, a history of sleeping under a bed net was found to protect against malaria.[37]

Enteric Fever

Enteric fever, an infection caused by *Salmonella enterica* serotype *typhi* (typhoid fever) or *S enterica* serotype *paratyphi* A, B, C (paratyphoid fever), is a frequent cause of morbidity and mortality in many parts of the world. Most infections occur in Southern and Southeast Asia. Parts of Africa and Latin America are affected but at a lower frequency. In Asia, it is estimated that the incidence approximates 100 cases per 100,000 population. It is estimated that 22 million cases occur worldwide each year, of which more than 200,000 deaths result.[38,39] Travelers to endemic regions are at risk; it is estimated that approximately 3 to 30 cases per 100,000 travelers are affected by this febrile ailment each year.[40]

The major factor responsible for the magnitude of this problem is poor sanitary infrastructure resulting in substandard drinking water and contaminated food. Person-to-person transmission from chronic asymptomatic infections among inhabitants also contributes to the infection of susceptible individuals. Travelers visiting friends and relatives are at the highest risk of infection.

While fever, gastrointestinal symptoms (eg, vomiting, severe diarrhea, abdominal distension, pain), cough, relative bradycardia, rose spots, and splenomegaly are frequently regarded as features of typhoid and paratyphoid fever, many patients lack these, making diagnosis difficult if solely based on clinical features. Blood cultures are frequently positive; stool, less so. While liver enzymes are frequently elevated, leukocytosis is not always observed. However, leukocytosis is more frequently observed in children than adults.[41] Leukopenia and anemia are frequently associated with enteric fevers. Many suggest that bone marrow cultures have a higher sensitivity; however, obtaining this type of specimen is more invasive and impractical under most circumstances in a developing country. Jaundice is frequently observed among children. In a study of travelers with enteric fever, clinical and laboratory features were indistinguishable between S typhi and S paratyphi, which suggests that milder disease is not always observed with S paratyphi as originally thought.[38]

In studies from Pakistan, children younger than 5 years had more severe disease. More than 95% of these children had fever; 20% to 41% had hepatomegaly; 5% to 20% had splenomegaly; 19% to 28% had abdominal pain; and 8% to 35% had diarrhea.[41,42] Severe disease resulted in more hospitalizations. Intestinal perforation was a rare complication observed in fewer than 1% of children. Cough was observed in approximately 15% of patients.[41] Thrombocytopenia and intravascular disseminated coagulation are markers of severe disease.[43]

Relative bradycardia and rose spots are seldom observed in children. Febrile convulsions have been reported in children with enteric fever[44] and may be the presenting symptom in many children.[45]

The Widal test, a classical test that measures antibodies against O and H antigens of S typhi, was associated with the diagnosis of typhoid fever; however, it lacks sensitivity and specificity and should no longer be performed. A false-positive test may lead to overtreatment and a delay in considering other conditions.[43,46] Use of the Widal test led to many unnecessary treatments in rural Kenya, where typhoid fever is still rare among children and significantly less frequent than other bacterial pathogens.[47]

While pathogen-specific serologic and PCR assays are the preferred methods for diagnosing enteric fever, diagnosis is still made using clinical criteria in most lower-income countries. Unfortunately, early features of enteric fever mimic other conditions such as pneumonia, malaria, sepsis, dengue, acute hepatitis, and rickettsial infections.

Chloramphenicol, amoxicillin, and trimethoprim-sulfamethoxazole are no longer recommended as first-line agents because of a high frequency of treatment failures, resistance, and high relapse rates. Relapse rates in children are only 2% to 4% after therapy, while carrier rates occur in fewer than 2% of infected children.[43] Antimicrobial resistance observed in many countries has influenced the choice of agent for treating typhoid and paratyphoid fevers. Ceftriaxone remains the recommended agent in the most severe cases in which parenteral therapy is indicated. While fluoroquinolones, such as ciprofloxacin, are generally associated with high cure rates, defervescence within a week, and lowered relapse and fecal carriage rates, isolates from many Asian countries demonstrate resistance, rendering them ineffective. Azithromycin appears favorable in the treatment of these; however, ciprofloxacin remains the drug of choice for Africa.[48] For obvious reasons, attention to proper hydration, perfusion, and fever control are integral components of treating enteric fever.

Undoubtedly, improving the quality of drinking water and food will lead to the prevention of disease, but other strategies may be of benefit. Vaccinating those older than 2 years dwelling in slums in India with the Vi capsular polysaccharide typhoid vaccine demonstrated a 61% protective effectiveness compared with a placebo. In children 2 to 5 years of age, the protective effect was 80%. Of interest, the level of protection was 44% among unvaccinated members of Vi vaccinee clusters.[49]

A multidrug-resistant *S enterica* serotype *paratyphi* A emerged as an important pathogen in Asia. Azithromycin was found to be an effective alternative for non-severe disease in this region.[50] Infections from *S paratyphi* A are becoming more frequent than *S typhi* among travelers.[51] A similar trend has been observed in Nepal.[52]

Mixed infections with multiple pathogens do occur in tropical endemic countries. Treatment against enteric fever should be considered for children with unremitting fevers after completing adequate antimalarial therapy.[53]

Ileal perforations in the tropics are frequently considered to be associated with enteric fever. In one study, only 4.2% and 6.3% of ileal perforations were associated with *S typhi* and *S paratyphi* A, respectively.[54]

In Nigeria, 50% of all admissions for typhoid-related ileal perforation were in children, with 62.5% of these occurring between the ages of 5 and 6 years.[55]

Fever, vomiting, and abdominal tenderness and distension are suggestive of ileal perforation. Postoperative complications are common, such as surgical wound infection, intra-abdominal abscesses, ileus, and re-perforation. Mortality is high in children—40.9% in those younger than 5 years and close to 20% in children older than 5 years.[56]

Non-typhoidal Salmonellosis

It is important not to forget that non-typhoidal salmonellosis remains a frequent cause of invasive disease in many regions of the world, especially sub-Saharan Africa. Children younger than 3 years and those infected with HIV have the greatest burden. Mortality remains high, especially in children with bacteremia and meningitis. Seasonal peaks of disease correlate well with the rainy season, which leads to fecal contamination of drinking water. In many countries, investigators found an association of malaria and non-typhoid salmonellosis, which may lead to delays in treatment resulting in a rise in morbidity and mortality. Clinical features, such as fevers, anemia, and splenomegaly, are frequent findings in both conditions.[57]

Leptospirosis

Leptospirosis is becoming an important cause of febrile disease in urban communities within developing countries. Urine from wild and domestic animals is the source of human infection. Contact with infected animals, poor sanitation and water quality, flash flooding, and overcrowding are contributing to an increase in cases. Approximately 268 pathogenic serovars of *Leptospira* were identified. *Leptospira interrogans* is the primary pathogenic species.[58] Jaundice and renal failure, known as hepatorenal syndrome or Weil disease, is the stereotypical presentation associated with leptospirosis; however, this condition represents just a smaller number of cases. Hemorrhagic pneumonia and meningitis are also described with the infection and high mortality is associated with these. *Leptospira* causes a nonspecific febrile illness in most cases. It mimics other diseases such as malaria and dengue.[59] In a low-income region of Dhaka, Bangladesh, leptospirosis accounted for 2% to 8% of acute outpatient febrile episodes.[60] Eighteen percent of dengue-negative individuals were found to have leptospirosis during a dengue outbreak in the same region in 2001.[61]

Visualization of leptospires by dark field microscopy, detection of specific antibody in serum, or DNA by PCR are the most frequently used methods for diagnosis. Unfortunately, most are impractical in regions with limited resources.

Penicillin for 5 days is the agent of choice for treatment. Erythromycin (5 days) and doxycycline (10 days) are alternative agents.

Dengue

Dengue is an acute febrile illness caused by a flavivirus transmitted by the mosquitoes *Aedes aegypti* and *A albopictus*. Disease is frequently associated with high fever and intense joint and muscle pain. Hemorrhagic complications and shock have also been reported. Dengue remains a common cause of hospitalizations in Southeast Asia. In a study in Vietnam, dengue was responsible for one third of febrile illnesses presenting to a public primary care clinic. The presentations were highly nonspecific; most were not suspected clinically. Approximately 32% of the cases without a clinical diagnosis were positive by serologies; this was mostly among children younger than 15 years. In patients with acute dengue, other diseases were suspected clinically, such as pharyngitis, typhoid fever, tonsillitis, leptospirosis, and hepatitis.[62] Febrile seizure, macular rash, petechiae, and thrombocytopenia were presenting clinical features of infants with dengue virus infection. However, asymptomatic infections were 6-times higher than symptomatic cases.[63]

Clinicians caring for children in the tropics where dengue is endemic should become familiar with WHO guidelines on the management of dengue, dengue hemorrhagic fever (DHF), and dengue shock syndrome (DSS).[64] Dengue hemorrhagic fever and DSS are frequent severe complications. Promptly recognizing signs of DHF and DSS and initiating appropriate treatment is critical for reducing fatalities. Massive capillary leak is usually observed after the child becomes afebrile (days 3 to 6). Close monitoring is appropriate at this stage of the illness. A drop in platelet count accompanied by rising hematocrit usually precedes shock. Persistent vomiting along with abdominal pain are signs of impending shock. Thrombocytopenia less than 100,000 with a hematocrit rise of 20% or more, with spontaneous bleeding, is indicative of DHF (grade 2 using a dengue classification scale). Signs of circulatory failure and shock confirm DSS (grade 3-4). The use of crystalloid oral and IV fluids, and colloids when indicated, are critical components of this management.[65]

Dengue is frequently characterized by acute onset of fever and 2 of the following: retro-orbital pain, rash, headaches, myalgias, arthralgias, leukopenia, or hemorrhagic manifestations, such as positive tourniquet test, bleeding gums, thrombocytopenia, petechiae, or purpura or ecchymoses.[66]

Mixed infections with dengue do occur in endemic regions. Of 602 children admitted to a hospital in Mumbai, India, 30 had malaria, 11 had enteric fever, and 7 had mixed infections; 27 children had leptospirosis. Clinical features were shared among these infections. However, contact with floodwater, myalgia, and conjunctival suffusion were more associated with leptospirosis. Abdominal pain, rash, and bleeding manifestations were more associated with dengue.[67]

Dengue is frequently undiagnosed in parts of south Texas along the US-Mexico border where vectors are found. In addition, imported cases are frequently reported in mainland United States.[68,69]

■ OTHER CAUSES OF FEVER IN THE TROPICS

Acute Rheumatic Fever

The incidence of acute rheumatic fever remains high in many lower-income countries. In a study from Lebanon, carditis was present in 93% of patients, followed by arthritis in about 40%.[70] In many developing countries, acute rheumatic fever remains a common cause of acquired heart disease. The presence of fever along with signs of carditis, arthritis, and Sydenham chorea is seen. Fever, arthralgias, and congestive heart failure are frequently the first evidence of the disease.[70] Children younger than 5 years frequently present with severe carditis. Moderate to severe carditis with arthritis or erythema marginatum are common presentations. Rheumatic fever in this age group is somewhat challenging because many clinicians would not consider it; a high degree of suspicion would be needed.[71]

Rickettsial Infections

Scrub and murine typhus in children is frequently misdiagnosed as enteric fever because children frequently lack classical features. Nonspecific features, such as fever, tachypnea, and hepatosplenomegaly, are reported.[72]

Community-Acquired Bacteremias

Community-acquired bloodstream infections are common in Africa. In a meta-analysis of studies from 1984 to 2006, in infants younger than 1 year, the incidence of community-acquired bacteremia (CAB) was estimated at 1,457 cases per 100,000 children; 100 in children younger than 2 years; and 505 in children younger than 5 years. Twenty-six percent of all in-hospital deaths were in children with CAB, with 70.5%

of these occurring in the first 2 days of hospitalization.[73] HIV infection and malnutrition may have been contributing factors. Bacteremia was responsible for more deaths in young infants than malaria. Twenty-nine percent of infections were caused by *S enterica;* approximately 58% of these were non-typhoidal. The most isolate in children was *Streptococcus pneumoniae* (18.3%). Other common pathogens were *Staphylococcus aureus* and *Escherichia coli.* In HIV patients, *Mycobacterium tuberculosis* was isolated when mycobacterial culture techniques were used.[73]

E coli and *Streptococcus agalactiae* (group B streptococcus) were the most frequently isolated pathogens in infants younger than 60 days in a rural hospital in Kilifi, Kenya. *S pneumoniae*, non-typhoidal *Salmonella* species, *Haemophilus influenzae,* and *E coli* were common in children older than 60 days.[74]

Blood cultures should be obtained in all febrile children with malaria. In a study in Nigeria, bacteremia was detected in 38.2% of infants and malaria parasitemia was found in 46.1%. *E coli, S aureus*, and *Klebsiella* were most commonly isolated.[75] Empiric antibacterial therapy should be administered to all children being treated for malaria when laboratory facilities are not available.

Fifty percent of febrile individuals had a positive blood culture, when malaria was excluded, in a study from 3 rural hospitals in Ghana. The median age was 15 years. *Salmonella* was the most frequently isolated pathogen—59% were *S typhi*. Most isolates were resistant to chloramphenicol, trimethoprim-sulfamethoxazole, and ampicillin.[76] Similar findings were found in a study from Mozambique.[77]

Familial Mediterranean Fever

Familial Mediterranean fever (FMF) is frequently observed in the Middle East. This autosomal-recessive disorder is not limited to any given part of the world and is estimated to affect more than 10,000 individuals worldwide. A high number of individuals are of Romanian or Jewish ancestry. Episodic fever attacks are accompanied by evidence of peritonitis, pleuritis, and arthritis. Symptoms may last for a few hours or up to 3 to 4 days. A large percentage of patients complain of abdominal pain as well as arthritis and chest pain, indicating pleuritis. Evidence of acute scrotal swelling and tenderness has been reported. If undiagnosed, some of the affected individuals may develop amyloidosis, resulting in chronic renal disease. In some countries individuals are empirically treated with colchicine without genetic testing. Genetic testing for the FMF gene is commercially available but expensive.[78]

Fever of Unknown Origin

Fever of unknown origin (febrile illness lasting more than 2 weeks) is also recognized in tropical countries. Enteric fever is a common cause. In India, visceral leishmaniasis and tuberculosis are frequently the cause.[79]

Miscellaneous Causes

Clinicians should not forget that common infections, such as acute otitis media, can cause fever in young children in the tropics.[80] Infections in aboriginal communities in tropical north-central Australia presenting with fever frequently had respiratory infections such as acute otitis media or influenza, bacterial pneumonia, and tuberculosis. Infectious diarrheas caused by *Salmonella, Shigella,* or *Campylobacter,* and skin infections such as impetigo and staphylococcal furunculosis, were also frequently diagnosed. Pyogenic arthritis and pyomyositis, osteomyelitis, rheumatic fever, and meningitis were seen. Respiratory syncytial virus was a common cause of severe pneumonia in Kenya.[81] Hospitalized febrile children with a history of travel to the tropics were frequently found to have nonspecific fever. Malaria, bacillary dysentery, dengue, and typhoid occurred less frequently.[82]

■ KEY POINTS

- Febrile illnesses remain important causes of morbidity and mortality in children around the world.
- Prompt recognition of etiology and the institution of appropriate supportive care or antimicrobial therapy are critical as the means of improving prognosis.
- Improving quality of water, food, and environment will ultimately have a greater effect.
- Cosmopolitan causes of fever, such as otitis media, pharyngitis, cellulitis, and sinusitis, are also frequent.

■ REFERENCES

1. Black RE, Cousens S, Johnson HL, et al. Global, regional, and national causes of child mortality in 2008: a systematic analysis. *Lancet.* 2010;375:1969–1987
2. Stanfield JP. Fever in children in the tropics. *BMJ.* 1969;1:761–765
3. West NS, Riordan FAI. Fever in returned travelers: a prospective review of hospital admissions for a 2 ½ year period. *Arch Dis Child.* 2003;88:432–434
4. Hagmann S, Neugebauer R, Schwartz E, et al. Illness in children after international travel: analysis from the Geosentinel Surveillance Network. *Pediatrics.* 2010;125: e1072–e1080
5. World Health Organization, United Nations Children's Fund. Integrated management of childhood illness. http://www.emro.who.int/cah/pdf/IMCI-Adaptation-yem.pdf. Accessed June 17, 2011

6. Factor SH, Schillinger JA, Kalter HD, et al. Diagnosis and management of febrile children using the WHO/UNICEF guidelines for IMCI in Dhaka, Bangladesh. *Bull WHO.* 2001;79:1096–1105

7. Nadjim B, Amos B, Mtove G, et al. WHO guidelines for antimicrobial treatment in children admitted to hospital in an area of intense *Plasmodium falciparum* transmission: prospective study. *BMJ.* 2010;340:c1350

8. Bottieau E, Clerinx J, Schrooten W, et al. Etiology and outcome of fever after a stay in the tropics. *Arch Intern Med.* 2006;166:1642–1648

9. Sripanidkulchai R, Lumbiganon P. Etiology of obscure fever in children at a university hospital in Northeast Thailand. *Southeast Asian J Trop Med Public Health.* 2005;36:1243–1246

10. Manock SR, Jacobsen KH, Brito de Bravo N, et al. Etiology of acute undifferentiated febrile illness in the Amazon basin of Ecuador. *Am J Trop Med Hyg.* 2009;81:146–151

11. Uzochukwu BSC, Onwujekwe EO, Onoka CA, Ughasoro MD. Rural-urban differences in maternal responses to childhood fever in South East Nigeria. *PLoS ONE.* 2008;3:e1788

12. Kazembe LN, Appleton CC, Kleinschmidt I. Choice of treatment for fever at household level in Malawi: examining spatial patterns. *Mal J.* 2007;6:40

13. Kandala NM, Ji C, Stallard N, Stranges S, Cappuccio FP. Morbidity from diarrhoea, cough and fever among young children in Nigeria. *Ann Trop Med Parasitol.* 2008; 102:427–445

14. Cox-Singh J, Davis TME, Lee KS, et al. *Plasmodium knowlesi* malaria in humans is widely distributed and potentially life threatening. *Clin Infect Dis.* 2008;46:165–171

15. Daneshvar C, Davis TME, Cox-Singh, et al. Clinical and laboratory features of human *Plasmodium knowlesi* infection. *Clin Infect Dis.* 2009;49:852–860

16. Crawley J, Chu C, Mtove G, Nosten F. Malaria in children. *Lancet.* 2010;375:1468–1481

17. Fuehrer HP, Starzengruber P, Swoboda P, et al. Indigenous *Plasmodium ovale* malaria in Bangladesh. *Am J Trop Med Hyg.* 2010;83:75–78

18. MacKenzie G, Ceesay SJ, Hill PC, et al. A decline in the incidence of invasive non-typhoidal *Salmonella* infection in The Gambia temporally associated with a decline in malaria infection. *PLoS.* 2010;5:e10568

19. Tripathy R, Parida S, Das L, et al. Clinical manifestations and predictors of severe malaria in Indian children. *Pediatrics.* 2007;120:e454–e460

20. Poespoprodjo JR, Fobia W, Kenangalem E, et al. Vivax malaria: a major cause of morbidity in early infancy. *Clin Infect Dis.* 2009;48:1704–1712

21. Dondorp AM, Lee SJ, Faiz MA, et al. The relationship between age and the manifestations of and mortality associated with severe malaria. *Clin Infect Dis.* 2008;47:151–157

22. Komba AN, Makani J, Sadarangani M, et al. Malaria as a cause of morbidity and mortality in children with homozygous sickle cell disease on the coast of Kenya. *Clin Infect Dis.* 2009;49:216–222

23. McAuley CF, Webb C, Makani J, et al. High mortality from *P. falciparum* malaria in children living with sickle cell anemia on the coast of Kenya. *Blood.* 2010;116:1663–1668

24. Joshi R, ColfordJr JM, Reingold AL, Kalantri S. Nonmalarial acute undifferentiated fever in a rural hospital in Central India: diagnostic uncertainty and over-treatment with antimalarial agents. *Am J Trop Med Hyg.* 2008;78:393–399

25. Ansah EK, Narh-Bana S, Epokor M, et al. Rapid testing for malaria in settings where microscopy is available and peripheral clinics where only presumptive treatment is available: a randomised controlled trial in Ghana. *BMJ.* 2010;340:c930

26. Stauffer WM, Cartwright CP, Olson DA, et al. Diagnostic performance of rapid diagnostic tests versus blood smears for malaria in US clinical practice. *Clin Infect Dis.* 2009;49:908–913

27. Hawkes M, Katsuva JP, Masumbuko CK. Use and limitations of malaria rapid diagnostic testing by community health workers in war-torn Democratic Republic of Congo. *Mal J.* 2009;8:308

28. Yukich J, D'Acremont V, Kahama J, Swai N, Lengeler C. Cost savings with rapid diagnostic tests for malaria in low-transmission areas: evidence from Dar es Salaam, Tanzania. *Am J Trop Med Hyg.* 2010;83:61–68

29. Pöschl B, Waneesorn J, Thekisoe O, Chutiponguivate S, Panagiotis K. Comparative diagnosis of malaria infection by microscopy, nested PCR and LAMP in northern Thailand. *Am J Trop Med Hyg.* 2010;83:56–60

30. Nkrumah B, Agyekum A, Acquah SE, et al. Comparison of the novel Partec Rapid Malaria Test to the conventional Giemsa stain and the gold standard real time PCR. *J Clin Microbiol.* 2010

31. World Health Organization. *Guidelines for the Treatment of Malaria.* 2nd ed. Geneva, Switzerland: World Health Organization. http://www.who.int/malaria/publications/atoz/9789241547925/en/index.html

32. Sowunmi A, Gbotosho GO, Happi C, et al. Therapeutic efficacy and effects of artesunate-mefloquine and mefloquine along on malaria-associated anemia in children with uncomplicated *Plasmodium falciparum* malaria in Southwest Nigeria. *Am J Trop Med Hyg.* 2009;81:979–986

33. Keiser J, N'Guessan NA, Adoubryn KD, et al. Efficacy and safety of mefloquine, artesunate, mefloquine-artesunate, and praziquantel against *Schistosomahaematobium*: randomized, exploratory open-label trial. *Clin Infect Dis.* 2010;50:1205–1213

34. Thriemer K, Starzengruber P, Khan WA, et al. Azithromycin combination therapy for the treatment of uncomplicated falciparum malaria in Bangladesh: an open-label randomized, controlled clinical trial. *J Infect Dis.* 2010;202

35. Kyu HH, Fernández E. Artemisinin derivatives versus quinine for cerebral malaria in African children: a systematic review. *Bull WHO.* 2009;87:896–904

36. PrayGod G, de Frey A, Eisenhut M. Artemisinin derivatives versus quinine in treating severe malaria in children: a systematic review. *Mal J.* 2008;7:210

37. NNedu ON, Rimel B, Terry C, et al. Syndromic diagnosis of malaria in rural Sierra Leone and proposed additions to the National Integrated Management of Childhood Illness guidelines for fever. *Am J Trop Med Hyg.* 2010;82:525–528

38. Patel TA, Armstrong M, Morris-Jones SD. Imported enteric fever: case series from The Hospital for Tropical Diseases, London, United Kingdom. *Am J Trop Med Hyg.* 2010; 82:1121–1126

39. Bhutta ZA. Current concepts in the diagnosis and treatment of typhoid fever. *BMJ.* 2006;333:78–82

40. Steffen R, Richenbach M, Wilhelm U, Helminger A, Schar M. Health problems after travel to developing countries. *J Infect Dis.* 1987;156:84–91

41. Siddiqui FJ, Rabbani F, Hasan R, Nizami SQ, Bhutta ZA. Typhoid fever in children: some epidemiological considerations from Karachi, Pakistan. *Int J Infect Dis.* 2006;10:215–222

42. Bhutta ZA. Impact of age and drug resistance on mortality in typhoid fever. *Arch Dis Child.* 1996;75:14–17

43. Bhutta ZA. Current concepts in the diagnosis and treatment of typhoid fever. *BMJ.* 2006;333:78–82

44. Yaramis A, Yildirim I, Katar S, et al. Clinical and laboratory presentation of typhoid fever. *Int Pediatr.* 2001;16:227–231

45. Laditan AA, Alausa KO. Problems in the clinical diagnosis of typhoid fever in children in the tropics. *Ann Trop Paediatr.* 1981;1:191–195

46. Adeleke SI, Nwokedi EE. Diagnostic value of Widal test in febrile children. *Afr Scient.* 2008;9:5–8

47. Mweu E, English M. Typhoid fever in children in Africa. *Trop Med Int Health.* 2008;13:532–540

48. Thaver D, Zaidi AKM, Critchley J, et al. A comparison of fluoroquinolones versus other antibiotics for treating enteric fever: meta-analysis. *BMJ.* 2009;338:b1865

49. Sur D, Ochiai RL, Bhattacharya SK, et al. A cluster-randomized effectiveness trial of Vi typhoid vaccine in India. *N Engl J Med.* 2009;361:335–344

50. Crump JA, Mintz ED. Global trends in typhoid and paratyphoid fever. *Clin Infect Dis.* 2010;50:241–246

51. Meltzer E, Sadik C, Schwartz E. Enteric fever in Israeli travelers: a nationwide study. *J Travel Med.* 2005;12:275–281

52. Maskey AP, Basnyat B, Thwaites GE, et al. Emerging trends in enteric fever in Nepal: 9124 cases confirmed by blood culture 1993–2003. *Trans R Soc Trop Med Hyg.* 2008;102:91–95

53. Uneke CJ. Concurrent malaria and typhoid fever in the tropics: the diagnostic challenges and public health implications. *J Vector Borne Dis.* 2008;45:133–142

54. Capoor MR, Nair D, Chintamani MS, et al. Role of enteric fever in ileal perforations: an overstated problem in tropics? *Indian J Med Microbiol.* 2008;26:54–57

55. Uba AF, Chirdan LB, Ituen AM, Mohammed AM. Typhoid intestinal perforation in children: a continuing scourge in a developing country. *Pediar Surg Int.* 2007;23:33–39

56. Ekenze SO, Ikefuna AN. Typhoid intestinal perforation under 5 years of age. *Ann Trop Pediatr.* 2008;28:53–58

57. Morpeth SC, Ramadhani HO, Crump JA. Invasive non-typhi *Salmonella* disease in Africa. *Clin Infect Dis.* 2009;49:606–611

58. Vijayachari P, Sugunan AP, Shiriam AN. Leptospirosis: an emerging global public health problem. *J Biosci.* 2008;33:557–569

59. Bruce MG, Sander EJ, Leake JA, et al. Leptospirosis among patients presenting with dengue-like illness in Puerto Rico. *Acta Trop.* 2005;96:36–46

60. Kendall EA, LaRocque RC, Bui DM, et al. Short report: leptospirosis as a cause of fever in urban Bangladesh. *Am J Trop Med Hyg.* 2010;82:1127–1130

61. LaRocque RC, Breiman RF, Ari MD, et al. Leptospirosis during dengue outbreak, Bangladesh. *Emerg Infect Dis.* 2005;11:766–769

62. Phuong HL, de Vries PJ, Nga TTT, et al. Dengue as a cause of acute undifferentiated fever in Vietnam. *BMC Infect Dis.* 2006;6:123

63. Capeding RZ, Brian JD, Caponpon MM, et al. The incidence, characteristics, and presentation of dengue virus infections during infancy. *Am J Trop Med Hyg.* 2010;82: 330–336

64. World Health Organization. Dengue, dengue haemorrhagic fever and dengue shock syndrome in the context of the Integrated Management of Childhood Illness. http://whqlibdoc.who.int/publications/2009/9789241547871_eng.pdf

65. Rocha C, Silva S, Gordon A, et al. Improvement in hospital indicators after changes in dengue case management in Nicaragua. *Am J Trop Med Hyg.* 2009;81:287–292

66. Gregory CJ, Santiago LM, Argüello DF, Hunsperger E, Tomashek KM. Clinical and laboratory features that differentiate dengue from other feasible illnesses in an endemic area-Puerto Rico, 2007–2008. *Am J Trop Med Hyg.* 2010;82:922–929

67. Zaki SA, Shanbag P. Clinical manifestations of dengue and leptospirosis in children in Mumbai: an observational study. *Infection.* 2010

68. Courtney M, Shetty AK. Imported dengue fever. An important reemerging disease. *Pediatr Emer Care.* 2009;25:769–772

69. Neitzel D, Fisher R, Crimmings K, et al. Dengue fever among US travelers returning from the Dominican Republic—Minnesota and Iowa, 2008. *MMWR.* 2010;59:654–656

70. Bitar FF, Hayek P, Obeid M, et al. Rheumatic fever in children. A 15-year experience in a developing country. *Pediatr Cardiol.* 2000;21:119–122

71. Abdin ZH, Eissa A. Rheumatic fever and rheumatic heart disease in children below the age of 5 years in the tropics. *Ann Rheum Dis.* 1965;24:389–391

72. Silpapokakul K, Chupuppakarn S, Yuthasompob S, et al. Scrub and murine typhus in children with obscure fever in the tropics. *Pediatr Infect Dis J.* 1991;10:200–203

73. Reddy EA, Shaw AV, Crump JA. Community-acquired bloodstream infections in Africa: a systematic review and meta-analysis. *Lancet Infect Dis.* 2010;10:417–432

74. Berkley JA, Lowe BS, Mwangi I, et al. Bacteremia among children admitted to a rural hospital in Kenya. *N Engl J Med.* 2005;352:39–47

75. Ayoola OO, Adeyemo AA, Osinusi K. Concurrent bacteraemia and malaria in febrile Nigerian infants. *Trop Doctor.* 2005;35:34–36

76. Zimmerman O, de Ciman R, Gross U. Bacteremia among Kenyan children. *N Engl J Med.* 2005;352:1379–1381

77. Mandomando I, Sigaúque B, Morais L, et al. Antimicrobial drug resistance trends of bacteremia isolates in a rural hospital in southern Mozambique. *Am J Trop Hyg.* 2010;83:152–157

78. Padeh S. Periodic fever syndromes. *Pediatr Clin North Am.* 2005;52:577–609

79. Joshi N, Rajeshwari K, Dubey AP, Singh T, Kaur R. Clinical spectrum of fever of unknown origin among Indian children. *Ann Trop Paediatr.* 2008;28:261–266

80. Alabi BS, Abdulkarim AA, Olatoke F, Suleiman OA. Acute otitis media—a common diagnosis among febrile children in the tropics. *Trop Doctor.* 2006;36:31–32

81. Berkley JA, Munywoki P, Ngama M, et al. Viral etiology of severe pneumonia among Kenyan infants and children. *JAMA.* 2010;303:2051–2057

82. Klein JL, Millman GC. Prospective, hospital based study of fever in children in the United Kingdom who had recently spent time in the tropics. *BMJ.* 1998;316:1425

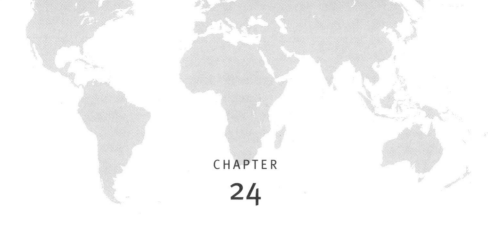

CHAPTER

24

Gastrointestinal Infections

John C. Christenson, MD, FAAP

■ INTRODUCTION

Respiratory and diarrheal infections, malaria, and tuberculosis are among the most common causes of morbidity and mortality in children in developing countries. Five of the 10 leading causes of death around the world affect children.[1] Only neonatal deaths and respiratory infections surpass gastrointestinal (GI) infections as causes of infant mortality.[2] Diarrhea is the main reason for hospitalization in pediatric age groups. It is estimated that more than 1 billion cases of diarrhea occur each year in developing countries.[3,4] Approximately 2 million children younger than 5 years die each year from GI infections caused by rotavirus, cholera, diarrheagenic *Escherichia coli,* typhoid fever, and dysentery; this represents approximately 19% of total child deaths. The World Health Organization (WHO) Africa and southeast regions combined contain 78% of all diarrheal deaths, with 73% of them concentrated within 15 developing countries.[5] Malnutrition, immune deficiencies such as HIV/AIDS, dehydration, malaria, pneumonia, and infection by invasive enteropathogens such as *Shigella, Salmonella,* and *Entamoeba histolytica* are considered risk factors for fatal diarrhea. Fortunately, through improvements in infrastructure and rotavirus vaccination programs, many developing countries are seeing decreases in GI infections. The introduction and use of oral rehydration solution (ORS) has also contributed to a decrease in mortality.

Because most morbidity and mortality associated with diarrheal disease relates to dehydration, recurrent disease, and malnutrition, this chapter presents a comprehensive understanding of the epidemiology and appropriate management of diarrheal disease in the developing world and the means to prevent it.

■ EPIDEMIOLOGY OF ACUTE DIARRHEA IN CHILDREN

Rotavirus, enterotoxigenic *E coli* (ETEC), and *Shigella* are the most important pediatric enteropathogens.[3,4] They are frequently associated with acute diarrhea, resulting in the passage of loose stools for fewer than 14 days. Other organisms, such as *Salmonella,Campylobacter,* adenovirus (40 and 41), *Clostridium difficile,* norovirus, astrovirus, *Cryptosporidium,* and *Giardia,* are associated with acute disease in the immunocompetent and well-nourished host.[6] With the exception of rotavirus, most other viruses are infrequent causes of acute diarrhea. While norovirus-related outbreaks are well described in magnitude of numbers, rotavirus dwarfs all other viral enteropathogens.[7]

Community outbreaks of non-typhoid salmonellosis and shigellosis are common because both have low infective doses at approximately 100 and less than 200 colony-forming units (CFU), respectively.[6] Norovirus attack rates can be high because they cause vomiting and produce large-volume stools that contain large amounts of the virus and can spread easily in areas with poor hygiene. In addition, the low inoculum (less than 100 viral particles) required to produce infection also facilitates new cases.

Mortality is much higher in younger children. As previously stated, the availability of ORS significantly diminished the mortality observed in high-risk groups. While the incidence of diarrhea has not changed in some regions, mortality clearly has. Invasive pathogens, such as *Shigella, Salmonella, Campylobacter,*and *E histolytica,*are more prone to cause mortality than organisms that are traditionally responsible for dehydration, such as rotavirus, cholera, and diarrheagenic *E coli.*

Dysentery remains a common problem in the tropics. The most common causative organism is *Shigella dysenteriae* type 1. The organism readily spreads from person to person through fecal-oral transmission. *S flexneri* is also frequently isolated. Mortality has been reported as high as 15% in some Latin America communities.

Vibrio cholerae O1 continues to cause worldwide disease. Mortality for this organism is estimated to be 3% to 4%. Large epidemics still occur in many places of the developing world, including circulation of new strains, such as O139. Cholera remains endemic in portions of India,

Pakistan, Bangladesh, Afghanistan, and many countries of Southeast Asia. Outbreaks of cholera among poverty-stricken and displaced people in Zimbabwe and Haiti have been ongoing in recent months.[8,9] In 2005, 78% of countries reporting indigenous cases of cholera were in sub-Saharan Africa.[10] The number of cases in Africa is close to 100 times higher than those reported in Asia and 16,600 times higher than incidences in Latin America. In that same year, case fatalities in Africa were 3 times higher than in Asia with no reported deaths in Latin America. As of December 17, 2010, 121,518 cases of cholera had been reported in Haiti, resulting in 63,711 hospitalizations and 2,591 deaths.[9] Farming and disruptions in sanitation in impoverished environments, such as refugee camps full of displaced people caused by economic or political turmoil, are frequent associations.

Cholera has always served as an indicator of unsafe drinking water, poor sanitation, and inadequate health care.[10] In Latin America, investments to improve drinking water, sanitation, and health care not only reduced the number of cases and associated mortality but also decreased hepatitis A and typhoid fever cases. In addition to clean water, access to ORS significantly decreased the mortality rate associated with this infection. The introduction of ORS in South Asia decreased the case fatality rate from 30% to less than 1%.[7,9] If cholera is to be eliminated, improvements in sanitation and water quality must occur in Africa. It is estimated that approximately 17% of the world's population lacks access to safe water and 42% lacks proper sanitary facilities. While vaccination has not succeeded in preventing all cases of cholera, improvements in sanitation have had demonstrable beneficial effects. Other pathogens, such as *Shigella, Salmonella, Campylobacter, Aeromonas,* and *Plesiomonas,* protozoa and helminthic parasites commonly occur in impoverished areas with poor environmental sanitation.[11]

Studies demonstrate that the lack of micronutrients, such as zinc, which is extensively lost in the stool of cholera victims, may lead to acrodermatitis enteropathica. While zinc supplementation will prevent this complication, it also reduces stool volume and shortens the duration of diarrhea.[12,13]

Accessibility to ORS, zinc supplementation, and basic health care will need to be enhanced. Along with these improvements, increased breast-feeding and measles vaccination rates contributed to the decrease in diarrhea-related infant mortality in Brazil.[14] Brazil can serve as a model to other countries. Before these interventions, infants exclusively receiving powdered milk or cow's milk were approximately 14 times more likely to die from diarrhea than those who were exclusively breastfed.[15]

In addition, mass vaccination programs with effective vaccines against cholera will have beneficial effects, especially in regions with a high prevalence of HIV infection.[10]

While it is well known to parents that ORS and feedings are essential for children with diarrhea, many affected children are still not receiving them. In a recent study, 52% of children received reduced or no food during diarrheal episodes.[16] This was frequently observed in children younger than 3 years. This trend appears to be increasing. In recent years, the percentage of children receiving ORS, recommended home fluids, and receiving increased fluids during illness (as recommended by WHO guidelines) was 68% overall in surveyed countries.[16] However, of greater concern, ORS use in Rwanda was less than 1% and was 32% in Kenya and Nigeria. The reason for this decline in appropriate diarrheal management appears to be multifactorial. A recent shift in attention toward HIV/AIDS, malaria, and tuberculosis treatment and prevention strategies may have diminished the focus on diarrhea management. The creation of integrated approaches to care at the level of health care facilities and with health care workers appears to have resulted in gaps in the promotion of basic diarrhea management at the community level.[16] In addition, limited resources at home caused by an inability to work because of tuberculosis, malaria, or HIV/AIDS appears to be a contributing factor. Increased knowledge may be beneficial, but it does not always lead to better clinical practices.[7,16]

The vicious cycle of severe GI infections leading to malnutrition is frequently seen in the developing world. Maternal and childhood undernutrition leads to approximately 3.5 million deaths and is responsible for 35% of the disease burden in children younger than 5 years.[17] Gastrointestinal infections and diarrhea impair not only weight and height gains but also physical and cognitive development. Malnourished children will have a slower recovery from diarrheal episodes and will be unable to catch up with non-malnourished children in height and weight. Malnourished children will have lower IQ scores compared with non-malnourished children.[17,18] This cognitive impairment due to diarrhea equates to nearly 10 IQ points. A decrease in cognitive abilities, as well as disease burden, affects the individual's ability to benefit from education and dramatically affects disability-adjusted life year (DALY) rates. Fitness impairment leads to approximately 17% decreased work productivity.[18]

It is estimated that 34% of disease burden in children is attributable to the environment. Globally, it is estimated that 24% of the disease burden is due to environmental risk factors. Most disease burden is associated with contaminated water and poor sanitation.[19] Environmental contributors to diarrheal diseases are closer to 94%. In rural Pakistan, higher prevalence of diarrhea was associated with lack of maternal education, lack of exclusive breastfeeding, roundworm infection, and multiple young children in the home. Among predictors of mortality, severe malnutrition and non-breastfeeding are the most common.[20] Child mortality secondary to diarrheal diseases in Matlab, Bangladesh, was lowest in the postharvest months of February, March, and August compared with the "hungry" months of September and October.[21] This effect was only observed in homes with no maternal schooling. Additional studies from the same region showed diarrheal deaths peaking in the hot-wet season.[22]

It is not uncommon to find patients infected with multiple pathogens at the same time. In a study in Mexico City, 52% of patients were infected with more than one enteropathogen, notably E histolytica, E dispar, and Salmonella.[23] In Nigeria, approximately 36% of patients had multiple pathogens; among these were ETEC, enterohemorrhagic E coli, enteroaggregative E coli (EAEC), Salmonella, Shigella, and E histolytica.[24]

■ CHILDREN WITH PERSISTENT OR CHRONIC INFECTIONS

Diarrhea

Children with persistent diarrhea and malnutrition were more likely to die during their third year of life. *Persistent diarrhea* is defined as a diarrheal episode that lasts 14 days or more.[25]

In Matlab, Bangladesh, 49% of diarrheal deaths were in malnourished children with persistent diarrhea.[26] Most enteropathogens, bacterial, viral, or parasitic, are associated with persistent diarrhea and enteropathy. Prior malnutrition, recurrent infections, suboptimal or delayed diarrhea treatment, and micronutrient malnutrition are all contributing factors for persistent diarrhea.[25,27] Postinfectious malabsorption syndromes are partially responsible for the malnutrition and failure of growth in young infants. This is prominently observed once mothers stop breastfeeding and exclusively rely on farmed or purchased goods and contaminated water for hydration.

Patients infected with *Salmonella typhi* and *S paratyphi* are likely to develop prolonged infections and suffer from severe enteric fever.[28] Parasitic infections from *Cryptosporidium* and *Giardia* frequently lead to chronic diarrhea in the immunocompromised and malnourished host.

Enteroaggregative *E coli* has emerged as an important diarrheal pathogen. Acute and persistent diarrhea, and even asymptomatic infections, have been reported with this enteropathogen.[29,30] Community and nosocomial outbreaks have also been reported. It appears that a large amount of bacteria (at least 10^{10} CFU) is required for diarrheal illness. The incubation period is approximately 8 to 18 hours. The illness is self-limiting in most hosts and only requires ORS and supportive care. Ciprofloxacin and a poorlyabsorbable antibiotic, rifaximin, are shown to be effective against EAEC among travelers. Unfortunately, multidrug-resistant isolates of EAEC have been recognized in Africa.[31]

In populations with moderate malnutrition, low weight for age and diarrhea itself are risk factors for recurrent and persistent diarrheal diseases.[16] Recurrent diarrhea is not infrequent. Children may experience an average of 3 to 10 episodes per year.[4] Persistent diarrhea may occur in some children, prolonging increased stool output for more than 14 days; this can be observed mainly with parasitic infections and in immuno-compromised children. Pathogens, such as measles, and enteric viruses, such as norovirus, are also responsible for malabsorption problems.

Gastritis

In spite of *Helicobacter pylori* not being known as a diarrheal pathogen, it is a common cause of gastric and peptic ulcer disease. The prevalence in lower-income countries is much higher than in higher-income countries—80% to 90% versus 10% to 50%, respectively. Infection rates are closely associated with low economic status, poor sanitation, over-crowding, and poor hygiene. Of interest, infected children are more often infected with other enteral pathogens. This supports a fecal-oral route of transmission. A recent study from Bangladesh confirms these findings. Not surprisingly, the infections by this organism appear to occur more often in children after they are weaned from breast milk.[32]

Enteric Fever

Enteric fever is a common systemic infection observed in the developing world. It can be caused by *Salmonella enterica,* which includes 2 serotypes, *S typhi* and *S paratyphi* A, B, or C. *S typhi* is estimated to cause approximately 22 million worldwide infections every year with 200,000 deaths; *S paratyphi* is responsible for 5.4 million illnesses.[33] While it was initially thought that *S paratyphi* caused a milder disease than typhoid fever, recent experiences confirm that this is not the case. The area with the highest incidence of enteric fever is the India sub-continent. Enteric fever is prevalent worldwide, but it is only in those countries where improvements in public health and sanitation have been implemented where the incidence of typhoid and paratyphoid fever is low.

Tropical Enteropathy

Contaminated environments and recurrent GI infections will lead to chronic enteropathies and malabsorption syndromes such a tropical enteropathy (tropical sprue).[34-37] These lead to vitamin (B_{12}), fat, amino acid, and micronutrient deficiencies.[38] Most of these enteropathies are subclinical.[39]

In developing countries, 26% of preschool children are underweight. More than 50% of childhood deaths are associated with being underweight.[40-42] These children are more likely to die from pneumonia, measles, malaria, and diarrhea.[43] This is frequently associated with infections caused by a multiplicity of different viral, bacterial, and parasitic pathogens. No single organism can be identified as a cause in all cases. Reports from parts of South America, the Caribbean, and Southeast Asia have enteropathy rates much higher than areas of Northern Africa, Southern Europe, and parts of Africa.[36,37]

While infectious agents are a frequent trigger of this condition, there appears to be a genetic predisposition for the condition, specifically in the presence of histocompatibility antigens AW19 or AW31.[36] Bacterial colonization through the adhesive properties of bacteria, such as *E coli*, *Salmonella*, and *V cholerae*, is responsible for much of the observed disease, especially the blunting of intestinal villi with increased lymphocytic and plasma cell infiltrations. The blunting of villi is in part responsible for the malabsorption observed in these patients. Patients with more of a colonic involvement are unable to absorb the necessary fluids to prevent diarrhea, which makes chronic diarrhea common. As a consequence of malabsorption, weight loss is a prominent feature, followed by malnutrition and vitamin B_{12} and folate deficiencies. With the mucosal injury to the bowel, there is an increase of gut hormones such as enteroglucagon, which is responsible for reduced small intestine transit time, leading to further intraluminal bacterial colonization, perpetrating further mucosal injury.[36] This vicious cycle can be eliminated by eradicating the bacterial overgrowth with antimicrobial agents and healing the mucosal lining with folates. In addition, an adequate diet, in combination with antimicrobial therapy and folates, is usually necessary.

Other Bacterial Pathogens

Malabsorption is frequently observed in the immunocompromised host, such as those affected by HIV, because chronic infections with organisms such as *Cryptosporidium parvum*, *Isospora belli*, and *Giardia* occur often in this population. While rare, intestinal tuberculosis may also be responsible for chronic diarrhea and malabsorption.

■ PARASITES AND OTHER GASTROINTESTINAL PATHOGENS

Parasites

Parasites frequently cause diarrhea in developing countries. Recurrent infections may lead to chronic diarrhea, malabsorption, anemia, micronutrient deficiencies, and malnutrition.[44] Chronic infections are common in the immunocompromised host with HIV/AIDS and in malnourished children. Intestinal parasites were observed in 46.5% of children with diarrhea in Delhi. *Cryptosporidium,Giardia intestinalis,* and *E histolytica* were the most commonly found.[45] Intestinal parasites were found in 19% of the examined population in a national prevalence study from Iran; *Giardia lamblia* was the most common. The highest infection rates were found in rural children between the ages of 2 and 14 years.[46] Helminths, such as *Ascaris lumbricoides* and *Trichuris trichiura,* were found less frequently.[45-47] Additional studies confirmed the importance of *Giardia* and *Cryptosporidium* as parasitic enteropathogens.[48-52] The prevalence of hookworms, *Schistosoma mansoni,* and *Ascaris lumbricoides* was 15% or higher in displacement camps within Sierra Leone.[49] In Tanzania, in addition to *Shigella, E histolytica, G lamblia,* and *S mansoni* were frequently found in the stool of patients with bloody diarrhea.[53] Among children with parasitic infections, Nigerian children with large parasite burdens were shorter in height and had lower weights than noninfected children.[54] As in most countries, geophagia or pica is associated with nematode intestinal parasitic infections.[55]

Parasitic infections associated with chronic inflammation are also associated with cancer. Chronic infections of the urinary bladder with *S haematobium,* the portal venous system of the liver with *S mansoni* and *S japonicum,* and the hepatobiliary tract with *Opisthorchis* or *Clonorchis* may lead to various types of malignancies. Early diagnosis and treatment and measures to prevent infection will help reduce the incidence of these cancers.[56]

Hepatic and Biliary Infections

Hepatic and biliary infections are frequently associated with poor sanitation and contaminated food and water. A diverse number of pathogens, such as hepatitis A and hepatitis E viruses, are frequently associated with these conditions. Hepatitis B and C viruses are frequently transmitted perinatally but are also transmitted through contact with contaminated body fluids. These agents can be responsible for jaundice seen in acute infections. Dengue, acute schistosomiasis (Katayama fever), herpes simplex virus, and enteroviruses could also be responsible for acute jaundice. Infections such as leptospirosis, typhoid fever, syphilis, and malaria are also responsible for jaundice in the tropics. In some instances, chronic liver disease will develop specifically in those with hepatitis B and C. Venoocclusive and portal hypertension have been observed in patients with chronic infections with schistosomiasis. Splenomegaly and bleeding varices will be ultimate complications. Biliary tract disease is usually related to parasitic organisms, such as ascariasis, clonorchiasis, and opisthorchiasis. Early diagnosis is imperative because chronic infections of the biliary tract may lead to pancreatic carcinomas and cholangiocarcinomas. Organisms such as *E histolytica* can also cause liver abscesses that would present with right upper-quadrant pain, hepatomegaly, and fever. These patients may have a history of a preceding diarrheal illness, fever, or jaundice.

■ APPROACHING THE CHILD WITH DIARRHEA

Oral Rehydration Fluids

Dehydration is responsible for most morbidity associated with acute diarrhea. Prompt replacement of fluid and electrolytes is critical in the management of this condition by reversing dehydration but also replacing ongoing fecal losses. Fluids can be administered intravenously in the severely dehydrated child or with ORS. Different ORS formulations have been suggested, but because glucose-based ORS (G-ORS) is inexpensive and easy to prepare, it remains the standard recommended ORS for managing the dehydrated child with diarrhea. Rice-flour–based ORS preparations have demonstrated a slightly better reduction in stool output than G-ORS in the first 6 hours of treatment, but this benefit did not persist after 12 hours of treatment. Overall, they appear to have an efficacy similar to G-ORS.[57]

Since 1978, the recommended WHO and United Nations Children's Fund (UNICEF) ORS preparation was a formulation containing 90 mEq/L sodium with an osmolarity of 311 mOsm/L. While effective in replacing fluid losses, the preparation had no effect on stool volume or duration. The formulation was considered hyperosmolar because of its sodium content and, thus, hypernatremia was a great concern. This was particularly so in young infants and children with non-cholera diarrhea. So work on a new formulation was deemed necessary.

In a clinical trial in Bangladesh, a formulation containing 60 mmol/L sodium with an osmolarity of 250 mOsm/L (reduced-osmolarity solution) was found to be equally effective as the WHO solution containing 90 mEq/L sodium, but with no significant hyponatremia in any treated patients.[58] In a similar study, using a 75 mmol/L sodium formulation (245 mOsm/L) for patients with acute diarrhea resulted in a 33% reduction in the need for intravenous (IV) fluids; results were similar to the standard WHO formulation at the time.[59] In a meta-analysis of existing studies, reduced-osmolarity ORS, when compared with standard WHO ORS, was associated with fewer unscheduled IV fluid infusions, reduced stool volumes, and less vomiting with no increase in hyponatremia episodes.[60] Since 2002, the WHO formulation has contained 75 mEq/L sodium and 75 mmol/L glucose with an osmolarity of 245 mOsm/L. [61-63]

In the United States, maintenance ORS such as Pedialyte containing 45 mmol/L sodium with an osmolarity of 250 mOsm/L is frequently used as ORS in children with diarrhea. Although the sodium content is lower than the WHO formulations, they were found to be as effective as ORS in a non-comparative study.[64] When used appropriately, ORS effectively corrects mild to moderate dehydration in infants and children with acute gastroenteritis. Oral rehydration solution can minimize the need for IV fluid infusions even in higher-income countries with good access to health care.

■ ASSESSING AND TREATING DEHYDRATION

In the child with diarrhea, the initial step in management is to quickly assess the degree of dehydration. Important questions to ask include, how many stools per day? What is the volume of the stools? Is the child vomiting? Clinicians caring for infants and children with diarrhea in lower-income countries will find excellent resources to assist them in the care of these patients. [61,62] Most children could be treated at home; however, medical evaluation of an infant or child with acute diarrhea is recommended if the infant is younger than 6 months, has preexisting medical conditions, or is highly febrile (39°C or higher); there is visible blood in the stool; and there are signs of toxicity or severe dehydration (Table 24-1). Mental status changes (eg, lethargy, irritability, unresponsiveness), persistent vomiting that interferes with taking oral fluids, and a suboptimal response to or an inability to take ORS should also trigger a medical evaluation.[61]

The management of acute diarrhea is based on the degree of dehydration. Oral rehydration solution can be used for rehydration but should be initiated promptly after the onset of diarrhea (within 3 to 4 hours). Once dehydration is corrected, an age-appropriate diet should be restarted. Breastfeeding should not be interrupted. If diarrhea continues, an appropriate amount of fluid should be given to match ongoing losses.[61] In the child with minimal or no dehydration, treatment is targeted at providing adequate fluid while continuing age-appropriate diet. In general, for each gram of stool output, 1 mL of fluid should be

SYMPTOM	MINIMAL OR NO DEHYDRATION (<3% LOSS OF BODY WEIGHT)	MILD TO MODERATE DEHYDRATION (3%–9% LOSS OF BODY WEIGHT)	SEVERE DEHYDRATION (>9% LOSS OF BODY WEIGHT)
Table 24-1. Assessment of Dehydration for Infants and Children			
Mental status	Well; alert; interactive	Normal, fatigued or restless, irritable	Apathetic, lethargic, unconscious
Thirst	Drinks normally; might refuse liquids	Thirsty; eager to drink	Drinks poorly; unable to drink
Heart rate	Normal	Normal to increased	Tachycardia, with bradycardia in most severe cases
Quality of pulses	Normal	Normal to decreased	Weak, thready, or non-palpable
Breathing	Normal	Normal; fast	Deep
Eyes	Normal; tears present	Slightly sunken; tears decreased	Deeply sunken; tears absent
Oral mucous membranes	Moist	Dry	Parched
Skin turgor	Instant recoil	Recoil in <2 seconds	Recoil in >2 seconds
Capillary refill	Normal	Prolonged	Prolonged; minimal
Extremities	Warm	Cool	Cold; mottled; cyanotic
Urine output	Normal to decreased	Decreased	Minimal

Adapted from Hahn S, Kim S, Garner P. Reduced osmolarity oral rehydration solution for treating dehydration caused by acute diarrhoea in children. *Cochrane Database Syst Rev.* 2002;(1):CD002847; and King CK, Glass R, Bresee JS, Duggan C, Centers for Disease Control and Prevention. Managing acute gastroenteritis among children: oral rehydration, maintenance, and nutritional therapy. *MMWR Recomm Rep.* 2003;52(RR-16):1–16

administered. Alternatively, 60 to 120 mL of ORS should be given for each diarrheal stool or vomiting episode if the child is less than 10 kg body weight. In the child weighing more than 10 kg, 120 to 140 mL ORS is needed. In the child with mild to moderate dehydration, at least 50 to 100 mL/kg body weight of ORS should be given within 2 to 4 hours to replace existing fluid deficit. Additional amount is given to replace on-going losses. In the severely dehydrated child, a 20 mL/kg body weight IV bolus of lactated Ringer solution or normal saline should be given until perfusion and mental status normalize, followed by appropriate fluids (5% dextrose, half normal saline) at twice the maintenance fluid rates. If IV access is not available and child is unable to drink, ORS can be administered by nasogastric tube for the child who needs fluids to replace losses (20 mL/kg/hour for 6 hours, for a total of 120 mL/kg).[62] Intravenous fluids of 5% dextrose, one fourth normal saline, with 20 mEq/L potassium chloride can also be administered. Oral rehydration solution can be initiated if the health care facility is more than 30 minutes away.

The US Agency for International Development (USAID) micronutrient program offers a simplified method of computing fluid needs for the first 4 hours of treatment in infants and children with diarrhea (Table 24-2). After the first 4 hours of rehydration, the child is reassessed for signs of dehydration and additional fluid needs are calculated. Health care professionals and families need to be educated on the proper use of ORS.[65]

The child with severe dehydration needs to receive fluids promptly—preferably IV fluids. While referral to a health care facility with the capability to administer IV fluids is indicated, fluid administration should not be delayed. Whenever possible, give more fluids than needed. If the infant can breastfeed, continue to do so, but do so more frequently and for longer periods. Oral rehydration solution or clean water (previously boiled) can be given to older children. Approximately 50 to 100 mL of fluid (¼ large cup) should be given with each loose stool in children younger than 2 years; older children can receive double that amount. [62] Soft drinks, sweetened tea, juices, and coffee should not be given, as they are likely to increase stool output. Caregivers need to monitor adequacy of fluid intake in children who are sent home. Children should return to the clinic for reevaluation if they are passing more stools, are persistently thirsty, have sunken eyes, have decreased urine output, do not seem to be getting better, are febrile, and are not eating or drinking well.

Diagnostic Testing

Once the correction of dehydration is underway, carefully assessing stool characteristics (ie, watery versus bloody) and other clinical features (eg, high fevers, abdominal pain) will help determine the cause of the diarrhea, which will dictate additional therapies if needed.[62] The use of

Table 24-2. US Agency for International Development Micronutrient Program Fluid Needs for the First 4 Hours of Treatment for Dehydration

AGE	≤4 MO	4 TO 12 MO	1 TO 2 Y	2 TO 5 Y
Body weight, kg	<6	6–<10	10–<12	12–19
Amount of fluid, mL	200–400	400–700	700–900	900–1,400

smears for fecal leukocytes as an initial screen has been recommended. Patients with positive smear results would be more likely to have a bacterial pathogen for which a stool culture would be ordered. Unfortunately, studies have demonstrated variable results in patients with bacterial enteric infections. The sensitivity of the fecal leukocyte test in patients with shigellosis was 73%, while for most other bacterial pathogens it was approximately 50% at best.[66] Bacterial stool cultures, rotavirus, and *Giardia* or *Cryptosporidium* antigen detection assays, and materials for the examination of other fecal parasites, are commercially available in most countries.[67] However, some health care facilities within developing countries may lack these because of limited resources; clinical assessments of the patient will usually dictate the management pathway.

Antimicrobial Therapy

Overemphasis on antimicrobial therapy and other medications will have limited effect on infantile diarrhea-related mortality. In developing countries, most patients with diarrhea do not require antimicrobial therapy. Most guidelines recommend antimicrobial therapy only in suspected cases of cholera or dysentery. [62,68] In most instances, an ongoing outbreak leads to treatment recommendations. The majority of diarrheal illnesses are self-limiting, and antibiotic therapy is costly and leads to resistance or infections with *C difficile.*

In addition to hydration fluids, the patient with bloody stools (when dysentery is suspected in an area) should receive 5 days of antibacterial therapy against *Shigella.*[62] The precise cause of bloody diarrhea would require a stool culture with at least 2 to 3 days of incubation and workup for results. The identification of diarrheagenic *E coli,* with the exception of Shiga toxin-producing *E coli* (STEC), requires the use of polymerase chain reaction technology. [67,69]

While routine use is generally discouraged, certain infections should be treated with antimicrobial therapy. [61,62] In addition to shigellosis, antimicrobial treatment of the following should also be considered: giardiasis, cholera, amebiasis, salmonellosis in the young febrile infant or infant with a positive blood culture and signs of dissemination, or the compromised host with *Campylobacter* or certain types of diarrheagenic *E coli* (eg, ETEC, EAEC).[70]

Widespread use of antibiotics leads to resistance. In a study from rural western Kenya, among stool specimens from 3,445 persons, 32% yielded at least one bacterial pathogen.[71] *Shigella,* the most commonly isolated pathogen (16% of all illnesses), was susceptible to frequently used agents in the community in less than 25% of occasions. Most persons were treated with an antibiotic to which their isolate was resistant. In data from an active surveillance community-based study in the Peruvian Amazon, *Shigella,* the most common cause of symptomatic disease, was resistant to ampicillin in 73% of isolates; 62% to chloramphenicol; 79% to trimethoprim-sulfamethoxazole (TMP-SMX); and 83% to tetracycline.[72] Ninety-seven percent of isolates were susceptible to ceftriaxone; 84% to azithromycin; and 97% to ciprofloxacin. In a similar study from Gaza, Palestine, high-level resistance was observed among isolates of *Salmonella* and *Shigella.*[73] In this region, ampicillin and TMP-SMX were no longer recommended agents for the empiric treatment of childhood diarrhea. Similar high-level resistance has been reported in Nepal and Tanzania.[53,74]

In Thailand, most isolates of *Campylobacter* are resistant to ciprofloxacin and more than 90% of *Shigella* isolates are resistant to TMP-SMX.[75] While azithromycin has become the recommended agent for treating *Campylobacter,* resistance to this agent is increasing. Similar findings have been observed among children with *Campylobacter* diarrhea in rural Egypt.[76]

In uncomplicated *Salmonella* enteritis, treatment is not routinely indicated.[77] When necessary, azithromycin or a third-generation cephalosporin such as ceftriaxone is the agent of choice for treating diarrhea, especially in children.[78,79] A single dose of azithromycin is effective for treating cholera.[80-82] A fluoroquinolone, such as ciprofloxacin or levofloxacin, is considered an alternative in patients with shigellosis, ETEC, or EAEC.[68,83]

The treatment of rotavirus gastroenteritis has been supportive with emphasis on correcting and preventing dehydration. There are no existing antiviral agents effective against this pathogen or any other virus responsible for diarrhea. However, in a double-blind, placebo-controlled trial from Egypt, a 3-day course of nitazoxanide was found to significantly reduce the duration of rotavirus disease in hospitalized pediatric patients.[84] Nitazoxanide is an anti-infective medication with broad activity against *Giardia, Cryptosporidium,* and *C difficile.* In vitro, the agent inhibits replication of various types of viruses, including rotavirus.[84] The findings of this small clinical trial deserve further study.

Antibiotics and Hemolytic Uremic Syndrome

In the United States and other higher-income countries, clinicians are advised not to give antibiotics empirically to children with bloody diarrhea because this therapy may increase the risk of hemolytic uremic syndrome (HUS) if the child is infected with *E coli* O157:H7 (also known as STEC O157). In a study by Wong and associates in Seattle, WA, antibiotic treatment of children with *E coli* O157:H7 infection increased their risk for HUS (relative risk, 17.3).[86] This study prompts the questions: Should a practitioner in a developing country have the same concern when evaluating a child with bloody diarrhea? Is there STEC O157 in developing countries? While the precise prevalence is not well known, data are available from some countries.

In Thailand, approximately 7% of food samples yielded STEC O157 but with no isolations from diarrheal specimens.[87] In 1992 in Swaziland in southern Africa, there was a large outbreak of bloody diarrhea by *E coli* O157:H7, which was associated with drought, carriage of the organism by cows, and heavy rains contaminating surface water.[88] In 1996, an outbreak of hemorrhagic colitis occurred in the Central African Republic. Initially it was suspected to be caused by viral hemorrhagic fever; however, an enterohemorrhagic strain of *E coli* (STEC) was implicated after further investigation.[89] The major contributing risk factor was the consumption of locallymade meat pies made with smoked zebu meat.

In spring 2011, an epidemic of STEC O104:H4 was observed throughout Europe. As of July 14, 2011, 3,867 cases of STEC were reported in the European Union, with Germany and France being the most affected countries. Several imported cases were reported in other non-European countries, including the United States. Hemolytic uremic syndrome, a complication of STEC, was observed in 762 cases. Forty-four infected persons have died of the infection and its complications. Asymptomatic infection appears to be the common event. Contaminated bean sprouts appear to be the source of the epidemic.[90]

Without proper microbiologic laboratory surveillance, clinicians may assume *Shigella* dysentery is the cause of bloody diarrhea and treat the child with an antimicrobial agent. Making the distinction from cholera is not difficult, as profuse watery diarrhea is characteristic of cholera, while bloody stools and severe abdominal pain are uncharacteristic. Empiric use of antibiotics without laboratory confirmation may lead to HUS if the patient is infected with STEC. Most US laboratories test for *E coli* O157:H7. Non-O157 STEC is being reported more often. Hemolytic uremic syndrome has also been associated with these strains.[91] Unfortunately, not all laboratories routinely test for these organisms. Hemolytic uremic syndrome is not only limited to STEC, as cases have been reported after infections by *S dysenteriae*.[92,93]

Zinc Supplementation

Increased stool zinc loss is frequently observed in patients with diarrhea. Studies link milder zinc deficiencies with childhood diarrhea. Patients receiving supplementation have improved outcomes in acute or chronic diarrhea. Zinc supplementation may even have a prophylactic effect. In randomized, controlled trials from Bangladesh, India, and Nepal, children with cholera or other causes of acute diarrhea who received zinc supplementation had significantly shorter durations of diarrhea and reduced stool output.[14,94]

In a review paper by Scrimgeour and Lukaski, the authors argue that in light of rising antimicrobial resistance around the world, along with a lack of effective antidiarrheal vaccines, the use of zinc supplementation could have a beneficial effect in diminishing morbidity associated with diarrheal disease.[12] The current USAID, UNICEF, and WHO recommendations for zinc supplementation are based on an analysis of available randomized, controlled trials.[62] Children with acute diarrhea should receive 20 mg per day of zinc for 10 to 14 days. Infants younger than 6 months should receive 10 mg per day.[12,62] There is evidence that zinc supplementation may prevent certain parasitic infections as well. In Sazawal and associates' trial in India, the clinical benefit of zinc supplementation was greater in children with stunted growth than in those with normal growth.[93] The use of zinc supplementation was found to be highly cost-effective. In contrast, the role of zinc supplementation in children with acute diarrhea in the developed world requires further study.[94]

Conflicting data have emerged in recent years. In a study from South Africa, the use of zinc alone or in combination with vitamin A or other micronutrients did not reduce diarrhea or morbidity related to respiratory infections.[95] Years earlier, a study from Tanzania demonstrated that vitamin A significantly reduces the risk of severe watery diarrhea but only among children with HIV-related wasting disease and malnourishment. An increased risk of diarrhea was observed in normally nourished children.[96]

Probiotics

Probiotics, such as human *Lactobacillus casei* strain GGand *Saccharomyces boulardii*, have demonstrable beneficial effects in treating rotavirus gastroenteritis.[94,97] Analysis of many randomized, placebo-controlled trials confirms that probiotics significantly reduce antibiotic-associated diarrhea and acute diarrhea caused by multiple organisms.[98] However, most of these studies were performed in higher-income countries. It is unclear how beneficial these supplements would be in malnourished children. More studies are needed before they can be recommended for use in children with diarrhea from lower-income countries.

Antidiarrheal Medications

Antidiarrheal agents such as kaolin-pectin and diphenoxylate-atropine (Lomotil) have been used in children with acute diarrhea. However, no beneficial therapeutic effect was observed in a placebo-controlled trial in Guatemala.[99] Similar results were noted in a study from Sweden.[100] Diphenoxylate-atropine use in young children has been associated with severe complications, such as paralytic ileus, vomiting, abdominal discomfort, and lethargy—its use in children should be avoided.[101–103]

Bismuth subsalicylate (BSS) has been shown to decrease the duration of diarrhea in children.[104,105] In a randomized, placebo-controlled study from Peru, infants with acute diarrhea who received BSS had significant reductions in total stool output, total intake of ORS, and hospitalization.[105] A similar study from Chile demonstrated identical findings.[104] In both studies, blood levels of bismuth and salicylates were measured and found to be below toxic levels. In patients with diarrheal infections caused by ETEC, BSS was found to be very effective in diminishing the duration of diarrhea and reducing symptoms such as nausea and abdominal pain.[104,105] In addition, BSS-treated individuals cleared ETEC from their intestinal tracts quicker than untreated persons.[106] Of interest, even BSS-treated university students with shigellosis did not experience a prolonged course of diarrhea.[107] Children with chronic diarrhea have also benefited from BSS.[108,109] This raises the question of why BSS is not used more often for treating diarrhea. The relationship between the use of salicylates (especially aspirin) and Reye syndrome dampened any desire for using this medication in children.

Adults frequently use loperamide for relief of diarrheal symptoms. It is generally well tolerated. In young children with acute diarrhea, especially those younger than 3 years, loperamide use has been associated with paralytic ileus, drowsiness and lethargy, and even death.[110,111] It appears that a malnourished, moderately to severely dehydrated, systemically ill child with or without bloody stools is at the highest risk for these adverse events. However, despite its known safety profile, some children have benefited from the medication.[112,113] However, at this time, risks outweigh potential benefits and its use is not recommended for young children.

■ PREVENTING GASTROINTESTINAL INFECTIONS

Rotavirus

While improvements in the quality of water, housing, and sanitary infrastructures and the use of antimicrobial therapy have reduced the frequency of GI disease caused by other enteric pathogens, the magnitude of rotavirus infection has remained unchallenged. However, in recent years, the introduction of live, attenuated rotavirus vaccines has resulted in a significant reduction in the number of cases of severe gastroenteritis in countries where the vaccine has been introduced. A decrease in infant deaths secondary to gastroenteritis has already been observed in some developing countries.

The first rotavirus vaccine (RotaShield) was licensed in the United States in 1998 but was withdrawn a year later because of concerns over increased risks of intussusception. Currently there are 2 vaccines available commercially in the United States and many other countries. A pentavalent vaccine (RV5), RotaTeq, and a monovalent vaccine (RV1), Rotarix, were found to be highly effective (98%–100%) in preventing severe gastroenteritis; both demonstrated reductions in diarrhea-related hospitalizations.[114,115] No increase in cases of intussusception was observed in these randomized, placebo-controlled studies.

In 2006, the WHO recommended use of the rotavirus vaccines in the United States and Europe. In the 2007–2008 season, despite there not being a full year of vaccination, reduction in diagnosed cases of rotavirus were greater than expected, indicating that any degree of vaccination may induce some herd immunity. Based on these findings, in 2009 the WHO extended its recommendations for rotavirus vaccine to be included in all national vaccination programs around the world. The WHO prioritized efforts in nations where diarrheal disease accounts for more than 10% of childhood mortality. Studies from Latin America and Africa have demonstrated significant reductions in hospitalizations, diarrhea-related health care visits, and in one study, diarrhea-related deaths.[116,117]

Rotavirus Vaccines and Adverse Events

Adverse events from vaccination are very few. The major concern—a possible increase in intussusceptions—has been the most discussed and studied. Recently, post-licensure surveillance from Brazil and Mexico demonstrated a slight increase in cases of intussusception in association with receipt of RV1.[116] The combined annual excess of 96 cases of intussusception in these countries (with 5 deaths of intussusception) needs to be put in perspective with the fact that the vaccine prevented approximately 80,000 hospitalizations and 1,300 death attributed to diarrhea each year.

Vaccination in immunocompromised hosts, especially those with severe combined immunodeficiency, has been shown to cause severe gastroenteritis with protracted viral shedding.[118] In the HIV-positive patients, no increase in adverse events was seen in comparison with the general population, and the maximum time of viral shedding post-vaccination was approximately 7 days, the same as in HIV-negative patients. There was no effect on the immunosuppressive effects of primary HIV disease.

Vaccine Use in Developing Countries

In resource-limited settings, there have been concerns that the vaccine may not be as immunogenic as in the developed world. This may be due in part to host and environmental factors, such as malnutrition with poor absorptive capacity, interference by breast milk antibodies, or concurrent enteric infections. However, studies in El Salvador have shown that one dose confers approximately 50% protection and would have its greatest effect in the 2- to 6-month age range when the risk of death is greatest. Overall vaccination programs there showed 40% to 50% reduction in admits for gastroenteritis from rotavirus in the 2008–2009 season and overall, approximately 76% protection.[119] Additional studies in India, which accounts for 23% of worldwide deaths due to rotavirus, have shown that 44,000 deaths, 293,000 admissions, and 328,000 outpatient visits are prevented by the national rotavirus immunization program, saving about US $20.6 million per year.[120] Additional studies have confirmed the benefits of vaccination.[121–123]

Reducing the need for hospitalization by half still has a significant effect on the disease and health care expenditures. It should be the priority of health care systems worldwide to develop vaccines that will prevent enteric infections. Vaccines against ETEC, *Shigella,* and *Campylobacter* and a more effective vaccine against typhoid fever and cholera would have significant effects on disease burden. These are high priorities within the WHO.[124]

Building well-maintained water treatment plants, installing sewage systems, and providing clean water will significantly reduce the number of diarrheal cases. Chlorine disinfection, solar disinfection, ceramic infiltration, and concrete biosand filters can help reduce the number of diarrheal cases in children.[125] It is estimated that 24% of the global burden of disease is attributable to environmental factors; 94% in the case of diarrheal disease. This is in contrast with respiratory infections and malaria, in which the percentages are 41% and 42%, respectively.[19]

Appropriate management of animal feces and agriculture practices would also have an effect. In preventing schistosomiasis, teaching people to minimize contact with freshwater by using rubber boots when working in irrigation canals would be beneficial. Proven strategies in reducing the incidence of diarrheal disease include provision of safe and clean water, availability of sewage systems, improvements in personal and food hygiene, and avoiding the use of human manure for fertilizing fields and crops.[126,127] Extending the duration of breastfeeding in young infants and controlling the fly population will also help reduce the frequency of diarrheal disease.

The migration of rural inhabitants to frequentlyovercrowded impoverished urban or suburban areas creates favorable conditions for the spread of parasites and other enteric pathogens. Strategies to periodically reduce parasitic burden through deworming, especially school-aged children, should be implemented.[128-131] In the urban slums of Lucknow, India, 17.5% of preschool children had intestinal parasites.[132] People also need to be taught good food safety and distribution measures. Food handlers at a municipal market had one or more parasitic infections.[133] Of greater concern, meat and vegetables sold at the market were frequently contaminated with parasites (more than 65% of samples).

Chronic or recurrent infections with EAEC, *Cryptosporidium,* and *Giardia* have a great effect over malnutrition, growth, and development. An increase in the quality and amounts of nutrients improves intestinal growth and barrier function of the GI tract, hence reducing the likelihood of future enteric infections. Supplements of glutamine, arginine, vitamin A, zinc, and other micronutrients enhance gastrointestinal tract health.

Early childhood diarrhea has greater disabling effects on children, leading to growth and fitness impairment, which leads to decreased work productivity later in life. Populations with moderate malnutrition, low weight for age, and diarrhea itself are associated with increased diarrhea risk. Studies from Egypt validated these findings.[134]

Once again the vicious circle of malnutrition and diarrhea becomes evident. Preventing diarrhea prevents malnutrition; preventing malnutrition prevents diarrhea. In most tropical lower-income nations, the peak of diarrheal disease is usually during the summer months, which is related to the warmest rainy seasons. Lower maternal education, use of untreated water sources, poor water storage practices, and underweight are key determinants for the risk of shigellosis. A reduction in diarrheal disease in the developing world could be achieved through the implementation of a community education program emphasizing the benefits of vaccination, providing information to parents and health care professionals on how to use ORS, and introducing a zinc supplementation program.

Various typhoid fever vaccines are commercially available around the world. An injectable formulation such as Vi capsular polysaccharide vaccine and an oral form of the live, attenuated vaccine (Ty21a) are available in the United States. Vaccine efficacy has been extremely variable, ranging from 19% to 96% with an average vaccination efficacy closer to 50%.[34] Many endemic countries have vaccination programs targeting typhoid fever. To maintain immunity, revaccination every 2 to 3 years limits their clinical utility in countries with limited resources. Many countries lack the necessary funds to maintain an active immunization program. However, if made available, effective vaccines against rotavirus, typhoid fever, ETEC, and *Shigella* would significantly affect the morbidity and mortality of young children around the world.[124]

Mass-scale campaigns focused on hygiene and preventive health could potentially help reduce parasitic infections. In developed nations, the routine treatment of immigrants from developing countries with albendazole would reduce DALYs and health costs and prevent hospitalizations and deaths.[135]

In contrast with higher-income countries, enteropathogens still pose a great challenge to health care professionals and promoters, governmental officials, and the population at large. Preventive measures do work. Building infrastructure and educating people on how to prevent disease is still the way to achieve success.

■ KEY POINTS

- Diarrhea and other gastrointestinal infections are a leading cause of morbidity and mortality among young children around the world.
- Poor sanitation, contaminated water sources, inadequate access to primary health care, lack of maternal education, and lack of breastfeeding are major risk factors for diarrheal disease.
- Oral rehydration solution and zinc supplements are major components for treating acute diarrhea in lower-income countries.
- Antimicrobial therapy is only useful in shigellosis, parasitic infections, cholera, and immunocompromised hosts.

■ REFERENCES

1. Murray CJL, Lopez AD. Mortality by cause for eight regions of the world: global burden disease study. *Lancet.* 1997;349:1269–1276
2. Elliott EJ. Acute gastroenteritis in children. *BMJ* 2007;334:35–40
3. DuPont HL. Diarrheal diseases in the developing world. *Infect Dis Clin North Am.* 1995;9:313–324
4. Boschi-Pinto C, Velebit L, Shibuya K. Estimating child mortality due to diarrhea in developing countries. *Bull World Health Organ.* 2008;86:710–717
5. Musher DM, Musher BL. Contagious acute gastrointestinal infections. *N Engl J Med.* 2004;351:2417–2427
6. Mathews MS, Pereira SM, Kirubakaran C, et al. Role of viruses in acute gastroenteritis in infants and young children at Vellore, South India. *J Trop Pediatr.* 1996;42:151–153
7. Mintz ED, Guerrant RL. A lion in our village-the unconscionable tragedy of cholera in Africa. *N Engl J Med.* 2009;360:1060–1063
8. Centers for Disease Control and Prevention. Update on cholera-Haiti, Dominican Republic, and Florida, 2010. *MMWR.* 2010;59:1637–1641
9. Gaffga NH, Tauxe RV, Mintz ED. Cholera: a new homeland in Africa? *Am J Trop Med Hyg.* 2007;77:705–713
10. Lucas MES, Deen JL, von Seidlein L, et al. Effectiveness of mass oral cholera vaccination in Beira, Mozambique. *N Engl J Med.* 2005;352:757–767
11. O'Ryan M, Prado V, Pickering LK. A millennium update on pediatric diarrheal illness in the developing world. *Semin Pediatr Infect Dis.* 2005;16:125–136
12. Scrimgeour AG, Lukaski HC. Zinc and diarrheal disease: current status and future perspectives. *Curr Opin Clin Nutr Metab Care.* 2008;11:711–717
13. Roy SK, Hossain MJ, Khatun W, et al. Zinc supplementation in children with cholera in Bangladesh: randomised controlled trial. *BMJ.* 2008;336:266–268
14. Victora CG. Diarrhea mortality: what can the world learn from Brazil? *J Pediatr (Rio J).* 2009;85:3–5
15. Victora CG, Smith PG, Vaughan JP, et al. Infant feeding and deaths due to diarrhea. A case-control study. *Am J Epidemiol.* 1989;129:1032–1041
16. Ram PK, Choi M, Blum LS, et al. Declines in case management of diarrhoea among children less than five years old. *Bull World Health Organ.* 2008;86:E–F
17. Guerrant RL, Oriá RB, Moore SR, et al. Malnutrition as an enteric infectious disease with long-term effects on child development. *Nutr Rev.* 2008;66:487–505
18. Guerrant RL, Oria R, Bushen OY et al. Global impact of diarrheal diseases that are sampled by travelers: the rest of the hippopotamus. *Clin Infect Dis.* 2005;41:S524–S530
19. Prüss-Üstün A, Corvalán C. How much disease burden can be prevented by environmental interventions? *Epidemiology.* 2007;18:167–178
20. Durley A, Shenoy A, Faruque ASG, et al. Impact of a standardized management protocol on mortality of children with diarrhoea: an update of risk factors for childhood death. *J Trop Pediatr.* 2004;50:271–275
21. Muhuri PK. Estimating seasonality effects on child mortality in Matlab, Bangladesh. *Demography.* 1996;33:98–100
22. Becker S, Weng S. Seasonal patterns of deaths in Matlab, Bangladesh. *Int J Epidemiol.* 1998;27:814–823
23. Paniagua GL, Monroy E, García-González O, et al. Two or more enteropathogens are associated with diarrhoea in Mexican children. *Ann Clin Microbiol Antimicrob.* 2007;6:17
24. Okeke IN, Ojo O, Lamikanra A, Kaper JB. Etiology of acute diarrhea in adults in southwestern Nigeria. *J Clin Microbiol.* 2003;41:4525–4530

25. World Health Organization. Persistent diarrhoea in children in developing countries: memorandum from a WHO meeting. *Bull WHO.* 1988;66:709–717

26. Fauveau V, Henry FJ, Briend A, et al. Persistent diarrhea as a cause of childhood mortality in rural Bangladesh. *Acta Paediatr Suppl.* 1992;381:12–14

27. Bhutta ZA. Persistent diarrhea in developing countries. *Ann Nestlé.* 2006;64:39–47

28. Crump JA, Mintz ED. Global trends in typhoid and paratyphoid fever. *Clin Infect Dis.* 2010;50:241–246

29. Huang DB, Mohanty A, DuPont HL, et al. A review of an emerging enteric pathogen: enteroaggregative *Escherichia coli. J Med Microbiol.* 2006;55:1303–1311

30. Villaseca JM, Hernández U, Sainz-Espuñes TR, et al. Enteroaggregative *Escherichia coli* an emergent pathogen with different virulence properties. *Rev Latinoam Microbiol.* 2005;47:140–159

31. Sang WK, Oundo JO, Mwituria JK, et al. Multidrug-resistant enteroaggregative *Escherichia coli* associated with persistent diarrhea in Kenyan children. *Emerg Infect Dis.* 1997;3:373–374

32. Bhuiyan TR, Qadri F, Saha A, Svennerholm AM. Infection by *Helicobacter pylori* in Bangladeshi children from birth to two years. Relation to blood group, nutritional status, and seasonality. *Pediatr Infect Dis J.* 2009;28:79–85

33. Whitaker JA, Franco-Paredes C, del Rio C, Edupuganti S. Rethinking typhoid fever vaccines: implications for travelers and people living in highly endemic areas. *J Travel Med.* 2009;16:46–52

34. Fagundes-Neto U, Viaro T, Wehba J, et al. Tropical enteropathy (Environmental enteropathy) in early childhood: a syndrome caused by contaminated environment. *J Trop Pediatr.* 1984;30:204–209

35. Walker-Smith JA. Paediatric problems in tropical gastroenterology. *Gut.* 1994;35:1687–1689

36. Haghighi P, Wolf PL. Tropical sprue and subclinical enteropathy: a vision for the nineties. *Crit Rev Clin Lab Sci.* 1997;34:313–341

37. Mathan VI. Tropical sprue. *Springer Semin Immunopathol.* 1990;12:231–237

38. Rhodes AR, Shea N, Lindenbaum J. Malabsorption in asymptomatic Liberian children. *Am J Clin Nutr.* 1971;24:574–577

39. Baker SJ. Subclinical intestinal malabsorption in developing countries. *Bull WHO.* 1976;54:485–494

40. Humphrey JH. Underweight malnutrition in infants in developing countries. An intractable problem. *Arch Pediatr Adolesc Med.* 2008;162:692–694

41. Pelletier DL, Frongillo EA Jr, Habicht J-P. Epidemiologic evidence for a potentiating effect of malnutrition on child mortality. *Am J Public Health.* 1993;83:1130–1133

42. Pelletier DL, Frongillo EA Jr, Schroeder DG, Habicht J-P. The effects of malnutrition on child mortality in developing countries. *Bull WHO.* 1995;73:443–448

43. Caulfield LE, de Onis M, Blössner M, Black RE. Undernutrition as an underlying cause of child deaths associated with diarrhea, pneumonia, malaria and measles. *Am J Clin Nutr.* 2004;80:193–198

44. Amuta EU, Olusi TA, Houmsou RS, et al. Relationship of intestinal parasitic infections and malnutrition among school children in Makurdi, Benue State-Nigeria. *Internet J Epidemiol.* 2009;7

45. Kaur R, Rawat D, Kakkar M, et al. Intestinal parasites in children with diarrhea in Delhi, India. *Southeast Asian J Trop Med Public Health.* 2002;33:725–729

46. Sayyari AA, Imanzadeh F, Bagheri Yazdi SA, et al. Prevalence of intestinal parasitic infections in the Islamic Republic of Iran. *East Med Health J.* 2005;11:377–383

47. Menezes AL, Lima VMP, Freitas MTS, et al. Prevalence of intestinal parasites in children from public daycare centers in the city of Belo Horizonte, Minas Gerais, Brazil. *Rev Inst Med Trop S Paulo.* 2008;50:57–59

48. Wongstitwilairoong B, Srijan A, Serichantalergs O, et al. Intestinal parasitic infections among pre-school children in Sangkhlaburi, Thailand. *Am J Trop Med Hyg.* 2007;76:345–350

49. Gbakima AA, Konteh R, Kallon M, et al. Intestinal protozoa and intestinal helminthic infections in displacement camps in Sierra Leone. *Afr J Med Med Sci.* 2007;36:1–9

50. Wadood A, Bari A, Rhman A, Qasim KF. Frequency of intestinal parasite infestation in children hospital Quetta. *Pakistan J Med Res.* 2005;44:87–88

51. Mosier DA, Oberst RD. Cryptosporidiosis. A global challenge. *Ann NY Acad Sci.* 2000;916:102–111

52. Savioli L, Smith H, Thompson A. *Giardia* and *Cryptosporidium* join the "neglected diseases initiative." *Trends Parasitol.* 2006;22:203–208

53. Temu MM, Kaatano GM, Miyaye ND, et al. Antimicrobial susceptibility of *Shigella flexneri* and *S. dysenteriae* isolated from stool specimens of patients with bloody diarrhoea in Mwanza, Tanzania. *Tanzan Health Res Bull.* 2007;9:186–189

54. Adelunle L. Intestinal parasites and nutritional status of Nigerian children. *Afr J Biomed Res.* 2002;5:115–119

55. Glickman LT, Camara AO, Glickman NW, McCabe GP. Nematode intestinal parasites of children in rural Guinea, Africa: prevalence and relationship to geophagia. *Int J Epidemiol.* 1999;28:169–174

56. Khurana S, Dubey ML, Malla N. Association of parasitic infections and cancers. *Indian J Med Microbiol.* 2005;23:74–79

57. Molina S, Vettorazzi C, Peerson JM, et al. Clinical trial of glucose-oral rehydration solution (ORS), rice dextrin-ORS, and rice fluor-ORS for the management of children with acute diarrhea and mild or moderate dehydration. *Pediatrics.* 1995;95:191–197

58. Alam NH, Yunus M, Faruque ASG, et al. Symptomatic hyponatremia during treatment of dehydrating diarrheal disease with reduced osmolarity oral rehydration solution. *JAMA.* 2006;296:567–573

59. CHOICE Study Group. Multicenter, randomized, double-blind clinical trial to evaluate the efficacy and safety of a reduced osmolarity oral rehydration salts solution in children with acute watery diarrhea. *Pediatrics.* 2001;107:613–618

60. Hahn S, Kim S, Garner P. Reduced osmolarity oral rehydration solution for treating dehydration caused by acute diarrhoea in children. *Cochrane Database Syst Rev.* 2002;1:CD002847

61. King CK, Glass R, Bresee JS, et al. Managing acute gastroenteritis among children: oral rehydration, maintenance, and nutritional therapy. *MMWR.* 2003;52(RR-16):1–16

62. US Agency for International Development, United Nations Children's Fund, World Health Organization. *Diarrhoea Treatment Guidelines Including New Recommendations for the Use of ORS and Zinc Supplementation for Clinic-Based Healthcare Workers.* Arlington, VA: US Agency for International Development, United Nations Children's Fund, World Health Organization; 2005. http://whqlibdoc.who.int/publications/2005/a85500.pdf. Accessed June 17, 2011

63. World Health Organization, United Nations Children's Fund. *Oral Rehydration Salts (ORS): A New Reduced Osmolarity Formulation.* Geneva, Switzerland: World Health Organization, United Nations Children's Fund; 2002. http://www.emro.who.int/CAH/pdf/ors_reduced_osmolarity.pdf. Accessed June 17, 2011

64. Cohen MB, Mezoff AG, Laney DW, et al. Use of a single solution for oral rehydration and maintenance therapy of infants with diarrhea and mild to moderate dehydration. *Pediatrics.* 1995;95:639–645

65. Jousilahti P, Madkour SM, Lambrechts T, Sherwin E. Diarrhoeal disease morbidity and home treatment practices in Egypt. *Public Health.* 1997;111:5–10

66. Hines J, Nachamkin I. Effective use of the clinical microbiology laboratory for diagnosing diarrheal diseases. *Clin Infect Dis.* 1996;23:1292–1301

67. Christenson JC, Korgenski EK. Laboratory diagnosis of infection due to bacteria, fungi, parasites, and rickettsia. In: Long SS, Prober CG, Pickering LK, eds. *Principles and Practice of Pediatric Infectious Diseases.* 3rd ed. Philadelphia, PA: Churchill Livingstone/Elsevier; 2008:1341–1352

68. Guerrant RL, Van Gilder T, Steiner TS, et al. Practice guidelines for the management of infectious diarrhea. *Clin Infect Dis.* 2001;32:331–350

69. Nguyen TV, Van PL, Huy CL, et al. Detection and characterization of diarrheagenic *Escherichia coli* from young children in Hanoi, Vietnam. *J Clin Microbiol.* 2005;43:755–760

70. Davidson G, Barnes G, Bass D, et al. Infectious diarrhea in children: Working Group Report of the First World Congress of Pediatric Gastroenterology, Hepatology, and Nutrition. *J Pediatr Gastroenterol Nutr.* 2002;35(suppl 2):S143–S150

71. Brooks JT, Ochieng JB, Kumar L, et al. Surveillance for bacterial diarrhea and antimicrobial resistance in rural Western Kenya, 1997–2003. *Clin Infect Dis.* 2006;43:393–401

72. Kosek M, Yori PP, Pan WK, et al. Epidemiology of highly endemic multiply antibiotic-resistant shigellosis in children in the Peruvian Amazon. *Pediatrics.* 2008;122:e541–e549

73. Abu Elamreen FH, Sharif FA, Deeb JE. Isolation and antibiotic susceptibility of *Salmonella* and *Shigella* strains isolated from children in Gaza, Palestine from 1999 to 2006. *J Gastroenterol Hepatol.* 2008;23:e330–e333

74. Kansakar P, Malla S, Ghmire GR. *Shigella* isolates of Nepal: changes in the incidence of *Shigella* subgroups and trends of antimicrobial susceptibility pattern. *Kathmandu Univ Med J.* 2007;5:32–37

75. Hoge CW, Gambel JM, Srijan A, et al. Trends in antibiotic resistance among diarrheal pathogens isolated in Thailand over 15 years. *Clin Infect Dis.* 1998;26:341–345

76. Avery ME, Snyder JD. Oral therapy for acute diarrhea: the underused simple solution. *N Engl J Med.* 1990;323:891–894

77. Chiu CH, Lin TY, Ou JT. A clinical trial comparing oral azithromycin, cefixime and no antibiotics in the treatment of acute uncomplicated *Salmonella* enteritis in children. *J Paediatr Chil Health.* 1999;35:372–374

78. Niyogi SK. Increasing antimicrobial resistance—an emerging problem in the treatment of shigellosis. *Clin Microbiol Infect.* 2007;13:1141–1143

79. Adachi JA, Ericsson CD, Jiang ZD, et al. Azithromycin found to be comparable to levofloxacin for the treatment of US travelers with acute diarrhea acquired in Mexico. *Clin Infect Dis.* 2003;37:1165–1171

80. Khan WA, Saha D, Rahman A, et al. Comparison of single-dose azithromycin and 12-dose, 3-day erythromycin for childhood cholera: a randomized, double-blind trial. *Lancet.* 2002;360;1722–1727

81. Saha D, Karim MM, Khan WA, et al. Single-dose azithromycin for the treatment of cholera in adults. *N Engl J Med.* 2006;354:2452–2462

82. Bhattacharya MK, Dutta D, Ramamurthy T, et al. Azithromycin in the treatment of cholera in children. *Acta Paediatr.* 2003;92:676–678

83. Leibovitz E, Janco J, Piglansky L, et al. Oral ciprofloxacin vs. intramuscular ceftriax-one as empiric treatment of acute invasive diarrhea in children. *Pediatr Infect Dis J.* 2000;19:1060–1067

84. Rossignol JF, Abu-Zekry M, Hussein A, et al. Effect of nitazoxanide for treatment of severe rotavirus diarrhoea: randomised double-blind placebo-controlled trial. *Lancet.* 2006;368:124–129

85. Wong CS, Jelacic S, Habeeb RL, et al. The risk of the hemolytic-uremic syndrome after antibiotic treatment of *Escherichia coli* O157:H7 infections. *N Engl J Med.* 2000;342:1930–1936

86. Voravuthikunchai SP, Keisaku O, Iida T, Honda T. Surveillance of enterohaemorrhagic *Escherichia coli* O157:H7 in Southern Thailand. *J Health Popul Nutr.* 2002;20:189–191

87. Effler P, Isaäcson M, Arntzen L, et al. Factors contributing to the emergence of *Escherichia coli* O157 in Africa. *Emerg Infect Dis.* 2001;7:812–819

88. Germani Y, Soro B, Vohito M, et al. Enterohaemorrhagic *Escherichia coli* in Central African Republic. *Lancet.* 1997;349:1670

89. Johnson KE, Thorpe CM, Sears CL. The emerging clinical importance of non-O157 Shiga toxin-producing *Escherichia coli*. *Clin Infect Dis.* 2006;43:1587–1595

90. International Society for Infectious Diseases. ProMED-mail. E Coli O104—European Union (33): Update, Asymptomatic Infection. Archive number 20110714-2132. Published July 14, 2011. http://promedmail.org

91. Bin Saeed AAA, El Bushra HE, Al-Hamdan NA. Does treatment of bloody diarrhea due to *Shigella dysenteriae* type 1 with ampicillin precipitate hemolytic uremic syndrome? *Emerg Infect Dis.* 1995;1:134–137

92. Bhimma R, Rollins NC, Coovadia HM, Adhikari M. Post-dysenteric hemolytic uremic syndrome in children during an epidemic of *Shigella* dysentery in Kwazulu/Natal. *Pediatr Nephrol.* 1997;11:560–564

93. Sazawal S, Black RE, Bhan MK, et al. Zinc supplementation in young children with acute diarrhea in India. *N Engl J Med.* 1995;333:839–844

94. Salvatore S, Hauser B, Devreker T, et al. Probiotics and zinc in acute infectious gastro-enteritis in children: are they effective? *Nutrition.* 2007;23:498–506

95. Luabeya KK, Mpontshane N, Mackay M, et al. Zinc or multiple micronutrient supple-mentation to reduce diarrhea and respiratory disease in South African children: a randomized controlled trial. *PLos ONE.* 2007;2:e541

96. Fawzi WW, Mbise R, Spiegelman D, et al. Vitamin A supplements and diarrheal and respiratory tract infections among children in Dar es Salaam, Tanzania. *J Pediatr.* 2000;137:660–667

97. Isolauri E, Juntunen M, Rautanen T, et al. A human *Lactobacillus* strain (*Lactobacillus casei* sp strain *GG*) promotes recovery from acute diarrhea in children. *Pediatrics.* 1991;88:90–97

98. Santosham M, Keenan EM, Tulloch J, et al. Oral rehydration therapy for diarrhea: an example of reverse transfer of technology. *Pediatrics.* 1997;100:e10

99. Portnoy BL, DuPont HL, Pruitt D, et al. Antidiarrheal agents in the treatment of acute diarrhea in children. *JAMA.* 1976;236:844–846

100. Alestig K, Trollfors B, Stenqvist K. Acute non-specific diarrhoea: studies on the use of charcoal, kaolin-pectin and diphenoxylate. *Practitioner.* 1979;222:859–862

101. Bargman GJ, Gardner LI. Near fatality in an infant following "Lomotil" poisoning. *Pediatrics.* 1969;44:770–771

102. Harries JT, Rossiter M. Fatal "Lomotil" poisoning. *Lancet.* 1969;1(7586):150

103. Rosenstein G, Freeman M, Standard AL, Weston N. Warning: the use Lomotil in children. *Pediatrics*. 1973;51:132–134

104. Soriano-Brücher H, Avendano P, O'Ryan M, et al. Bismuth subsalicylate in the treatment of acute diarrhea in children: a clinical study. *Pediatrics*. 1991;87:18–27

105. Figueroa-Quintanilla D, Salazar-Lindo E, Sack RB, et al. A controlled trial of bismuth subsalicylate in infants with acute watery diarrheal disease. *N Engl J Med*. 1993;328:1653–1658

106. Graham DY, Estes MK, Gentry LO. Double-blind comparison of bismuth subsalicylate and placebo in the prevention and treatment of enterotoxigenic *Escherichia coli*-induced diarrhea in volunteers. *Gastroenterology*. 1983;85:1017–1022

107. DuPont HL, Sullivan P, Pickering LK, et al. Symptomatic treatment of diarrhea with bismuth subsalicylate among students attending a Mexican university. *Gastroenterology*. 1977;73:715–718

108. Gryboski JD, Hillemeier AC, Grill B, Kocoshis S. Bismuth subsalicylate in the treatment of chronic diarrhea of childhood. *Am J Gastroenterol*. 1985;80:871–876

109. Gryboski JD, Kocoshis S. Effect of bismuth subsalicylate on chronic diarrhea in childhood: a preliminary report. *Rev Infect Dis*. 1990;12:S36–S40

110. Motala C, Hill ID, Mann MD, Bowie MD. Effect of loperamide on stool output and duration of acute infectious diarrhea in infants. *J Pediatr*. 1990;117:467–471

111. Li ST, Grossman DC, Cummings P. Loperamide therapy for acute diarrhea in children: systematic review and meta-analysis. *PLoS Med*. 2007;4:e98

112. Sandhu BK, Tripp JH, Milla PJ, Harries JT. Loperamide in severe protracted diarrhoea. *Arch Dis Child*. 1983;58:39–43

113. Diarrhoeal Diseases Study Group. Loperamide in acute diarrhoea in childhood: results of a double blind, placebo controlled multicentre clinical trial. *BMJ*. 1984;289:1263–1267

114. Ruiz-Palacios GM, Pérez-Schael I, Velázquez FR, et al. Safety and efficacy of an attenuated vaccine against severe rotavirus gastroenteritis. *N Engl J Med*. 2006;354:11–22

115. Vesikari T, Matson DO, Dennehy P, et al. Safety and efficacy of a pentavalent human-bovine (WC3) reassortant rotavirus vaccine. *N Engl J Med*. 2006;354:23–33

116. Patel MM, Lopez-Collada VR, Bulhoes MM, et al. Intussusception risk and health benefits of rotavirus vaccination in Mexico and Brazil. *N Engl J Med*. 2011;364(24):2283–2292

117. Madhi SA, Cunliffe NA, Steele D, et al. Effect of human rotavirus vaccine on severe diarrhea in African infants. *N Engl J Med*. 2010;362(4):289–298

118. Bakare N, Menschik D, Tiernan R, et al. Severe combined immunodeficiency (SCID) and rotavirus vaccination: reports to the Vaccine Adverse Events Reporting System (VAERS). *Vaccine*. 2010;28:6609–6612

119. De Palma O, Cruz L, Ramos H et al. Effectiveness of rotavirus vaccination against childhood diarrhoea in El Salvador: case-control study. *BMJ*. 2010;341:c2825

120. Esposito DH, Tate JE, Kang G, et al. Projected impact and cost-effectiveness of a rotavirus vaccination program in India, 2008. *Clin Infect Dis*. 2011;52:171–177

121. Patel M, Pedreira C, De Oliveira LH, et al. Association between pentavalent rotavirus vaccine and severe rotavirus diarrhea among children in Nicaragua. *JAMA*. 2009;301:2243–2251

122. Yen C, Armero Guardado JA, Alberto P, et al. Decline in rotavirus hospitalizations and health care visits for childhood diarrhea following rotavirus vaccination in El Salvador. *Pediatr Infect Dis J*. 2011;30(1 Suppl):S6–S10

123. Becker-Dreps S, Paniagua M, Dominik R, et al. Changes in childhood diarrhea incidence in Nicaragua following 3 years of universal infant rotavirus immunization. *Pediatr Infect Dis J*. 2011;30(3):243-247

124. Levine MM. Enteric infections and the vaccines to counter them: future directions. *Vaccine*. 2006;24:3865–3873

125. Stauber CE, Ortiz GM, Loomis DP, Sobsey MD. A randomized controlled trial of the concrete biosand filter and its impact on diarrheal disease in Bonao, Dominican Republic. *Am J Trop Med Hyg*. 2009;80:286–29

126. World Health Organization. Food and Nutrition Programme. Food Safety Unit. Contaminated food: a major cause of diarrhoea and associated malnutrition among infants and young children. *Facts Infant Feed*. 1993;3:1–4

127. Shah SM, Yousafzai M, Lakhani NB, et al. Prevalence and correlates of diarrhea. *Indian J Pediatr*. 2003;70:207–211

128. Crompton DWT, Savioli L. Intestinal parasitic infections and urbanization. *Bull WHO*. 1993;71:1–7

129. Mehraj V, Hatcher J, Akhtar S, et al. Prevalence and factors associated with intestinal parasitic infection among children in an urban slum of Karachi. *PLos ONE*. 2008;3:e3680

130. Chandrashekhar H. Food- and water-borne parasites. *Proc ASEAN Congr Trop Med Parasitol*. 2008;3:43–46

131. Stephenson LS. Helminth parasites, a major factor in malnutrition. *World Health Forum*. 1994;15(2):169–172

132. Awasthi S, Pande VK. Prevalence of malnutrition and intestinal parasites in preschool slum children in Lucknow. *Indian Pediatr*. 1997;34(7):599–605

133. Nyarango RM, Aloo PA, Kabiru EW, et al. The risk of pathogenic intestinal parasite infections in Kisii Municipality, Kenya. *BMC Public Health*. 2008;8:237.

134. Wierzba TF, El-Yazeed RA, Savarino SJ, et al. The interrelationship of malnutrition and diarrhea in a periurban area outside Alexandria, Egypt. *J Pediatr Gastroenterol Nutr*. 2001;32(2):189–196

135. Muennig P, Pallin D, Sell RL, et al. The cost effectiveness of strategies for the treatment of intestinal parasites in immigrants. *N Engl J Med*. 1999;340(10):773–779

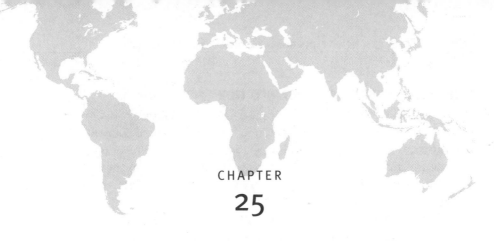

CHAPTER

25

Respiratory Conditions

James T. McElligott, MD, MSCR
Andrea P. Summer, MD, MSCR, FAAP

■ INTRODUCTION

Respiratory disease is a major cause of morbidity and mortality for all children but disproportionately burdening those in the developing world. As many as 95% of all clinical pneumonias may occur in developing countries.[1] In 2004 the World Health Organization (WHO) reported that nearly one fifth of all deaths in children younger than 5 years are attributable to pneumonia, making pneumonia the single leading cause of death. Many experts believe that gains can be made toward reducing the burden of respiratory disease through improving the provision and distribution of existing prevention and treatment techniques that are validated and proven effective. However, many challenges hinder receipt of these interventions at the local level in much of the developing world.

Major population-specific barriers include recognition of the severity of disease, timely access to care, and availability of preventive measures, which include addressing vaccination use, malnutrition and micronutrient deficiencies, the effect of air pollution, and the burden of coinfection. Barriers specific to the delivery of health care include the assessment of disease severity, appropriate provision of effective antibiotics, and when possible, provision of supportive care for dehydration, malnutrition, and hypoxemia. Addressing these barriers in a resource-poor setting is a daunting task. Fortunately, the international research community provided guidelines for care that, when tailored to the local situation, have the potential to save millions of lives.

■ UPPER RESPIRATORY TRACT INFECTION

Children presenting with new-onset cough or increased work of breathing present a treatment dilemma in many lower-income countries. Delay in appropriate treatment for children who may have a lower respiratory tract infection can lead to a life-threatening situation. On the other hand, many children with respiratory symptoms are uninfected or will have a self-limited course.

As in higher-income countries, most viral upper respiratory infections are likely to be self-limited, although malnutrition and concurrent infections (eg, diarrhea, malaria) can weaken a child's immune system and predispose him to more significant diseases. Viruses, such as respiratory syncytial virus (RSV) and parainfluenza viruses, typically begin as an upper respiratory process but can quickly progress to involve the lower respiratory tract, resulting in significant signs and symptoms of distress (eg, wheezing, stridor, retractions), even in otherwise healthy children.

Because there is minimal research on respiratory infections that are managed in the outpatient setting in the developing world, health care professionals must rely on a careful clinical assessment combined with a standardized management approach to maximize identification and timely treatment of the child who will progress to severe disease. The WHO published guidelines for first-level health practitioners that rely on observers' ability to measure respiratory rate and the presence of lower chest wall in-drawing (retractions specific to the lower chest).

When tachypnea is absent, the WHO recommends symptomatic care only with instructions for the caregiver to watch for danger signs. The presence of tachypnea (respiratory rate greater than 50 for infants 2 to 12 months of age, greater than 40 for children 1 to 5 years of age) defines pneumonia, while the addition of lower chest in-drawing or stridor in a calm child represents severe pneumonia. The Integrated Management of Childhood Illness (IMCI) danger signs (ie, unable to drink or breastfeed, vomits everything, convulses, lethargic or unconscious) should also prompt referral (WHO).[2]

These signs have been shown to have good sensitivity as well as reduce mortality in resource-poor settings by prompting early initiation of antibiotics and referral.[3-6] However, there is concern that the guidelines are likely to lead to overuse of antibiotics and undertreatment of reactive airways disease.[7,8] Other factors to consider when basing management decisions on respiratory rate are fever and high altitude, which may elevate the rate, and poor nutritional status, which may depress the rate.[9]

■ LOWER RESPIRATORY TRACT INFECTION

Bacterial pneumonia leads to significant morbidity and mortality in children, particularly for those younger than 5 years. *Streptococcus pneumoniae, Haemophilus influenzae* type b, and *Staphylococcus aureus* are the 3 most important pathogens leading to hospitalization and death for children with pneumonia.[10]

Vaccination against *S pneumoniae* and *H influenzae* type b has led to a substantial reduction in invasive disease with these pathogens in developed countries and has also shown promise in reducing infections in resource-poor settings where the distribution of these immunizations is still limited primarily due to vaccine costs.[11] In high endemic areas, tuberculosis is a significant contributor to childhood pneumonia, comprising approximately 8% of cases and a higher proportion that lead to death.[12–14]

Among hospitalized children, studies have shown evidence of a viral etiology in about two thirds of illnesses that WHO criteria classify as pneumonias.[15,16] Of these, RSV, influenza, and rhinovirus are the most common. Less is known about viral infections that do not lead to hospitalization. Other viruses commonly implicated for lower respiratory tract infections are metapneumovirus (now suspected to be a frequent cause of childhood lower respiratory infection after RSV), adenovirus, and parainfluenza.[13,17] Seasonal and pandemic influenza are major health threats throughout the world. Vaccination coverage is variable throughout the developing world and it is likely that despite strong recommendations, coverage will remain inadequate without major funded initiatives.[18]

In lower-income countries, a significant proportion of viral pneumonia is complicated by concurrent bacterial infection, as a viral infection itself predisposes an individual to bacterial pneumonia.[19] Influenza infection is also shown to interact with *S pneumoniae* and exacerbate severe pneumonia.[20] Studies in developing countries report variable rates of mixed bacterial and viral pathogens of 8% to 40%. Prolonged or more severe symptoms warrant consideration of a mixed infection.

Bronchiolitis, most often from RSV, can be difficult to manage in a resource-poor setting and continues to contribute to childhood death from respiratory causes.[21] Even though much research focuses on bronchiolitis in higher-income countries, adequate research on its effect in the developing world is lacking.[21] The presence of viral symptoms and wheezing on auscultation can help differentiate viral bronchiolitis from pneumonia and potentially avoid overuse of antibiotics.[19] However, health care practitioners must be aware of the major complications of dehydration, hypoxemia, and superimposed bacterial infection, with predisposition to reactive airways disease and recurrent infections as delayed consequences.[22]

Laboratory evaluation (eg, complete blood cell counts, erythrocyte sedimentation rate, C-reactive protein) and chest radiography are useful when available for improving diagnostic accuracy, although their ability to improve sensitivity and specificity of a pneumonia diagnosis may not be large enough to warrant the excess cost.[23] Their value is increased for cases in which important management decisions must be made, such as when anemia or tuberculosis is suspected.

Management

Non-severe Pneumonia

Given the significant morbidity and mortality attributed to pneumonia, the efforts of the last 2 decades largely focused on the identification and management of severe pneumonia. Recently there has been a helpful focus on managing non-severe pneumonia for first-level providers. The most recent recommendations take into account the need for improved diagnostic accuracy, an increased knowledge of antibiotic effectiveness, and the influence of HIV, tuberculosis, and malaria on outcomes.

The WHO recommendation for first-line therapy for non-severe pneumonia is amoxicillin at 50 mg/kg per day in 2 divided doses for 3 days. This recommendation is based on strong evidence that considers cost and effectiveness. The authors of the WHO panel suggest a 5-day course in areas with high HIV prevalence. An alternative first-line treatment is co-trimoxazole (8 mg/kg of trimethoprim in 2 divided doses), although resistance is an emerging concern with this agent.[24] Treatment failure is defined as "lower chest-wall in-drawing, central cyanosis, stridor while calm, or IMCI-defined danger signs (the child being unable to drink or breastfeed, vomits everything, has convulsions, is lethargic or unconscious) at any time during a child's illness or a persistently raised respiratory rate at 72 hours (48 hours in an area of high HIV prevalence)."[24] This recommendation provides a more objective means of defining failure that has some validation; however, more research is needed.[24,25]

In the event of treatment failure, the health care practitioner should first determine if referral for more intensive care is necessary. Children with a persistently elevated respiratory rate but who do not need immediate referral should be assessed for the cause of treatment failure. A systematic approach using a defined algorithm has proven benefit, although there is currently not a validated algorithm to address treatment failure. The authors of the WHO recommendations suggest an algorithm that includes assessing delivery barriers of the medication, the need for bronchodilators, and the presence of tuberculosis, HIV, and malnutrition. Other factors should also be considered, such as anemia, reactive airway disease, cardiac conditions, foreign bodies, nonsusceptible pathogens, and complications of pneumonia, such as empyema.[7,24]

The recommendations for second-line antibiotic treatment for those children who do not require a referral are directed toward broadening coverage and addressing common resistance mechanisms. Changing therapy to amoxicillin-clavulanic acid at 80 to 90 mg/kg of amoxicillin in 2 divided doses for 5 days is recommended with suspected antibiotic failure. Alternatively, erythromycin may be added for children older than 3 years at 50 mg/kg in 4 divided doses for 5 to 7 days. Children who received co-trimoxazole as a first-line treatment should be switched to amoxicillin for a 5-day course. While these recommendations are logical, they are not validated.[24]

Severe Lower Respiratory Tract Infections

When possible, timely referral for more intensive treatment has the potential to save many lives.[5] Clinicians should be aware that tachypnea is the most sensitive means of diagnosing severe pneumonia in developing countries, with additional signs of chest in-drawing and auscultory findings enhancing specificity.[26] The clinician caring for children who have not responded to initial therapy must keep in mind a broader differential diagnosis, reasons for antibiotic failure, and special considerations for children with HIV and other coinfections.[24]

Timely referral of children with severe lower respiratory tract infection to a clinical location that can provide supportive care is of primary importance. These children often have expanded needs for hydration, nutritional support, and supplemental oxygen. Failure of first-line therapy warrants re-evaluating the child's condition and considering a change in therapy. A Cochrane review found that antibiotic treatment with a combination of penicillin and gentamicin intravenously was more efficacious for severe illness than chloramphenicol alone. The review also demonstrated evidence that high-dose (80 to 90 mg/kg/d) oral amoxicillin is as effective as injectable penicillin for those who can tolerate the oral route.[27]

For pneumonia, hypoxemia is known to be a predictor of severe disease and a risk factor for death. Supplemental oxygen has been shown to save lives but unfortunately is not routinely available to many children admitted to hospitals with severe respiratory illness.[28-30] Providing supplemental oxygen is a difficult task in many parts of the world, but the increased attention on reducing mortality related to respiratory illness could potentially improve its availability. In a systematic review by Subhi and colleagues, the median prevalence of hypoxemia among hospitalized children with acute lower respiratory tract infection was 13%; however, there was wide variation among the studies, with more severe disease consistently correlated to hypoxemia.[30] The best clinical predictor of hypoxemia is the presence of lower chest in-drawing,[31] supporting the use of WHO classification of severity.

Monitoring pulse oximetry has been shown to improve mortality compared with clinical signs alone,[32] but availability limits its use. The use of nasal prongs is the preferred oxygen delivery method for children when considering effectiveness, safety, cost, and availability; however, nasopharyngeal catheters are acceptable with adequate nursing supervision.[33] Oxygen concentrators play an increasingly important role in areas where oxygen cost and availability are concerns; however, their use is limited because they require electrical power. Appropriate and timely referral to centers that have the ability to provide oxygen may be the only option for many health care practitioners.

Pleural effusions are a relatively common complication of severe pneumonia and are associated with poor social conditions.[34] A Brazilian study found radiologically determined pleural involvement in 25% of children younger than 5 years who were hospitalized with severe pneumonia.[35] There is controversy, even in higher-income countries, over the management of significant intrathoracic complications of infections, such as empyema, although a procedural approach (ie, chest tube placement or operative management) is preferred when possible.[36]

Differential Diagnosis

While bacterial and viral pathogens are the most common cause of respiratory symptoms in children, other, more unusual pathogens, as well as noninfectious etiologies, must also be considered.

Parasitic Infections

Parasitic infections may manifest with respiratory symptoms by direct pulmonary involvement with the organism (eg, *Echinococcus,* amebiasis), by inducing an inflammatory response during the migratory phase through the lungs (eg, ascariasis, hookworms), or with a hypersensitivity syndrome, such as tropical pulmonary eosinophilia (eg, *Wuchereria bancrofti, Brugia malayi*). The potential organisms vary by geographic region. Treatment may be possible with appropriate antimicrobials, although surgical cyst resection is often necessary for a cure with certain pathogens.[37]

Pertussis

The typical persistent cough is a common presentation of *Bordetella pertussis* infection in older children. While whooping cough is often self-limited and preventable by vaccination, it does lead to 300,000 deaths per year. Many older children and adults carry the infection symptomatically or asymptomatically. Younger children are at higher risk of complications from the disease, such as post-tussive vomiting, seizures, encephalopathy, brain damage, conjunctival hemorrhage, and rectal prolapse. Young infants sometimes present only with apnea or sudden death and are at particular risk for pulmonary hypertension.

Prevention has been successful with vaccination; however, infections persist even in communities with high vaccination rates. Waning post-vaccination immunity is felt to be the reason for continued transmission despite good vaccine coverage in young children. As a result, many countries instituted a booster dose in adolescence to improve control.

Antibiotic treatment for active infection is helpful if provided in the first week after onset of illness. Macrolides (eg, azithromycin, erythromycin) are the antibiotics of choice; trimethoprim-sulfamethoxazole is an alternative agent. Prophylaxis with a macrolide antibiotic is warranted for vulnerable individuals, such as young infants and pregnant women, provided the antibiotic course is initiated within 3 weeks of exposure to the index case.[38]

Atypical Bacterial Infections

Atypical bacterial organisms such as *Mycoplasma pneumoniae, Moraxella catarrhalis,* and *Klebsiella pneumoniae* are each believed to account for less than 10% of pneumonias; however, this speculation is based on limited research in resource-poor settings.[24] These organisms should generally be considered when first-line therapy fails, assuming adequate adherence to the regimen.

Asthma

The prevalence of asthma varies widely throughout the world.[39] With the exception of Latin America, higher-income countries have higher asthma rates than lower-income countries, which has been attributed to the effects of an overly clean environment (hygiene hypothesis). However, there is evidence that the prevalence of asthma is increasing worldwide.[7] The prevalence of reactive airway disease in Latin America nears that of higher-income countries and appears to be a different epidemic with non-atopic phenotypes predominating, which may be a result of previous viral or parasitic infections.[40]

A history of previous respiratory disease and audible wheeze should prompt consideration of a bronchodilator trial, particularly in the absence of fever.[7] A child who responds to bronchodilator treatment is likely to benefit from treatment of the reactive component and avoidance of inciting exposures. Excess antibiotics may be avoided, although the possibility of superimposed infection should be considered with persistent symptoms.

Stridor

A child presenting with respiratory distress and extrathoracic noisy breathing that worsens on inspiration (ie, stridor) suggests an upper airway obstruction. Viral-induced croup is the most common cause in children between the ages of 3 months and 3 years, affecting 3% of children a year.[41] Treatments with proven benefit for viral croup include dexamethasone 0.6 mg/kg intramuscularly or orally and nebulized epinephrine. Humidified air is also commonly used, but no benefits were shown in studies within emergency departments, which suggests that severe illness may not respond.[42]

The introduction of the *H influenzae* type b vaccine markedly reduced the incidence of epiglottitis. It remains a concern in under-vaccinated areas and can be life threatening. Epiglottitis classically presents with severe stridor in an ill-appearing child. The airway may be significantly compromised and instrumentation of the oropharynx should be avoided. When possible, sedation and intubation is the recommended course of management of severe epiglottitis.[43] Bacterial tracheitis is also a serious respiratory infection that can become severe enough to require lifesaving airway management. From a study in Taiwan, the most common presenting symptoms were cough, fever, dyspnea, and hoarseness. The most common etiologies were alpha-hemolytic strep, *Pseudomonas*, and *S aureus*. One fifth of the children required intubation.[44]

Stridor in young children, especially infants, may indicate an anatomical or neuromuscular predisposition to respiratory compromise. In resource-poor settings, this evaluation may rely on clinical suspicion, although examination for dysmorphisms, abnormal airway anatomy, neuromuscular tone, and assessment of development are helpful. Finally, clinical suspicion for a foreign body as a cause of stridor or respiratory distress is important to avoid delays in diagnosis and management. A chest radiograph, including inspiratory and expiratory films, should be obtained to look for air trapping. Lateral films are an alternative option for young infants suspected of having a foreign body and may demonstrate air trapping in the dependent lung (ie, the side with the foreign body will not deflate when placed in the dependent position).

Non-respiratory Etiologies

Cardiac Disease

Heart disease is often difficult to manage in lower-income countries and may go undetected until a child presents with respiratory symptoms. In higher-income countries, rheumatic heart disease remains a major threat to children and young adults, comprising up to 60% of cardiac disease for these age groups. Good progress has been made in reducing mortality in a few locations (eg, Cuba, Egypt, Martinique, Guadalupe) that instituted prevention programs. However, significant mortality, morbidity, and economic burden are persistent worldwide. Congenital heart disease and sequelae from other infectious diseases, such as myocarditis, pericarditis, and those related to Kawasaki disease, may also lead to pulmonary manifestations.[45]

Other

Ingestions (eg, aspirin, hydrocarbons), pneumothoraces, and metabolic or endocrine causes (eg, acidosis, fever) should remain on the clinician's differential to avoid misdiagnosis and delay in management.

Risk Factors for Increased Morbidity and Mortality

Malnutrition

Malnourished children are at higher risk of death from lower respiratory tract infections. A weakened immune system and respiratory drive contribute to this higher mortality. Children with malnutrition are also more likely to have gram-negative bacteria or tuberculosis as the causative agents.[46] As such, it is prudent to refer malnourished children to a hospital for parenteral antibiotics and the consideration of tuberculosis infection.[47]

Young Infants

In addition to vulnerabilities associated with age, a broader range of bacterial pathogens are implicated in lower respiratory tract infections in infants younger than 3 months. Antibiotic coverage for gram-positive (S aureus, S pneumoniae, S pyogenes, group B streptococcus) and gram-negative (E coli, Salmonella, H influenzae, Klebsiella) organisms is indicated. The combination of ampicillin and gentamicin provides adequate coverage in most cases. A concern with this regimen is poor efficacy against S aureus, and an anti-staphylococcal antibiotic should be added to the treatment regimen in the event of treatment failure after 48 hours.[47]

HIV

The presence of coinfection with HIV may predispose children to more severe disease and infection with atypical organisms. The HIV epidemic greatly increased the burden of respiratory disease, particularly in sub-Saharan Africa.[10] The pneumonia mortality rate for children with HIV is 3 to 6 times greater than in children who are uninfected.[34] These children have a higher percentage of bacterial pneumonia and are more likely to be infected with atypical organisms such as *Pneumocystis jiroveci* and gram-negative organisms, although the most common bacterial etiology remains *S pneumoniae*.[14] In addition, those with HIV are also more likely to have severe disease from viral infections.[13] Therefore, children with HIV must be given special consideration for broader antimicrobial coverage and more aggressive supportive care when initial treatment fails.[47] Co-trimoxazole prophylaxis is recommended for children with HIV and children born to HIV-infected mothers.[48]

Malaria

A fever often warrants treatment for malaria in endemic areas. The presenting symptoms of malaria may also include cough and increased work of breathing, making a single diagnosis difficult. Research in regions with a high rate of malaria indicates that ill children with this presentation may often have both infections, suggesting that treatment for both conditions is a reasonable consideration.[48,49]

Measles

Pneumonia is a well-known and severe complication of measles. A Cochrane review indicates that antibiotic treatment can decrease the incidence of pneumonia; however, guidelines for the type of antibiotic or duration of treatment cannot be derived from this review.[50] Vitamin A supplementation has also shown to improve outcomes for children infected with measles and the complication of pneumonia.[51] Therefore, it is prudent to treat children infected with measles with antibiotics and vitamin A supplementation.

Chronic Cough

The WHO defines *chronic cough* as a cough that is present for 2 to 3 weeks.[52] Common causes of chronic cough in higher-income countries, such as rhinosinus disease (postnasal drip), asthma, and gastroesophageal reflux, are also likely to be common in lower-income countries. These conditions may be elucidated with a thorough history; however, the differential can be quite broad when diagnostic capabilities are limited. Toddlers and older children with a persistent cough warrant consideration for infectious causes such as rhinosinus disease (viral and bacterial), pneumonia, and B pertussis infection.

Tuberculosis should always be considered in endemic areas, as it is associated with high morbidity and mortality. Children comprise one fifth to a quarter of tuberculosis cases in resource-poor countries, which results in significant morbidity and mortality because of the increased propensity for disseminated disease in children younger than 5 years. Diagnosing tuberculosis in children is problematic because they are more likely to present with an extrapulmonary manifestation and are rarely sputum positive. Gastric aspirates, chest radiographs, and a placed purified protein derivative are helpful when results are positive, although false negatives are common. The combination of infection with HIV and tuberculosis has led to a synergistic increase in mortality. It is prudent to maintain a high level of suspicion in tuberculosis-endemic areas.[53]

Geographic-specific fungal and parasitic organisms should be considered as causative agents. As discussed, asthma, allergic rhinitis, irritants (eg, passive smoke, indoor use of fossil fuels), chemical aspiration, foreign bodies, and heart disease may present with a prolonged cough. Patients refractory to treatment also warrant consideration for systemic disease, such as immunodeficiency, cystic fibrosis, and sickle cell.

The young infant with a persistent cough may have infectious causes with greater morbidity and mortality in this age group. Viral disease may be more severe (eg, RSV, metapnuemovirus) and lead to prolonged symptoms. B pertussis infection may present with severe coughing spells and their associated complications, although infants 3 months and younger sometimes present with only apnea or sudden death. The severity of this infection in infants underlines the importance of immunization for all who are in contact with them. The newborn with persistent symptoms should also be considered for anatomic abnormalities such as vascular anomalies, laryngeal cleft, and pulmonary malformations. Gastroesophageal reflux is a common etiology of chronic cough for infants but usually a diagnosis of exclusion.

Prevention

As is true in much of the practice of medicine, adequate preventive methods exist that could greatly reduce the burden of respiratory disease in the world if adequately used. Preventive education efforts on awareness of the presence and severity of disease, vaccination, attention to nutrition, micronutrient supplementation, and prevention of HIV transmission all have the potential to reduce mortality related to respiratory disease.

Seeking Care Early

Delay in seeking care occurs for multiple reasons, including geography, cost, cultural beliefs, and awareness. A joint statement by the United Nations Children's Fund and the WHO reports evidence that a large percentage of ill children present late for care or not at all throughout the world.[54,55] Early intervention with case management by community health workers shows impressive reductions in childhood mortality.[5,54] To be successful, local health workers should be able to recognize and treat uncomplicated pneumonia and know when to refer for higher care.

Education efforts were also extended to the family level with a focus on cough and fast or difficult breathing. Caregivers often have diverse interpretations of signs of respiratory distress in various cultural settings. Education efforts for these caregivers show good short-term retention, particularly if local terminology is used. There are multiple reports on the success of interventions to improve the management of pneumonia based on the education of primary caregivers. The use of respiratory timers is helpful in these efforts.[48,54]

Vaccinations

Highly effective vaccines exist for many infectious etiologies that lead to the high death toll related to pneumonia. Knowledge of local population immunization coverage is essential for a clinician to provide adequate care. Vaccinations for diphtheria, pertussis, and tetanus; measles; *H influenzae* type b; and pneumococcal conjugate vaccines all greatly reduce the effect of childhood pneumonia.[56,57]

Coverage is variable throughout the world, particularly for the newer *H influenzae* type b and pneumococcal conjugate vaccines.[58] As discussed, pneumonia is the most common cause of death in children with measles.[48] Reducing measles with vaccination will also reduce mortality from pneumonia, yet population vaccination rates required to prevent this highly infectious organism have been difficult to obtain despite a long-standing effective vaccine.

Nutrition

As noted previously, nutritional support is necessary for the acutely ill child to overcome the infection, and addressing nutritional needs for all children in the community will decrease the risk of mortality related to pneumonia overall.[59]

Breastfeeding

The WHO reports that infants who are exclusively breastfed for the first 6 months of life are 5 times less likely to die from pneumonia. Extended breastfeeding continues to offer protection beyond 6 months of life.[48] The excellent nutrition and strengthened immune system that breastfeeding provides are incredibly valuable to the infant in this critical period.

Micronutrient Deficiencies

Zinc and vitamin A are the 2 micronutrients that have adequately been shown to reduce the burden of disease caused by pneumonia. Zinc intake early in the course of severe pneumonia decreases the duration, severity, and number of treatment failures in children with pneumonia.[60] Vitamin A supplementation only improves outcomes for pneumonia associated with measles. No effect is seen with pneumonia not associated with measles.[51]

Reducing Exposures

Indoor air pollution from heating and cooking fires is a common environmental exposure that contributes to respiratory problems such as asthma. Biomass fuel is common in developing countries; many lower-income families use biomass fuel for indoor heating and cooking without adequate ventilation. These fuels cause more than 1.5 million premature deaths worldwide and disproportionately affect women because of traditional occupational roles. Exposure to cooking smoke from biomass combustion is linked to many conditions, including asthma and acute lower respiratory tract infections. A WHO review estimates that indoor air pollution accounts for 3.7% of disease in lower-income countries with high mortality, making it one of the top 10 contributors to disease.[61]

Outdoor air pollution is also a growing problem in large urban areas of lower-income countries and for those who live close to roads.[62] As in higher-income countries, atmospheric pollution has a greater visible effect on the young, elderly, and ill. Strong associations have been made between air pollution metrics and respiratory symptoms.[63,64] The burden of respiratory disease on a community correlates with worsening air pollution.[65] The growing evidence on the health effects of air quality in the dense cities of the developing world indicates that it is a major contributor to morbidity and mortality.[66] Special attention should be given to the management of chronic respiratory disease for travelers to urban areas as even short-term exposure can have detrimental health effects.[67]

Tobacco smoke exposure is also a growing concern in lower-income countries. The relative burden of disease related to tobacco is likely to increase with expanded marketing.

Fungus in the home contributes to respiratory disease as a causative or exacerbating agent for rhinitis, asthma, hypersensitivity pneumonitis, and allergic bronchopulmonary aspergillus.

Hand Washing

Attention should be given to techniques aimed at reducing physical transmission of inciting organisms. Hand-washing programs are shown to reduce respiratory tract infections as well as diarrhea and other infections in high-risk settings.[68] Minimizing transmission is an important educational focus for health care professionals, caregivers, and children.

■ KEY POINTS

- Respiratory conditions are a major cause of death in children younger than 5 years.
- Tachypnea is the most sensitive means of diagnosing childhood pneumonia in developing countries (more than 50 resp/min for infants and more than 40 for children 1 to 5 years).
- Retractions or stidor are a key indication of severe pneumonia.
- First-line therapy for typical pneumonia is amoxicillin 50 mg/kg/d divided in 2 doses for 3 days.
- First-line therapy for severe pneumonia is amoxicillin-clavulanate 80 mg/kg/d divided in 2 doses for 5 days or erythromycin 50 mg/kg/d divided into 4 doses for 5 to 7 days.
- Children who die from respiratory infections are often malnourished.
- Improved preventive efforts (ie, vaccinations and timely access to medical care) could potentially reduce many deaths from respiratory illness.
- Differential diagnosis of respiratory symptoms should include atypical infections as well as noninfectious etiologies.
- Health care professionals on the front line are essential to reducing deaths from respiratory illness by recognizing the importance of respiratory symptoms and following a systematic approach to management.

■ REFERENCES

1. Rudan I, et al. Global estimate of the incidence of clinical pneumonia among children under five years of age. *Bull WHO.* 2004;82(12):895–903
2. World Health Organization. *Integrated Management of Childhood Illness.* Geneva, Switzerland: World Health Organization; 2005
3. Berman S, Simoes EA, Lanata C. Respiratory rate and pneumonia in infancy. *Arch Dis Child.* 1991;66(1):81–84
4. Harari M, et al. Clinical signs of pneumonia in children. *Lancet.* 1991;338(8772): 928–930
5. Sazawal S, Black RE. Effect of pneumonia case management on mortality in neonates, infants, and preschool children: a meta-analysis of community-based trials. *Lancet Infect Dis.* 2003;3(9):547–556
6. Shann F, et al. Aetiology of pneumonia in children in Goroka Hospital, Papua New Guinea. *Lancet.* 1984;2(8402):537–541
7. Savitha MR, Khanagavi JB. Redefining the World Health Organization algorithm for diagnosis of pneumonia with simple additional markers. *Indian J Pediatr.* 2008;75(6):561–565
8. Scott JA, et al. Pneumonia research to reduce childhood mortality in the developing world. *J Clin Invest.* 2008;118(4):1291–1300
9. Pio A. Standard case management of pneumonia in children in developing countries: the cornerstone of the acute respiratory infection programme. *Bull WHO.* 2003; 81(4):298–300
10. Zar HJ, Madhi SA. Childhood pneumonia—progress and challenges. *S Afr Med J.* 2006; 96(9 Pt 2):890–900
11. Madhi SA, et al. Vaccines to prevent pneumonia and improve child survival. *Bull WHO.* 2008;86(5):365–372
12. Jeena P, Pillay P, Adhikari M. Nasal CPAP in newborns with acute respiratory failure. *Ann Trop Paediatr.* 2002;22(3):201–207
13. Madhi SA, et al. Increased disease burden and antibiotic resistance of bacteria causing severe community-acquired lower respiratory tract infections in human immunodeficiency virus type 1-infected children. *Clin Infect Dis.* 2000;31(1):170–176
14. Zar HJ. Respiratory infections in children in developing countries. *Pediatr Ann.* 2002; 31(2):133–138
15. Cevey-Macherel M, et al. Etiology of community-acquired pneumonia in hospitalized children based on WHO clinical guidelines. *Eur J Pediatr.* 2009
16. Nascimento-Carvalho C, Ribeiro C, Cardoso M. The role of respiratory viral infections among children hospitalized for community-acquired pneumonia in a developing country. *Pediatr Infect Dis J.* 2008;27(10):939–941
17. Berman S. Epidemiology of acute respiratory infections in children of developing countries. *Rev Infect Dis.* 1991;13(Suppl 6):S454–S462
18. de Lataillade C, Auvergne S, Delannoy I. 2005 and 2006 seasonal influenza vaccination coverage rates in 10 countries in Africa, Asia Pacific, Europe, Latin America and the Middle East. *J Public Health Policy.* 2009;30(1):83–101
19. Stein RT, Marostica PJ. Community-acquired pneumonia. *Paediatr Respir Rev.* 2006;7(Suppl 1):S136–S137
20. O'Brien KL, et al. Severe pneumococcal pneumonia in previously healthy children: the role of preceding influenza infection. *Clin Infect Dis.* 2000;30(5):784–789
21. Fischer GB, Teper A, Colom AJ. Acute viral bronchiolitis and its sequelae in developing countries. *Paediatr Respir Rev.* 2002;3(4):298–302

22. Klig JE, Chen L. Lower respiratory infections in children. *Curr Opin Pediatr.* 2003;15(1):121–126

23. Greenberg D, Leibovitz E. Community-acquired pneumonia in children: from diagnosis to treatment. *Chang Gung Med J.* 2005;28(11):746–752

24. Grant GB, et al. Recommendations for treatment of childhood non-severe pneumonia. *Lancet Infect Dis.* 2009;9(3):185–196

25. Hazir T, et al. Can WHO therapy failure criteria for non-severe pneumonia be improved in children aged 2-59 months? *Int J Tuberc Lung Dis.* 2006;10(8):924–931

26. Ayieko P, English M. Case management of childhood pneumonia in developing countries. *Pediatr Infect Dis J.* 2007;26(5):432–440

27. Kabra SK, Lodha R, Pandey RM. Antibiotics for community acquired pneumonia in children. *Cochrane Database Syst Rev.* 2006;3:CD004874

28. Duke T, et al. Improved oxygen systems for childhood pneumonia: a multihospital effectiveness study in Papua New Guinea. *Lancet.* 2008;372(9646):1328–1333

29. English M, et al. Assessment of inpatient paediatric care in first referral level hospitals in 13 districts in Kenya. *Lancet.* 2004;363(9425):1948–1953

30. Subhi R, et al. The prevalence of hypoxaemia among ill children in developing countries: a systematic review. *Lancet Infect Dis.* 2009;9:219–227

31. Basnet S, Adhikari RK, Gurung CK. Hypoxemia in children with pneumonia and its clinical predictors. *Indian J Pediatr.* 2006;73(9):777–781

32. Duke T, Mgone J, Frank D. Hypoxaemia in children with severe pneumonia in Papua New Guinea. *Int J Tuberc Lung Dis.* 2001;5(6):511–519

33. Muhe L, Webert M. Oxygen delivery to children with hypoxaemia in small hospitals in developing countries. *Int J Tuberc Lung Dis.* 2001;5(6):527–532

34. Stein RT, Marostica PJ. Community-acquired pneumonia: a review and recent advances. *Pediatr Pulmonol.* 2007;42(12):1095–1103

35. Pinto KD, Maggi RR, Alves JG. [Analysis of social and environmental risk for pleural involvement in severe pneumonia in children younger than 5 years of age]. *Rev Panam Salud Publica.* 2004;15(2):104–109

36. Avansino JR, et al. Primary operative versus nonoperative therapy for pediatric empyema: a meta-analysis. *Pediatrics.* 2005;115(6):1652–1659

37. Ranganathan SC, Sonnappa S. Pneumonia and other respiratory infections. *Pediatr Clin North Am.* 2009;56(1):135–156

38. Crowcroft NS, Pebody RG. Recent developments in pertussis. *Lancet.* 2006;367(9526):1926–1936

39. Patel SP, Jarvelin MR, Little MP. Systematic review of worldwide variations of the prevalence of wheezing symptoms in children. *Environ Health.* 2008;7:57

40. Pitrez PM, Stein RT. Asthma in Latin America: the dawn of a new epidemic. *Curr Opin Allergy Clin Immunol.* 2008;8(5):378–383

41. Johnson DW. Croup. *Clin Evid (Online).* 2009

42. Moore M, Little P. Humidified air inhalation for treating croup: a systematic review and meta-analysis. *Fam Pract.* 2007;24(4):295–301

43. Acevedo JL, et al. Airway management in pediatric epiglottitis: a national perspective. *Otolaryngol Head Neck Surg.* 2009;140(4):548–551

44. Huang YL, et al. Bacterial tracheitis in pediatrics: 12 year experience at a medical center in Taiwan. *Pediatr Int.* 2009;51(1):110–113

45. World Health Organization. *Rheumatic Fever and Rheumatic Heart Diseases. Report of a WHO Expert Consultation.* Geneva, Switzerland: World Health Organization; 2001. http://www.who.int/cardiovascular_diseases/resources/en/cvd_trs923.pdf. Accessed June 17, 2011

46. Adegbola RA, et al. The etiology of pneumonia in malnourished and well-nourished Gambian children. *Pediatr Infect Dis J.* 1994;13(11):975–982

47. Rasmussen Z, Pio A, Enarson P. Case management of childhood pneumonia in developing countries: recent relevant research and current initiatives. *Int J Tuberc Lung Dis.* 2000;4(9):807–826

48. United Nations Children's Fund, World Health Organization. *Pneumonia: The Forgotten Killler of Children.* Geneva, Switzerland: United Nations Children's Fund, World Health Organization; 2006. http://www.unicef.org/mdg/mortalitymultimedia/Pneumonia_The_Forgotten_Killer_of_Children.pdf. Accessed June 17, 2011

49. Kallander K, Nsungwa-Sabiiti J, Peterson S. Symptom overlap for malaria and pneumonia—policy implications for home management strategies. *Acta Trop.* 2004;90(2):211–214

50. Kabra SK, Lodha R, Hilton DJ. Antibiotics for preventing complications in children with measles. *Cochrane Database Syst Rev.* 2008;3:CD001477

51. Huiming Y, Chaomin W, Meng M. Vitamin A for treating measles in children. *Cochrane Database Syst Rev.* 2005;4:CD001479

52. World Health Organization. *Respiratory Care in Primary Care Services: A Survey in 9 Countries.* Geneva, Switzerland: World Health Organization; 2004

53. Adams LV. Childhood turberculosis in the developing world. *Pediatr Ann.* 2004;33(10):685–690

54. World Health Organization, United Nations Children's Fund. *WHO/UNICEF Joint Statement: Managment of Pnuemonia in Community Settings.* Geneva, Switzerland: World Health Organization, United Nations Children's Fund; 2004. http://whqlibdoc.who.int/hq/2004/WHO_FCH_CAH_04.06.pdf. Accessed June 17, 2011

55. Schellenberg JA, et al. Inequities among the very poor: health care for children in rural southern Tanzania. *Lancet.* 2003;361(9357):561–566

56. Pertussis vaccines. WHO position paper. *Wkly Epidemiol Rec.* 2005;8(28):29–40

57. Pneumococcal conjugate vaccine for childhood immunization. WHO position paper. *Wkly Epidemiol Rec.* 2007;12(82):93–104

58. Mahoney RT, et al. The introduction of new vaccines into developing countries. IV: global access strategies. *Vaccine.* 2007;25(20):4003–4011

59. Victora CG, Kirkwood BR, Ashworth A, et al. Potential interventions for the prevention of childhood pneumonia in developing countries: improving nutrition. *Am J Clin Nutr.* 1999;70(3):309–320

60. Haider BA, Bhutta ZA. The effect of therapeutic zinc supplementation among young children with selected infections: a review of the evidence. *Food Nutr Bull.* 2009;30(1 Suppl):S41–S59

61. World Health Organization. *Indoor Air Pollution: National Burden of Disease Estimates.* Geneva, Switzerland: World Health Organization; 2007. http://www.who.int/indoorair/publications/indoor_air_national_burden_estimate_revised.pdf. Accessed June 17, 2011

62. Venn A, et al. Proximity of the home to roads and the risk of wheeze in an Ethiopian population. *Occup Environ Med.* 2005;62(6):376–380

63. Mansourian M, Javanmard SH, Poursafa P, et al. Air pollution and hospitalization for respiratory diseases among children in Isfahan, Iran. *Ghana Med J.* 2010;44(4):138–143

64. Vichit-Vadakan N, Ostro BD, Chestnut LG, et al. Air pollution and respiratory symptoms: results from three panel studies in Bangkok, Thailand. *Environ Health Perspect.* 2001;109(Suppl3):381–387

65. Roy A, Sheffield P, Wong K, et al. The effects of outdoor air pollutants on the costs of pediatric asthma hospitalizations in the United States, 1999 to 2007. *Med Care.* 2011; in print

66. Hedley AJ, Wong CM, Thach TQ, et al. Cardiorespiratory and all-cause mortality after restrictions on sulphur content fuel in Hong Kong: an intervention study. *Lancet.* 2002;360(9346):1646–1652

67. Sanford C. Urban medicine: threats to health of travelers to developing world cities. *J Travel Med.* 2004;11(5):313–327

68. Luby SP, et al. Effect of handwashing on child health: a randomised controlled trial. *Lancet.* 2005;366(9481):225–233

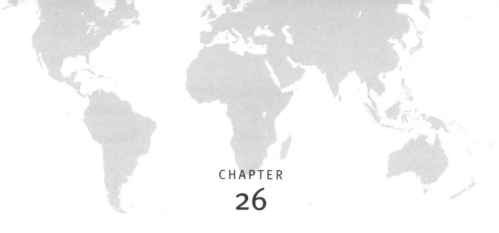

CHAPTER

26

Dermatology

Gregory Juckett, MD, MPH

■ INTRODUCTION TO DERMATOLOGIC DIAGNOSIS

Rash Classification

Dermatologic diagnosis is largely a process of complex pattern recognition, similar to that employed by a naturalist using a field guide. Of course, the landmarks in question differ, but mastering a differential diagnosis for each classic rash will facilitate quick identification. Although this diagnostic approach must be learned in stages, the process eventually becomes more intuitive with experience. Once the diagnosis is established, any standard reference provides treatment guidelines.

The correct use of terminology in describing the primary lesion is essential, not just for better communication but also for better comprehension. Several key pairs of useful descriptive terms exist that are defined, in part, by their relative size (5 to 10 mm, depending on reference). *Macules* are flat, discolored lesions up to 10 mm in size, whereas *patches* are larger macules greater than 10 mm. Likewise, *elevated lesions* (ie, papules and plaques), and *deeper solid lesions* (ie, nodules and tumors) may also be distinguished by being less or greater than 10 mm. On the other hand, *blisters* (ie, vesicles and bullae) and *subcutaneous blood deposits* (ie, petechiae and purpura) may be demarcated by whether they measure less or greater than 5 mm (Table 26-1). Many skin presentations necessitate the use of multiple descriptive terms (eg, maculopapular, papulovesicular, papulosquamous). Secondary features require additional terminology (eg, scaling, crusting, lichenification) that further describes the primary lesion (Table 26-2).

Table 26-1. Dermatologic Terminology for Primary Lesions

DESCRIPTION	SMALLER SIZE	EXAMPLES	LARGER SIZE	EXAMPLES
Flat, circumscribed spot	Macule <10 mm	Freckle (lentigo)	Patch >10 mm	Vitiligo
Raised lesion, circumscribed, superficial	Papule <5 mm	Wart, nevus, acne, insect bite	Plaque >5 mm	Psoriasis patch Mycosis fungoides
Solid lesion with depth below surface	Nodule <5 mm	Dermatofibroma	Tumor >5 mm	Lipoma
Raised blister(s) with serous fluid	Vesicle <5 mm	Chickenpox, contact dermatitis, HSV	Bulla >5 mm	Second-degree burn, blister
Blood deposit	Petechia <5 mm	Insect bite	Purpura >5 mm	Ecchymosis

Abbreviation: HSV, herpes simplex virus.

Taking a Dermatologic History

The history of the rash is important. As in journalism, who, what, when, where, why, and how are the usual questions to ask. *Who* did the patient contact (eg, people, animals, things)? *What* precipitated the rash's appearance? *When* did it start? *Where* did it spread? The answer to *"Why* did you get the rash?"* will reflect the patient's own theory of causation and provide insight into how he views the problem. The questions *"How* has the rash changed over time?"* and *"How* has it been managed?"* provide the most useful information. Certain therapies may obfuscate the original cause (eg, steroids on a fungal infection) or even provoke a secondary allergic response (eg, sensitizing products ending in -caine or -dryl, topical antibiotics such as Neosporin).

The symptoms, location, and seasonality of the rash provide additional clues. *Pruritic* lesions suggest an allergic reaction. Tender lesions and rashes associated with fever are obviously more likely infectious in origin. *Centrifugal* rashes start centrally and spread to the periphery (eg, varicella, rubella), while the reverse is true for *centripetal* rashes (eg, dengue, Rocky Mountain spotted fever [RMSF]). Outside the tropics, incidence of skin disease changes with the seasons, with eczematous conditions worsening in winter and fungal infections and contact reactions increasing in summer. Acne tends to flare in spring and fall. Even within the tropics, the wet season is much more likely to be associated with fungal and insect-borne diseases such as dengue.

Table 26-2. Secondary and Descriptive Dermatologic Terminology

Alopecia	Loss of hair or baldness. Pediatric causes include alopecia areata (autoimmune), traction alopecia, tinea capitis, telogen effluvium (stress shedding), and trichotillomania (self-induced from twisting or pulling).
Atopy	Allergy-mediated eczematous reactions causing dry, rough skin patches and itching (may be associated with asthma or hay fever)
Atrophy/Striae	Thinning of susceptible skin, often caused by prolonged steroid therapy; striae are stretch marks, a characteristic hallmark of atrophic skin.
Crust	Scab or dried exudate over damaged skin
Cyst	Enclosed cavity with a lining containing a liquid or semisolid
Erosion	Superficially denuded epidermis that usually heals without scarring
Exanthem versus Enanthem	Exanthems describe a generalized skin eruption; erythematous (macular), vesicular, and papular subtypes are recognized. Enanthems are mucous membrane eruptions.
Excoriation versus Abrasion	Traumatic skin loss due to scratching versus scraping
Fissure	Skin split extending into dermis
Hypopigmentation/ Hyperpigmentation	Loss of skin pigmentation (eg, pityriasis alba, vitiligo, tinea versicolor) versus increased skin pigmentation (café au lait macule)
Keloid versus Hypertrophic Scar	Exaggerated scarring. Hypertrophic scars appear earlier (within 1 min), remain confined to original scar, and regress with time. They are also less associated with skin pigmentation than keloids.
Lichenification	Leatherlike thickening of skin with accentuated skin markings because of chronic rubbing or scratching (eg, atopic eczema, lichen simplex chronicus)
Pustule	Papule containing pus (acne pustule)
Scale	Accumulation of desquamated stratum corneum (eg, seborrhea, psoriasis)
Telangiectasias	Dilated superficial blood vessels, often associated with skin atrophy
Ulcers	An area of destroyed dermis, resulting in a sunken sore. Deeper than an erosion and may result in scarring. Decubitus ulcers or bedsores are secondary to pressure-induced skin necrosis.
Wheal	Edematous smooth pink to red migratory papule, usually with pruritus (hives or urticaria)

Several noninfectious skin conditions deserve special mention because they mimic many other rashes. Allergic contact dermatitis, perhaps the most common pediatric diagnosis, is a delayed cell-mediated hypersensitivity response to various allergens. Itching and erythema appear within 24 hours to several days post-allergen exposure, and the rash often becomes papular or vesicular. Poison ivy *(Toxicodendron)* is the best known example, but there are many tropical plant allergens—mango rind, cashew sap, poisonwood *(Toxicodendron),* and carrot weed *(Parthenium).* Photodermatitis causes rash only in areas exposed to sunlight; it is triggered by certain drugs (eg, tetracycline, thiazides) and plants (eg, fig, citrus juices, rue). Polymorphous light eruption (sun allergy) presents as pruritic papules or plaques after an unaccustomed exposure to ultraviolet (UV) A light. Lastly, there are numerous drug eruptions, including generalized maculopapular rashes, urticarial reactions (hives), lichenoid reactions (eg, flattop, itchy, red papules), and fixed drug eruption (local plaques). Erythema multiforme (target lesions evolving into bullae) may be caused by drugs or recent infection (eg, herpes simplex). Erythema multiforme reactions are part of a spectrum, including Stevens-Johnson syndrome or erythema multiforme major (with mucous membrane involvement), and life-threatening toxic epidermal necrolysis (TEN).

When confronted by a new rash, the following questions should be asked: What is the primary lesion (macule, papule, etc.)? What are its secondary characteristics (scaly, blanching if red)? Where on the body is it located (central or peripheral distribution)? What are the associated symptoms (itching, fever, tenderness)? The answers will usually point in the right direction. Also, remember that uncommon presentations of common conditions (eg, contact dermatitis, eczema) are much more likely than common presentations of uncommon conditions; hence, this chapter will focus on the most common infectious pediatric conditions found in the tropics.

Physical Examination

The examination should be conducted with most of the patient's clothing off to avoid missing lesions of which she may be unaware. Scalp, genital, foot, and mouth lesions are most easily missed. The oral examination is especially useful and may confirm conditions such as lichen planus. Nevi of concern and congenital lesions should be measured, and even diagramed if possible, so they can be followed over time. Photography provides the best documentation because photos can be dated and placed in the chart.

Physical examination of dark-skinned individuals poses additional challenges, especially for physicians new to the tropics who are accustomed to caring for whites. Although darkly pigmented skin has the same number of melanocytes as white skin, these melanocytes are far more efficient at producing pigment, which provides much better protection from UV radiation and reduces the risk of sunburn and skin malignancies (excepting more vulnerable areas such as fingernails, lips, and palms and soles). Post-inflammatory hyperpigmentation (post-acne) and hypopigmentation (post-cryotherapy) are less-desirable consequences. Pityriasis alba, which describes diffusely hypopigmented macules on the cheeks or arms subsequent to dry skin or eczema, is very common with darker skin. Vitiligo, well-demarcated immune-mediated pigment loss, is present in all skin types but is much more conspicuous with dark skin. Erythema is masked by skin pigment, although it can still be detected with experience. Palpation of the skin often assists in detecting warmth and induration. Cyanosis can be identified by viewing lips and oral mucosa, while jaundice is apparent in the sclera, palms, and soles. Severe anemia causes an ashen appearance in black patients and a yellowish-brown shade in brown-skinned individuals.

Birthmarks are more prevalent (up to a 20% incidence) in blacks compared with whites (2% to 3%). Mongolian spots (often over the sacrum but occurring in other locations) are blue-gray macules present in up to 90% of blacks at birth and in a majority of Latino (70%) and Asian (80%) children.[1] Almost 10% of white infants are also affected. The spots usually resolve by age 4 years but may last longer; their resemblance to bruises may lead to false suspicions of child abuse, as can real but benign bruises from the Asian folk practices of coining and cupping. More efficient collagen production following trauma results in exuberant scarring or keloid formation. Sternal areas, upper arms, shoulders, and earlobes are most vulnerable. Many keloids are entirely preventable if unnecessary procedures, such as ear piercing, are avoided in high-risk individuals.

Basic Laboratory Assessment

Laboratory facilities are often quite limited in developing countries; however, scalpel blades, glass slides, a Wood lamp, and a microscope are helpful diagnostic tools. Diascopy, pressing a glass slide over an erythematous lesion, checks for blanching; inflamed capillaries transiently disappear with pressure while petechiae do not. Scraping scaly lesions with a number 15 scalpel and adding a drop of 20% potassium hydroxide (KOH) to the resulting specimen will permit microscopic examination for fungal hyphae. Florescence with a Wood lamp can help distinguish erythrasma (coral red) from *Microsporum* tinea infections (green). Finally, shave or ellipse biopsies of unusual lesions provide a definitive diagnosis as well as therapeutic guidance (or even cure) for skin malignancies. Web-based pathologic services have vastly improved the availability and reliability of these services in recent years.

Treatment Principles

Treatment involves knowing proper indications for topical preparations as well as standard oral therapies. The choice of which topical vehicle to use should be based on the condition's moisture content, its location, and its susceptibility to therapy. Tapes and patches provide optimal occlusion and coverage for small lesions. Occlusion with tape increases the penetration and potency of a topical steroid treatment. Ointments provide moisture to dry lesions and excellent occlusion but may be messy to apply. Water-based creams are the most popular for typical use due to their ease of application. Lotions and sprays are more practical to apply to extensive or hair-covered areas. Alcohol-based gels may be the most suitable for wet lesions because of their drying effect. It makes sense to dry wet lesions and moisten dry ones.

The potency of steroid preparations may be rated from 1 (most potent) to 7 (least potent), or perhaps more usefully as strong (high potency: classes 1–2), moderate (intermediate: 3–5), and weak (low potency: 6–7) as shown in Box 26-1. Areas of thin delicate skin, such as the face, genitalia, axillary and inguinal areas, and young children's skin in general, are subject to permanent atrophy and stretch marks (striae) if excessively potent steroids are prescribed for too long. Therefore, the lowest effective strength should be used and even this should be modified as the condition improves.

Mild steroids should be used on the face or genital areas and more potent ones for palms and plantar surfaces. More refractory skin conditions, such as contact dermatitis and psoriasis, mandate potent therapy to be effective. It is helpful to become familiar with an affordable generic option in each of the 3 categories, eg, hydrocortisone 1% (mild), triamcinolone 0.1% (moderate), and betamethasone dipropionate 0.05% (potent). For most given agents, potency may be adjusted up or down with choice of vehicle (in order of potency): tape, ointment, cream, lotion, and gel. The amount of steroid is also critical. A fingertip unit, the amount of cream from the tip of the index finger to the first (distal) crease, will be enough to treat an area the size of an adult's palm. Without parental instruction it is likely that far too much medicine will

Box 26-1. Topical Steroid Potency Ratings

LOW POTENCY (EG, FACE, GENITALS)
Hydrocortisone acetate 0.5%, 1%, 2.5% (Cortisporin, Hytone, Vytone)
Alclometasone dipropionate 0.05% (Aclovate)
Fluocinolone acetonide 0.01% (Synalar Solution)
Triamcinolone acetonide 0.025% (Kenalog, Aristocort)

INTERMEDIATE POTENCY (MOST USES, EG, ECZEMA)
Desonide cream 0.05% (DesOwen)
Desoximetasone 0.05% (Topicort)
Fluocinolone acetonide 0.025% (Synalar)
Flurandrenolide 0.025%, 0.05% (Cordran SP)
Fluticasone propionate 0.005%, 0.05% (Cutivate)
Hydrocortisone valerate 0.2% (Westcort)
Hydrocortisone probutate 0.1% (Pandel)
Hydrocortisone butyrate 0.1% (Locoid)
Mometasone furoate 0.1% (Elocon)
Prednicarbate 0.1% (Dermatop E)
Triamcinolone acetonide 0.1% (Kenalog, Aristocort)

HIGH POTENCY (EG, PSORIASIS, LICHEN, CONTACT DERMATITIS)
Amcinonide 0.1% (Cyclocort)
Betamethasone dipropionate 0.05% (Diprolene)
Clobetasol propionate 0.05% (Temovate, Temovate E)
Desoximetasone 0.05% (Topicort Gel)
Desoximetasone 0.25% (Topicort Cream, Topicort Ointment)
Diflorasone diacetate 0.05% (Psorcon E cream, Psorcon Ointment)
Fluocinonide 0.05% (Lidex, Lidex-E)
Flurandrenolide 4 μg/cm^2 (Cordran Tape)
Halcinonide 0.1% (Halog, Halog-E)
Halobetasol propionate 0.05% (Ultravate)
Triamcinolone acetonide 0.5% (Kenalog, Aristocort)

be applied. The duration of therapy should also be discussed to prevent indefinite use. High-potency steroids should be limited to fewer than 2 weeks of use.

The use of oral steroids is a double-edged sword; they dramatically improve symptoms for conditions such as contact dermatitis, but rebound occurs if the treatment is terminated too quickly, as happens with many dose packs. Rebounding psoriasis often ends up far worse than it was at the beginning—a good reason to avoid any systemic steroid use for this condition. Steroid injections in the wrong areas (eg, arms) may induce permanent tissue atrophy. Psychiatric symptoms such as insomnia, anxiety, and even psychosis may be provoked at higher doses (greater than 40 mg) in susceptible patients. Chronic use results in steroid dependency, glucose intolerance, cataracts, ulcers, osteoporosis, and immune deficiency. In the developing world, prolonged use may unwittingly activate latent tuberculosis (TB) in malnourished, infected patients.

■ VIRAL SKIN INFECTIONS

Papular Presentations of Viral Infections

Molluscum Contagiosum

Molluscum contagiosum presents as characteristic 2 to 8 mm, often umbilicated shiny papules, sometimes with surrounding erythema. This harmless poxvirus is easily spread by skin-to-skin contact in children between the ages of 2 and 12 years; lesions may appear 2 weeks to as long as 6 months postexposure.[2] The infection usually resolves within 4 to 6 months unless there is immune compromise, in which case unusually numerous or large (giant molluscum) or difficult-to-treat lesions occur. In children, molluscum usually appears on the trunk, face, or extremities. In sexually active teens, a genital presentation is more common (although this area can also be infected by scratching). Treatment involves destruction of lesions through curettage, application of trichloroacetic acid, or cryotherapy (freezing). Cryotherapy may produce areas of persistent hypopigmentation in dark-skinned patients. Lesions too numerous to treat individually respond to imiquimod 5% cream, although this indication is not yet approved by the Food and Drug Administration (FDA).[3]

Human Papillomavirus

Human papillomavirus (HPV) consists of more than 70 genotypes clinically presenting as common, flat, plantar, and genital warts. They are ubiquitous with an estimated 10% incidence in childhood, but two thirds spontaneously resolve within 2 years.[4] Common warts (types 1, 2, 4, and 7) are flesh-colored, rough dome-shaped, or filiform papules that commonly affect the dorsum of the hands and periungual areas of fingers. Oral mucosal involvement is rare. Flat warts (types 5, 8, and 17) are tiny, 2- to 5-mm flat papules occurring in colonies and easily spread though skin trauma or shaving. Plantar warts (type 1) are ingrown, often painful lesions, sometimes forming colonies or mosaics, on the soles of the feet. Genital warts occur on genital or perianal areas as multiple soft, verrucous papules. Human papillomavirus types 6 and 11 commonly cause genital warts, but other types (most notably 16 and 18) pose an increased risk of cervical cancer. In children, genital warts raise the additional possibility of sexual abuse; however, vertical (maternal) transmission may also occur.[5] An effective quadrivalent HPV vaccination

(Gardasil) is now approved for girls and young women 9 to 26 years of age. In 2009, approval was extended to include males in the same age range.

Warts are diagnosed by appearance; they are usually flesh-colored, verrucous papules. Plantar warts often require paring with a number 15 scalpel to distinguish them from calluses or "black heel" secondary to trauma. Dark specks or "seeds" (thrombosed capillaries) and interrupted skin lines distinguish warts from other lesions.

Treatment may be with cryotherapy (difficult and painful for children), salicylic acid liquids and plasters, topical cantharidin, or imiquimod 5% cream. For recalcitrant common or plantar warts, injection with *Candida* antigen (0.1 mL of a 1:1,000 solution, same as used for dermal immune testing) with added lidocaine 1% is a non–FDA-approved option that is effective 74% of the time, often with concomitant disappearance of non-injected warts.[6] Cimetidine oral therapy, thought to stimulate T cells, has produced mixed results and may be no more effective than placebo.[7] Duct tape occlusion may also be ineffective. Surgical therapy or electrocautery should be avoided because it can result in permanent scarring and it is usually better to wait for natural resolution. Tretinoin cream, imiquimod 5% creams, or gentle cryotherapy are effective options for flat warts. Genital warts may be treated with cryotherapy, podofilox gel, or imiquimod 5% cream, although the latter 2 therapies are unapproved in children.

Vesicular Presentations of Viral Disease

Herpes Simplex Virus

Herpes simplex virus (HSV), types 1 (oral) and 2 (genital), are a common cause of recurrent oral and genital vesicles. Herpes simplex virus is capable of persisting in nerve ganglia in a dormant state where it cannot be reached by therapy. Primary herpes gingivostomatitis, usually from HSV type 1, causes oral and perioral lesions with stomatitis, sore throat, and cervical lymphadenopathy, most commonly in children younger than 5 years. While many primary infections are asymptomatic, severe cases can last 2 weeks and result in dehydration. The recurrent vesicles of herpes labialis, known as cold sores or fever blisters, appear in clusters on the vermilion border of the lip following a brief prodrome of tingling. They often become secondarily infected (impetiginized) and are precipitated by stress, illness, or excess sun exposure. Herpetic whitlow occurs when a finger (the patient's or a caregiver's) is inoculated with the virus, causing a painful fingertip swelling for several weeks. Herpes keratoconjunctivitis may cause recurrent conjunctivitis (red eye) with corneal opacification, leading to permanent vision loss. Steroid eyedrops are notorious for exacerbating this condition, and ocular HSV should be excluded by slit lamp examination prior to their use. Herpes gladiatorum describes clustered vesicles on the trunk or extremities in wrestlers or athletes exposed to infected secretions. In patients with atopic dermatitis, eczema herpeticum (Kaposi varicelliform eruption) may produce a generalized vesicular outbreak due to the loss of a normal skin barrier. Erythema multiforme, with target lesions, is a secondary immune response often following an outbreak of labial herpes.

Genital herpes (usually HSV type 2) also cause primary and secondary infections. Primary outbreaks occur 2 to 8 days after sexual exposure with painful genital vesicles and inguinal adenopathy. Scrapings from the base of fresh ulcers, as in HSV type 1, are positive for multinucleated giant cells on Tzanck preparations. Secondary outbreaks are milder and more frequent in the first years following infection. Those with frequent episodes also have a higher risk for asymptomatic viral shedding, which renders them contagious between symptomatic outbreaks.[8] Treatment for either type of HSV is oral acyclovir, famciclovir, or valacyclovir started within 24 hours, although beneficial even 2 to 3 days later. Antiviral therapy can also be used to reduce genital recurrences and suppress HSV shedding indefinitely. Topical antiviral creams for cold sores are much less effective, although they may reduce symptoms and shedding by a day or 2 if started promptly.

Recurrent aphthous stomatitis (RAS) is sometimes confused with oral herpes. These "canker sores" are painful, shallow, gray ulcerations of the oral mucosa, not involving the vermilion border, that last for 1 to 2 weeks. Their etiology is poorly understood and they are thought to be related to stress, minor trauma, or an autoimmune response. Minor RAS (few small lesions) is very common, but occasionally major RAS (with larger lesions) is noted. Treatment is symptomatic, often with topical lidocaine, amlexanox, or steroids in denture paste.

Varicella Zoster (Shingles)

Varicella zoster or shingles is a vesicular eruption caused by reactivation of latent varicella (chickenpox) virus in the sensory ganglia. The vesicles are clinically similar to those of herpes simplex (positive Tzanck preparation) but are characteristically unilateral and limited to a specific dermatome. The rash is preceded by hyperesthesia or discomfort in the involved area. The vesicles erupt over a period of 1 week, then take another week to crust over and heal.

Varicella zoster is usually associated with advanced age or immune compromise (frequently a presenting condition in AIDS), but it also occurs in children and teens, including healthy children immunized with attenuated varicella vaccine.[9] Common dermatomes infected include C2-L2 and the trigeminal (fifth) and facial (seventh) cranial nerves. Hutchinson sign is vesicular involvement of the tip of the nose, which indicates ophthalmic branch involvement of cranial nerve V (impending keratitis) and should prompt an immediate ophthalmology referral. Ramsay Hunt syndrome describes Bell palsy, auditory canal shingles, and disturbed hearing and balance. Abdominal shingles presents with severe abdominal pain, which sometimes leads to surgery, prior to any appearance of rash.

Treatment is with high-dose antiviral therapy, such as acyclovir, ideally started within 72 hours of rash onset. Post-herpetic neuralgia, characterized by burning, persistent nerve pain, is uncommon in children but increases with age and delayed treatment.

Viral Exanthems of Childhood With Fever

At the start of the 20th century, Filatov described 6 rashes of childhood, including rubeola (measles), scarlet fever or scarlatina (nonviral, due to group A beta-hemolytic streptococci [GABHS]), rubella (German measles), Duke disease (fourth disease, now obsolete but believed to be related to staphylococcal infection), erythema infectiosum (fifth disease), and erythema subitum or roseola (sixth disease). Other childhood rashes include chickenpox (varicella), mumps, coxsackievirus, mononucleosis, Kawasaki disease, and assorted nonspecific viral exanthems. Dengue is a major cause of rash and fever in the tropics and the leading cause of fever with rash in returning travelers. Fortunately, the ancient scourge of smallpox (variola) is now extinct outside the laboratory, but a similar-appearing, albeit milder rash, monkeypox, occasionally occurs as a zoonotic infection in Africa.

Rubeola

Rubeola (measles) is a well-known contagious viral childhood illness that is now rare in the United States because of vaccination but is still common worldwide. Its prodrome consists of fever and the 3 Cs—cough, coryza, and conjunctivitis, along with characteristic Koplik spots (whitish papules on the buccal mucosa). The classic morbilliform or measles-like (red, maculopapular) exanthem starts on the face about 4 days after the start of the prodrome and spreads to the body and extremities. Atypical measles can cause a petechial rash mimicking

RMSF or meningococcemia. Measles is infectious from 1 day prior to the start of the prodrome to 4 days after the rash appears. Incubation period is about 10 days. The diagnosis is clinical, but initial laboratory findings include leukopenia and the detection of measles IgM antibody within 4 days of illness.[10]

A live measles vaccine (now administered as part of the measles, mumps, rubella [MMR] vaccine) was introduced in the United States in 1963 for children 12 to 15 months of age. After a US measles outbreak in 1989 and 1990, a second dose of vaccine was recommended at 4 to 6 years of age (with revaccination at 11 to 12 years or older for children who needed it). Americans born before 1956 usually have had wild measles, while those born after 1956 need 2 doses of MMR for lasting immunity. Measles complications include pneumonia, encephalitis, and the rare (1 in 100,000) delayed neurologic disease, subacute sclerosing panencephalitis.[10] Malnutrition, particularly vitamin A deficiency, significantly increases measles mortality; thus, vitamin A supplementation (200,000 IU orally) is critical if deficiency is suspected or if the region's measles mortality rate is greater than 1%.[11] Prompt vaccination efforts in overseas refugee populations can prevent devastating measles epidemics. Measles therapy is mostly supportive, although measles immunoglobulin can reduce symptoms if given within 6 days of exposure.[12]

Rubella

Rubella (German or 3-day measles) is a much milder measles-like illness characterized by a pink macular eruption starting on the face and spreading onto the trunk and later to the extremities. The rash fades within 48 hours and is indistinguishable from many other viral exanthems. An estimated half of all cases are subclinical. The child usually appears well despite mild fever and posterior cervical lymph nodes that precede the rash. Infectivity begins a week prior to rash onset and lasts for 4 days afterward (although infants with congenital rubella syndrome can shed the virus for months). The incubation period is 14 to 21 days. Laboratory confirmation involves finding rubella IgM antibody within 28 days of rash.[10] A monoarticular arthritis may also occur (more likely in females), outlasting the rash by weeks. This complex presentation—sore throat, arthritis, rash (STAR)—may be seen in rubella and parvovirus infections, among others. Rubella is notorious for causing congenital rubella syndrome in infants born to mothers infected in the first trimester (microcephaly, deafness, mental retardation, and hepatomegaly). The best protection is through live, attenuated rubella vaccination prior to pregnancy.

Erythema Infectiosum

Erythema infectiosum (fifth disease) is a mild childhood illness caused by parvovirus B19. The rash begins with redness of one or both cheeks (75% of cases), the classic slapped-cheek presentation, which is followed by a lacy reticular macular rash for 3 to 5 days, although this rash may transiently reappear with heat or exercise for up to 4 months. Palmar rash is common. Some patients may develop purple hands and feet (gloves-and-socks syndrome). Fever is present only in 20% of cases. The rash's appearance usually signals the end of infectivity, so these children may attend school and no treatment is necessary. However, like rubella, erythema infectiosum can present as the STAR complex (albeit with symmetrical arthritis) and even cause fetal death if women in the first half of pregnancy are infected. The precaution of avoiding contact with pregnant women for 2 weeks may be overkill, as the diagnostic rash coincides with loss of infectivity. Exceptions would be rubella aplastic crisis cases (seen in sickle cell disease) in which the patient may be contagious for a week after symptoms, and immunocompromised patients who may shed the virus for months.[10]

Roseola Infantum

Roseola infantum (erythema subitum) is a human herpesvirus 6 (or 7) infection in children younger than 2 years. Classically, there are 3 days of sustained high fever followed by the appearance of an erythematous macular rash that fades in 24 hours. Febrile seizures may occur, but the condition is otherwise benign. Echovirus 16 (Boston exanthem) may mimic roseola in preschool children, although it can also cause petechial eruptions on the extremities and the fever may overlap with the rash.

Varicella

Varicella (chickenpox) is a common contagious childhood illness, peaking in late winter, with a prodrome of fever, chills, and myalgia followed within 48 hours by crops of vesicles on an erythematous base ("dewdrops on rose petals"). The centrifugal rash first appears on the trunk, face, and scalp, then spreads to the extremities. New crops of vesicular lesions continue appearing and crusting over for 3 to 4 days, so it is usually possible to find lesions in all stages of development. Residual scarring often occurs, but infection results in lifelong immunity. The patient is infectious for 1 to 2 days before the prodrome starts until the last crusts form at about 5 days. The incubation period is about 14 to 21 days.[10] Most childhood chickenpox cases are uneventful, but adolescents older than 12 years and adults are prone to more severe illness and should be treated with antivirals such as acyclovir. Aspirin exposure in chickenpox and influenza must be avoided because of the risk of Reye syndrome, acute encephalopathy, and fatty degeneration of the liver.

Live, attenuated varicella vaccine (Varivax) has been recommended for children aged 12 to 18 months since 1996. A second dose is now recommended 1 month after the first for children and susceptible adults.

Once infected (or vaccinated), the varicella-zoster virus remains dormant in sensory ganglia, from which it can later emerge to cause varicella zoster (shingles).

Dengue

Dengue (breakbone fever) is a mosquito-borne illness of the tropics and subtropics characterized by high (often biphasic) fever for 5 to 7 days, headache, retro-orbital pain, myalgia, arthralgia, and rash in 50%. Four dengue flavivirus serotypes (dengue 1–4) cause the condition with very little cross-protection among the 4 serotypes. The generalized maculopapular rash, often with islands of spared skin, usually appears when the fever subsides, but this is often difficult to appreciate in dark-skinned patients. Complications include dengue hemorrhagic fever (DHF), which is characterized by increased vascular permeability, thrombocytopenia, fever, and hemorrhage. The related dengue shock syndrome (DSS) describes DHF complicated by shock and carries a 12% mortality rate even with good care.[13] Secondary infection by another dengue serotype is considered the likely cause of DHF and DSS.

Dengue is usually diagnosed clinically, but reverse-transcriptase polymerase chain reaction (RT-PCR) testing for viremia can confirm the diagnosis within the first 5 days of infection. An IgM antibody capture enzyme-linked immunosorbent assay test (eg, DENV Detect IgM Capture ELISA), turning positive 1 week postinfection, may help distinguish dengue from other tropical febrile illnesses such as leptospirosis, malaria, typhoid, and the very similar chikungunya fever.[14] A 4-fold increase in hemagglutination inhibition antibody titer between acute and convalescent serum specimens is also diagnostic. In the United States, dengue testing is performed by the Centers for Disease Control and Prevention (CDC) Dengue Branch. Leukopenia and thrombocytopenia are common findings. A positive result from a tourniquet test (greater than 20 petechiae per square inch of skin) after 5 minutes of blood pressure cuff inflation, midway between diastolic and systolic pressures, indicates hemorrhagic risk. Abdominal pain and vomiting in children with a sudden drop in temperature also presages DSS.

Dengue often occurs in epidemics due to high numbers of infected *Aedes* mosquitoes, which bite for several hours after dawn and before dusk. The illness usually starts 4 to 7 days after being bitten. The best protection is insect repellent, as there is no effective vaccine or medical prophylaxis. Treatment is supportive with hydration to prevent shock. Corticosteroids are ineffective.

Hand-Foot-and-Mouth Disease

Hand-foot-and-mouth disease is a common viral illness of young children (often younger than 5 years) that causes deep vesicles on the palms and soles with painful oral vesicles. Malaise and fever may also be present. The disease is usually caused by coxsackieviruses A or B and is self-limited. However, enterovirus 71 epidemics may produce more severe hand-foot-and-mouth disease with death. Coxsackieviruses may also cause herpangina in somewhat older children with painful throat vesicles and fever. Hydration and pain relief is important. Herpangina resolves in 1 week without specific treatment.

Infectious Mononucleosis

Infectious mononucleosis is a several week syndrome of fatigue, sore throat (75%), fever, and anterior and posterior cervical adenitis in children and adolescents that is usually followed by extreme fatigue. Childhood infections are much milder than those of college-aged students. Most children in developing countries are infected by 5 years of age, but those in higher-income countries are infected later in life. Epstein-Barr virus causes 85% of mononucleosis-like presentations; the remainder are caused by cytomegalovirus, human herpesvirus 6, toxoplasmosis, and others. Acute retroviral syndrome, the initial infection of HIV, may mimic mononucleosis symptoms before entering the latent phase of infection.

About 5% to 15% of mononucleosis patients develop a transient macular skin eruption. Prescribing amoxicillin (and occasionally other antibiotics) for sore throat causes a delayed red morbilliform rash in most of these patients that lasts for at least 1 week. This is thought to be caused by an amoxicillin-antibody immune complex rather than a true amoxicillin allergy. Jaundice from mononucleosis hepatitis occurs in 4% of young adults, although a majority may have mild liver enzyme elevation.[10]

Mononucleosis is spread through saliva (eg, kissing, sharing beverages); the saliva continues to be infectious for 6 to 18 months. The incubation period is 2 to 7 weeks. A heterophile IgM antibody test (monospot) confirms the diagnosis, but 15% of patients may have negative test results until the second or third week of illness. Atypical lymphocytes are also common. Leukocytosis is common at first, but neutropenia and thrombocytopenia often develop later in the illness. Upper airway obstruction (preventable with oral steroids), mild hepatitis, and splenic rupture are other potential complications. Treatment is mostly supportive.

Nonspecific Viral Exanthems

Nonspecific viral exanthems may be described by their primary lesion as vesicular, papular (or maculopapular), petechial, or urticarial. They may also be described by the rash they resemble—morbilliform (measles-like), scarlatiniform (scarlatina-like), or rubelliform (rubella-like). These rashes are usually erythematous macular or maculopapular rashes without distinguishing features but are usually associated with respiratory or gastrointestinal illness. Most resolve in 1 week without treatment. Enteroviruses are common causes of exanthems in summer months, whereas respiratory viruses (eg, adenovirus, respiratory syncytial virus) are more common in the winter.

Variola Major (Smallpox) and Monkeypox

Smallpox was eradicated in 1980, with the last case occurring in Somalia in 1977. However, the virus is still maintained in high-security laboratories in the United States and Russia, and there is some concern that it might be used in future bioterrorism. The characteristic centrifugal rash is pustular, starting on the face and spreading to the rest of the body, with the extremities becoming extensively involved. The rash is preceded a few days prior by high fever, myalgia, and red oral macules. Mortality used to be around 30% and survivors were often scarred for life. No specific treatment exists. Malignant (vesicular) and hemorrhagic variants were usually fatal.

A much milder form of smallpox, variola minor, was also recognized. Vaccination against smallpox with cowpox (Dryvax live vaccinia vaccine) was sometimes complicated by eczema vaccinatum in atopic children with vaccinia immunoglobulin being the treatment of choice. The FDA licensed a new live vaccine for smallpox (ACAM2000) in 2007, which the CDC now distributes.[15] Although routine smallpox vaccination in the United States ended in 1972, ACAM2000 vaccine is being stockpiled out of concern for bioterrorism.

Monkeypox is a zoonotic infection that resembles smallpox and is occasionally reported from West and Central Africa. It is spread to humans from rodents (or from eating monkeys infected by rodents). It made headlines in 2003 when a brief US outbreak was triggered by pet prairie dogs that were infected by an imported Gambian rat. Fortunately, it is much milder and less contagious than smallpox.

Hemorrhagic Fevers

Fever and hemorrhage (including skin manifestations) are principal symptoms of various Old and New World hemorrhagic fever viruses. *Arenavirus* includes multiple types, including lymphocytic choriomeningitis virus and Lassa virus (West Africa), which are zoonotic infections from rodents. *Filovirus* includes the rare but dreaded Ebola and Marburg hemorrhagic fevers of Africa that infect nonhuman primates and humans, although the animal source of these viruses remains unknown. *Bunyavirus* includes Rift Valley fever (*Aedes* mosquito bites) and Congo-Crimean hemorrhagic fever (tick bites). There are multiple *Hantavirus* associated with rodents (worldwide), of which the Sin Nombre virus, described after a 1993 US outbreak, is representative. *Flaviviruses* include yellow fever and DHF, which are arthropod-borne viral infections with hemorrhagic manifestations. Bacterial infections, notably meningococcal meningitis, may also cause rash and hemorrhage.

Jaundice and Fever

Yellow fever, malaria, infectious hepatitis, and leptospirosis are potential causes of febrile jaundice and can have clinically similar presentations. Scleral icterus, nausea, and dark urine are classic symptoms. Hepatitis A is usually less symptomatic in children and is unlikely to cause jaundice in the very young. Yellow fever, spread by *Aedes* mosquitoes, is characterized by fever, myalgias, and vomiting, with 15% of cases progressing to a toxic, often fatal, phase with jaundice, abdominal pain, hemorrhage, and hematemesis (black vomit).[16] Nonviral causes of febrile jaundice include leptospirosis (secondary to the *Leptospira* spirochete) and malaria. Malaria may cause hemolysis with resultant unconjugated hyperbilirubinemia and jaundice. Leptospirosis may present with fever, jaundice, renal failure, and hemorrhagic lesions (Weil disease) or as an anicteric illness with fever, headache, conjunctival hyperemia, hepatosplenomegaly, and an erythematous maculopapular or urticarial rash. The face and extensor surfaces are often spared.[17]

HIV and AIDS-Related Skin Disease

HIV is associated with a great many different skin manifestations. Acute retroviral syndrome occurs 2 to 4 weeks after infection and often resembles clinical mononucleosis with a nonspecific erythematous maculopapular rash and lymphadenopathy. A high viral load is present, but antibody testing results are negative at this stage of the disease. Later,

AIDS-related rashes include herpes zoster (a prime indicator of AIDS in high-incidence areas), intractable seborrheic dermatitis (ie, scaly red rash of the scalp and face), oral candidiasis (thrush), severe tinea infections, cutaneous histoplasmosis, oral hairy leukoplakia (white lesions on the lateral tongue borders secondary to Epstein-Barr virus), eosinophilic folliculitis, cutaneous tuberculosis, and scrofula (TB adenitis). Bacillary angiomatosis *(Bartonella)* and Kaposi sarcoma (human herpesvirus 8) manifest as purple-red skin papules. Giant molluscum, cryptococcosis, and coccidioidomycosis may all present as papules that may be difficult to distinguish clinically. Penicilliosis *(Penicillium marneffei)* is the third most common AIDS-related opportunistic infection in Southeast Asia. It presents with umbilicated papules closely resembling those of molluscum contagiosum.[18] AIDS-related hair changes include loss of normal curliness, alopecia, elongated eyelashes, and premature graying. Drug eruptions, especially those from sulfa, also occur more frequently.

Pityriasis Rosea

Pityriasis rosea is a common childhood and adolescent rash of probable viral origin (human herpesvirus 6 and 7 were found in some studies), although there may well be other causative agents.[19] Most cases start with an oval, scaly herald patch that closely resembles tinea corporis. The herald patch is followed by a secondary outbreak of multiple smaller, scaly oval papules (often with a collarette of scale) that follow the lines of skin cleavage. Itching may occur during the outbreak but is usually minimal. Classically, a Christmas tree pattern may appear on the back when the rash is fully developed. Most of the rash is on the trunk and proximal extremities, usually sparing the face. Sometimes there is an inverse distribution affecting the arms, inguinal area, and lower extremities (sparing much of the trunk). Black children have a higher incidence of this variant and sometimes have more atypical-appearing (rounder, more papular) lesions. Any atypical case or the presence of distal lesions should prompt syphilis serology testing. Fortunately this rash is self-limited and requires no treatment.[20] Sunlight exposure appears to hasten resolution of the rash, as may erythromycin.[21]

Kawasaki Disease

The etiology is still unknown for this acute febrile mucocutaneous lymph node syndrome. This childhood disease should be considered whenever there is sustained fever (more than 5 days), red eyes (non-exudative conjunctivitis), and a maculopapular erythematous rash (especially pronounced at the skin folds). Most cases occur in children younger than 5 years; Asians are at increased risk. Red, crusted lips and a strawberry tongue are common. Hands and feet become swollen and develop red palms and soles that later desquamate. More than half of affected children have cervical lymphadenopathy. The diagnosis is basically clinical and there are no confirmatory laboratory tests. Other conditions possibly resembling Kawasaki disease include scarlet fever, toxic shock syndrome, drug reactions, and RMSF. Serious vasculitic complications may occur, particularly occlusion of the coronary arteries, which can cause sudden death even months after apparent recovery. Treatment is with aspirin (ideally started within 10 days of illness onset and continued for 2 months) along with intravenous (IV) immunoglobulin.[10]

■ BACTERIAL, TREPONEMAL, AND RICKETTSIAL SKIN INFECTIONS

Bacterial Skin Infections

Pyodermas

Pyodermas are ubiquitous in the tropics. Impetigo (summer sores) is a common, contagious, superficial skin infection of children presenting in non-bullous (crusted) and bullous forms. The hallmark of the more common non-bullous impetigo is a honey-colored crust that develops on an erythematous base. *Staphylococcus aureus* and GABHS are the principal causes. Bullous impetigo is characterized by small blisters due to *S aureus*. These bacteria often colonize the nasal mucosa (or genitalia) and are spread by scratching insect bites or traumatized skin with dirty hands. Mupirocin cream or ointment is an effective topical treatment for staphylococcal impetigo (including that caused by methicillin-resistant *S aureus* [MRSA]) and may also be used to reduce nasal carriage, albeit with less than permanent results.[22] Oral therapy for more extensive impetigo is accomplished with erythromycin, azithromycin, dicloxacillin, amoxicillin-clavulanate, or cephalexin. Methicillin-resistant *S aureus* infections respond to sulfamethoxazole-trimethoprim, doxycycline, vancomycin, or clindamycin. Although most impetigo is now staphylococcal-related, nephritogenic streptococcal skin infections may still occasionally result in outbreaks of post-streptococcal nephritis and scarlet fever, despite appropriate antibiotics.

Ecthyma is a deeper form of GABHS impetigo, penetrating the epidermis to form deep, punched-out ulcers that heal slowly with scarring. A hemorrhagic ulceration, ecthyma gangrenosum, is caused by *Pseudomonas* infection in immunocompromised children. Superficial folliculitis, or staphylococcal hair follicle infection, typically appears as small pustules with central hairs (Bockhart impetigo) and usually responds to topical antibiotic treatment. Hot tub or pseudomonal folliculitis occurs 1 to 2 days after exposure to a hot tub or pool with inadequate chlorination. Lesions are often on the trunk in areas covered by the swimsuit. They usually resolve in a week without any antibiotic treatment. Pseudofolliculitis (razor bumps) is an inflammatory condition caused by ingrown curly hairs, which is managed by growing the hair out or avoiding close shaves.

Deeper, more painful lesions include furuncles (boils or abscesses) and the larger aggregates of furuncles called carbuncles. Both are caused by S aureus and may be misdiagnosed as spider bites in early stages. These lesions present as red, tender nodules that soon become fluctuant and filled with pus. Adequate incision and drainage is optimal treatment, and often incision and drainage alone is sufficient to resolve the problem, although in practice, systemic anti-staphylococcal antibiotics are often added. In recent years, culture and sensitivity testing has become much more important because of the increasing incidence of MRSA infection.

Cellulitis is an acute infection of the subcutaneous tissue with tender erythema and swelling that often follows skin trauma. It is usually caused by S aureus or GABHS but occasionally may be caused by streptococcal pneumonia or Haemophilus influenzae type b. Systemic anti-staphylococcal drugs are effective for most cases. Erysipelas is a cellulitis variant, usually caused by GABHS, characterized by shiny red plaques with sharply demarcated margins on the head or hands. Penicillin is the drug of choice. Necrotizing fasciitis (flesh-eating bacteria) is a life-threatening GABHS or polymicrobial infection that rapidly destroys tissue and requires immediate surgical debridement and multiple systemic antibiotics (including clindamycin).

Staphylococcal scalded skin syndrome is caused by an epidermolytic toxin-producing a strain of S aureus that causes diffuse skin erythema and blistering in young children. Hospital outbreaks are common. The blisters are caused by the toxin, not the bacteria, and are followed by skin exfoliation. A first-generation cephalosporin or clindamycin may be used for treatment. Staphylococcal scalded skin syndrome is distinguishable from the similar TEN because the latter involves mucus membranes and is usually drug induced. Toxic shock syndrome (TSS) is caused by toxin-producing S aureus strains that cause fever, rash, and hypotensive shock. A scarlatiniform erythroderma develops with a strawberry tongue followed by skin desquamation. While first associated with superabsorbent tampons, TSS may occur with nasal packing or indeed any toxin-producing staphylococcal infection. A streptococcal shock syndrome has also been identified.

Corynebacterial Kytococcus *Skin Infections*

Erythrasma *(Corynebacterium minutissimum)* is a superficial gram-positive bacterial skin infection closely resembling tinea but distinguishable by a coral-red fluorescence on Wood lamp examination. It usually appears as an asymptomatic scaly red-brown patch, often in the groin or axilla. Topical antibiotics, such as erythromycin and clindamycin, are effective, as are oral antibiotics. Another corynebacterial infection is trichomycosis axillaris *(C tenuis),* which causes yellowish axillary or pubic hair nodules and reddish perspiration. Treatment involves shaving the infected hair. Pitted keratolysis was formerly considered a corynebacterial infection but is now reclassified as *Kytococcus (Micrococcus) sedentarius.* Topical antibiotics (ie, erythromycin, clindamycin, or mupirocin) are curative, but the condition can also be controlled with aluminum chloride antiperspirants.

Bartonella *Skin Infections*

Bartonella species are gram-negative bacteria that may cause cat scratch disease, bacillary angiomatosis, trench fever, and Carrion disease (including Oroya fever and verruga peruana). *Bartonella henselae* causes cat scratch disease. A small papule soon develops at the scratch site (usually from a kitten) and is followed by enlargement of regional lymph nodes, which occasionally become fluctuant. Cat scratch disease is self-limited in immune-competent children and lymph nodes usually start to subside after several months. Azithromycin or ciprofloxacin are recommended for at least 1 month in immunocompromised patients.[10]

In immunocompromised patients, usually with AIDS, *B henselae* (from cat fleas) and *B quintana* (from lice) may cause bacillary angiomatosis, which presents as purplish, 1 to 2 cm skin papules. Biopsy distinguishes these from Kaposi sarcoma and pyogenic granulomas. The lesions resolve with prolonged erythromycin or doxycycline treatment.

Trench or shinbone fever is caused by *B quintana* and is spread by lice. It is currently associated with homelessness but was also common in wartime. High fever recurring about every 5 days (fifth day is quintana) is associated with leg shin pain and a central maculopapular rash (80%). Tetracycline or chloramphenicol are quickly curative.[10]

Bartonellosis may manifest as a severe, often fatal hematogenous infection, termed Oroya fever, or as a milder cutaneous eruption known as verruga peruana (Peruvian wart). Both of the hematogenous and cutaneous manifestations of infection are now recognized as different manifestations of the same disease. It is named after Peruvian medical student Daniel Carrión, who died from Oroya fever after a friend inoculated him with material from a wart, thereby proving these 2 conditions were linked. The disease is spread by *Lutzomyia* sandfly bites, which take several months to become symptomatic. Oroya fever is characterized by fever, headache, arthralgia, and hemolytic anemia, which persist for 2 to 4 weeks and are often fatal without treatment. Peripheral blood smears show the bacteria inside red blood cells. Verruga peruana is an angiomatous eruption on the extremities of children and may take 3 forms: miliar (multiple small, reddish papules), nodular (larger, skin-covered nodules), and mular (larger but open nodules). It is best diagnosed by biopsy with Warthin-Starry staining. Both manifestations of Carrion disease can be treated with ciprofloxacin.[23]

Cutaneous Anthrax

Cutaneous anthrax is a gram-positive, spore-forming infection of herbivores that incidentally infects humans. Contact with spores on infected hides or meat is the usual source of infection, although bioterrorism has become an additional concern. Most cases are the cutaneous form starting as a malignant pustule that turns into a black eschar surrounded by non-pitting edema. The lesion usually heals in 2 to 6 weeks with scarring; however, 20% of treated lesions may turn into a systemic fatal bacteremia.[24] The oropharyngeal and inhalation forms of anthrax are usually fatal without prompt therapy. A Gram stain from the ulcer documents anthrax bacteria, which can also be readily cultured. Ciprofloxacin is the usual therapy if bioterrorism is suspected, but penicillin or doxycycline is effective for usual cases. A military vaccination is available, although it is not licensed for commercial use.

Meningococcemia

Meningococcemia is a flu-like, frequently fatal illness with headache, fever, nausea, and a grayish or purpuric petechial rash; the rash occurs in half to two thirds of patients. The neck may be stiff in only half of patients at the time of initial presentation. A transient nonspecific maculopapular exanthem, very different from the petechial rash, may also appear for 1 or 2 days.

Meningitis is spread via droplet contact by *Neisseria meningitidis,* a gram-negative diplococcus with 5 different serogroups: A, B, C, Y, and W-135. Outbreaks in the African meningitis belt occur in the dry season (December through June) and are mostly due to serogroup A (or sometimes C). Outbreaks in Asia are usually serogroup A and recent outbreaks related to the Hajj religious pilgrimage were W-135. Serogroup B tends to be more common in higher-income nations because it is not amenable to prevention through vaccination. Two conjugate quadrivalent meningitis vaccines (Menactra and Menveo) are now available and recommended for travelers to areas of risk, military recruits, and freshman college students.

Ceftriaxone treatment should be started even while arranging for lumbar puncture because deterioration with fatal shock may occur extremely rapidly. Intravenous penicillin G is the standard treatment once diagnosis is confirmed. Cultures will likely be positive if cerebrospinal fluid (CSF) is obtained within an hour of antibiotic administration.[25] Prophylaxis for close contacts is usually with ciprofloxacin or rifampin.

Melioidosis

Melioidosis *(Burkholderia pseudomallei)* is a Southeast Asian gram-negative infection that is usually acquired from soil or water. It is especially common in rice paddy workers but is often subclinical in healthy patients. Diabetics and immunocompromised patients are likely to become very ill with fever, anemia, and jaundice. Subcutaneous abscesses or pustules develop in 10% to 20%, and children are likely to develop a parotid abscess. Treatment is with amoxicillin-clavulanate or ceftazidime.[26]

Erysipeloid

Erysipeloid *(Erysipelothrix rhusiopathiae)* is a gram-positive bacterial infection that closely resembles erysipelas, a streptococcal infection. Within a week of handling infected meat or shellfish, a painful, violet-red, well-demarcated hand rash develops. Occasionally erysipeloid is complicated by systemic infection with endocarditis. Treatment is with systemic antibiotics such as penicillin, erythromycin, or doxycycline. Untreated cases usually resolve spontaneously.

Tropical Ulcer

Tropical ulcer (phagedenic ulcer) is a bacterial ulceration of the lower extremity caused by poor hygiene and malnutrition in moist tropical areas. In the initial stages the ulcer is quite painful and foul smelling, with 2 organisms usually found: *Fusobacterium fusiformis* and *Borrelia vincentii*. The round or oval ulcer passes through acute, subacute, and chronic stages; in the chronic stage it may be painless with a mixed bacterial flora. The edges are not undermined as they are in Buruli ulcer. Although healing eventually occurs with proper care with antibiotics and nutrition, many of these ulcers require skin grafting and some develop osteomyelitis or malignancies (Marjolin ulcer).

Noma

Noma (cancrum oris) is a rare gangrenous anaerobic infection of the mouth and cheek that is associated with *Fusobacterium* and *Borrelia*. Like the phagedenic ulcer, this disease only occurs with malnutrition and starts with a painful lesion that soon ulcerates. Periodontal disease, poor hygiene, and malnutrition (often exacerbated by a recent infection) appear to be necessary prerequisites. Antibiotics, surgical debridement, nutritional support, and reconstructive surgery are essential if the patient is to survive.

Noma neonatorum is a gangrenous *Pseudomonas aeruginosa* infection of the face or anogenital area of low birth weight infants. It may be a form of ecthyma gangrenosum.

Treponemal Infections (Spirochetes)

Syphilis

Syphilis, the best-known treponemal infection, is a sexually transmitted infection with primary (chancre), secondary (latent), and tertiary stages. The syphilis rash is polymorphic with multiple presentations that can mimic many other conditions. Children become infected through maternal-fetal transmission. Other tropical treponemal infections, such as pinta and yaws, are non-venereal.

Congenital Syphilis

Congenital syphilis *(Treponema pallidum)* is maternal syphilis transmitted via placenta to the fetus. Although many babies with this condition are stillborn, two thirds of surviving newborns appear normal at delivery but become ill several months later. The syphilitic umbilical cord may be streaked with red, white, and blue colors (a barber pole cord). Early congenital syphilis (up to 2 years of age) is characterized by hepatosplenomegaly, fever, rhinitis ("snuffles"), and rash. The infectious rash is similar to secondary syphilis in adults with a papulosquamous pink eruption often involving the palms and soles (which are often red and shiny) and later fading to a more coppery brown color. The plantar spots may blister (syphilitic pemphigus). Other lesions include genital condyloma lata, mucous patches around the lips (later forming scar-like fissures termed rhagades or Parrot lines), skin desquamation, and severe diaper rash. Late congenital syphilis (after 2 years) is characterized by various stigmata such as Hutchinson incisors (notched, peg-like front teeth), mulberry molars (malformed lower first molars), and paroxysmal cold hemoglobinuria (dark urine and chills after cold exposure). The classic but uncommon Hutchinson triad is Hutchinson incisors, interstitial keratitis, and eighth nerve deafness. Saber shins, saddle nose, frontal skull bossing, Higoumenakia sign (thickened inner third of clavicles), gemmae, and mental retardation are other signs of late congenital disease.[27] Maternal screening and treatment for syphilis should be routine. Suspected newborns should be screened with serum and CSF-Venereal Disease Research Laboratory tests. Parenteral penicillin G is the treatment of choice.

Pinta

Pinta *(Treponema carateum)* is a rare non-venereal treponemal infection found in isolated indigenous peoples in Central and South America. The disease is spread by skin contact. In primary pinta, red papules at inoculation sites develop into erythematous, scaly plaques that may resemble psoriasis. Pintids (multiple scaly reddish papules later enlarging into multicolored scaly plaques) develop in the secondary stage. In tertiary pinta (2 to 5 years postinfection), abnormal skin pigmentation develops over bony prominences with spotty areas of hypopigmentation. The painted appearance is responsible for the Spanish name. Syphilis serology is positive in pinta cases. Penicillin is the treatment of choice.

Yaws

Yaws *(Treponema pertenue)* is a more widespread non-venereal infection spread by skin contact. It usually starts in childhood and, like other treponemal infections, has primary, secondary, and tertiary stages. A papular mother yaw occurs at the inoculation site and develops satellite lesions before ulcerating and healing months later. The secondary stage (framboesiform yaws) begins with multiple smaller daughter yaws or framboesias (from their resemblance to raspberries). A rash on the palms and soles develops into painful fissures and a crab-like gait (crab yaws). Destructive skin and bone lesions (gemmae) develop in the uncommon tertiary stage. Diagnosis and treatment is the same as for syphilis.

Lyme Disease

Lyme disease *(Borrelia burgdorferi)* is a spirochetal infection spread through the bite of tiny *Ixodes* (deer or black-legged) ticks, although the tick bite is often not recalled. Ticks must be attached for 24 hours to transmit the disease and routine antibiotic prophylaxis for tick bites is not recommended. Lyme disease is common in the United States, Europe, and North Asia. The characteristic erythema migrans rash starts with a red papule at the site of the bite that enlarges into a red, round patch. As the patch continues to expand it often develops central clearing before gradually fading. Multiple patches can be present in this early localized Lyme disease, but serologic testing results at this stage may still be negative.

In early disseminated disease, headache, myalgias, arthralgias, lymphadenopathy, and Bell palsy (seventh cranial nerve paralysis) may develop. Arthritis, meningitis, and myocarditis with heart block are more serious Lyme sequelae. Late disease is characterized by arthritis (often knees), encephalitis, or neuropathy. Lyme antibody testing results are positive in disseminated disease. Treatment of Lyme disease is with doxycycline for 14 to 21 days in children older than 8 years. Younger children are treated with amoxicillin, erythromycin, or clarithromycin. Late disease with arthritis or encephalitis should be treated with ceftriaxone for 21 days.[10]

Rickettsial Diseases

Rickettsiae are obligate, intracellular gram-negative bacteria. Rickettsial infections are traditionally divided into spotted and typhus fevers.

Spotted Fevers

Rocky Mountain Spotted or Brazilian Spotted Fever

Rocky Mountain spotted fever or Brazilian spotted fever is caused by *Rickettsia rickettsii*. Despite its name, RMSF is most common in the southeastern United States in spring and summer when it is spread by dog ticks *(Dermacentor)*. The same disease occurs in Central and South America and is known in Brazil as Brazilian spotted fever. A classic triad of fever, headache, and rash occurs within 1 to 2 weeks of tick bite but may not be evident early in the infection. Unfortunately, many patients fail to recall a tick bite, which makes diagnosis even more difficult. The centripetal rash (red, blanching macules or papules) begins on the extremities 2 to 3 days after the start of symptoms and spreads centrally before turning into petechial macules. About 10% of cases lack any rash. An indirect fluorescent antibody (IFA) test is positive 10 to 14 days postinfection, but empirical treatment with doxycycline for 7 to 10 days (or until afebrile for 3 days) is usually necessary while awaiting confirmation. Rocky Mountain spotted fever is an exception to the rule that doxycycline be avoided in children younger than 8 years because risk of this potentially fatal disease far outweighs the small risk of dental staining.

Mediterranean Spotted or Boutonneuse Fever

Mediterranean spotted or boutonneuse fever *(Rickettsia conorii)* is spread by the brown dog tick *(Rhipicephalus sanguineus)* in Mediterranean countries, North Africa, the Middle East, and India. The site of the bite develops a small, 1 cm black eschar or tache noire. Fever, headache, and an eventual centripetal spotted rash occur in most patients. Thrombocytopenia is common. As in RMSF, IFA serology confirms the diagnosis and doxycycline is the best treatment.

North Asian Tick Typhus, Queensland Tick Typhus, and Oriental Spotted Fever

North Asian tick typhus *(R siberica)*, Queensland tick typhus *(R australis)*, and oriental spotted fever *(R japonica)* are similar tick-borne rickettsial infections with headache, myalgias, fever, eschar(s), and centripetal spotted rash best treated with doxycycline.

Rickettsialpox

Rickettsialpox *(R akari)* is spread by biting mites that normally feed off house mice. A papule, soon to be an eschar, develops at the site of the bite, followed a week later by fever and generalized papulovesicular rash (papules with central vesicles) for 1 to 2 weeks. Rickettsialpox may resemble chickenpox, but bite eschars and the lack of giant cells distinguish this infection. The infection is self-limited but may be treated with doxycycline for 2 to 5 days (brief 2-day courses in children). Rodent control prevents outbreaks.

Epidemic, Murine, and Scrub Typhus

Epidemic Typhus

Epidemic typhus *(R prowazekii)* is spread by body lice infestations, commonly in crowded refugee populations or in wartime. The organism multiplies in the louse gut (eventually killing it) and is excreted in its feces. Scratching introduces typhus into the bites. Contact with southern flying squirrels, an animal reservoir, may also cause sporadic cases of typhus. Headache, fever, and an erythematous macular or petechial rash (developing around the fifth day) are key symptoms. Unlike spotted fevers, the centrifugal rash of typhus develops on the trunk and spreads to the extremities, sparing the palms and soles. Most cases resolve in 2 weeks, but vasculitis and gangrene are potential complications. Brill-Zinsser disease is a milder form of recurrent typhus, sometimes occurring many years later. Polymerase chain reaction (PCR) testing is now the preferred method of diagnosis, replacing the older, less-specific

Weil-Felix agglutination reaction.[28] Treatment for typhus is doxycycline 200 mg once daily for 5 days. Doxycycline can also be used as prophylaxis in an outbreak until delousing removes the source of infection.

Murine or Endemic Typhus

Murine or endemic typhus *(R typhi)* is a milder, worldwide form of typhus spread by fleas. In the United States, cases occur in southern California and Texas. Infected flea droppings are inoculated into bites by scratching. Fever, headache, nausea, and a maculopapular, usually truncal, rash (less than 50%) develop 1 to 2 weeks after flea contact. Treatment is similar to that of typhus.

Scrub Typhus

Scrub typhus *(Orientia tsutsugamushi)* is an Asian typhus that is spread by infected trombiculid mites (chiggers). A papule develops at the chigger bite evolving into an eschar with regional lymphadenopathy. Fever, headache, and a maculopapular truncal (centripetal) rash follow. Neurologic symptoms (eg, obtunded mental state, deafness), meningitis, and vasculitis may occur. Untreated cases may have a 50% mortality.[29] Travelers returning from endemic areas with headache, fever, and rash therefore warrant empiric treatment with doxycycline 200 mg per day for 14 days.

Q Fever

Q fever *(Coxiella burnetii)* is a widespread zoonotic infection from farm animals that is spread by inhaled aerosols. It recently received attention as a possible bioterrorism agent. Flu-like illness with fever and persisting malaise are the usual symptoms. While often undiagnosed and self-limited, Q fever may cause serious myocarditis or central nervous system involvement. A nonspecific variable rash may occur in 20% of cases. Diagnosis is by serology or PCR. Doxycycline or quinolone therapy is recommended.

Ehrlichiosis

Ehrlichiosis describes 2 different diseases with very similar symptoms: human monocytic ehrlichiosis (caused by *Ehrlichia chaffeensis)* and human granulocytic ehrlichiosis (caused by *Anaplasma phagocytophilia)*. Human monocytic ehrlichiosis is spread by the bite of the lone star tick in southeastern United States. Anaplasmosis or human granulocytic ehrlichiosis is spread by deer or dog ticks in much of the United States. Both diseases produce the usual rickettsial symptoms of fever, headache, fatigue, and nausea. Lymphopenia and thrombocytopenia are common. Human monocytic ehrlichiosis may be associated with hepatosplenomegaly and elevated liver tests. Rash is less common than in other rickettsial infections and is variable in appearance. Diagnosis, if accomplished, is often through paired serology (initial and recovery). Doxycycline is the usual therapy, although rifampin has been proposed for children.[30]

■ MYCOBACTERIAL INFECTIONS

Leprosy or Hansen Disease

Leprosy or Hansen disease *(Mycobacterium leprae)* is becoming rare, with more than 80% of cases occurring in just 6 countries: India (number 1), Brazil, Madagascar, Mozambique, Nepal, and Tanzania.[31] Much of the world's population (95%) appears to be naturally immune, with less than 1% truly susceptible.[32] Deficient cell-mediated immunity is associated with the development of illness. Cases are most common between 10 and 15 and 30 and 60 years of age. Spread is through airborne droplets or contact with skin lesions, but the incubation period may last many years. In addition to infected humans and primates, the 9-banded armadillo may host leprosy.

Ridley-Jopling classification divides leprosy into 5 subtypes depending on host immune response. From greater to lesser response, these include tuberculoid (TT), borderline tuberculoid (BT), borderline (BB), borderline lepromatous (BL), and lepromatous (LL) (Figure 26-1). Yet another category, indeterminate leprosy, presents with only a few hypopigmented lesions but no sensory loss or nerve hypertrophy. The World Health Organization (WHO) considers tuberculoid leprosy as paucibacillary (TT, BT) and borderline to lepromatous leprosy (BB, BL, LL) as multibacillary.

Tuberculoid leprosy has a high cell-mediated immunity and consequently few bacteria. It presents with fewer than 5 well-demarcated anesthetic hypopigmented or red plaques. Peripheral nerve enlargement is common. Borderline leprosy has more but less well-defined lesions with punched-out centers. Lepromatous leprosy, the leprosy of popular imagination, is associated with low cell-mediated immunity and high number of bacteria. Bilateral infiltration of the earlobes and facial skin create the so-called Leonine (lionlike) facies. Nasal destruction (saddle nose), neuropathy, inability to close the eyes (lagophthalmos), and multi-organ system involvement occur. Nosebleeds and nasal congestion are common. Motor and sensory neuropathy develop in all subtypes of untreated leprosy, resulting in a loss of sensation and repeated injury and infection, which cause the dreaded digit loss and deformities associated with the disease.

Figure 26-1. Ridley-Joplin Spectrum of Leprosy

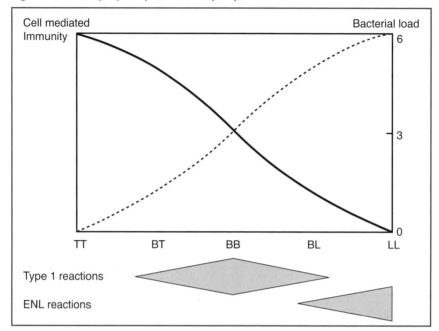

From Lockwood D. Leprosy. In: Warrell DA, Cox TM, Firth JD, Benz EJ, eds. *Oxford Textbook of Medicine.* 4th ed. Oxford, United Kingdom: Oxford University Press; 2003

The WHO definition of *leprosy* is a patient with one of the following conditions: an anesthetic skin lesion, a hypertrophic peripheral nerve, and positive skin slit smears (usually obtained from the earlobe). Punch biopsies of the lesion border are also helpful.

There are 4 reactions in leprosy that may occur before, during, or after treatment. Type 1, reversal or upgrading reaction, occurs in borderline (BT, BB, BL) leprosy when there is an increase in cell-mediated immune response. It usually occurs 6 to 12 months after starting therapy and presents with a hypersensitivity reaction (lesion redness and swelling or hand/foot edema, sometimes with nerve damage). Type 2 reaction, erythema nodosum leprosum, is caused by antigen antibody immune complexes in BL and LL. It produces multiple red papules or nodules, fever, myalgia, and hand/foot edema. Type 3 is a downgrading reaction caused by a loss in cell-mediated immunity marked by new lesions in untreated or non-adherent patients. Type 4, usually found in Mexico and Central America, is Lucio vasculitic reaction in untreated Lucio leprosy (diffuse lepromatous skin infiltration), which manifests as tender purpura (later ulcerating) on the extremities.

Leprosy treatment is with dapsone and rifampin per WHO recommendations. Paucibacillary disease is treated with dapsone 100 mg daily for 6 months and supervised monthly rifampin 600 mg for 6 months. Multibacillary disease is treated with daily dapsone 100 mg and clofazimine 50 mg and supervised monthly rifampin 600 mg and clofazimine 300 mg for 12 months. National Hansen's Disease Program recommendations are available for US cases.[32] Bacille Calmette-Guérin (BCG) vaccine appears to be partially protective against leprosy.

Tuberculosis Skin Manifestations

Cutaneous Tuberculosis Infection
Lupus vulgaris, describing infection of the skin, appears as soft red-brown papules that have a characteristic apple-jelly appearance when compressed by a glass slide (diascopy). It is slow growing, but papules can develop into plaques with time. *Mycobacterium tuberculosis* can also cause scrofuloderma, a painless cervical lymphadenopathy that drains through the skin. Treatment is the same as for uncomplicated pulmonary TB—isoniazid, rifampin, and pyrazinamide for 2 months, followed by isoniazid and rifampin for 4 months.

Tuberculid Hypersensitivity Reactions
Tuberculid hypersensitivity reactions include papulonecrotic tuberculid, erythema induratum of Bazin, and lichen scrofulosorum. All are characterized as inflammatory hypersensitivity reactions from the dissemination of TB to the skin. Tuberculids appear as red papules or nodules on elbows, knees, or buttocks that often ulcerate. Erythema induratum is a recurring reddish-purple panniculitis affecting posterior calves, which later heal as atrophic scars. Lichen scrofulosorum describes flattop, shiny, red-brown papules, usually on the trunk, associated with TB lymph node infection.

Mycobacterium Marinum
Mycobacterium marinum, an atypical TB organism usually affecting saltwater or freshwater fish, is frequently inoculated into minor wounds or abrasions. It is often acquired from fish tanks or ponds, hence the term *fish tank granuloma*. It starts as a firm red area that develops into a slow-growing reddish brown nodule that may later develop satellites or ulcerate. Hands, feet, and extensor surfaces are commonly affected. Diagnosis is usually through biopsy. Treatment is with prolonged doxycycline or rifampin (with or without ethambutol). Without treatment, the granuloma may take several years to resolve. Many other atypical

mycobacteria can cause similar skin lesions (ie, *M kansasii, M szulgai, M fortuitum-chelonae*) or cervical adenopathy (ie, *M avium-intracellulare, M scrofulaceum*).

Buruli Ulcer

Buruli ulcer *(M ulcerans)* is another atypical mycobacterium. It is a common cause of pediatric skin ulcers in West Africa and other humid tropical areas. A skin nodule often starts at a traumatized site and evolves into a painless ulcer with characteristically undermined borders. The ulcer enlarges and causes extensive scarring and deformity. Purified protein derivative skin testing results are often negative until the ulcer is healed. Although rifampin can help small lesions, most ulcers require surgical removal with skin grafting. Hyperthermic water baths or hyperbaric oxygen are experimental therapies.

Bacille Calmette-Guérin Reactions

In many countries, BCG, an attenuated strain of *M bovis*, is used in infants for the prevention of TB. As BCG is a live vaccine with variable regional strains, it may create larger than usual local ulcerations that may later be complicated by keloid formation. Erythema nodosum, a hypersensitivity reaction with red, tender nodules on the anterior legs, may occur after BCG, although streptococcal infections, drug reactions, and sarcoidosis are classically associated. BCG may occasionally spread to cause axillary lymphadenitis in an infant. Dactylitis (finger inflammation) is a rare complication.

■ FUNGAL SKIN INFECTIONS

Superficial

Tinea Infections (Ringworm)

Dermatophytic fungi can be classified as anthropophilic, geophilic, and zoophilic depending on whether they are acquired from people, soil, or animals. Anthropophilic species include *Trichophyton tonsurans* (by far the most common) and *Microsporum audouinii* (now rare due to treatment). Zoophilic species include *M canis* from pets and *T verrucosum* from cattle. These "alien" species provoke a more intense immune response. Classic scaly patches with central clearing and raised annular borders suggest the diagnosis, although it is occasionally confused with the herald patch of pityriasis rosea. Diagnosis is confirmed by seeing hyphae on microscopic examination of skin scrapings (best from the lesion border) with a drop of 20% KOH.

Tinea Capitis

Tinea capitis (scalp ringworm) is common in children. It forms scaly scalp patches with hair loss and may also involve the eyebrows and lashes. Black dot ringworm, wherein hairs break off at the surface, is caused by *T tonsurans* and *T violaceum*. Gray patch ringworm is caused by *M canis*. A Wood lamp causes *Microsporum* to fluoresce green, whereas *Trichosporum* does not. Potassium hydroxide examination can also help speciate the fungus by identifying hair shaft involvement—ectothrix (outside, as in *Microsporum)* or endothrix (inside, as in *T tonsurans).* Favic hair invasion causes air bubbles in the hair shaft. Kerion (inflamed boggy scalp) is usually due to zoophilic infection. Dandruff in young children is highly unusual, so ringworm should be suspected. Treatment is with an extended course of systemic antifungals, such as griseofulvin, fluconazole, or itraconazole.[33]

Tinea Corporis

Tinea corporis (body ringworm) affects the body and is most commonly caused by *T rubrum* and *T mentagrophytes*. Steroid therapy alters the classic appearance (tinea incognito). The ring-shaped lesions gradually expand outward. Treatment is with topical antifungal creams for several weeks. A tropical species, *T concentricum,* causes tinea imbricata, which produces annular concentric rings. Oral treatment with griseofulvin or terbinafine is necessary.

Tinea Cruris

Tinea cruris (jock itch) is tinea of the groin, usually in young men. Itching is a common symptom. It is occasionally confused with monilia *Candida* infection but unlike monilia, it never involves the scrotum. Treatment is with topical antifungals.

Tinea Pedis

Tinea pedis (athlete's foot) is a common cause of foot itching and odor by the same organisms that cause tinea corporis. Interdigital, moccasin-type, and vesicobullous presentations are known. Treatment is with topical antifungal creams and antiperspirants. Tinea pedis can be mimicked by pompholyx (dyshidrotic eczema) of the feet.

Onychomycosis

Onychomycosis (tinea unguium or nail fungus) causes unsightly thickened yellow or white nails, often due to *T rubrum,* although non-dermatophytes like *Candida* may also be involved. Distal nail involvement is much more common than the proximal subungual type. Proximal white superficial onychomycosis is often associated with immune deficiency. Psoriatic nail involvement can look similar to fungal infection except for characteristic pitting. Nail trauma can cause similar nail deformities. Fungal culture or 20% KOH nail scrapings confirm the diagnosis of onychomycosis. Daily oral terbinafine for 6 weeks (fingernails) or 12 weeks (toenails) is first-line therapy to clear this infection, although itraconazole and fluconazole are also effective.[34] Topical therapy usually fails to penetrate the nail matrix, but ciclopirox topical solution for 1 year may be considered if systemic therapy is not an option.

Candida *(Monilia) Infections*

Candida albicans and other *Candida* species are ubiquitous yeasts that cause a variety of skin infections. Scrapings of the lesions show pseudohyphae or budding yeast. Oral candidiasis (thrush) is mucous membrane involvement in infants or immunocompromised adults that appears as adherent white oral plaques. *Candida* diaper dermatitis is characterized by a red base (involving skin folds) and erythematous satellite pustules that differentiate it from more common irritant diaper dermatitis, which lacks these features. Intertrigo describes weeping erythematous yeast infections of moist skin folds. *Candida* vulvovaginitis is a curd-like white discharge with vaginal itching frequently following antibiotic therapy. Diabetics are particularly prone to recurrent infections. *Candida* balanitis describes tender red papules of the (usually) uncircumcised glans penis. Nail involvement (onychomycosis and paronychia) and perlèche (infections of the corners of the mouth where moisture accumulates) are other candidal syndromes. Treatment for *Candida* infections is with miconazole, ketoconazole, clotrimazole, or econazole creams, usually for 10 days. Terbinafine may be ineffective for yeast.[35] Fluconazole single-dose therapy is especially convenient for vaginal yeast infections.

Miscellaneous Fungal Infections

Pityriasis Versicolor

Pityriasis versicolor *(Malassezia furfur)* is a lipophilic yeast that colonizes the stratum corneum, producing scaly hypopigmented or hyperpigmented macules that often coalesce. *M pachydermatis* of animals can also infect humans. This unsightly fungal condition is widespread in young people, especially in humid, warm climates. The fungus is more conspicuous in summer months because it inhibits tanning. Skin scrapings (with added potassium hydroxide) show characteristic clumps of spores and hyphae, the classic spaghetti-and-meatball pattern. Treatment is with antifungal creams (ie, terbinafine 1%, ketoconazole 2%, or fluconazole 2%) or selenium sulfide lotion. Unfortunately, this yeast appears to survive in the pores and eventually recurs. Oral ketoconazole 200 mg as a 2-tablet single dose (or fluconazole 300 mg with a repeated dose in 2 weeks) is therefore even more effective.[36]

Piedra

Piedra is a tropical fungal hair infection that comes in black and white varieties. Black piedra *(Piedraia hortae)* produces black, firmly adherent nodules on the hair shaft. White piedra *(Trichosporon beigelii)* produces white lesions, somewhat similar to lice nits, which are easy to remove. Cutting the hair is usually curative and no medication is required.

Tinea Nigra Palmaris

Tinea nigra palmaris *(Hortae werneckii)* is another tropical or subtropical fungus presenting as a brown, stain-like macule affecting the palms or soles, and occasionally on the neck or trunk. It also has been reported in the southeast United States. It is easily treated with one of the azole antifungal creams or Whitfield ointment (6% salicylic acid, 12% benzoic acid).

Subcutaneous Fungal Infections

Sporotrichosis

Sporotrichosis *(Sporothrix schenckii)* is a saprophytic fungus that can be inoculated into wounds by minor trauma. Rose thorn injuries and working with sphagnum moss are classically associated. A nodular inoculation chancre develops at the site, which is sometimes followed by a line of other nodules that develop along superficial lymphatics (lymphocutaneous sporotrichosis). Biopsy identifies the fungus. Treatment is with a saturated solution of potassium hydroxide given orally for 2 to 3 months. Children use half the adult dose.

Mycetoma or Madura Foot

Mycetoma or Madura foot is a chronic tropical infection from actinomycetes (filamentous bacteria, including *Nocardia* and others) or various fungi *(Madurella* and others) that is introduced into tissue by traumatic inoculation. Rural farmers are commonly affected. Nodules and draining fistulae appear in the extremity, followed by a tumorlike swelling (mycetoma). Drainage granules enable identification of the specific actinomycete, and culture may identify the fungus. Treatment depends on the organism involved and is lengthy and complex. *Nocardia* is treated with sulfamethoxazole-trimethoprim for 2 to 3 years. Fungal Madura foot (eumycetoma) is even more difficult to treat with current protocols, including itraconazole (or ketoconazole) for 1 to 2 years, surgery, and topical negative-pressure therapy.[37]

Chromoblastomycosis

Chromoblastomycosis is a third fungal infection introduced by skin trauma, usually to the legs. Dematiaceous (black mold) saprophytic fungi produce a plaque at the inoculation site that later enlarges into a warty growth. Diagnosis is by biopsy or microscopic examination of the exudate, which shows classic thick-walled (muriform) fungal cells. Treatment is difficult and early lesions should be excised. Prolonged azole or terbinafine antifungal therapy yields unpredictable results.

Lobomycosis

Lobomycosis *(Lacazia loboi)* is a very rare Amazonian fungal disease presenting with impressive keloid-like nodules. Diagnosis is confirmed by biopsy, but there is no effective treatment besides excision. It has also been found in dolphins and nonhuman primates.[38]

Systemic Fungal Infections

Systemic fungal infections include histoplasmosis, North American blastomycosis, South American blastomycosis (paracoccidioidomycosis), coccidioidomycosis, and penicilliosis marneffei, an opportunistic infection of AIDS patients in Southeast Asia. Most produce various granulomatous skin lesions in addition to systemic disease but are beyond the scope of this chapter.

■ PARASITIC INFECTIONS

Endoparasites

Leishmaniasis

The term leishmaniasis *(Leishmania)* describes cutaneous, mucocutaneous, and visceral diseases caused by obligate intracellular protozoan parasites. There exists a confusing array of Old and New World *Leishmania* species. The vector is sandflies—*Phlebotomus* in the Old World or *Lutzomyia* in the New World.

Cutaneous leishmaniasis (CL) is known by multiple names depending on geographic location—uta, bay sore, oriental sore, Baghdad boil, and Chiclero ulcer. A papule develops at the site of the sandfly bite, followed by a persistent shallow ulcer with raised margins. In Asia, CL may present as wet ulcers (the oriental sore of *L major)* or crusted dry ulcers *(L tropica)*. Chiclero ulcer develops on the ears of rubber tappers working in New World jungles. Occasionally these ulcers may develop an atypical (eg, lichenoid, nodular, impetiginous) appearance, making diagnosis more difficult. Untreated lesions usually heal with scarring, but this takes many months and certain species may recur to involve the mucus membranes.

Mucocutaneous leishmaniasis (MCL), sometimes known as espundia, is a much more invasive infection that causes facial ulcerations and deformities (eg, tapir nose). New World species such as *L (Viannia) braziliensis* are most often associated with espundia, sometimes many years after the initial cutaneous infection resolves, with the presenting symptoms usually being nasal congestion and bleeding.[39] Diagnosis of CL and MCL is usually from biopsy of the ulcer margin.

Visceral leishmaniasis (kala-azar or black disease or fever in Hindi) is less important for this chapter, as it often lacks dermatologic features. Only some patients develop the darkened skin on the abdomen and extremities that gives this disease its name. It is usually treated with miltefosine in south Asia due to widespread antimonial resistance there.

Treatment of CL and MCL depends on the extent of lesions and the causative organism. Many ulcers eventually heal without therapy. Multiple or persistent lesions warrant pentavalent antimony compounds, eg, sodium stibogluconate (IV or intramuscular) for 20 days. Treatment is also indicated for *L braziliensis* and related New World forms associated with mucocutaneous disease. Intralesional pentavalent antimony, heat, pentamidine, and paromomycin sulfate ointment (available in Israel for *L major)* are alternative regimens.[40] Leishmaniasis is amenable to prevention through vaccination, but no commercial vaccine is currently available.

Filarial Infections

Filarial infections are blood and tissue nematode infections that have specific skin manifestations. Insect vectors spread the disease. The adult filarial worms inhabit the host lymphatics or subcutaneous tissue. Their progeny, termed microfilaria, are transmitted to other people via insect bites or, in the case of *Dracunculus,* by ingesting infected water fleas.

Onchocerciasis

Onchocerciasis is popularly known as African river blindness, crawcraw, or sowda. It is prevalent in West Africa and localized areas of Latin America, where it is known to produce eye inflammation leading to blindness. The vector is the blackfly *Simulium,* which breeds near streams. Adult worms inhabit subcutaneous nodules called onchocer-coma. The microfilaria are found in subcutaneous tissue, where they produce chronic itching and atrophic skin changes (eg, depigmentation of the shins, hanging groin), and in the anterior chamber of the eye (where they are visible with slit lamp examination). Skin snips from the iliac crest area are placed in saline to examine for characteristic micro-filariae. Ivermectin kills the microfilariae but not the adults, requiring periodic re-treatment to control or prevent symptoms.[41] There is risk of encephalitis from ivermectin if coinfected with *Loa loa*. Adjunctive ther-apy with doxycycline 100 mg daily for 6 weeks kills *Wolbachia* bacteria required for *Onchocerca* fertility.

Loa Loa

Loa loa is a West African filarial nematode that migrates through the subcutaneous tissue. It is known as the African eye worm because it occasionally appears beneath the conjunctiva of the eye, causing tempo-rary eye irritation and conjunctivitis. The vector is the *Chrysops* deer or antelope fly. *Loa loa* microfilariae are active in the blood stream by day (when the vector is biting) but retreat into the lymphatics at night. The identification of loa microfilaria on a blood smear confirms the diagno-sis. Skin manifestations are Calabar or fugitive swellings that appear to be localized allergic reactions to the migrating worm. Treatment is with diethylcarbamazine (DEC) with escalating doses and steroids to prevent encephalopathy from dying microfilariae.[42] However, because of the rar-ity of this condition in the United States, DEC is only available from the CDC. Excision of adult worms, when visible, is also an option, although there may be 4 to 6 adult worms in the average patient.

Elephantiasis

Elephantiasis (lymphatic filariasis) describes lymphatic obstruction produced by *Wuchereria bancrofti* or *Brugia malayi* filarial worms. Both are transmitted by several species of night-feeding mosquitoes, so the microfilariae are present in the blood only at night. Adult worms residing in the lymphatics result in inflammation followed by obstruc-tion and lymphedema of the scrotum or leg. The term *elephantiasis* refers to the elephant-like skin changes and swelling of the extremity. Podoconiosis (non-filarial elephantiasis) is a similar-appearing condition caused by lymphatic scarring from chronic silicate exposure in barefoot people. It is preventable by wearing shoes. Treatment of true filariasis is accomplished with cautious use of DEC for 3 weeks. Unfortunately, this treatment will not undo prior damage, so later procedures to improve lymphatic drainage and surgical reduction may be necessary.

Dracunculiasis

Dracunculiasis (guinea worm) is a tissue infection by *Dracunculus medinensis* found in Africa and (previously) South Asia. The adult worm resides in the subcutaneous tissues of an extremity. When female worms mature (after about 1 year), they protrude to form a painful subcutaneous nodule. Intense burning at this site causes the patient to immerse the lesion in water and this, in turn, stimulates the female to release her larvae. Copepods (water fleas) consume these and people inadvertently ingest the infected fleas in drinking water, thus completing the cycle. Fortunately, humans are the only host and the cycle is easily interrupted by filtering copepods out of drinking water with cheesecloth. Guinea worm is on the verge of eradication and only persists in remote African areas, particularly in Sudan and Nigeria. Treatment is manually extracting the worm by coiling it around a matchstick at the rate of 2 to 5 mm per day.

Trypanosomiasis

African Trypanosomiasis

African trypanosomiasis (African sleeping sickness) is primarily a neurologic disease caused by *Trypanosoma brucei* and is transmitted by the tsetse fly (glossina). There are 2 forms, *T brucei gambiense* of West Africa and the more virulent *T brucei rhodesiense* of East Africa. The bite of an infected tsetse fly produces a boil-like trypanosomal chancre within 48 hours, especially with the East African variety. Fever, headache, and transient papular rashes follow the waves of parasitemia. Posterior cervical adenopathy (Winterbottom sign) develops in the West African variety. Psychiatric symptoms are also common. The final stages of the disease involve meningoencephalitis and coma. Treatment is complex, depending on the type (West or East African) and stage (early or late) of the infection.[42]

South American Trypanosomiasis

South American trypanosomiasis (Chagas disease) is found in rural Central and South America. *Trypanosoma cruzi* is transmitted by reduviid or kissing bugs *(Triatoma* or *Rhodnius)* that reside in the palm thatch or cracked walls of substandard housing. These bloodsucking insects defecate near their bite and the infection is inoculated into the wound by scratching. A few cases have been transmitted by drinking asai (palm fruit) juice contaminated by these insects.[43] If the eye is the site of inoculation, unilateral periorbital swelling occurs (Romana sign). Other sites of infection result in chagomas, furuncle-like lesions at the inoculation site, usually with regional lymphadenopathy. After a latent period, cardiac, esophageal, and intestinal disease (megacolon) develop. Treatment is with benznidazole or nifurtimox for several months.[42]

Cutaneous Larva Migrans

Cutaneous larva migrans (CLM) (creeping eruption) is mostly caused by *Ancylostoma braziliense,* the dog or cat hookworm, although other parasites and migratory myiasis occasionally produce a similar picture. The infection is often acquired while walking barefoot on a beach where dogs have defecated. The hookworm larva penetrates the skin, causing considerable itching, and then creates a serpiginous wandering track under the skin. Cutaneous larva migrans is self-limited in humans because the parasite cannot escape from the skin and eventually dies. The clinical appearance is diagnostic. Usual treatment is with oral mebendazole, albendazole, or ivermectin. Thiabendazole ointment is very effective if it can be locally compounded.[44] Single lesions can sometimes be cured with cryotherapy if this is directed ahead of the advancing margin.

Ectoparasites and Insect Bites and Stings

Scabies or Itch Mite

Scabies or itch mite *(Sarcoptes scabiei)* is a common human infestation that causes intense itching, particularly at night. The female mite burrows into the stratum corneum, producing a hypersensitivity reaction with characteristic burrows, papules, and excoriations. Finger webs, the flexor aspect of wrists, axillae, breasts, belt line, buttocks, and genitals (where it often appears as a nodular variant) are common areas of involvement. Infants often develop scabies papules on the palms and soles. The face is usually spared, except in infants. Scabies is easily spread through any skin contact, often as a sexually transmitted infection. Thus, it is important to treat sexual partners and any close contacts. Crusted scabies is a severe, highly infectious form often found in institutionalized or immunocompromised patients. Sarcoptic mites from dogs or other animals (the cause of mange) may cause itching but are unable to reproduce on human hosts.

Careful skin inspection may reveal characteristic burrows, but these are often obscured by excoriation. A wash of diluted india ink painted over affected skin will help visualize burrows. Microscopic examination of scrapings obtained from the end of the burrow with a number 15 blade usually reveals mites or their eggs and feces.

Treatment is usually with permethrin 5% cream applied over the entire body from the neck down and left on overnight. The cream is showered off the next morning and all bedding and clothing must be washed. Treatment is ideally repeated in 7 to 14 days to ensure eradication.[45] A similar regimen with gamma-benzene hexachloride lotion (lindane) is more toxic and is being abandoned for safety and environmental reasons. It is contraindicated in infants and pregnancy. Under less unhygienic conditions, oral ivermectin 200 μg/kg may be given as a single dose and, if possible, repeated in 2 weeks.[46] This off-label use of ivermectin for scabies is safe in patients without concomitant filarial infection. With any of these treatments, itching from the dead mites persists for 1 to 2 weeks posttreatment.

Pediculosis

Pediculosis (lice) describes an infestation by bloodsucking insects that include head or body lice (both subspecies of *Pediculus humanis)* or crab lice *(Pthirus pubis)*. Itching is the primary symptom. Head lice are the most common and are usually diagnosed by nits (eggs), which are most evident on hairs behind the ears or on the nape of the neck. African head lice are adapted to flat hair shafts, whereas their European cousins prefer round hair shafts. This explains why African American children are often spared head lice in the United States, where the European variety predominates. Nits hatch within 1 week and lice mature in 15 days. Nits further out on the hair shaft (more than 5 mm from scalp) are usually nonviable and no-nit school policies are unnecessary.[47]

Crab lice are spread through sexual contact affecting pubic and body hair. In addition to nits, an associated skin finding is maculae caeruleae (blue spots), which probably represents hemosiderin deposits. Body lice are uncommon except in conditions of poverty. Nits are deposited on the clothing instead of body hair.

Topical treatment is with pyrethrins, synthetic pyrethroids (permethrin), gamma-benzene hexachloride (lindane), and 50% isopropyl myristate (Resultz). The latter treatment damages the louse exoskeleton, causing dehydration. Shaving the scalp is useful but nit combs, used after a vinegar rinse, are an alternative. Malathion 0.5% lotion application (Ovide) applied for 8 hours is a more toxic second-line therapy for resistant infections approved for children older than 6 years. Ivermectin also seems to work at the same dosage as for scabies. All family members and close contacts should be treated, even if asymptomatic.

Because of increasing resistance to pyrethrins, newer treatments such as spinosad (Natroba), benzyl alcohol (Ulesfia), or heat (LouseBuster) are gaining popularity.

Other Insects

Fleas include the human flea *(Pulex irritans)* and dog and cat fleas *(Ctenocephalides canis, C felis)*. Pruritic ankle papules from fleabites are the usual presentation. Fleas occasionally act as vectors for plague and endemic typhus. Flea traps and sprays, oral and systemic flea treatments for pets, and topical insect repellents are all effective.

The chigoe or jigger flea *(Tunga penetrans)* is a burrowing flea found in tropical South America, Africa, and south Asia. The female burrows between the toes or on the feet, producing an inflamed pea-sized nodule in which she produces eggs. Sometimes, small white eggs may be seen being extruded from these lesions. The nodules frequently become secondarily infected. Treatment consists of removing the lesion and updating tetanus if necessary.[45]

Myiasis

Myiasis describes infection by human botfly larvae. Perhaps the best known species is *Dermatobia hominis,* the common botfly of Central and South America. This fly captures biting insects, attaches its eggs to them, and releases the insects to find new animal or human hosts. When eggs reach their destination, the larvae hatch, penetrate the skin, and create small furuncles, each having a tiny central breathing pore. In Africa, the tumbu *(Cordylobia anthropophaga)* lays its eggs on clothing hung out to dry. The eggs hatch once the clothing is worn, after which they develop into numerous furuncles. Fortunately, ironing clothes will kill the eggs. This species produces multiple furuncles that mature in 2 to 3 weeks, whereas *Dermatobia* lesions are few but last 6 weeks. The African Lund's fly *(C rhodaini)* places its eggs on the ground, where they infest the feet. The Congo floor maggot does not burrow but feeds on humans sleeping on dirt floors at night.

Patients often report a crawling sensation with furuncular myiasis. Surgical excision is an option, but this can be facilitated by first applying Vaseline over the furuncle. This occludes the larvae spiracle (breathing apparatus), forcing it to partially emerge. Applying raw bacon or fatback over the furuncle causes larva to migrate upward, facilitating easy removal with forceps a few hours later.[45]

Chigger Bites

Chigger bites are caused by larval trombiculid mites or red bugs *(Trombicula alfreddugesi)* that inject an irritant when they bite. Lesions are usually large, itchy papules that develop on areas where clothing is tight, such as sock and belt lines. Straw itch mites and avian mites can produce similar lesions. Treatment is symptomatic.

Insect Bites

Insect bites (eg, bedbugs, mosquitoes, sandflies, gnats, blackflies, deer-flies, horseflies) appear as erythematous itchy papules, often with a central punctum. Bedbugs *(Cimex lectularius)* are oval, 3 to 5 mm flat reddish-brown insects that feed at night, producing itchy papules. Often there are several lesions in a row—the classic breakfast, lunch, and dinner sign. Tropical bedbugs *(Cimex hemipterus)* are longer insects but otherwise similar. Although there has been much speculation that these insects could act as disease vectors, clinical evidence for this is lack-ing, although some may be colonized with antibiotic-resistant bacteria. Lesion treatment is symptomatic, but eradication to prevent further bites is essential.[48]

Insect bites are treated with cool compresses, oral antihistamines, and stronger steroid creams. Prevention is with insect repellents ideally con-taining DEET 30% or picaridin 20%.[49] Both are applied to exposed skin and are safe in children older than 2 months (avoiding the hands and lips). Permethrin 0.5% spray (Permanone) may be applied to clothing to repel ticks and insects.

Insect Stings

Insect *(Hymenoptera)* stings from bees *(Apidae)*, wasps, hornets and yellow jackets *(Vespidae)*, and stinging ants *(Formicidae)* produce an immediate reaction with a painful papule that usually resolves within a few hours. Cold compresses, sometimes with baking soda or papain meat tenderizer, are used with variable success. Calamine lotion and oral antihistamines also help. Late-phase local hypersensitivity reactions closely resemble cellulitis with a red, warm area appearing around the sting site within 48 hours and lasting up to a week. Local hypersensitivity reactions are best treated with oral steroids or antihistamines rather than antibiot-ics. Anaphylactic reactions involve generalized urticaria (hives), hypo-tension, and possible airway obstruction and cardiovascular collapse. Subcutaneous or intramuscular epinephrine (1:1,000) is the immedi-ate therapy, with diphenhydramine and systemic steroids preventing relapse. Anaphylaxis cases should be observed for a minimum of 6 hours because relapses are common.[50] An epinephrine injection device (EpiPen, EpiPen Jr) and insect sting desensitization should be recommended for those with a history of generalized hives or anaphylactic reaction to stings.

■ KEY POINTS

Diagnosis

- First try to identify the primary skin lesion (eg, macule versus patch, papule versus plaque, vesicle versus bullae).
- Are there any secondary characteristics present (eg, scaling, crusting, excoriations)?
- Pruritus suggests allergy, while tenderness suggests infection.
- Did the rash start on the trunk and spread to the extremities (centrifugal) or did it spread from the extremities (centrifugal) to the trunk?
- Always ask what the patient has been using on the rash, as it may now be contributing to it.
- Always take a thorough drug and travel history.
- Uncommon presentations of common conditions are more likely than common presentations of uncommon ones.
- Have the patient disrobe for the examination and do not forget to examine the mouth.

Treatment

- Instruct the patient or parent on the correct amount of the topical agent (in fingertip units) to apply and how to apply it. Discuss duration and conclusion of therapy.
- Avoid high-potency steroids on the face, genitals, and axillary and inguinal areas.
- Avoid systemic steroid use in psoriasis because of the risk of a flare on discontinuation.

Viral Infections

- Removing a viral skin lesion with a number 15 scalpel to check its gross or microscopic appearance often aids diagnosis (eg, molluscum lesions, HSV vesicles).
- Cryotherapy frequently results in hypopigmentation in dark-skinned patients.
- Viral exanthems can be differentiated by age of onset, site of onset, rash progression, and appearance.

Bacterial Infections

- Honey-colored crusts and erosions are typical findings in impetigo. Topical mupirocin is usually effective.
- Skin pyodermas may initially resemble spider bites. Methicillin-resistant *S aureus* often presents this way.
- Abscesses should always be drained of pus, not just treated with antibiotics. Usually, thorough drainage is sufficient treatment in immune-competent patients.

Fungal Infections

- Classic tinea appears as a scaly pruritic patch with annular margins and central clearing.
- Diagnosis of fungal infection is confirmed by obtaining a skin scraping with a number 15 scalpel and examining it for hyphae under a drop of 20% KOH.
- Use of topical steroids on fungal skin lesions alters their appearance and may confuse diagnosis (tinea incognito).
- Most tinea infections do not fluoresce with Wood lamp illumination. *Microsporum* infections fluoresce green (but are now rare) and erythrasma, a bacterial infection resembling tinea, fluoresces coral red.

Rickettsial Infections

- Fever, headache, and (often) rash are characteristic of rickettsial infections. Doxycycline is the best therapy.

Parasitic Infections

- Eosinophilia is associated with helminthic tissue infection in immunocompetent hosts.
- Eosinophilia is usually absent in protozoal infections.
- A travel history is essential in determining the differential diagnosis for parasitic infection.

Ectoparasitic Infestations

- Patients should be counseled that pruritus from scabies is slow to resolve after treatment and antihistamines may be helpful in the interim.
- Increasing pyrethrin resistance in head lice mandates newer treatments such as spinosad, benzyl alcohol, and heat treatments.

■ REFERENCES

1. Cordova A. The Mongolian spot: a study of ethnic differences and a literature review. *Clin Pediatr (Phila)*. 1981; 20(11):714–719

2. Braue A, Ross G, Varigos G, et al. Epidemiology and impact of childhood molluscum contagiosum: a case series and critical review of the literature. *Pediatr Dermatol*. 2005;22(4):287–294

3. Hengge U, Eser S, Schultewolter T, et al. Self-administered topical 5% imiquimod for the treatment of common warts and molluscum contagiosum. *Br J Dermatol*. 2000;143(5):1026–1031

4. Massing A, Epstein W. Natural history of warts: a two year study. *Arch Dermatol*. 1997;12:141–167

5. Siegfried E, Frasier L. Anogenital warts in children. *Adv Dermatol*. 1997;12:141–167

6. Stulberg D, Galbraith Hutchinson A. Molluscum contagiosum and warts. *Am Fam Phys*. 2003;67(6):233–240

7. Rogers CJ, Gibney MD, Siegfried E, et al. Cimetidine therapy for recalcitrant warts in adults: is it any better than placebo? *J Am Acad Dermatol*. 1999;41:123–127

8. Wald A, Zeh J, Selke S, et al. Virologic characteristics of subclinical and symptomatic genital herpes. *N Engl J Med*. 1995;333:770–775

9. Uebe B, Sauerbrei A, Burdach S, Horneff G. Herpes zoster by reactivated vaccine varicella virus in a healthy child. *Eur J Pediatr*. 2002;161(8):442–444

10. Heyman D, ed. *Control of Communicable Diseases Manual*. 18th ed. Washington, DC: American Public Health Association; 2004

11. Villamor E, Fawzi W. Vitamin A supplementation: implications for morbidity and mortality in children. *J Infect Dis*. 2000;192(Suppl):S12–S133

12. American Academy of Pediatrics. *Red Book: 2003 Report of the Committee on Infectious Diseases*. Pickering LK, ed. 26th ed. Elk Grove Village, IL: Am Academy of Pediatrics; 2003

13. Tassniyom S, Vasanawathana S, Chirawatkul A, et al. Failure of high dose methylprednisolone in established dengue shock syndrome; a placebo controlled double blind study. *Pediatrics*. 1993;92:111

14. Rigau-Perez J, Gubler G, Vorndam A, et al. Dengue surveillance—United States, 1986–92. *MMWR CDC Surveill Summ*. 1994;43:7

15. Notice to readers: newly licensed smallpox vaccine licensed to replace old smallpox vaccine. *MMWR*. 2008;57(8):20–208

16. Lupi O, Tyring S. Tropical dermatology: viral tropical diseases. *J Am Acad Dermatol*. 2003;49:975–1000

17. Younes-Ibrahim M, da Rosa Santos O. Leptospirosis. In: Tyring SK, Lupi O, Hennge UR, eds. *Tropical Dermatology*. Philadelphia, PA: Elsevier; 2006:352–358

18. Maniar J, Kamath R. HIV and HIV-associated disorders. In: Tyring SK, Lupi O, Hennge UR, eds. *Tropical Dermatology*. Philadelphia, PA: Elsevier; 2006:93–124

19. Kosuge H, Tanaka-Taya K, Miyoshi H, et al. Epidemiologic al study of human herpesvirus-6 and human herpesvirus-7 in pityriasis rosea. *Br J Dermatol*. 2000;143(4):795–798

20. Hartley A. Pityriasis rosea. *Pediatr Rev*. 1999;20(8):266–269

21. Sharma P, Yadav T, Gautam R, et al. Erythromycin in pityriasis rosea: a double-blind placebo controlled clinical trial. *J Am Acad Dermatol*. 2000;42:241–244

22. McGinigle K, Gourlay M, Buchanan I. The use of active surveillance cultures in adult intensive care units to reduce methicillin-resistant Staphylococcus aureus–related morbidity, mortality, and costs: a systematic review. *Clin Infect Dis*. 2007;44:186–189

23. Bravo FG. Bartonellosis. In: Tyring SK, Lupi O, Hennge UR, eds. *Tropical Dermatology.* Philadelphia, PA: Elsevier; 2006:303–312

24. Sanderson W, Stoddard R, Echt A, et al. Bacillus anthracis contamination and inhalational anthrax in a mail processing distribution center. *J Appl Microbiol.* 2004;96:1048–1056

25. Hoyne A, Brown R. 727 meningococcal cases, an analysis. *Ann Intern Med.* 1948;28:248–259

26. Tyring SK. Miscellaneous bacteria. In: Tyring SK, Lupi O, Hennge UR, eds. *Tropical Dermatology.* Philadelphia, PA: Elsevier; 2006:372–374

27. Paller AS, Mancini AJ. Cutaneous disorders of the newborn. In: Paller AS, Mancini AJ, eds. *Hurwitz Clinical Pediatric Dermatology.* 3rd ed., Philadelphia, PA: Elsevier Saunders; 2006:17–47

28. Jiang J, Temenak J, Richards A. Real time duplex PCR assay for Rickettsia prowazekii and Borrelia recurrentis. *Ann NY Acad Sci.* 2003;990:757–764

29. Watt G, Strickman D. Life-threatening scrub typhus in a traveler returning from Thailand. *Clin Infect Dis.* 1994;18:624–626

30. Lantos P, Krause P. Ehlichosis in children. *Semin Pediatr Infect Dis.* 2002;13(4):249–256

31. World Health Organization. *World Health Organization Leprosy Elimination Project. Status Report 2003.* Geneva, Switzerland: World Health Organization; 2004. http://www.who.int/lep/resources/StatusRpt01.pdf. Accessed June 17, 2011

32. National Hansen's Disease Programs. *Standards of Care for Hansen's Disease in the United States.* Louisiana, USA: 2003

33. Patteron T, McGinnis M. Tinea capitus and Tinea favosa. Doctor Fungus. http://www.doctorfungus.org/mycoses/human/other/tinea_captius_favosa.htm. Accessed June 26, 2009

34. Krob A, Fleisher A Jr, D'Agostino R Jr, et al. Terbinafine is more effective than itraconizole in treating toenail onychomycosis: results from a meta-analysis of randomized controlled trials. *J Cutan Med Surg.* 2003;149(suppl 65):15–18

35. Gupta A, Ahmad I, Summerbell R. Fungicidal activities of commonly used disinfectants and antifungal pharmacologic spray preparations against clinical strains of Aspergillis and Candida species. *Med Mycol.* 2002;40(2):201–208

36. Yazdanpanak M, Azizi H, Suizi B. Comparison between fluconazole and ketoconazole effectivity in the treatment of Pityriasis versicolor. *Mycoses.* 2007;50(4):311–314

37. Estrada-Chavez G, Vega-Mernijie M, Arenas R, et al. Eumycotic mycetoma caused by Madurella mycetomatis successfully treated with antifungals, surgery and topical negative pressure therapy. *Int J Dermatol.* 2009;48(4):401–403

38. Ali-Daraji W. Cutaneous lobomycosis: a delayed diagnosis. *Am J Dermatopathol.* 2008;30(6):575–577

39. Lessa M, Lessa H, Castro T, et al. Mucosal leishmaniasis: epidemiological and clinical aspects. *Braz J Otorhinol.* 2007;73(6):843–847

40. Minodier P, Parola P. Cutaneous leishmaniasis treatment. *Travel Med Infect Dis.* 2007;5(3):150–158

41. Stingl P. Onchocerciasis: developments in diagnosis, treatment and control. *Int J Dermatol.* 2009;48(4):393–396

42. Drugs for parasitic infections. *Treat Guidel Med Lett.* 2007;5(Suppl):e1–e11

43. Pereira K, Schmidt F, Guaraldo A, et al. Chagas disease as a food-borne illness. *J Food Prot.* 2009;72(2):441–446

44. Heukelbach J, Feldmeier H. Epidemiological and clinical characteristics of hookworm-related cutaneous larva migrans. *Lancet Infect Dis.* 2008;8(5):302–309

45. Davis R, Johnston G, Sladden M. Recognition and management of common ectoparasitic diseases of travelers. *Am J Clin Dermatol.* 2009;10(1):1–8

46. Abedins S, Narang M, Gandhi V, Narang S. Efficacy of permethrin cream and oral ivermectin in the treatment of scabies. *Indian J Pediatr.* 2007;74(10):915–916

47. Mumcuoglu K, Meinking T, Burkhart CN, Burkhart CG. Head louse infestations: the "no nit" policy and its consequences. *Int J Dermatol.* 2006;45(8):891–896

48. Goddard J, deShazo R. Bedbugs (Cimex lectularius) and clinical consequences of their bites. *JAMA.* 2009;301(13):1358–1366

49. Katz T, Miller J, Herbert A. Insect repellents: historical perspectives and new developments. *J Amer Acad Dermatol.* 2008;58(5):865–871

50. Liberman D, Teach S. Management of anaphylaxis in children. *Pediatr Emerg Care.* 2008;24(12):861–866

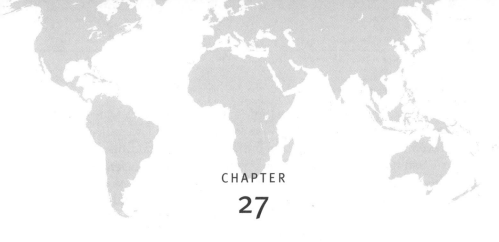

CHAPTER

27

Bites and Stings

Gregory Juckett, MD, MPH

■ INTRODUCTION

Travel to the tropics invariably raises concerns about deadly snakebites, insatiable insects, and malign infestations. Fortunately, these fears are almost always exaggerated. For travelers, snakebites are extremely rare events that can usually be avoided with a few simple precautions. While insect bites and stings are another matter, even in the tropics they usually are only a nuisance. The exception, of course, is anaphylaxis from bee and wasp stings. Anaphylaxis represents a true medical emergency that may occur anywhere. Because emergency care is far less available in lower-income countries, the most important medical item to bring along is epinephrine 1:1,000 in a self-injectable form. Epinephrine remains the key intervention in anaphylaxis and will outperform all other medical options (eg, steroids, diphenhydramine) for life-threatening allergic reactions.

In contrast with travelers, residents of the tropics are confronted by the local fauna on a daily basis and lack many of the resources (eg, footwear, bed nets, insect sprays) insulating the more affluent from their environment. Snakebites usually affect agricultural workers, making it an occupational, rather than a recreational, disease in these settings. Once bitten, there may be far less access to care; therefore, morbidity and mortality rates for residents are much higher.[1]

■ SPIDER BITES

Most spider bites are relatively harmless. For example, only widow *(Latrodectus)*, recluse *(Loxosceles)*, and South American bird spiders *(Phoneutria)* are causes for concern in the Americas. Worldwide, the Australian funnel web spiders *(Atrax)* rank as the most dangerous. However, other much-feared spiders, such as the tarantula, pose very little threat to human health, although they can certainly bite and are even known to flick urticating hairs if annoyed. Most tarantula bites hurt, but they do not require any medical care.

In general, spider bites tend to be over-dreaded and overdiagnosed. Patients and physicians falsely attribute many unexplained skin lesions, usually pyodermas, to spiders. In fact, many of these lesions appear to be caused by methicillin-resistant *Staphylococcus aureus* (MRSA).[2]

Widow spiders *(Latrodectus)* are distributed worldwide, but the best-known species is the black widow *(L maculans)*, famous for its characteristic red hourglass mark on the ventral abdomen. It possesses a very potent neurotoxic venom known as alpha-latotoxin. Black widow bites are usually felt as a mild pinprick (often presenting with a halo around the site) followed within an hour by severe pain and muscle cramping. Systemic symptoms such as nausea, vomiting, and sweating may also occur. Upper extremity bites produce chest pain, while those on the lower extremity mimic an acute abdomen. Fatal respiratory arrest has occurred in children.

Widow bites are treated with local application of ice and intravenous (IV) diazepam to reduce muscle spasm. Traditionally, 10% calcium carbonate was used to treat muscle cramps, but benzodiazepines and narcotics have replaced this as standard therapy.[3] An equine *Latrodectus* antivenom (1 vial diluted in 50 mL normal saline) is available but is usually reserved for pediatric envenomations. The antivenom is also very effective at relieving pain.

Brown recluse or fiddleback spiders *(Loxosceles reclusa)* of the south-central United States are the most important American cause of necrotic arachnidism or skin necrosis caused by spider bites. Brown recluse venom contains sphingomyelinase-D. These spiders are readily identifiable by an inverted violin-shaped marking on the dorsal thorax and by having only 6 eyes (most spiders have 8). Even more dangerous is the larger South American *Loxosceles* relative, the Chilean recluse *(L laeta)*, which has established limited colonies in parts of the United States. Recluse spiders usually live in homes where they seek out dry, dark locations such as inside clothing or behind picture frames. Bites may not be painful at first, but a painful blister with a multicolored halo (red, white, and blue sign) usually forms within 6 hours. The skin around the bite sloughs off after several days, leaving a very slow-healing ulcer.

Most recluse bites clear up with the initial application of ice, routine wound care, and antihistamines. Routinely cutting out the bite site is no longer recommended.[4] However, skin grafting may eventually be required in the rare severe case. Transdermal nitroglycerin has been tried on bites to prevent skin necrosis. Although dapsone (to limit neutrophil degranulation within the first 48 to 72 hours) is still sometimes recommended, there is little conclusive evidence confirming its effectiveness; as such, dapsone is no longer standard therapy.[5] Steroid use is also controversial. There is little evidence-based research with which to guide therapy.

The Brazilian wandering spider or banana spider *(Phoneutria nigriventer)* can cause severe pain requiring local anesthetic injection. Narcotics may increase the risk of respiratory arrest and should be avoided. The male funnel web spider *(Atrax robustus)* is probably the most dangerous spider in the world but is limited to eastern Australia. Its neurotoxic bites are treated with a compression and immobilization dressing, atropine, and *Atrax* antivenom.

■ SCORPION STINGS

Scorpions are nocturnal arachnids that often enter homes in hot climates where they can be easily spotted with a black (ultraviolet) light. Their habit of seeking refuge in shoes results in many stings. While most scorpion stings are no more dangerous than bee stings, a few can be life threatening. Many small-clawed scorpions have a tendency to compensate with much more potent venom in their tail stinger (telson). The *Buthidae* family of scorpions, characterized by small claws and a triangular sternal plate, are notorious for severely neurotoxic stings that cause an autonomic storm (Box 27-1). A few non-buthid scorpions, such as *Hemiscorpius lepturus,* may also inflict serious stings; however, their venom results in local skin necrosis.[6]

The bark scorpion *(Centruroides exilicauda [sculpturatus])* of Arizona and Mexico is the most dangerous US buthid. Its sting is painful and causes local paresthesia, violent neuromotor hyperactivity, cholinergic symptoms (eg, nausea, sweating, salivation), tachycardia, hypertension, and respiratory complications. Stings are treated with local ice, IV diazepam, atropine, and careful blood pressure control in an intensive care unit setting. An experimental F (ab) antivenom (University of Arizona) appears quite effective in severe envenomations[7] and may replace a goat-derived scorpion antivenom that is no longer manufactured.

Box 27-1. Most Dangerous Scorpions

BUTHIDAE FAMILY: NEUROTOXIC VENOMS

Tityus—Caribbean, South America

Androctonus australis (yellow scorpion)—North Africa

Buthus—North Africa

Leiurus quinquestriatus (5-keeled yellow scorpion)—North Africa and Middle East

Mesobuthius tumulus (red scorpion)—India

Centruroides exilicauda (bark scorpion)—southwest United States and Mexico (cholinergic toxicity)

Parabuthius—South Africa (cholinergic toxicity)

SCORPIONIDA FAMILY: CYTOTOXIC VENOM

Hemiscorpion lepturus—Middle East (sting site necrosis)

■ STINGING CATERPILLARS

Many caterpillars possess venomous spines or hairs for defense. The US saddleback caterpillar *(Acharia [Sibine] stimulea)* and the Io moth *(Automeris io)* are typical species producing severe stings on contact. The puss moth, wooly slug, or asp caterpillar *(Megalopyge opercularis)* is also capable of producing long-lasting pain. Tape application may remove adherent spines, and ice compresses with local anesthetic injection help alleviate pain.

Some tropical caterpillars are much more serious. *Lonomia* caterpillars from South America are probably the most dangerous, with venom that activates prothrombin, causing a persistent coagulopathy.

■ HYMENOPTERA STINGS

Hymenoptera stings (ie, bees, wasps, and ants) are responsible for more fatalities than any other venomous animal. Anaphylaxis with shock is the usual cause of death. Bee venom appears to be the most allergenic; however, yellow jackets, a type of wasp, actually cause more fatalities because of their aggression. Wasps are also capable of stinging repeatedly, whereas bees, with barbed stingers, do so only once—their venom sacs and stingers remain in the victim as the bee flies off to die. Typical immediate sting reactions involve short-lived pain and swelling that is usually treated with ice, antihistamines, or compresses of baking soda or papain (meat tenderizer). Late phase reactions (48 hours to a week later) appear as local areas of redness, heat, and swelling that closely mimic cellulitis. A short course of antihistamines or prednisone is the most effective treatment. Antibiotics are frequently prescribed but are seldom needed. Prednisone is also very useful for the serum sickness–like reaction (eg, fever, arthralgia, urticaria) that may sometimes follow a sting.

Honeybee *(Apis mellifera)* venom consists largely of melittin (50%) with highly allergenic phospholipase A, adolapin (an anti-inflammatory peptide), and hyaluronidase.[8] Africanized "killer" bee venom is no more toxic than the European variety, but the bees are far more aggressive. Swatting bees causes them to release pheromones that provoke an even more aggressive attack. Wasps or vespids include paper wasps *(Polistes),* bald-faced hornets *(Dolichovespula),* European hornets *(Vespa),* and yellow jackets *(Vespula).* The intense pain of wasp stings is caused by the serotonin in its venom.

Fire ants *(Solenopsis invicta)* are an imported Argentine species that are widespread throughout the southern United States. Their nests are conspicuous mounds of dry earth that must be avoided at all costs. Attacking fire ants anchor themselves to their victim by biting and then stinging repeatedly. These painful stings soon develop into clusters of sterile white pustules.

The samsum ant *(Pachycondyla)* in Africa and the Middle East is the equivalent of the fire ant. In tropical Latin America, the bullet or 24-hour ant *(Paraponera)* has the most dreaded sting, which often requires anesthetic injection at the sting site. The local name, 24-hour ant (hormiga veinticuatro), refers to the 24 hours of pain it causes. However, symptomatic therapy (eg, ice, antihistamines) suffices for most ant stings.

Anaphylaxis is a life-threatening emergency that usually occurs within 30 minutes (occasionally longer) after an allergenic exposure. Generalized urticaria, intense anxiety, shortness of breath, and weakness are usually evident. Death often occurs within 1 hour and is precipitated by airway obstruction or cardiovascular collapse. A biphasic pattern occurs in 20% of cases in which an apparent remission is followed by another episode 3 to 5 hours later. Therefore, it is imperative that every suspected case of anaphylaxis be observed for at least 6 hours before discharge.[9]

The cornerstone of anaphylaxis therapy is intramuscular or subcutaneous epinephrine (1:1,000) injection at a dosage of 0.01 mL/kg (0.3 mL maximum) repeated every 15 to 20 minutes until improvement. Diphenhydramine is also useful, but relapse with diphenhydramine alone is very common. Antihistamines alone should never be depended on to reverse anaphylaxis. Airway intubation, bronchodilators, IV steroids, and normal saline are all part of standard care. Patients on beta-blockers are notoriously refractory to epinephrine and require IV glucagon for effective treatment.[9]

Anaphylaxis is mimicked by many other conditions—anaphylactoid events (non-IgE mediated but managed the same way), certain drug reactions, panic attacks, and vasovagal episodes. Tryptase, released from mast cells, peaks within 1 hour of true anaphylaxis and remains elevated for at least 24 hours. Patients with systemic reactions should be prescribed an epinephrine injection device (eg, EpiPen, EpiPen Jr) and referred for insect sting desensitization. Venom immunotherapy should continue until repeat skin results are negative, usually at 3 to 5 years.[10]

■ INSECT BITES

Dipteran insects, such as mosquitoes, blackflies, and gnats, commonly cause allergic reactions at the bite site. These itchy red papules typically have a minute central punctum, but their severity and duration depend on individual sensitivity. While responding well to antihistamine therapy, they are best prevented by the judicious use of insect repellents. DEET-containing repellents up to 50% concentration are now considered safe in children older than 2 months.[11]

Similar itchy papules on the ankles suggest an allergic reaction to fleabites, which are usually from a cat or dog flea *(Ctenocephalides canis)*. This flea is especially prone to attack humans if its preferred host is temporarily unavailable. Human fleas *(Pulex irritans)* occur in less hygienic situations. Bed bugs *(Cimex)* cause clusters or short lines of large pruritic papules on the trunk or extremities. These clustered 3 to 4 lesions are sometimes termed the breakfast, lunch, and dinner sign. Extermination is the only effective solution.

Chiggers or red bugs are harvest mite *(Trombicula)* larvae that live in dry grass and migrate up the body until clothing constriction stops them, which explains why their large, intensely itchy bites often occur at sock or belt lines. Contrary to popular opinion, these itchy bites are allergic reactions to the mite's feeding, not to the mite itself.

The tropical burrowing flea *(Tunga penetrans)* actually embeds itself in the tissues of the toes or feet where it provokes severe inflammation and sometimes secondary infections. Diagnosis is often confirmed by observing the discharge of tiny white eggs from the skin lesion. Proper footwear is critical in preventing infestation. The best therapy is surgical removal.

■ MYIASIS (HUMAN BOTFLY INFESTATION)

Several species of botflies attack humans in addition to animals. In Central and South America, the human botfly, *Dermatobia hominis*, captures mosquitoes or other biting insects on which to attach its eggs. When these released insects reach their victim, the eggs hatch and infest the host, producing a small furuncle. Over the next 6 weeks, the maggot develops within the skin to eventually emerge as an adult fly.

In Africa, the tumbu or putzi fly *(Cordylobia anthropophaga)* lays its eggs on damp or sweat-stained clothing, especially clothing that is hung up to dry. Unless these clothes are thoroughly ironed before being worn, eggs will hatch on contact with skin to produce multiple boils, which develop much faster than the prior species (often within several weeks). The patient's perception of motility within the lesion suggests the correct diagnosis. Lund fly *(Cordylobia rodhaini)* is a similar species that infests the feet. There is even a free-living Congo floor maggot *(Auchmeromyia)* that feeds on people sleeping on the ground.

Fly larvae of many species can infest necrotic wound tissue. Less commonly, screwworm larvae may attack viable tissue of humans and animals; these can be paralyzed with topical 5% chloroform in olive oil and removed manually. *Hypoderma* fly larvae may tunnel through human skin to produce lesions closely resembling those of cutaneous larva migrans (creeping eruption); ivermectin clears this infection.[12]

Surgically excising or ejecting botfly larvae by injecting 2 mL local anesthetic into the lesion base is curative. Traditionally, applying fatback (raw bacon) or any occlusive material over the larval spiracle (breathing aperture) encourages the maggot to migrate upward, making removal much easier. Usually larvae can be removed with forceps several hours after bacon therapy.

■ VENOMOUS SNAKEBITES

There are 4 principal venomous snake families in the world: vipers, elapids (including *Hydrophis* and *Laticauda* sea snakes), colubrids (mostly nonvenomous but including some rear-fanged species such as the boomslang), and burrowing asps of Africa (Box 27-2). Most important are the vipers, usually fat, thick-bodied snakes with broad heads and cytotoxic or hemotoxic venom that digests tissue and breaks down blood. American pit vipers (ie, rattlesnakes, copperheads, and cotton-mouths) are crotalid representatives of the viper family. Elapids (including mambas, cobras, kraits, coral snakes, and sea snakes) are slender tropical and subtropical species with mostly neurotoxic venom that paralyzes respiratory muscles. Thus, elapid snakes can kill within hours, whereas most vipers, with rare exceptions, take days to kill their victims. Sea snakes are mostly neurotoxic but frequently produce rhabdomyolysis. Other exceptions include Mojave rattlesnake venom (neurotoxic and mycotoxic effects) and cobra venom, which can attack muscles and the nervous system.

Box 27-2. Venomous Snake Families

Viperidae (vipers and pit vipers: mostly hemotoxic venom)
True vipers include the European adder, saw-scaled, or carpet viper (Africa and Asia); puff adder (Africa); Gaboon viper (Africa); Russell viper (Asia). The crotalid or pit viper subfamily include rattlesnakes (Americas), copperheads (North America), water moccasins or cottonmouths (North America), fer-de-lance (Central and South America), bushmaster (South America), Malayan pit viper (Asia), Temple viper (Asia).

Elapidae (elapids: mostly neurotoxic venom)
Typical elapids include black and green mambas (Africa), cobras (Africa and Asia), spitting cobras (Africa and Asia), king cobra (Asia), kraits (Asia), coral snakes (Americas), taipans (Australia), and the misleadingly named death adder of Australia (all venomous Australian snakes are elapids).

The sea snake subfamily *(Hydrophis)* includes many aquatic species living in the Indian and Pacific oceans such as the beaked sea snake and annulate sea snake. These seldom bite in the water but often do so when captured.

The *Laticauda* subfamily includes the yellow-lipped sea krait, which may be found on shore rocks or in the ocean.

Colubridae (colubrids: mostly nonvenomous snakes but includes venomous rear-fanged species as well)
Venomous colubrids include the boomslang *(Dispholidus)* and twig snakes *(Thelotornis)* of Africa and the Asian red-necked keelback *(Rhabdophis)*.

Atractaspididae (African burrowing asps): uncommon causes of snakebite, but these are the only snakes unable to be held safely behind the head because they are capable of rotating their fangs sideways or backward to inflict bites.

First aid for snakebite depends on the snake type. Viper or pit viper bites (including nearly all US snakebites) are treated with a lymphatic constriction band loose enough to allow a finger to slide beneath, and rapid transport to a nearby hospital where antivenom can be administered. Tourniquets do more harm than good. Rings and jewelry should be removed before swelling starts. Ice packs, fang mark cutting, wound suction, and electric shock therapy should all be avoided. Stun guns and other forms of shock do not neutralize venom and may be harmful. Venom extraction devices are probably of no benefit, even if used within the necessary 3-minute window, because the high viscosity of snake venom makes removal difficult.[13]

Envenomated elapid bites are very different from those of vipers and often have little, if any, local reaction. Because there is less local destruction of tissue, the entire extremity should be immobilized and wrapped in a lymphatic constriction band; this effectively traps the neurotoxic venom in the limb lymphatics, keeping it from reaching the central nervous system. Antivenom must be given for some elapid bites (eg, coral snakes, kraits) even when there may be minimal signs of local envenomation. Elapid neurologic symptoms, once begun, are quite difficult to reverse. Respirations should be closely monitored and ventilator support should be available.

Pit viper bite envenomation usually produces a significant local reaction with immediate pain and swelling. Table 27-1 lists the common symptoms of envenomation. Classically, 2 fang marks are present; rarely there may be 1 to 4 fang marks because of fang loss or the presence of replacement fangs. Many bites turn out to be dry with no appreciable venom. It is estimated that 20% to 30% of pit viper bites are dry compared with more than 50% of elapid and 75% of sea snake.[14] Any suspected dry pit viper bites should be observed a minimum of 8 hours before discharge versus 24 hours for elapids.[13] Basic laboratory tests should be performed as soon as possible before venom effects interfere with typing and crossing blood, and repeated within 12 hours to monitor bleeding parameters and renal function (Table 27-2). Bites should also be graded at the time of admission and periodically thereafter because severity determines the starting dose of antivenom (Table 27-3).

Swelling of the bitten extremity is usually dramatic in pit viper or viper bites and is often quite persistent, notably so even in the otherwise less venomous American copperhead. Swelling frequently mimics a compartment syndrome, but unless measured compartment pressures are truly elevated, fasciotomy usually causes more harm than good. Most swelling proves to be superficial.[15]

Table 27-1. Symptoms of Snakebite Envenomation

Hemotoxic Symptoms	Neurotoxic Symptoms
Intense pain	Minimal pain
Edema	Ptosis
Weakness	Weakness
Swelling	Paresthesia (often numb at bite site)
Numbness or tingling	Diplopia
Rapid pulse	Dysphagia
Ecchymoses	Sweating
Muscle fasciculation	Salivation
Paresthesia (oral)	Diaphoresis
Unusual metallic taste	Hyporeflexia
Vomiting	Respiratory depression
Confusion	Paralysis
Bleeding disorders	

Adapted from Juckett G, Hancox JG. Venomous snakebites in the United States: management review and update. *Am Fam Physician.* 2002;65(7):1367–1374. Reprinted with permission from American Academy of Family Physicians.

Table 27-2. Laboratory Evaluation in Snakebite

Complete blood cell count with platelets and differential[a]	Blood urea nitrogen
Prothrombin time[a]	Platelet count
Partial thromboplastin time[a]	Liver function tests
Fibrinogen[a]	Bilirubin
Fibrin degradation products[a]	Creatine phosphokinase
Blood type and cross match	Creatinine urinalysis[b]
Serum electrolytes	Stool hemoccult
Glucose	Electrocardiography[c]
	Arterial or capillary blood gas[d]

[a]Should be performed as soon as possible and repeated within 12 hours.
[b]Including free protein, hemoglobin, and myoglobin.
[c]Suggested for patients older than 50 years and patients with a history of heart disease.11
[d]Should be tested if any signs or symptoms of respiratory compromise are evident.

Adapted from Juckett G, Hancox JG. Venomous snakebites in the United States: management review and update. *Am Fam Physician.* 2002;65(7):1367–1374. Reprinted with permission from American Academy of Family Physicians.

Table 27-3. Grading Scale for Severity of Pit Viper Bites and CroFab Antivenom Administration[a]

DEGREE OF ENVENOMATION	PRESENTATION	TREATMENT
0. None	Punctures or abrasions; some pain or tenderness at the bite	Local wound care, no antivenom[b]
I. Mild	Pain, tenderness, edema at the bite; perioral paresthesias may be present.	If antivenin is necessary, administer about 4 vials CroFab.
II. Moderate	Pain, tenderness, erythema, edema beyond the area adjacent to the bite; often, systemic manifestations and mild coagulopathy	Administration of 4 to 6 vials of CroFab
III. Severe	Intense pain and swelling of entire extremity, often with severe systemic signs and symptoms; coagulopathy	Administer more than 6 vials of CroFab.

[a]Modified to include recommended CroFab dosages.
[b]Because of their less potent venom, grade I (mild) copperhead bites are often not treated with antivenom.

Adapted from Juckett G, Hancox JG. Venomous snakebites in the United States: management review and update. *Am Fam Physician.* 2002;65(7):1367–1374. Reprinted with permission from American Academy of Family Physicians.

Antivenom is the most effective therapy for a venomous snakebite and should ideally be administered within 4 to 6 hours but may be helpful for up to 72 hours if coagulopathy is evident. Specific antivenom (made for one particular species) is most effective, but polyvalent antivenom is often the most practical solution because it covers many related snakes. Children need the same antivenom dose as adults (or more) because the amount of venom to be neutralized may be the same with a much smaller body size. Common errors include giving too little antivenom too late or, in the case of viper bites, giving antivenom without any sign of envenomation. If death occurs from viper bites, it is usually delayed (taking several days) and occurs from bleeding disorders or delayed renal failure from myoglobinuria.

Most antivenom worldwide is made by injecting escalating doses of snake venom into horses and harvesting the antibody. Horse serum antivenom sometimes provokes anaphylactic or anaphylactoid reactions and should be given by a physician with epinephrine and antihistamines available at bedside. Manufacturers recommend prior skin testing for horse serum allergy, but this is notoriously unreliable and some experts dispense with it. Even if a skin test result is positive, there may be no alternative except to pre-medicate the patient with IV steroids and diphenhydramine. Equine antivenom administration is complicated by serum sickness 1 to 4 weeks later in approximately 50% of cases and should be treated with oral prednisone therapy.

New, much more expensive non-equine F (ab) antivenom is being developed because whole IgG equine antivenom is associated with allergic reactions. This new antivenom lacks the more antigenic antibody "tail" (Fc portion) and is consequently much safer. CroFab antivenom is replacing antivenom (Crotalidae) polyvalent for US pit viper bites. CroFab is made from injecting sheep with the venom of western and eastern diamondback rattlesnakes, Mohave rattlesnakes, and cottonmouths. Skin testing is not recommended; however, papain allergy is a contraindication because papain is used to create the F (ab) fragments. Reconstitution of a vial of dried CroFab is accomplished in under 45 minutes compared with 60 minutes for the previous product.[16] Each antivenom vial should be diluted with 10 mL sterile water and then diluted in 250 mL normal saline for infusion over 60 minutes. The manufacturer recommends an initial infusion rate of 25 to 50 mL per hour for the first 10 minutes, all the while checking for signs of allergy. The infusion can be increased to 250 mL per hour until completion if allergy signs do not develop. Four to 6 vials are recommended for mild to moderate envenomations; more than 6 vials are recommended for severe envenomation.[17] Unfortunately, the current equine coral snake antivenom was discontinued (supplies expired in late 2009), but trials are underway to approve a Mexican F (ab) coral snake antivenom for use in the United States.

Most fatal snakebites occur in lower-income countries where barefoot farmers labor in fields. Proper footwear would prevent many of these bites. South Asia has the most fatalities, but southeast Asia, tropical Africa, and the Amazon are also considered moderate to high risk. Bites increase in the rainy season when flooding forces snakes onto higher ground. Although elapids are more dreaded because of their rapid-acting venom, the bulk of fatalities actually occur from rural viper bites, which result in coagulopathies or delayed renal failure. Bites of the irritable saw-scaled or carpet viper *(Echis carinatus)* of Africa, the Middle East, and South Asia cause severe coagulopathies and is perhaps the world's most dangerous snake, despite the fact that other species possess far more potent venom.[18] Although Australia is known for having many dangerous elapids, its mortality rate is remarkably low because of good footwear and prompt medical care.

Most snakebites can be prevented by wearing boots, avoiding tall grass and brush, and using a flashlight when on a path at night. Many so-called illegitimate snakebites occur while teasing or attempting to kill snakes; alcohol is often a contributing factor. Dead snakes are able to bite through reflex action for several hours even if decapitated. Children should thus be warned to leave even dead snakes alone. Bites from exotic snakes kept as pets are a growing concern in urban areas. Because crotalid antivenom is quite ineffective in such situations, the appropriate exotic antivenom must then be located through poison control or regional zoos or aquariums.[19] Further information may be obtained through Poison Help at 800/222-1222 or the Rocky Mountain Poison & Drug Center at 303/389-1100 or www.rmpdc.org.

■ KEY POINTS

- Widow spider bites result in intense muscle spasms and are usually managed with benzodiazepines or narcotics.
- Brown recluse spider bites result in local skin necrosis, but most can be managed conservatively with antihistamines. Outside of this spider's native range (south-central United States), most spider bites may actually be early MRSA infections.
- *Buthidae* scorpions, such as *Centruroides*, are characterized by small claws, triangular breastplates, and severely neurotoxic stings. Most other scorpion stings can be managed conservatively.
- Hymenoptera (ie, ant, bee, wasp) stings kill more people through anaphylaxis than any other type of envenomation.
- Epinephrine 1:1,000 injection is the drug of choice for anaphylaxis. Patients taking beta-blockers are resistant to epinephrine and may require IV glucagon.

- Observe all patients with anaphylaxis for at least 6 hours after treatment because 20% of cases may relapse in 3 to 5 hours.
- Vipers and pit vipers have mostly cytotoxic or hemotoxic venom, which causes severe local swelling and coagulopathy. Death usually takes days.
- Most elapids have rapidly acting neurotoxic venom that causes ptosis, respiratory paralysis, and death from respiratory failure. Cobra bites result in local swelling, but no swelling may occur even in serious coral snake and krait envenomations.
- Most traditional snakebite first aid does more harm than good. Immobilization and wrapping the affected extremity in a compression dressing are helpful in elapid bites. Tourniquets should be avoided, although a temporary compression band (restricting lymph but not blood flow) may be useful in viper bites.
- Avoid fasciotomy in snakebite unless critically elevated compartment pressures can be documented.
- Prompt antivenom administration is the key treatment for venomous snakebite. Dose is not reduced for children. Epinephrine should be available by the bedside in the event of an anaphylactic reaction.

■ REFERENCES

1. Cruz L, Vargas R, Lopes A. Snakebite envenomation and death in the developing world. *Ethn Dis.* 2009;19(1):S1-42–S1-46
2. Dominguez T. It's not a spider bite, it's community-acquired methicillin-resistant Staphylococcus aureus. *J Am Board Fam Pract.* 2004;17(3):220–226
3. Boyer LV, Binford GJ, McNally JT. Spider bites. In: Auerbach PS, ed. *Wilderness Medicine.* 5th ed. Philadelphia, PA: Mosby Elsevier; 2007:1008–1033
4. Carlton P. Brown recluse spider bite? Consider this uniquely conservative treatment. *J of Family Practice.* 2009;58(2):e1–e6
5. Vetter R, Bush S. Additional considerations in presumptive brown recluse bites and dapsone therapy. *Am J Emerg Med.* 2004;22(6):494–495
6. Radmanesh M. Clinical study of Hemiscorpius lepturus in Iran. *J Trop Med Hyg.* 1990;93:327
7. Boyer L, Theodorou A, Berg R, Mallie J. Antivenom for critically ill children with neurotoxicity from scorpion stings. *N Engl J Med.* 2009;360(20):2090–2098
8. Erickson TD. Arthropod envenomation and parasitism. In: Auerbach PS, ed. *Wilderness Medicine.* 5th ed. Philadelphia, PA: Mosby Elsevier; 2007:947–982
9. Liberman D, Teach S. Management of anaphylaxis in children. *Pediatr Emerg Care.* 2008;24(12):861–866
10. Arguin P, Steele. Chapter 2. The pretravel consultation (malaria). In: Health Information for International Travel. Centers for Disease Control and Prevention. 2010
11. Lerch E, Muller U. Long-term protection after stopping immunotherapy: results of re-stings in 200 patients. *J Allergy Clin Immunol.* 1998;101(5):
12. Jelinek T, Northdurft H, Rieder N, Loscher T. Cutaneous myiasis: review of 13 cases in travelers returning from tropical countries. *Int J Dermatol.* 1995;34:624–626

13. Norris RL, Bush SP. Bites by venomous reptiles in the Americas. In: Auerbach PS, ed. *Wilderness Medicine.* 5th ed. Philadelphia, PA: Mosby Elsevier; 2007:1051–1085

14. Kunkel D, Curry S, Vance M, Ryan P. Reptile envenomations. *Clin Toxicol.* 1983;21(4-5):5033–5526

15. Hall E. Role of surgical intervention in the management of crotaline snake envenomation. *Am Emerg Med.* 2001;31:175–180

16. Hill RE, Bogdan GM, Dart RC. Time to reconstitution: purified Fab antivenom vs unpurified IgG antivenom. *Toxicon.* 2001;39:729–731

17. Crofab: Crotalidae Polyvalent Immune Fab (Ovine). Packet insert; Savage Laboratories; 2000

18. Ali G, Kak M, Kmuar M, et al. Acute renal failure following echis carinatus (saw-scaled viper) envenomation. *Indian J Nephrol.* 2004;14:177–181

19. McNally J, Boesen K, Boyer L. Toxicologic information resources for reptile envenomations. *Vet Clinics N Am Exotic Animal Practices.* 2008;11(2):389–401

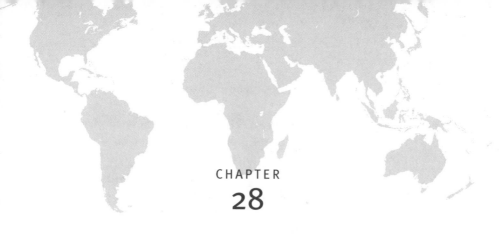

CHAPTER

28

HIV and AIDS

Michael A. Tolle, MD, MPH

■ INTRODUCTION

The global HIV pandemic has had a devastating effect on children. HIV is a major cause of death where prevalence is high (Figure 28-1)— more than 50% of child deaths are HIV related in some settings.[1] In addition, millions of children worldwide have been orphaned by HIV.

Figure 28-1. Global HIV Prevalence

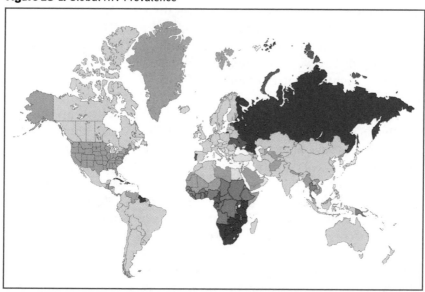

From Joint United Nations Programme on HIV/AIDS. *Global Report: UNAIDS Report on the Global AIDS Epidemic 2010.* Geneva, Switzerland: Joint United Nations Programme on HIV/AIDS; 2010:23. http://www.unaids.org/documents/20101123_2010_HIV_Prevalence_Map_em.pdf. Accessed March 25, 2011

HIV and its associated morbidities place a substantial strain on fragile health systems.

Pediatric HIV infections are rare in higher-income countries because of effective interventions to prevent mother-to-child transmission (MTCT); however, they remain common in many lower-income settings. Scaling up the prevention of MTCT and antiretroviral therapy (ART) programs for children is a global health priority, yet the uptake of several critical interventions remains low in many settings, particularly where health systems struggle to meet even basic maternal-child health needs and where stigma associated with HIV infection remains high.[2]

While tremendous strides have been made in the global response to pediatric HIV over the past few years, challenges persist and children remain underrepresented in care and treatment programs compared with adults.[2] In settings of high HIV prevalence, Millennium Development Goals (MDGs) related to child and maternal survival will not be met without further concerted efforts and progress toward making HIV prevention, care, and treatment universally available as part of community-level, primary health care.[1-3]

■ EPIDEMIOLOGY

While no country or region is spared the effects of HIV infection, its distribution is not uniform (Figure 28-1). Sub-Saharan Africa bears the largest burden with more than 90% (2.3 million) of the world's estimated 2.5 million HIV-infected children; nearly 90% (260,000) of the estimated 370,000 new HIV infections in children in 2009 occurred in sub-Saharan Africa.[4] Nearly 85% of the 16 million children orphaned by HIV worldwide live in sub-Saharan Africa, and in some high-prevalence countries, such as Zambia and Botswana, more than 15% of all children are orphans—the vast majority due to HIV.[5]

HIV accounts for a reasonably small proportion of global child deaths (less than 5% of deaths in children younger than 5 years); however, child mortality attributable to HIV may exceed 50% in areas of high prevalence. Thus, HIV-specific interventions form the cornerstone of attempts to reach MDG 4—a two-thirds reduction in child mortality by 2015 (from 1990 levels).[1,2] In regions of high HIV prevalence, progress toward reaching MDG 4 lags behind other regions; generalized HIV epidemics were noted in nearly 80% of countries where child mortality worsened between 1990 and 2006.[3,6]

Most pediatric HIV infections (more than 90%) are caused by MTCT (vertical transmission); accordingly, pediatric HIV infection is common where antenatal HIV prevalence is high.[2] The geographic focal effect of

HIV is noted in a total of 25 countries in sub-Saharan Africa and South, East, and Southeast Asia, accounting for more than 90% of the 1.4 million pregnant women needing antiretrovirals to prevent vertical transmission, as well as more than 90% of children younger than 15 years in need of ART (Table 28-1).[2]

Historically, children have been neglected in national responses to HIV infection for a myriad of reasons.[7] This remains the case today, when more than 50% of adults who need ART have access to it, compared with 28% of children.[2]

Health system approaches to pediatric HIV infection vary by particular prevalence within a given country. HIV services are, by necessity, delivered at the primary health care level where HIV is prevalent and affects a broad cross section of the population. Most countries with such a context place a high priority on making HIV services universally available via integration into national health services, particularly maternal and child health. The World Health Organization (WHO) produced detailed recommendations on prevention of MTCT and pediatric HIV care and treatment that are aligned to this paradigm and widely used in developing countries around the globe.[8,9]

■ PREVENTION OF HIV INFECTION IN CHILDREN

While not neglecting other routes of HIV transmission in children (eg, contaminated blood transfusions and injections, early sexual debut, sexual abuse), HIV prevention efforts in pediatric health care focus on prevention of MTCT given the dominant role of MTCT in HIV infection. At the population level, scaling up effective prevention programs yields benefits beyond preventing new infections to improving child survival, and is the most effective strategy for preventing HIV-attributable mortality in children.[2] Toward this end, the Joint United Nations Programme on HIV/AIDS set the goal of virtually eliminating MTCT by 2015.[2]

HIV MTCT may occur during pregnancy, labor and delivery, and breastfeeding. Risk factors are well defined and include prenatal maternal factors such as high viral load (the level of HIV RNA in the blood), low CD4 cell count (indicative of immune suppression caused by HIV), and advanced clinical stage (the progressive clinical deterioration of an individual infected with HIV), as well as obstetric factors such as prolonged membrane rupture, invasive obstetric procedures, and whether the child breastfeeds.[10]

Without any intervention, the risk of MTCT in a non-breastfeeding population is 15% to 30%. Approximately 70% of transmission in a non-breastfeeding population occurs before delivery, with roughly 30% of transmission occurring during delivery.[11]

Table 28-1. Twenty-five Low- and Middle-Income Countries With the Highest Estimated Numbers of Pregnant Women Living With HIV in Need of Antiretrovirals to Prevent Mother-to-Child Transmission of HIV and the Corresponding Number of Children in Need of Antiretroviral Therapy, 2009

RANK	COUNTRY	ESTIMATED NUMBER OF PREGNANT WOMEN IN NEED OF ANTIRETROVIRALS IN 2009 (OR [RANGE] WHERE DATA LACKING)	% OF TOTAL IN LMIC	ESTIMATED NUMBER OF CHILDREN IN NEED OF ANTIRETROVIRAL THERAPY IN 2009 (OR [RANGE] WHERE DATA LACKING)	% OF TOTAL IN LMIC
1	South Africa	210,000	15.6	160,000	12.5
2	Nigeria	210,000	15.0	180,000	14.5
3	Mozambique	97,000	7.1	66,000	5.2
4	Uganda	88,000	6.4	76,000	6.0
5	United Republic of Tanzania	84,000	6.1	75,000	5.9
6	Kenya	81,000	5.9	89,000	7.0
7	Zambia	68,000	5.0	59,000	4.7
8	Malawi	57,000	4.2	61,000	4.8
9	Zimbabwe	50,000	3.6	71,000	5.6
10	India	43,000	3.1	[30,000–76,000]	4.1
11	Democratic Republic of the Congo	[20,000–54,000]	2.6	[17,000–46,000]	2.4
12	Cameroon	34,000	2.5	28,000	2.2

Table 28-1. Twenty-five Low- and Middle-Income Countries With the Highest Estimated Numbers of Pregnant Women Living With HIV in Need of Antiretrovirals to Prevent Mother-to-Child Transmission of HIV and the Corresponding Number of Children in Need of Antiretroviral Therapy, 2009, continued

RANK	COUNTRY	ESTIMATED NUMBER OF PREGNANT WOMEN IN NEED OF ANTIRETROVIRALS IN 2009 (OR [RANGE] WHERE DATA LACKING)	% OF TOTAL IN LMIC	ESTIMATED NUMBER OF CHILDREN IN NEED OF ANTIRETROVIRAL THERAPY IN 2009 (OR [RANGE] WHERE DATA LACKING)	% OF TOTAL IN LMIC
13	Ethiopia	[17,000–51,000]	2.4	[27,000–74,000]	3.9
14	Côte d'Ivoire	20,000	1.5	29,000	2.3
15	Chad	16,000	1.2	12,000	1.0
16	Angola	16,000	1.2	12,000	0.9
17	Burundi	15,000	1.1	14,000	1.1
18	Sudan	14,000	1.0	8,700	0.7
19	Lesotho	14,000	1.0	13,000	1.1
20	Ghana	13,000	1.0	13,000	1.0
21	Botswana	13,000	0.9	9,400	0.7
22	Rwanda	11,000	0.8	11,000	0.9
23	Swaziland	9,300	0.7	6,800	0.5
24	Namibia	7,700	0.6	9,200	0.7
25	Burkina Faso	6,500	0.5	8,000	0.6

Abbreviation: LMIC, low- and middle-income countries.

From World Health Organization, Joint United Nations Programme on HIV/AIDS, United Nation Children's Fund. *Towards Universal Access: Scaling Up Priority HIV/AIDS Interventions in the Health Sector: Progress Report 2010*. Geneva, Switzerland: WHO Press; 2010. http://whqlibdoc.who.int/publications/2010/9789241500395_eng.pdf. Accessed June 23, 2011

In a breastfeeding population, an additional 5% to 20% of infants are at risk for postnatal HIV transmission, such that the total risk increases to as much as 50%.[11] An individual patient could have a substantially higher or lower risk depending on individual risk factors, such as the mother's health, viral load, and duration of breastfeeding.

There are opportunities to prevent perinatal HIV transmission at each point when it can take place—pregnancy, labor and delivery, and breastfeeding. The effectiveness of strategies to reduce perinatal transmission differs by setting. The risk of MTCT can be decreased to less than 2% in a non-breastfeeding population in a developed country by administering antiretroviral drugs to women during pregnancy and labor, obstetric interventions including cesarean delivery (prior to membrane rupture), complete avoidance of breastfeeding, and administering antiretrovirals to the neonate after birth.[12]

In developing countries, several of these interventions may prove difficult. Cesarean delivery is often not safely available, and while the WHO and United Nations Children's Fund (UNICEF) have defined criteria that must be present for formula-feeding to be considered safe (described on page 775), these criteria may be difficult for families to satisfy.

However, studies show that perinatal transmission rates comparable to higher-income settings can be achieved in lower-income countries, including high-prevalence, low-income settings in sub-Saharan Africa, without cesarean delivery and with breastfeeding.[9] For example, in a Mozambican cohort, only 0.8% of babies born to women who were given antiretrovirals (ie, zidovudine [AZT], lamivudine [3TC], and nevirapine [NVP]) from as early as the 25th week of pregnancy through 6 months of breastfeeding were HIV-infected at 6 months of age; similar results have been seen elsewhere.[9,13–15]

In response to the needs of developing countries, particularly where HIV prevalence is high, the WHO issued comprehensive MTCT prevention guidelines organized around a comprehensive strategic approach that includes the following 4 components[9]:

- Primary prevention of HIV infection among women of childbearing age
- Preventing unintended pregnancies among women living with HIV
- Preventing HIV MTCT
- Providing appropriate treatment, care, and support to mothers living with HIV and their children and families

The first 2 components, while broad, are surmountable. The WHO notes that minimally reducing the prevalence of HIV infection and moderately reducing the number of unintended pregnancies among

HIV-positive women of childbearing age can reduce infant HIV infection similarly to single-dose NVP–based prevention interventions.[16] This is a substantial effect given that such interventions (administering a single dose of NVP [a non-nucleoside reverse-transcriptase inhibitor] to a pregnant woman at the onset of labor and to the baby as close to birth as possible) can reduce perinatal transmission by approximately 40%.[17] Preventing HIV transmission from an HIV-infected woman to her newborn focuses on ensuring that she is able to access antiretrovirals early in her pregnancy. Paramount to this is awareness of one's HIV status, which is inextricably linked to the availability and uptake of HIV testing; the opportunity to access perinatal transmission prevention interventions will not be realized if HIV-infected status is not appreciated. Globally, HIV testing rates in pregnancy remain low—only 26% of pregnant women in developing countries received an HIV test in 2009.[2] Rates also vary by location, ranging from 75% in Europe and Central Asia, to near 0% in the Middle East and North Africa, and 35% in high-prevalence sub-Saharan Africa.[2]

Rates of retesting during pregnancy are much lower.[2] This has implications for perinatal transmission because women whose test results are negative early in pregnancy (per standard recommendations) may become infected later in pregnancy. Acute HIV infection is associated with high viral load and thus an increased risk of perinatal transmission.[12] A substantial number of perinatal transmissions occur after HIV infection during pregnancy in high-prevalence settings; thus, retesting in late pregnancy (or during labor or as soon as possible after delivery) is recommended.[2,9] In any setting (including pediatric testing), rates of accepting HIV testing are higher when suggested by health care professionals rather than relying on patients or families to seek testing on their own.[18] Instituting provider-initiated testing and counseling into standard maternal-child health packages (including antenatal care) is appreciated as a critical feature of programs in higher-income countries and resource-limited settings with high MTCT prevention coverage and pediatric HIV services.[2,18]

Revisions to the WHO prevention of MTCT guidelines in 2010 (Table 28-2) reflect new evidence on the efficacy of various interventions, particularly antiretroviral use during pregnancy. In discussing antiretroviral use in pregnant women, their use for the *treatment* of HIV infection (with triple-drug ART) in eligible women (as determined by clinical stage and CD4 count where available) must be distinguished from *prophylaxis* against HIV transmission.

Table 28-2. 2010 World Health Organization Prevention of Mother-to-Child Transmission Guidelines: Antiretroviral Prophylaxis Options Recommended for HIV-infected Pregnant Women Who Do Not Need Treatment for Their Own Health

OPTION A: MATERNAL AZT	OPTION B: MATERNAL TRIPLE ANTIRETROVIRAL PROPHYLAXIS
Mother • Antepartum AZT (from as early as 14 weeks' gestation) • Single-dose NVP at onset of labor[a] • AZT + 3TC during labor and delivery[a] • AZT + 3TC for 7 days postpartum[a]	**Mother** Triple antiretrovirals from 14 weeks until 1 week after all exposure to breast milk has ended • AZT + 3TC + LPV/r • AZT + 3TC + ABC • AZT + 3TC + EFV • TDF + 3TC (or FTC) + EFV
Infant *Breastfeeding* • Single-dose NVP at birth plus daily NVP from birth until 1 week after all exposure to breast milk has ended *Non-breastfeeding* • Single-dose NVP at birth plus AZT or NVP from birth until 4 to 6 weeks	**Infant** *Breastfeeding* • AZT or NVP from birth until 4 to 6 weeks *Non-breastfeeding* • AZT or NVP from birth until 4 to 6 weeks

Abbreviations: ABC, abacavir; AZT, zidovudine; EFV, efavirenz; FTC, emtricitabine; LPV/r, lopinavir/ritonavir; NVP, nevirapine; TDF, tenofovir disoproxil fumarate; 3TC, lamivudine.

[a]Single-dose NVP and AZT + 3TC may be omitted if mother receives > 4 weeks of AZT antepartum.

From World Health Organization. *Antiretroviral Drugs for Treating Pregnant Women and Preventing HIV Infection in Infants: Recommendations for a Public Health Approach: 2010 Version.* Geneva, Switzerland: WHO Press; 2010. http://whqlibdoc.who.int/publications/2010/9789241599818_eng.pdf. Accessed March 25, 2011

HIV-infected pregnant women should be assessed clinically for evidence of advanced HIV disease progression (WHO clinical stage 3 or 4 [Box 28-1]), as well as have a CD4 cell count to look for evidence of immunosuppression. Clinical assessment alone is insufficient because more than half of individuals in clinical stage 1 or 2 may have CD4 counts below 350 cells/µL.[3,9] Antiretroviral therapy should be initiated as early as possible in pregnant women in WHO clinical stage 3 or 4 or with CD4 counts below 350 cells/µL; ART should continue throughout life, including during breastfeeding, which will improve mother's health and reduce the risk of perinatal HIV transmission.

When HIV-infected pregnant women do not need ART for their own health (ie, WHO clinical stage is 1 or 2 and CD4 count is greater than 350 cells/µL), the WHO recommends antiretrovirals be provided as 1 of 2 options. Option A is "short-course zidovudine"; option B is triple antiretroviral prophylaxis (Table 28-2). This should be started as early

Box 28-1. World Health Organization Clinical Staging of HIV Infection

1. Asymptomatic
2. Mild signs and symptoms of HIV infection
3. Substantial signs and symptoms of HIV infection
4. Severe illness due to HIV infection, including most opportunistic infections

From World Health Organization. *WHO Case Definitions of HIV for Surveillance and Revised Clinical Staging and Immunological Classification of HIV-Related Disease in Adults and Children.* Geneva, Switzerland: WHO Press; 2007. http://www.who.int/hiv/pub/guidelines/HIVstaging150307.pdf. Accessed June 23, 2011

as 14 weeks of pregnancy; the decision should be made at the country level in response to local capacity and feasibility of implementation.

While both options are efficacious, clinical trial and observational data favor triple antiretroviral prophylaxis over AZT plus single-dose NVP in terms of HIV prevention rates.[9] Recent evidence from Botswana shows that the choice of specific ART makes little difference in transmission outcomes. In a comparison of 3 different triple antiretroviral combinations (AZT + 3TC + abacavir [ABC], AZT + 3TC + lopinavir/ritonavir [LPV/r], and AZT + 3TC + NVP) administered during pregnancy through planned weaning after 6 months of breastfeeding, all 3 regimens resulted in high rates of virologic suppression and a cumulative perinatal transmission rate of 1.1%.[14]

When option A is chosen, data from Botswana suggest that maternal NVP may be omitted if the mother received at least 4 weeks of antiretrovirals prior to delivery.[19] While administering AZT plus 3TC for 1 week is recommended to reduce NVP resistance (occurring in 25% to 50% of cases after a single dose of NVP) after single-dose NVP,[20] data from Zambia suggest a single dose of tenofovir-emtricitabine (Truvada) may provide nearly as much protection against NVP resistance.[21]

Safety of Antiretrovirals

In developing countries, health care practitioners and families commonly express concerns about antiretroviral safety in the developing fetus and newborn. While certain antiretroviral combinations have been shown unsafe for pregnant women (eg, stavudine plus didanosine is associated with lactic acidosis), they are generally felt to be safe for the fetus and newborn.[22-24] The Antiretroviral Pregnancy Registry longitudinally assesses the risk of birth defects associated with antiretrovirals. The prevalence of birth defects in babies exposed in utero to antiretrovirals does not differ significantly from birth defect rates in the general population.[25]

Zidovudine, as part of ART, may cause anemia in infants and children, but clinically significant anemia during newborn prophylaxis is rare.[26] In addition, NVP prophylaxis is well tolerated by babies; toxicity was uncommon in trials of extended NVP (through 14 weeks).[27,28] However, efavirenz caused teratogenic effects in monkeys[29] and case reports showed neural tube and other birth defects in human newborns who were exposed to efavirenz in utero,[30,31] which led to the recommendation that it not be used in the first trimester of pregnancy.[9] The WHO recommends that NVP be substituted for efavirenz if it is realized that a woman taking efavirenz is in the first trimester of pregnancy.[9] However, a recent meta-analysis found no overall increased risk of birth defects among women exposed to efavirenz during the first trimester of pregnancy compared with exposure to other antiretroviral drugs. In this study, overall prevalence of birth defects with first-trimester efavirenz exposure was similar to that of the general population but sample size was limited, preventing definitive conclusions as to the risk of neural tube defects and other rare outcomes.[32]

Infant Feeding

Avoidance of breastfeeding has long been part of standard approaches to prevention of MTCT, given that as much as 40% of perinatal HIV transmission may be because of breastfeeding.[11] This approach has proven successful in developed countries where perinatal HIV transmission has become rare,[12] as well as in many low- and middle-income settings. Thailand incorporated replacement feeding into its national approach to MTCT prevention since the 1990s, as did Botswana. Rates of perinatal transmission in both countries are now less than 5%,[33,34] with the success credited in part to national formula programs. However, providing free formula to infants as a part of MTCT prevention is not economically or logistically feasible in many developing countries. In addition, breastfeeding is recognized as one of the most powerful child survival interventions and a cornerstone to reduce younger-than-5-years mortality worldwide.[35]

The issue of infant feeding is further complicated, particularly in lower-income countries, in that prevention of HIV infection in an infant does not necessarily increase an infant's likelihood of survival. Studies in developing countries show serious morbidity and mortality risks associated with formula-feeding. In the Botswana Mashi trial, cumulative mortality from all causes at 7 months of age was significantly higher (9.3% versus 4.9%) in infants who were randomly assigned to formula-feeding versus those who were assigned to breastfeeding plus AZT. HIV-free survival at 18 months of age was equivalent between the 2 groups, showing that the early mortality increase seen with formula-feeding negates the benefits of reduced HIV transmission.[19]

A Kenyan study showed that formula-fed infants have higher early mortality than breastfed infants (11% versus 9%).[36] A South African study showed cumulative 3-month mortality of 15.1% in infants who were given replacement feedings, whereas the corresponding rate in exclusively breastfed infants was only 6.1%.[37] Additionally, more than 22,000 Botswanan infants experienced diarrhea (compared with a little more than 9,000 for the same period in 2005), and the number of deaths in children younger than 5 years increased 20-fold during an outbreak of diarrhea in early 2006.[38] Virtually all the deaths that occurred during the outbreak were in formula-fed infants, which suggests a lack of protective immunity in formula-fed versus breastfed infants. This finding is consistent with the long-appreciated immunologic benefits of breastfeeding. Malnutrition and growth failure are also more common in formula-fed versus breastfed HIV-exposed infants.[39]

Recognizing this, the recently revised WHO guidelines on HIV and infant feeding focus on the prevention of perinatal HIV transmission, as well as what strategy— breastfeeding or its avoidance—is most likely to result in HIV-free survival of those infants who are exposed to HIV. National health authorities are advised to make their decisions based on national epidemiologic trends, the coverage of prevention of MTCT and ART services, and the main local causes of maternal and child undernutrition and mortality.

This decision will favor breastfeeding in most lower-income countries. The WHO recently clarified the conditions required to formula-feed safely (Box 28-2); however, these conditions are difficult to satisfy in most developing countries. Even in relatively wealthy settings, such

---

Box 28-2. Conditions Needed for an HIV-Positive Woman to Safely Use Formula-Feeding

1. Safe water and sanitation are ensured at the household level and in the community.
2. The mother or other caregiver can reliably provide sufficient infant formula to support normal growth and development of the infant.
3. The mother or caregiver can prepare it cleanly and frequently enough so that it is safe and carries a low risk of diarrhea and malnutrition.
4. The mother or caregiver can, in the first 6 months, exclusively give infant formula.
5. The family is supportive of this practice.
6. The mother or caregiver can access health care that offers comprehensive child health services.

From World Health Organization. *Antiretroviral Drugs for Treating Pregnant Women and Preventing HIV Infection in Infants: Recommendations for a Public Health Approach: 2010 Version.* Geneva, Switzerland: WHO Press; 2010. http://whqlibdoc.who.int/publications/2010/9789241599818_eng.pdf. Accessed March 25, 2011

as South Africa, the unavailability of formula at clinics is common.[40] Studies show other factors not specifically included in the WHO criteria to be associated with safe formula-feeding, such as a mother's disclosure of her HIV status.[41]

Recent evidence shows that the likelihood of HIV transmission via breastfeeding is markedly reduced when a mother is receiving ART or infants receive extended courses of NVP while breastfeeding when ART is not available for this aspect of MTCT prevention. Indeed, the WHO recommends that all HIV-exposed infants who are breastfeeding receive prophylaxis (option A or B in Table 28-2). Exclusive breastfeeding is recommended for the first 6 months, after which complimentary foods are introduced and infants continue to breastfeed up to 12 months. Weaning, a time when the risk of the infant developing malnutrition rises precipitously, should occur over approximately 1 month, and breastfeeding should cease only when a safe diet and adequate nutrition without breast milk can be ensured.

■ FOLLOW-UP OF THE HIV-EXPOSED INFANT

Prevention of perinatal HIV transmission does not end when an infant completes postnatal antiretroviral prophylaxis or is successfully weaned. In concert with a longitudinal, family-centered approach to care, mothers must have postpartum care and ongoing management of HIV infection, while infants must receive an assessment of HIV status, clinical monitoring, co-trimoxazole preventive therapy (CPT), and general infant care.

Diagnosis of HIV infection in exposed infants is of particular importance, as mortality is high in untreated HIV-infected children—as much as 50% by 2 years of age and 80% by 5 years of age.[42] Antiretroviral therapy reduces pediatric mortality considerably. The South Africa "Children with HIV Early Antiretroviral Therapy" study demonstrated a 75% decline in mortality for infants initiated on ART immediately after diagnosis[43] and the WHO now recommends that all infants younger than 24 months, regardless of clinical stage or CD4 count, receive ART. However, about only 275,000 children worldwide currently receive ART.[42] Many of the estimated 2.3 million HIV-infected children remain unidentified, particularly in developing countries, including many of the nearly 500,000 children in urgent need of ART.[42] Increasing HIV testing opportunities for children is a critical priority in the global response to pediatric HIV, particularly in high-prevalence developing countries.

Antibody tests such as HIV enzyme-linked immunosorbent assay and rapid HIV tests are not suitable for diagnosing HIV in infants because maternal antibodies to HIV cross the placenta and are detectable in infants up to 18 months of age. Therefore, a positive HIV antibody test result in an infant younger than 18 months only indicates that an infant was perinatally exposed to HIV and may or may not be infected. A virologic polymerase chain reaction (PCR) test must be used instead. While HIV DNA PCR is the gold standard for infant diagnosis, HIV RNA PCR is also sensitive and specific.[12]

In most developing countries, the first HIV DNA PCR test is performed at 4 to 6 weeks postpartum via dried blood spot collected from the infant's heel; this initial visit is also used to initiate CPT as well as give first immunizations. While WHO guidelines allow for an infant who was never breastfed to be considered definitively HIV negative after a single negative HIV DNA PCR test result (sensitivity and specificity greater than 99% at age 6 weeks), some developing country guidelines require 2 negative tests. United States guidelines require 2 negative virologic test results at 1 month or older and 4 months or older.[12] Breastfeeding infants must have repeat HIV DNA PCR testing 6 weeks after breastfeeding cessation.

Because more than 90% of 9-month-old HIV-uninfected infants have lost their maternal antibodies,[44] many developing countries use rapid testing for infants 9 months or older, with HIV DNA PCR tests performed only on those who are still antibody positive. In children older than 18 months, rapid antibody tests can be used for definitive HIV diagnosis, and most developing countries use a confirmatory rapid test at 18 months of age, regardless of prior test results, to demonstrate seroreversion (definitively HIV uninfected) or definitive HIV-infected status.

As mentioned earlier, mortality is high for untreated HIV-infected infants. Rapid disease progression is not uncommon. *Pneumocystis jiroveci* pneumonia (formerly *Pneumocystis carinii* pneumonia) is often the first manifestation, which may occur before HIV infection is realized. Accordingly, all HIV-exposed infants should be placed on co-trimoxazole prophylaxis against *Pneumocystis* pneumonia until HIV infection is excluded and the infant is no longer at risk of HIV acquisition through breastfeeding. Co-trimoxazole, which is safe, inexpensive, and widely available, has benefits for HIV-infected children beyond *Pneumocystis* prevention, including prevention of *Toxoplasma* encephalitis (also seen with advanced HIV disease, usually in older children and adults), as well as non–HIV-related diseases, including malaria, severe bacterial infections, and diarrhea, which are responsible for much child mortality in developing countries.[45]

Data from Zambia show a 50% mortality reduction and significant reduction in children's hospital admissions when on CPT,[46] while Zimbabwean data demonstrate reduced deaths due to acute respiratory infection in HIV-infected infants younger than 6 months.[47] Accordingly, the WHO advises CPT for all HIV-exposed infants and all HIV-infected infants and children in settings with high HIV prevalence, high infant mortality from infectious diseases, or limited health infrastructure.[45]

Despite the evidence and recommendations for CPT use, only 14% of HIV-exposed infants globally received CPT in 2009, and only 18% in high-prevalence Eastern and Southern Africa.[2] A clear need exists for scaling up this critical survival intervention.

The first set of routine immunizations, all of which are given to HIV-exposed infants, takes place during the first visit at 6 weeks of age. Given the propensity for substantial reactions,[48,49] bacille Calmette-Guérin (BCG) immunization is withheld from ill-appearing HIV-exposed infants and from all HIV-infected infants. There is concern that immunizations given to HIV-infected infants prior to ART initiation (and subsequent immune reconstitution) may not generate long-lasting immunity. While recent data indicate children on ART may benefit from revaccination, more data from regions of high HIV prevalence are needed to determine the ideal timing and number of vaccine doses for each vaccine-preventable disease.[50]

HIV-exposed infants should be seen monthly during the first year of life, with repeat HIV testing at any point should HIV be suspected on clinical grounds. The WHO defined clinical criteria for presumptive diagnosis of severe HIV disease when virologic testing is not available.[51] Such a diagnosis is made when an infant is HIV antibody-positive and an AIDS-indicator condition is present or the infant is symptomatic with 2 or more of following: oral thrush, severe pneumonia, severe sepsis. Other factors supporting presumptive HIV diagnosis in an HIV-exposed infant include recent HIV-related maternal death, advanced maternal HIV disease, or a CD4 count less than 20%.

■ IDENTIFYING THE HIV-INFECTED CHILD NOT IDENTIFIED IN INFANCY

As mentioned, fewer than half of women globally, including in high-prevalence sub-Saharan Africa, are tested for HIV in pregnancy. It is likely that even today most HIV-infected babies are born to mothers who were never tested for HIV and thus did not receive MTCT prevention interventions.[42] Not placed into post-prevention follow-up, these infants are at great risk of remaining unidentified and succumbing to HIV-related conditions and complications at an early age. When these HIV-infected children are identified, substantial HIV-related conditions and complications are often present. Targeted HIV testing strategies for infants and children are of paramount importance, particularly in high-prevalence settings.

Provider-initiated testing and counseling has been shown in many developing countries to yield higher rates of pediatric testing than older approaches, such as relying on families to approach health care professionals asking to be tested.[52] Efforts to make HIV testing part of health care routines are also gaining ground in many lower-income countries. Whatever the baseline HIV prevalence in a community, prevalence will be higher in settings where children are seeking health care and particularly where they are ill. Routine testing in health care settings, including pediatric wards, malnutrition units, and even immunization clinics, yields large numbers of HIV-infected patients,[53–55] particularly in high-prevalence settings. The willingness of health care workers to promote testing is a key factor influencing its utilization.[56] Therefore, training health care workers to increase their comfort level in discussing pediatric HIV with families is crucial.

Creative approaches toward increasing the identification of HIV-exposed and HIV-infected children may pay dividends. For example, in Malawi, the innovative strategy of incorporating volunteer parents of HIV-infected children to promoting routine testing on a busy pediatrics ward was shown to markedly increase the number of children tested, identified, and enrolled into care compared with a standard approach using counselors.[57] Another program in Malawi uses health care workers to improve identifying HIV-infected and HIV-exposed children and referring them earlier to community health centers. In this program, the approach of assigning a dedicated worker to HIV-infected pregnant women in the community has been particularly effective in improving outcomes for HIV-exposed infants.[58]

Health care workers should operate with a high index of suspicion for HIV infection when encountering ill children in developing countries, particularly where HIV is prevalent. Certain clinical findings suggest HIV infection, especially when children were orphaned or have mothers with known HIV infection. Integrated Management of Childhood Illness (IMCI) is a WHO/UNICEF strategy directed at reducing mortality in children younger than 5 years by improving health care at a primary level.[59] The IMCI algorithm for suspected symptomatic HIV infection focuses on whether the child has 1 or more of 4 conditions (pneumonia, persistent diarrhea, ear discharge, very low weight for age) or 3 findings (oral thrush [in children older than 3 months], parotid enlargement [typically bilateral], generalized lymphadenopathy).[60] Positive findings direct the clinician into the algorithm where the likelihood of HIV infection is classified. It should be noted that in the absence of HIV testing, the IMCI algorithm is not a sensitive tool for diagnosing HIV infection in children[61] but is very useful as a prompt for clinicians to suggest testing. Table 28-3 lists several physical findings that suggest HIV infection in children.

Table 28-3. Association of Physical Findings With Likelihood of HIV Infection in a Child, Particularly in Settings of Moderate to High HIV Prevalence		
HIV VERY LIKELY	**SUGGESTIVE OF HIV INFECTION**	**SUSPICIOUS FOR HIV INFECTION BUT ALSO COMMONLY SEEN IN HIV-UNINFECTED CHILDREN**
Kaposi sarcoma	Generalized lymphadenopathy	Persistent or recurrent upper respiratory infections, including otitis media
Pneumocystis pneumonia	Hepatosplenomegaly[a]	
Severe retinitis	Parotid enlargement	Failure to thrive
Persistent, severe diarrhea	Persistent or recurrent fever	Tuberculosis
Esophageal candidiasis	Recurrent, severe bacterial infection	Recurrent diarrhea
Invasive salmonellosis		Severe pneumonia
Cryptococcal meningitis	Persistent or recurrent oral candidiasis	Unexplained sepsis
Herpes zoster (multi-dermatomal)	Persistent, unexplained dermatitis	
	Loss of milestones	
	Neurologic dysfunction	

[a]Areas non-endemic for malaria.

Adapted from African Network for the Care of Children Affected by AIDS (ANECCA). *Handbook on Paediatric AIDS in Africa.* Revised July 2006; and Baylor International Pediatric AIDS Initiative (BIPAI). *HIV Curriculum for the Health Professional.* 4th Ed. © 2010 Baylor College of Medicine.

■ STAGING, DETERMINING ELIGIBILITY FOR ANTIRETROVIRAL THERAPY, AND COMMON MANIFESTATIONS OF HIV INFECTION

Once a child is identified as HIV infected, the clinical approach focuses on determining the child's eligibility for ART. Current recommendations suggest that all children younger than 24 months be initiated on ART at the time of diagnosis regardless of clinical stage or CD4 count. Children older than 24 months must meet criteria based on clinical stage and CD4 count for ART initiation. Table 28-4 shows the WHO recommendations for initiating ART in children.

Generally, clinical stages as determined by the WHO (Box 28-1) reflect the natural history of HIV infection in an individual over time. Table 28-5 lists specific conditions included in each clinical stage. The Centers for Disease Control and Prevention uses a similar clinical staging system in which stages N, A, B, and C roughly correspond to WHO

Table 28-4. World Health Organization Recommendations for Initiating Antiretroviral Therapy in Children

AGE	CRITERIA TO INITIATE ANTIRETROVIRAL THERAPY
Younger than 24 mo	All irrespective of WHO clinical stage or CD4 count
24–59 mo	Whichever of the following is lower, irrespective of WHO clinical stage: WHO clinical stage 3 or 4 *or* CD4 count ≤750 cells/μL or CD4 percentage ≤25
5 y and older	Irrespective of CD4 count, WHO clinical stage 3 or 4 *or* CD4 count ≤350 cells/μL (as in adults)
Special circumstances	Younger than 18 mo with presumptive clinical diagnosis of HIV infection

Abbreviations: WHO, World Health Organization.

Adapted from World Health Organization. *Antiretroviral Therapy for HIV Infection in Infants and Children: Towards Universal Access: Recommendations for a Public Health Approach: 2010 Revision.* Geneva, Switzerland: WHO Press; 2010. http://whqlibdoc.who.int/publications/2010/9789241599801_eng.pdf. Accessed June 23, 2011

stages 1, 2, 3, and 4. Accurate clinical staging depends on the clinician taking a careful, detailed history and performing a thorough physical examination.

HIV pathophysiology centers on its effect on CD4⁺ T cells. HIV leads to CD4 reduction with concomitant immunosuppression through a variety of mechanisms. Stage 4 conditions are notable for the presence of opportunistic infections not generally seen in immunocompetent individuals. Whereas the mean time from infection to immunosuppression in adults is several years, HIV typically causes a much swifter drop in CD4 counts in children. This drop varies by age, with infants being notable for very early immunosuppression after infection (months) to older children where 1 to 3 years of age is more common. In all age groups, there are those who are slow in progressing who tolerate HIV infection for long periods without developing clinically advanced disease or immunosuppression; however, this is much less common in children than adults, and all of the factors influencing this phenomenon remain to be determined. Because absolute CD4 counts tend to vary considerably in children, particularly younger children, CD4 percentages are considered more reliable in younger children.[8] Where available, CD4 percentages are preferred for children younger than 5 years, and children 5 years and older are managed using absolute CD4 counts.[8]

Table 28-5. World Health Organization Clinical Staging of HIV/AIDS for Children With Confirmed HIV Infection

CLINICAL STAGE 1	CLINICAL STAGE 2	CLINICAL STAGE 3	CLINICAL STAGE 4
• Asymptomatic • Persistent generalized lymphadenopathy	• Unexplained persistent hepatosplenomegaly • Papular pruritic eruptions • Extensive wart virus infection • Extensive molluscum contagiosum • Fungal nail infections • Recurrent oral ulcerations • Unexplained persistent parotid enlargement • Lineal gingival erythema • Herpes zoster • Recurrent or chronic upper respiratory tract infections (otitis media, otorrhea, sinusitis, or tonsillitis)	• Unexplained moderate malnutrition not adequately responding to standard therapy • Unexplained persistent diarrhea (14 days or more) • Unexplained persistent fever (above 37.5°C intermittent or constant, for longer than 1 month) • Persistent oral candidiasis (after 6–8 weeks of life) • Oral hairy leukoplakia • Acute necrotizing ulcerative gingivitis or periodontitis • Lymph node tuberculosis • Pulmonary tuberculosis • Severe recurrent bacterial pneumonia • Symptomatic lymphoid interstitial pneumonitis • Chronic HIV-associated lung disease including bronchiectasis • Unexplained anemia (<8 g/dL), neutropenia (<0.5 × 10⁹ per L), or chronic thrombocytopenia (<50 x 10⁹ per L)	• Unexplained severe wasting, stunting, or severe malnutrition not responding to standard therapy • *Pneumocystis* pneumonia • Recurrent severe bacterial infections (eg, empyema or pyomyositis bone or joint infection, meningitis [excluding pneumonia] • Chronic herpes simplex infection (orolabial or cutaneous of more than 1 month's duration or visceral at any site) • Extrapulmonary tuberculosis • Kaposi sarcoma • Esophageal candidiasis (or candidiasis of trachea, bronchi, or lungs) • Central nervous system toxoplasmosis (after 1 month of life) • HIV encephalopathy • Cytomegalovirus infection: retinitis or cytomegalovirus infection affecting another organ, with onset at older than 1 month • Extrapulmonary cryptococcosis (including meningitis) • Disseminated endemic mycosis (extra-pulmonary histoplasmosis, coccidioi-domycosis)

Table 28-5. World Health Organization Clinical Staging of HIV/AIDS for Children With Confirmed HIV Infection, continued

CLINICAL STAGE 1	CLINICAL STAGE 2	CLINICAL STAGE 3	CLINICAL STAGE 4
			• Chronic cryptosporidiosis • Chronic isosporiasis • Disseminated non-tuberculous mycobacterial infection • Cerebral or B cell non-Hodgkin lymphoma • Progressive multifocal leukoencephalopathy • Symptomatic HIV-associated nephropathy or HIV-associated cardiomyopathy • Additional specific conditions are included in regional classifications (eg, reactivation of American trypanosomiasis [meningoencephalitis and/or myocarditis] in the WHO region of the Americas, penicilliosis in Asia, and HIV-associated rectovaginal fistula in Africa)

Abbreviation: WHO, World Health Organization.

Adapted from World Health Organization. *WHO Case Definitions of HIV for Surveillance and Revised Clinical Staging and Immunological Classification of HIV-Related Disease in Adults and Children.* Geneva, Switzerland: WHO Press; 2007. http://www.who.int/hiv/pub/guidelines/HIVstaging150307.pdf. Accessed June 23, 2011

The WHO produced guidelines for managing common illnesses, including HIV-associated conditions, in hospitals with limited resources; an excellent resource for those practicing in developing countries is *Pocket Book of Hospital Care for Children* (available at www.who.int/ child_adolescent_health/documents/9241546700/en/index.html). While details on the diagnosis and management of the many HIV-associated conditions listed in Table 28-5 are beyond the scope of this chapter, some particularly important conditions deserve mention.

Generalized lymphadenopathy, especially if persistent, suggests HIV infection and represents early HIV clinical manifestation in a child (stage 1). Stage 2 conditions are notable for being common and nonspecific and are certainly seen in non–HIV-infected children as well. However, their recurrence or persistence is notable with HIV infection. For example, it is not uncommon for an HIV-infected child's health record to note multiple outpatient visits for recurrent otitis media, sinusitis, or bronchitis prior to HIV infection ultimately being diagnosed. Persistent hepatosplenomegaly outside of malaria-endemic areas is also characteristic of HIV infection. Health care workers are taught to recognize such recurrent presentations as indicative of HIV infection and to offer testing accordingly in HIV-prevalent areas.

Several skin conditions are notable for the presence of HIV infection and are unusual in its absence. Papular pruritic eruptions, extensive plane warts, and angular cheilitis (in adolescents) are particularly characteristic; having 3 or more discrete skin conditions and a history of recurrent skin rashes or angular cheilitis have been associated with immunosuppression.[62]

Malnutrition is a very common and important feature of advancing HIV infection that is multifactorial in nature, including the additional metabolic demand HIV infection places on the child, malabsorption, and the synergistic effect of food insecurity all too common in HIV-prevalent areas. Clinicians should note that the presence of even just a moderate degree of otherwise unexplained malnutrition (ie, due to poor or inadequate feeding, food insecurity, or other infections, and not responding to standard management) makes a child clinical stage 3 and qualified for ART, regardless of age or CD4 counts. Moderate malnutrition is defined by low weight-for-age z scores between -2 and -3, while severe malnutrition (stage 4) is defined by weight-for-height z scores (wasting) or height-for-age z scores (stunting) less than -3, or edema in the presence of malnutrition.

The effect of HIV on a child's developing nervous system can be profound. While cognitive delay and difficulty with school are common findings in HIV-infected children, more serious conditions can occur. HIV encephalopathy (stage 4) is a severe manifestation of the effect of HIV on the brain and is heralded by several features, including failure to attain or loss of developmental milestones or intellectual ability, symmetric motor deficits accompanied by other neurologic findings (ie, ataxia, gait disturbances, abnormal reflexes, or paresis), and impaired brain growth. Loss of milestones in an infant or young child is a particularly common presentation of HIV encephalopathy in developing countries and while not specific to HIV infection, should raise a strong warning for the possibility in areas where HIV infection is common. It is not uncommon for signs and symptoms of HIV encephalopathy to resolve considerably with ART.

Many different opportunistic infections further characterize clinical stage 4 and represent the presence of severe immunocompromise—all are clinical indications for ART. While the highest incidence of *Pneumocystis* pneumonia is seen among HIV-infected infants, it is also common in immunocompromised HIV-infected children beyond infancy, particularly when CPT is not being taken. A normal chest radiograph is often seen, even when tachypnea, dyspnea, and hypoxia are prominent. Table 28-6 notes WHO recommendations for CPT use. Co-trimoxazole preventive therapy should be administered daily; intermittent CPT has been associated with higher rates of invasive bacterial disease than daily CPT.[63] *Pneumocystis* pneumonia treatment includes a 21-day course of high-dose CTX.

Cryptosporidium parvum causes severe and persistent diarrhea in immunocompromised children, and case fatality rates can be high. While nitazoxanide has been shown to effectively treat *Cryptosporidium* in immunocompetent children and adults,[64] response to nitazoxanide has not been consistently demonstrated in immunocompromised children. Even high doses given for up to 28 days have been ineffective in clinical trials in sub-Saharan Africa.[65] *Cryptosporidium* generally responds to the immune restoration effected by ART.

While rarer in children than adults, cryptococcal meningitis presents similarly in both groups as a subacute but severe meningitis and can be life threatening. Ideal treatment includes an initial therapy of amphotericin B plus 5-flucytosine (5FC) for 14 days, followed by oral fluconazole for 8 to 10 weeks, and then continuation therapy. Where 5FC is not available, oral fluconazole should be combined with amphotericin B in initial therapy.[66] Amphotericin B is not available in many

Table 28-6. World Health Organization Recommendations for Co-trimoxazole Preventive Therapy for HIV-Exposed and HIV-Infected Infants and Children

GENERAL RECOMMENDATION FOR MOST SETTINGS	IN SETTINGS WITH HIGH HIV PREVALENCE, HIGH INFANT MORTALITY FROM INFECTIOUS DISEASES, OR LIMITED HEALTH INFRASTRUCTURE
All exposed infants younger than 1 y regardless of clinical or immunologic staging, starting at 4 to 6 weeks of age HIV-exposed breastfeeding children, regardless of clinical or immunologic staging All children 1 to 5 y for clinical stages 2, 3, 4, or CD4 percentage <25 All patients older than 5 y if • Clinical stage 2, 3, 4 (if no CD4) • CD4 <350 cells/μL • Clinical stage 3 or 4 (regardless of CD4)	CPT for *all* children born to HIV-positive mothers CPT for *all* HIV-positive children younger than 5 y, regardless of symptoms CPT for *all* symptomatic HIV-positive children 5 y and older

Abbreviation: CPT, co-trimoxazole preventive therapy.

Adapted from World Health Organization, United Nations Children's Fund. *Co-trimoxazole Prophylaxis for HIV-Exposed and HIV-Infected Infants and Children: Practical Approaches to Implementation and Scale Up.* Geneva, Switzerland: WHO Press; 2009. http://www.unicef.org/aids/files/CotrimoxazoleGuide_2009.pdf. Accessed June 23, 2011

developing countries, and oral fluconazole is the only agent available to treat cryptococcal meningitis; case fatality rates tend to be higher with this approach.[66] Markedly increased intracranial pressure is common with cryptococcal meningitis, with opening pressure often quite high on initial lumbar puncture. Intracranial pressure should be monitored with repeated lumbar puncture, especially during the first 2 weeks of therapy. Fluconazole is continued as secondary prophylaxis after treatment until immune restoration takes place with ART and patients are stable on therapy for several months. Guidelines for primary prophylaxis in children and for discontinuation of secondary prophylaxis in children 5 years and younger are not clearly defined.

Kaposi sarcoma is an unusual but common (especially in sub-Saharan Africa) malignant manifestation of an infection with human herpesvirus 8, primarily involving skin but also associated with severe disease in the lungs, gastrointestinal tract, liver, and spleen. Mucocutaneous lesions are usually a ruddy brown or purple and may be flat, raised, or nodular on any skin surface or inside the mouth. Lymphadenopathic forms may also occur. Visceral disease is frequently fatal. Antiretroviral therapy is often effective for Kaposi sarcoma, but chemotherapy is frequently required, especially when there is visceral involvement.

Globally, for HIV-infected and uninfected children alike, severe bacterial infections such as diarrhea and pneumonia are responsible for the majority of child deaths outside the neonatal period. In a given area, rates of diarrhea tend to be more common in HIV-infected children than uninfected children, and bacterial etiologies are common. Interventions directed at diarrhea prevention may be particularly likely to benefit HIV-infected children.[67]

HIV-infected children experience pneumonia more frequently than uninfected children and have a higher risk of severe disease even when on ART and no longer immunocompromised.[68] Standard approaches to managing pneumonia in children require modification in areas of high HIV prevalence with the addition of *Pneumocystis* pneumonia treatment (high-dose CPT) to empiric broad-spectrum antibiotics for infants or children not taking *Pneumocystis* prophylaxis.[68]

While the duration of diarrhea and pneumonia episodes tends to be longer in HIV-infected children, short-term multi-micronutrient supplementation containing vitamins A B, C, D, E, and folic acid, along with iron, copper, and zinc, has been noted in HIV-infected children to reduce duration of illness and length of hospitalization associated with these 2 important diagnoses.[69]

■ ANTIRETROVIRAL TREATMENT

While nutritional support and prophylaxis against opportunistic infections are very important for HIV-infected children, effective ART is the key to restoring health and its long-term maintenance. Highly active ART has been available in developed countries since the latter part of the 1990s but only recently became freely available in many developing countries, including high-prevalence sub-Saharan Africa. Pediatric ART programs have generated notable successes across diverse developing countries.[70-73] Even in rural areas and primary care settings in resource-poor countries, good clinical outcomes of ART on HIV-infected children have been noted.[74,75] Antiretroviral therapy reduces incidences of osteogenesis imperfecta and tuberculosis (TB) in HIV-infected children[76] and assists in restoring normal growth.[77] As mentioned earlier, ART dramatically reduces the mortality for HIV-infected children.[2] In resource-limited settings, more than half of the deaths of children who were on ART occur in the first 3 months[73]; young age, malnutrition, and low CD4 counts are associated with a higher risk of early death when on ART.[72,78] Early HIV diagnosis and treatment are clearly important, but the number of infants and young children enrolled in most pediatric ART programs is low in developing countries[74]; therefore, early identification and follow-up of HIV-exposed infants is critical.

Antiretroviral therapy is not curative. Effective ART results in prolonged suppression of HIV replication, which allows immune function to be restored in most cases.

Antiretroviral therapy efficacy is measured through 3 parameters with many clinical benefits: clinical, immunologic, and virologic. Immunologically, CD4 counts generally rise, often to non-immunosuppressed levels. Virologically, HIV RNA levels decline and are ideally undetectable within the first 6 months of ART initiation. Therefore, failure to achieve these parameters or regression after initial response are the hallmarks of ART failure.

Eligibility and Choice of Regimen

Clinical and immunologic parameters are used to determine ART eligibility for children older than 24 months (Table 28-7), while it is recommended that ART be initiated in infants and children younger than 24 months at the time of diagnosis, given the unreliability of clinical and immunologic markers of disease progression in young children.

Based on the mechanism of action, there are multiple categories of antiretrovirals. Unfortunately, options for children remain limited compared with options for adults, particularly in developing countries. Many existing antiretrovirals do not have pediatric formulations or approval for use in children. The WHO has placed emphasis on increasing pediatric antiretroviral options.

To lower the chance of resistance, antiretrovirals are used in combination with at least 3 different antiretrovirals active at 2 or more distinct sites of action in the HIV life cycle. Standard ART combinations generally include a backbone of 2 nucleoside reverse-transcriptase inhibitors plus a non-nucleoside reverse-transcriptase inhibitor or a protease inhibitor. Based on availability and feasibility considerations in resource-limited settings, the WHO recommends one of the following 2 nucleoside reverse-transcriptase inhibitor backbones (in order of preference) as first-line therapy for infants and children: AZT + 3TC; ABC + 3TC or stavudine + 3TC. The third antiretroviral choice depends on specific criteria as outlined in Table 28-7.

Adherence

Adherence to therapy is the critical factor in determining how well a child does on ART. Adherence between 95% and 105% of expected doses is required to maintain effect without developing antiretroviral resistance (seen with lower rates of adherence) or toxicity (more likely with antiretroviral overdosing); adherence rates for each antiretroviral should be calculated and any discrepancies addressed at each visit.

Table 28-7. Preferred First-line Antiretroviral Therapy for Infants and Children

PATIENT GROUP	THIRD ANTIRETROVIRAL TO BE PAIRED WITH AZT + 3TC OR ABC + 3TC BACKBONES IN FIRST-LINE ANTIRETROVIRAL THERAPY
Infants	
Infant or child younger than 24 mo not exposed to antiretrovirals	NVP
Infant or child younger than 24 mo exposed to NNRTI (EFV or NVP)	LPV/r
Infant or child younger than 24 mo with unknown antiretroviral exposure	NVP
Children	
Children 24 mo to 3 y	NVP
Children older than 3 y	NVP or EFV (many country guidelines favor EFV)
Concomitant TB Treatment	
Child younger than 3 y with TB treatment	NVP
Child older than 3 y or adolescent with TB treatment	EFV

Abbreviations: ABC, abacavir; AZT, zidovudine; EFV, efavirenz; LPV/r, lopinavir/ritonavir; NNRTI, non-nucleoside reverse-transcriptase inhibitor; NVP, nevirapine; TB, tuberculosis; 3TC, lamivudine.

From World Health Organization. *Antiretroviral Therapy for HIV Infection in Infants and Children: Towards Universal Access. Recommendations for a Public Health Approach: 2010 Revision.* Geneva, Switzerland: WHO Press; 2010. http://whqlibdoc.who.int/publications/2010/9789241599801_eng.pdf. Accessed June 23, 2011

Achieving good adherence is not easy for children and families. Taking multiple medications at different times, sometimes in coordination with meals, on a perpetual basis is complex. Early and ongoing counseling is critical, as is the responsibility of the entire health care team. Problems with transportation to the clinic, lack of support systems, and stigma should ideally be addressed prior to initiating ART and anticipated during ongoing supportive adherence counseling for those patients on ART. An age-appropriate disclosure process is an important component of adherence support, particularly for older children.

Monitoring

Infants and children on ART are followed for clinical, immunologic, and virologic response at regular intervals. The potential for ART to cause toxicity is also monitored. Early responses to ART are especially important. A gain in CD4 percentage in the first 6 months of ART has shown to predict subsequent ART outcomes, as has weight gain; children who respond poorly in these parameters early on are at higher risk of viral non-suppression, treatment failure, and death.[79]

Ideally, baseline values for viral load, CD4, hemoglobin, liver enzymes, and blood urea nitrogen/creatinine should be obtained prior to ART initiation and followed on a regular basis at least every 6 months, often more frequently early on, and as determined by the presence of symptoms or need to follow up on any toxicity noted.

Antiretrovirals commonly used in developing countries have characteristic toxicities: anemia with AZT; hepatitis and allergic skin reactions, including Stevens-Johnson Syndrome (rarely), with NVP and efavirenz; lipodystrophy and peripheral neuropathy (less commonly in children than adults) with stavudine; severe systemic hypersensitivity (although very rarely in African children[80]) with ABC; dyslipidemia with LPV/r; renal insufficiency with tenofovir; and psychological side effects with efavirenz. Management of specific toxicities depends on their severity; single-drug substitutions (swaps) may be carried out when necessary, such as stavudine for AZT-associated anemia or NVP for efavirenz-associated psychological effects. Severe toxicity may merit complete ART suspension. Lactic acidosis can be seen with any ART regimen (generally after more than 4 months on ART) but is most common with regimens containing stavudine or didanosine. Management is supportive with substitution for stavudine or didanosine and complete ART suspension in more substantial cases.

Data from large pediatric treatment programs in resource-limited settings have shown toxicity-related ART regimen change to be uncommon, which generally suggests good tolerability of WHO-recommended first-line regimens, including those containing NVP.[81,82]

Treatment Failure

Therapy is changed to second-line treatments when first-line ART fails; however, these treatments are not consistently available in all developing countries. While national policies differ among developing countries, the WHO defines ART failure along clinical, immunologic, and virologic lines after at least 24 weeks on ART in a treatment-adherent child.

- *Clinical failure:* Appearance or reappearance of WHO stage 3 or 4 events (clinical manifestations)
- *Immunological failure:* Developing or returning to age-related immunologic thresholds
  - CD4 count less than 200 cells/µL or CD4 percentage less than 10 for children 2 to 5 years of age
  - CD4 count less than 100 cells/µL for a child 5 years or older
- *Virological failure:* Persistent viral load above 5,000 RNA copies per mL

The importance of ensuring treatment adherence for a child failing ART is vital. Most treatment failure is due to non-adherence, and many failing children's therapy can be effective (even on a current line of therapy) if adherence can be restored. Changing therapy lines when children are non-adherent will swiftly lead to failure of the second-line regimen, again due to non-adherence.

Treatment-adherent children who are failing therapy are presumed to have antiretroviral resistance. Proving this with a resistance test, while perhaps ideal, is not essential; effective second-line regimens can be predicted from first-line drug exposures, as resistance tests are not available in many resource-limited settings. Second-line therapies use at least 2 drugs expected to be effective with LPV/r generally included in place of NVP or efavirenz, and vice versa, and ABC or AZT in place of the other. Lamivudine is maintained, as most resistant viruses have a particular mutation to 3TC (known as M184V) that reduces their pathogenicity; maintaining 3TC will help maintain this less virulent-resistant strain of HIV. Newer antiretrovirals, such as darunavir (latest-generation protease inhibitor) and raltegravir (integrase inhibitor), while not part of standard ART approaches in developing settings, are used in some settings, where available, as part of salvage therapy after second-line ART failure.

Immune Reconstitution Syndrome

Immune reconstitution syndrome (IRS) is a common complication of ART in the developing world in which a patient develops a paradoxical worsening of symptoms soon after initiating ART. Immune reconstitution syndrome is caused by ART awakening the child's immune system in the presence of an occult infection (often an opportunistic infection) not clinically apparent at the time of ART initiation, to which the awakened immune system reacts. Immune reconstitution syndrome frequently resembles the naturally occurring infection itself, such that a reaction to occult pulmonary TB after initiating ART presents with pulmonary symptoms, to occult central nervous system (CNS) cryptococcal infection with neurologic symptoms, and so on. Other common underlying infections unmasked by ART are hepatitis C, cytomegalovirus, and varicella-zoster virus. Reactions to BCG vaccine are also common.[83]

Immune reconstitution syndrome occurs in as many as 40% of HIV-infected patients with ART initiations,[84] usually within 12 weeks of therapy initiation. Immune reconstitution syndrome is more common with advanced HIV disease, particularly when initial CD4 counts are quite low; improvement in CD4 count in concert with symptoms is a hallmark of IRS diagnosis. Immune reconstitution syndrome management depends on its severity; while generally mild and self-limited,

IRS can be life threatening. Treating the underlying infection (eg, TB, *Cryptococcus*) is essential. Antiretroviral treatment can be continued in most cases. Steroids to control IRS-associated inflammatory processes may be required in more serious cases; ART is discontinued when life-threatening IRS (particularly pulmonary and CNS) is present.

Scaling Up Pediatric Antiretroviral Therapy Programs

Children are generally underrepresented in ART programs in developing countries compared with adults. Children and those living in rural areas have been specifically identified as challenges to the goal of universal access to ART.[2,85] Particularly where there is high HIV prevalence and a limited number of practitioners, physician-based models of care are unlikely to provide the universal access to HIV care and treatment that is required. Task shifting is an increasingly used method for addressing such human-resource limitations and for facilitating decentralization of services. While legitimate concerns exist over the quality of task-shifted care,[86] many developing countries have few options other than task shifting for immediate rapid scale-up of care and treatment programs.[7,87] Recent shifting of tasks to nurses and other nonphysician clinicians in Africa in the care and treatment of HIV (especially ART initiation and monitoring) has generally been favorable[88] and shown to increase the number of patients on ART and aid decentralization of services[87–89]; however, appropriate training and support for task-shifted personnel is crucial. For example, in a South African study, ART monitoring by a trained nursing cadre was non-inferior to that monitored by physicians,[90] while the quality of HIV care provided by nonphysicians in Mozambique was substandard, leading to the revision of nonphysician scope of practice and training.[91] In high-prevalence settings of pediatric HIV, effective strategies to rapidly develop quality, sustainable, task-shifted capacity for care are urgently needed. Clinical side-by-side mentoring of nonphysicians by skilled practitioners is used in some developing countries, including rural primary health care clinics.[92,93]

■ IMPORTANT COINFECTIONS

Tuberculosis

Tuberculosis is by far the most important coinfection in HIV-infected individuals. After being on the retreat for decades in the face of improved public health conditions in many lower-income countries, TB has surged in recent years, particularly in areas of high HIV prevalence. Tuberculosis is well-adapted to take advantage of immunosuppressive effects of HIV on individuals and the strain placed on national health systems by the HIV epidemic; where resources are limited, health authorities struggle with the challenge of addressing twin epidemics. Consequently, TB coinfection with HIV is common. In some countries, HIV prevalence in newly diagnosed TB cases exceeds 50%, and in HIV prevalent areas it is recommended to screen all new TB diagnoses for the presence of HIV infection.[94]

HIV-infected children are particularly susceptible to severe forms of TB, including TB meningitis, which has a high mortality rate. Adding to this susceptibility is the fact that while BCG protects against severe forms of TB in young children, it is not given to HIV-infected infants because of the risks of disseminated BCG disease (which carries a mortality rate greater than 70%)[48]; data also suggest that due to HIV effect on T-cell response in infected infants, BCG may offer little, if any, benefit to HIV-infected infants.[49] Symptomatic HIV-exposed infants are also not offered BCG, while healthy appearing HIV-exposed infants are immunized.

While the treatment of TB in HIV-infected children is the same as in noninfected children, there are special considerations with the coadministration of ART with antituberculosis drugs. Tuberculosis is a WHO clinical stage 3 condition and an indication for ART initiation in children. Rifampicin can lower levels of NVP and LPV/r below therapeutic margins, increasing the chance of resistance developing to these antiretrovirals. Accordingly, when co-therapy is given, efavirenz is substituted for NVP (not for children younger than 3 years who weigh less than 10 kg, for whom efavirenz is not indicated) and LPV/r, if continued, is given at double dose. Close scrutiny for the development of hepatotoxicity is important given the propensity of antituberculosis therapy, efavirenz, and LPV/r to affect the liver. Table 28-7 reviews the preferred first-line ART when given with TB treatment.

The timing of ART initiation in patients coinfected with HIV and TB is important, with data showing a survival benefit when ART is initiated prior to the completion of antituberculosis treatment compared with waiting until after antituberculosis treatment is complete.[95] It is important to wait at least 2 weeks after initiation of antituberculosis treatment to begin ART because a substantial IRS reaction against surviving TB organisms is likely if ART is initiated too soon.

Extrapulmonary forms of TB (eg, lymph node, abdominal, CNS) are more common in HIV-infected children; clinicians practicing in HIV- and TB-prevalent areas should maintain a high index of suspicion for both. In many developing countries, diagnostic modalities for TB diagnosis are limited, and treatment is often initiated based on clinical diagnosis and supportive investigations.[96] Tuberculosis meningitis, in particular, carries a high fatality rate and risk of severe sequelae in survivors; empiric treatment when suspected may be lifesaving.

Isoniazid Preventive Therapy

In many areas, latent TB rates in HIV-infected children are high and often exceed 30%.[97] While tuberculin skin tests can identify many such children, their accuracy in HIV-infected children is often limited. Because active TB development is common in latently infected children, it is rational to use isoniazid preventive therapy (IPT), which has been shown to reduce active TB development and TB-associated mortality in HIV-infected children.[98] While studies have shown that the maximum benefits of IPT (lower risk of developing TB and lower mortality) are achieved in HIV-infected children with evidence of TB infection, as demonstrated by a positive tuberculin skin test, benefits have also been shown among HIV-infected children in general, regardless of the test result.[99] The WHO recommends IPT as a cornerstone of global TB control, especially in HIV-prevalent areas.[94]

Many developing countries use an approach to IPT similar to South Africa, where IPT is given for 6 months to all HIV-infected children at the time of HIV diagnosis, providing there is no clinical suspicion for active TB.[100] In the South Africa approach, prior to IPT initiation, children are screened for signs and symptoms of active TB disease.

- Current cough (24 hours or longer)
- Fever
- Weight loss
- Drenching night sweats

Children with one or more signs or symptoms are considered TB suspect, are further investigated for active TB disease, and are not eligible for IPT until active TB disease is excluded on the basis of staining for acid fast bacilli and mycobacterial culture (either from sputum, including nebulized saline-induced sputum, or gastric aspirate). Bronchoscopy for obtaining sputum is not included in the South Africa approach to IPT and is rarely available in national pediatric HIV programs in resource-limited settings. Chest radiographs are not required prior to IPT initiation.

Isoniazid preventive therapy can be coadministered with ART to children without increased risk of hepatotoxicity.[101] While there is concern that active TB, which develops after recent IPT, may be more likely to be drug resistant, recent data from South Africa suggest that this is not the case, supporting wider IPT implementation.[102]

Malaria

Malaria is more common and more severe in people with HIV infection.[103] Incidence in a given area may be as high as 2-fold or more in HIV-infected individuals, with higher parasitemias.[103] Mortality and severe morbidity tend to be more common among persons with HIV infections and more so in areas where malaria transmission is less intense and individual immunity to malaria may not be present.[104]

Co-trimoxazole preventive therapy is beneficial to HIV-infected children in malaria-endemic areas because in addition to protection against osteogenesis impefecta and serious bacterial infections, it also reduces the risk of malaria.[2] Co-trimoxazole preventive therapy remains very effective in preventing malaria even where anti-folate resistance-mediating mutations in *Plasmodium* are common.[105]

The use of insecticide-treated bed nets by all persons is critical in malaria-endemic areas because they reduce incidence, morbidity, and mortality of malaria in children and adults[106,107] and are a priority intervention for improving child survival.[35] Their use is particularly important for HIV-infected pregnant women, as placental malaria is associated with a substantial risk of HIV MTCT.[108] Intermittent preventive treatment with 2 doses of sulfadoxine-pyrimethamine during pregnancy has also been shown to reduce placental malaria but is less effective in HIV-infected than uninfected women; a higher sulfadoxine-pyrimethamine dosage (eg, monthly administration) is recommended for HIV-infected pregnant women.[109]

Hepatitis B and C

As many as 10% of HIV-infected children in developing countries are coinfected with hepatitis B virus (HBV), the vast majority infected through MTCT.[110] Administration of HBV vaccine at birth alone is 70% to 75% effective for preventing MTCT of HBV, and the addition of hepatitis B immunoglobulin at birth brings efficacy to 95%[111]; these have particular utility in HBV-prevalent settings. In areas of higher hepatitis B prevalence, HIV-infected infants and children should be screened for hepatitis B infection, as should all HIV-infected infants and children with otherwise unexplained liver enzyme elevations.

Diagnosis of hepatitis B coinfection has implications for ART. Lamivudine has activity against HBV and is part of all standard first- and second-line ART. As HBV may develop 3TC-resistance when 3TC is used without a second drug with anti-hepatitis B activity,[112] use of tenofovir (also active against HBV) as part of ART along with 3TC (or emtricitabine, also active against hepatitis B) is preferable for hepatitis

B–coinfected patients. While tenofovir is not an option for young children, it may be used with proper monitoring in older children and adolescents.

Another important reason for knowing hepatitis B status in managing children's ART is that hepatitis B–infected children are at risk for a flare of underlying quiescent hepatitis, including fulminant hepatic failure and death (in some cases) when ART containing antiretrovirals with anti-hepatitis B activity is suddenly withdrawn.[113]

Hepatitis C coinfection with HIV in children is uncommon. When present, management does not differ from that of non–HIV-infected children.

■ ADOLESCENCE AND PSYCHOSOCIAL ISSUES

The special needs of HIV-infected adolescents are attracting more attention in developing countries' responses to pediatric HIV.[114] As ART programs expand and fewer perinatally infected children die from HIV infection, countries are experiencing growth in adolescent HIV numbers, augmented by sexually-acquired infections among young persons.[115,116] In high-prevalence settings, undiagnosed HIV in adolescents is not uncommon,[117] and a high proportion of adolescents admitted to hospitals are HIV infected with common admission diagnoses including TB, cryptococcal infection, pneumonia, and sepsis.[118] A clear role can be seen for expanded efforts in high-prevalence settings to identify HIV-infected adolescents.

Data suggest that adolescents may be less likely to maintain effective responses to ART than younger children, which is generally related to problems with non-adherence to antiretrovirals[119] and psychosocial concerns, particularly depression.[114,120] Depression and anxiety are also common in caregivers of adolescents and are positively associated with adolescents' difficulties in psychosocial functioning.[120] A family-centered approach to HIV infection has been suggested to offer many benefits to caregivers and children alike, including the opportunity to offer family therapy or other group approaches to managing psychosocial difficulties.[120,121] It has been suggested that screening for and treating depression should be part of standardized packages of services offered for families coping with HIV infection in resource-limited settings.[121]

Disclosure of HIV status is a difficult issue in the field of pediatric HIV in higher-income and lower-income countries. Caregiver reluctance to disclose HIV status to a child or an adolescent is often related to fear of stigmatization and discrimination, which are powerful cultural issues in many developing countries.[114] However, disclosure is important for HIV-infected children and adolescents, as it is associated with elevated self-esteem, willingness to accept treatment, and adherence to ART.[114] Health care professionals are recommended to assist caregivers with a stepwise approach to disclosure from an early age using age-appropriate language and concepts.[114,118]

A holistic approach to developing life skills compatible with long-term health is important for HIV-infected adolescents. Generally, in developing countries there is a lack of accurate and youth-friendly information available to HIV-infected adolescents on how to live a healthy life. Efforts are underway in some settings to address this with culturally relevant, targeted informational materials.[122] Structured peer support groups are used in some adolescent treatment programs and offer a venue for developing confidence in disclosure and peer relationships, as well as an opportunity to deliver an educational program focused on life skills.[123] Such support may help ART programs in lower-income countries deliver better outcomes for this challenging group of patients. In a study comparing virologic responses of children and adolescents in Uganda with those in the United Kingdom and Ireland, the superior virologic response seen in Ugandan adolescents was attributed in large part to successful adolescent support programs.[124]

■ IN PERSPECTIVE: THE GLOBAL RESPONSE TO PEDIATRIC HIV IN DEVELOPING COUNTRIES

In recent years, major strides have been made in the effort to address the effect of the global HIV epidemic on children and families. It has been shown that perinatal transmission can be markedly reduced and children can be broadly enrolled into effective treatment programs, even in very resource-poor settings.

And treatment itself works in children. Around the world, hundreds of thousands of previously ill children have had their health restored and been able to resume normal lives. In Africa, many caregivers cite their child's ability to return to school as their greatest source of satisfaction with the child's care.

Yet HIV-infected children and their families remain among the most vulnerable members of our global community. Many countries where HIV is prevalent have multiple competing and critical priorities, of which HIV is one. Resources are limited and sustenance of current programs is a daunting challenge, never mind expansion to those still in need.

It is said that every nation walks on its children's fragile feet. This is perhaps nowhere more true than in the regions markedly affected by HIV. The continued effort to bring HIV prevention, care, and treatment to all children and families in need keeps the promise of an HIV-free generation, and a healthy future for children and families coping with HIV challenges.

■ KEY POINTS

- HIV is a major cause of death where prevalence is high—such as in sub-Saharan Africa, where more than 90% of HIV-infected children reside—and millions of children worldwide have been orphaned by HIV.
- Despite substantial progress in recent years, children remain under-represented in care and treatment programs compared with adults.
- The vast majority of pediatric HIV infections are due to MTCT, and with a strong MTCT prevention approach, including opt-out HIV testing in pregnancy and expanding availability of ART to all pregnant women, developing settings can realize rates of MTCT under 2%.
- Decisions on feeding modality (breastfeeding versus formula-feeding) should center on child survival considerations, rather than strictly on the likelihood of HIV transmission; HIV-exposed infants should only formula-feed if all of the WHO conditions needed for an HIV-positive woman to safely use formula-feeding are present.
- Co-trimoxazole preventive therapy is a key yet underused intervention for HIV-exposed and HIV-infected infants and children.
- Health care professionals in developing countries should maintain a high index of suspicion for clinical signs and symptoms indicative of HIV infection, particularly in HIV-prevalent settings; provider-initiated testing and counseling in health settings is a key strategy to increase identification of HIV-infected children.
- Antiretroviral therapy is effective and lifesaving in infants and children; HIV-infected infants and children younger than 24 months should be initiated on ART regardless of clinical stage or CD4 count.
- Adherence to therapy is the critical factor in determining how well a child does on ART; age-appropriate disclosure process is a critical component of adherence support, particularly for older children, and should be part of every clinic visit.
- Tuberculosis is the most important coinfection for HIV-infected individuals; HIV-infected children are particularly susceptible to severe forms of TB and should receive IPT when indicated.
- HIV-infected adolescents require special attention with a particular focus on psychosocial concerns.

■ REFERENCES

1. Black RE, Cousens S, Johnson HL, et al. Global, regional, and national causes of child mortality in 2008: a systematic analysis. *Lancet.* 2010;375:1969–1987

2. World Health Organization. *Towards Universal Access: Scaling-up Priority HIV/AIDS Interventions in the Health Sector. Progress Report, 2010.* http://www.who.int/hiv/pub/2010progressreport/en/index.html

3. Rajaratnam JK, Marcus JR, Flaxman AD, et al. Neonatal, postneonatal, childhood, and under-5 mortality for 187 countries, 1970–2010: a systematic analysis of progress towards Millennium Development Goal 4. *Lancet.* 375:1988–2008

4. Joint United Nations Programme on HIV/AIDS. *AIDS Today: 2010 UNAIDS Global Report.* http://www.unaids.org/GlobalReport.htm

5. Data, United States Agency for International Development, 2010. http://www.usaid.gov

6. Countdown Coverage Writing Group. Countdown to 2015 for maternal, newborn, and child survival: the 2008 report on tracking intervention coverage. *Lancet.* 2008; 371:1247–1258

7. Kline MW. Perspectives on the pediatric HIV/AIDS pandemic: catalyzing access of children to care and treatment. *Pediatrics.* 2006;117:1388–1393

8. World Health Organization. *Antiretroviral Therapy for HIV Infection in Infants and Children: Towards Universal Access. Recommendations for a Public Health Approach, 2010 Revision.* http://whqlibdoc.who.int/publications/2010/9789241599801_eng.pdf

9. World Health Organization. *Antiretroviral Drugs for Treating Pregnant Women and Preventing HIV Infection in Infants. Recommendations for a Public Health Approach. 2010 version.* http://whqlibdoc.who.int/publications/2010/9789241599818_eng.pdf

10. Jourdain G, Mary J, Le Coeur S, et al. Risk factors for in utero or intrapartum mother-to-child transmission of human immunodeficiency virus type 1 in Thailand. *J Infect Dis.* 2007;196:1629–1636

11. Kourtis AP, Lee FK, Abrams EJ, et al. Mother-to-child transmission of HIV-1: timing and implications for prevention. *Lancet Infect Dis.* 2006;6:726–732

12. Panel on Treatment of HIV-Infected Pregnant Women and Prevention of Perinatal Transmission. Recommendations for use of antiretroviral drugs in pregnant HIV-1-infected women for maternal health and interventions to reduce perinatal HIV transmission in the United States. May 24, 2010. http://aidsinfo.nih.gov/ContentFiles/PerinatalGL.pdf

13. Palombi L, Marazzi MC, Voetberg A, et al. Treatment acceleration program and the experience of the DREAM program in prevention of mother-to-child transmission of HIV. *AIDS.* 2007;21(suppl 4):S65–S71

14. Shapiro RL, Hughes MD, Ogwu A, et al. Antiretroviral regimens in pregnancy and breast-feeding in Botswana. *N Engl J Med.* 2010;362:2282–2294

15. Chasela CS, Hudgens MG, Jamieson DJ, et al. Maternal or infant antiretroviral drugs to reduce HIV-1 transmission. *N Engl J Med.* 2010;362:2271–2281

16. World Health Organization, United Nations Children's Fund, Interagency Task Team on Prevention of HIV Infection in Pregnant Women, Mothers and their Children. *Guidance on Global Scale-up of the Prevention of Mother-to-Child Transmission of HIV: Towards Universal Access for Women, Infants and Young Children and Eliminating HIV and AIDS Among Children.* 2007. http://www.unicef.org/aids/files/PMTCT_enWEBNov26.pdf. Accessed June 17, 2011

17. Guay LA, Musoke P, Fleming T, et al. Intrapartum and neonatal single-dose nevirapine compared with zidovudine for prevention of mother-to-child transmission of HIV-1 in Kampala, Uganda: HIVNET 012 randomised trial. *Lancet.* 1999;354:795–802

18. World Health Organization, United Nations Children's Fund. Policy requirements for HIV testing and counseling of infants and young children in health facilities. 2010. http://www.unicef.org/aids/files/WHO_UNICEF_Testing _Policy_web.pdf

19. Thior I, Lockman S, Smeatin LM, et al. Breastfeeding plus infant zidovudine prophylaxis for 6 months vs formula feeding plus infant zidovudine for 1 month to reduce mother-to-child HIV transmission in Botswana. A randomized trial: the Mashi study. *JAMA*. 2006;296:794–805

20. Lockman S, McIntyre JA. Reduction of HIV-1 drug resistance after intrapartum single-dose nevirapine. *Lancet*. 2007;370:1668–1670

21. Chi BH, Sinkala M, Mbewe F, et al. Single-dose tenofovir and emtricitabine for reduction of viral resistance to non-nucleoside reverse transcriptase inhibitor drugs in women given intrapartum nevirapine for perinatal HIV prevention: an open-label randomized trial. *Lancet*. 2007;370:1698–1705

22. Lorenzi P, Spicher VM, Laubereau B, et al. Antiretroviral therapies in pregnancy: maternal, fetal and neonatal effects. Swiss HIV Cohort Study, the Swiss Collaborative HIV and Pregnancy Study, and the Swiss Neonatal Study. *AIDS*. 1998;12:F241–F247

23. European Collaborative Study, Study SMaCHC. Combination antiretroviral therapy and duration of pregnancy. *AIDS*. 2000;14:2913–2920

24. Kourtis AP, Schmid CH, Jamieson DJ, Lau J. Use of antiretroviral therapy in pregnant HIV-infected women and the risk of premature delivery: a meta-analysis. *AIDS*. 2007;21:607–615

25. Antiretroviral Pregnancy Registry Steering Committee. *Antiretroviral Pregnancy Registry International Interim Report for 1 January 1989 Through 31 July 2010*. Wilmington, NC: Registry Coordinating Center; 2010. http://www.APRegistry.com. Accessed June 17, 2011

26. Pacheco SE, McIntosh K, Lu M, et al. Effect of perinatal antiretroviral drug exposure on hematologic values in HIV-uninfected children: an analysis of the women and infants transmission study. *J Infect Dis*. 2006;194:1089–1097

27. Kumwenda NI, et al. Extended antiretroviral prophylaxis to reduce breast-milk HIV-1 transmission. *N Engl J Med*. 2008;358:119–129

28. Six Week Extended-Dose Nevirapine Study Team. Extended-dose nevirapine to 6 weeks of age for infants to prevent HIV transmission via breastfeeding in Ethiopia, India and Uganda: an analysis of three randomized controlled trials. *Lancet*. 2008;372:300–313

29. Taylor GP, Low-Beer N. Antiretroviral therapy in pregnancy: a focus on safety. *Drug Saf*. 2001;24(9):683–702

30. Fundarò C, Genovese O, Rendeli C, Tamburrini E, Salvaggio E. Myelomeningocele in a child with intrauterine exposure to efavirenz. *AIDS*. 2002;16:299–300

31. Saitoh A, Hull AD, Franklin P, Spector SA. Myelomeningocele in an infant with intrauterine exposure to efavirenz. *J Perinatol*. 2005;25:555–556

32. Ford N, Mofenson L, Kranzer K, et al. Safety of efavirenz in first-trimester of pregnancy: a systematic review and meta-analysis of outcomes from observational cohorts. *AIDS*. 2010;24:1461–1470

33. Data, Ministry of Public Health, Thailand. http://eng.moph.go.th

34. Baleta A. Botswana reduces mother-to-child transmission of HIV. *Lancet*. 2010;375:1954

35. Jones G, Steketee R, Black R, Bhutta ZA, Morris SS. How many child deaths can we prevent this year? *Lancet*. 2003;362:65–71

36. Mbori-Ngacha D, Nduati R, John G, et al. Morbidity and mortality in breastfed and formula-fed infants of HIV-1-infected women: a randomized clinical trial. *JAMA*. 2001;286:2413–2420

37. Coovadia HM, Rollins NC, Bland RM. Mother-to-child transmission of HIV-1 infection during exclusive breastfeeding in the first 6 months of life: an intervention cohort study. *Lancet.* 2007;369:1107–1116

38. Creek TL, Kim A, Lu L, et al. Hospitalization and mortality among primarily non-breastfed children during a large outbreak of diarrhea and malnutrition in Botswana, 2006. *JAIDS.* 2010;53:14–19

39. Kuhn L, Aldrovandi G. Survival and health benefits of breastfeeding versus artificial feeding in infants of HIV-infected women: developing versus developed world. *Clin Perinatol.* 2010;37:843–862

40. Doherty T, Chopra M, Nkonki L, et al. Effect of the HIV epidemic on infant feeding in South Africa: "When they see me coming with the tins they laugh at me." *Bull WHO.* 2006;84:90–96

41. Doherty T, Chopra M, Jackson D, et al. Effectiveness of the WHO/UNICEF guidelines on infant feeding for HIV-positive women: results from a prospective cohort study in South Africa. *AIDS.* 2007;21:1791–1797

42. Kellerman S, Essajee S. HIV testing for children in resource-limited settings: what are we waiting for? *PLoS Med.* 2010;7:e1000285

43. Violari A, Cotton MF, Gibb DM, et al. Early antiretroviral therapy and mortality among HIV-infected infants. *N Engl J Med.* 2008;359:2233–2244

44. Sherman GG, Stevens WS, Stevens G, Galpin JS. Diagnosis of human immunode-ficiency virus infection in perinatally exposed orphaned infants in a resource-poor setting. *Pediatr Infect Dis J.* 2000;19:1014–1015

45. World Health Organization, United Nations Children's Fund. Co-trimoxazole prophylaxis for HIV-exposed and HIV-infected infants and children: practical approaches to implementation and scale up, 2009. http://www.who.int/hiv/pub/paediatric/cotrimoxazole.pdf

46. Chintu C, et al. Cotrimoxazole as prophylaxis against opportunistic infections in HIV-infected Zambian children (CHAP): a double-blind randomised placebo-controlled trial. *Lancet.* 2004;364:1865–1871

47. Marinda E, et al. Child mortality according to maternal and infant HIV status in Zimbabwe. *Pediatr Infect Dis J.* 2007;26:519–526

48. Hessling AC, Johnson LF, Jaspan H, et al. Disseminated bacilli Calmette-Guerin disease in HIV-infected South African infants. *Bull WHO.* 2009;87:485–564

49. Mansoor N, Scriba TJ, de Kock M, et al. HIV-1 infection in infants severely impairs the immune response induced by Bacille Calmette-Guérin vaccine. *J Infect Dis.* 2009;199:982–990

50. Sutcliffe CG, Moss WJ. Do children infected with HIV receiving HAART need to be revaccinated? *Lancet Infect Dis.* 2010;10:630–642

51. World Health Organization. *WHO Case Definitions of HIV for Surveillance and Revised Clinical Staging and Immunological Classification of HIV-related Disease in Adults and Children.* Geneva, Switzerland: World Health Organization; 2007. http://www.who.int/hiv/pub/guidelines/HIVstaging150307.pdf. Accessed June 17, 2011

52. Bolu OO, Allread V, Creek T, et al. Approaches for scaling up human immunodeficiency virus testing and counseling in prevention of mother-to-child human immunodeficiency virus transmission settings in resource-limited countries. *Am J Obstet Gynecol.* 2007;197(3 Suppl):S83–S89

53. Kansaka C, Carter RJ, Briggs N, et al. Routine offering of HIV testing to hospitalized pediatric patients at university teaching hospital, Lusaka, Zambia: acceptability and feasibility. *JAIDS.* 2009;51:202–208

54. Ferguson P, Tomkins A. HIV prevalence and mortality among children undergoing treatment for severe acute malnutrition in sub-Saharan Africa: a systematic review and meta-analysis. *Trans R Soc Trop Med Hyg.* 2009;103:541–548

55. Rollins N, Mzolo S, Moodley T, et al. Universal HIV testing of infants at immunization clinics: an acceptable and feasible approach for early infant diagnosis in high HIV prevalence settings. *AIDS.* 2009;23:1851–1857

56. Horwood C, Voce A, Vermaak K, et al. Routine checks for HIV in children attending primary health care facilities in South Africa: attitudes of nurses and child caregivers. *Soc Sci Med.* 2010;70:313–320

57. McCollum ED, Preidis GA, Kabue MM, et al. Task shifting routine inpatient pediatric HIV testing improves program outcomes in urban Malawi: a retrospective observational study. *PLoS ONE.* 2010;5:e9626

58. Ahmed S, Kanjelo K, Nanthuru D, et al. Using community health workers to improve identification, enrollment into care, and outcomes for HIV-exposed infants at the Kawale Health Centre in Lilongwe, Malawi. XVIII International AIDS Conference; Vienna; July 18–23, 2010

59. World Health Organization, United Nations Children's Fund. Integrated management of child illness. http://www.who.int/child_adolescent_health/topics/prevention_care/child/imci/en

60. World Health Organization, United Nations Children's Fund. Integrated management of childhood illnesses for high HIV settings. 2008. http://www.who.int/child_adolescent_health/documents/9789241597388/en

61. Horwood C, Liebeschuetz S, Blaauw D, et al. Diagnosis of paediatric HIV infection in a primary health care setting with a clinical algorithm. *Bull WHO.* 2003;81:858–866

62. Lowe S, Ferrand RA, Morris-Jones R, et al. Skin disease among human immunodeficiency virus-infected adolescents in Zimbabwe: a strong indicator of underlying HIV infection. *Pediatr Infect Dis J.* 2010;29:346–351

63. Zar HJ, Workman L, le Roux SM, et al. A randomized controlled trial of intermittent compared with daily cotrimoxazole preventive therapy in HIV-infected children. *AIDS.* 2010;24:2225–2232

64. Rossignol JF. Cryptosporidium and Giardia: treatment options and prospects for new drugs. *Exp Parasitol.* 2010;124:45–53

65. Amadi B, Mwiya M, Sianongo S, et al. High dose prolonged treatment with nitazoxanide is not effective for cryptosporidiosis in HIV positive Zambian children: a randomised controlled trial. *BMC Infectious Diseases.* 2009;9:195

66. Chimalizeni Y, Tickell D, Connell T. Evidence behind the WHO guidelines: hospital care for children: what is the most appropriate anti-fungal treatment for acute cryptococcal meningitis in children with HIV? *J Trop Pediatr.* 2010;56:4–12

67. Van Eijk AM, Brooks JT, Adcock PM. Diarrhea in children less than two years of age with known HIV status in Kisumu, Kenya. *Int J Infect Dis.* 2010;14:e220–e225

68. Gray DM, Zar HJ. Community-acquired pneumonia in HIV-infected children: a global perspective. *Curr Opin Pulm Med.* 2010;16:208–216

69. Mda S, van Raaij J, de Villiers F, et al. Short-term micronutrient supplementation reduces the duration of pneumonia and diarrheal episodes in HIV-infected children. *J Nutr.* 2010;140:969–974

70. Kline MW, Rugina S, Ilie M, et al. Long-term follow-up of 414 HIV-infected Romanian children and adolescents receiving lopinavir/ritonavir-containing highly active antiretroviral therapy. *Pediatrics.* 2007;119:e1116–e1120

71. Ciaranello AL, Chang Y, Margulis AV, et al. Effectiveness of pediatric antiretroviral therapy in resource-limited settings: a systematic review and meta-analysis. *Clin Infect Dis.* 2009;49:1915–1927

72. Leyenaar JK, Novosad PM, Ferrer KT, el al. Early clinical outcomes in children enrolled in human immunodeficiency virus infection care and treatment in Lesotho. *Pediatr Infect Dis J.* 2010;29:340–345

73. Sauvageot D, Schaefer M, Olson D, et al. Antiretroviral therapy outcomes in resource-limited settings for HIV-infected children <5 years of age. *Pediatrics.* 2010;125: e1039–e1047

74. Janssen N, Ndirangu J, Newell M-L, Bland RM. Successful paediatric HIV treatment in rural primary care in Africa. *Arch Dis Child.* 2010;95:414–421

75. Sutcliffe CG, van Dijk JK, Bolton-Moore C, et al. Differences in presentation, treatment initiation, and response among children infected with human immunodeficiency virus in urban and rural Zambia. *Pediatr Infect Dis J.* 2010;29:849–854

76. Edmonds A, Lusiama J, Napravnik S, et al. Anti-retroviral therapy reduces incident tuberculosis in HIV-infected children. *Int J Epidemiol.* 2009;38:1612–1621

77. Aurpibul L, Puthanakit T, Taecharoenkul S, et al. Reversal of growth failure in HIV-infected Thai children treated with non-nucleoside reverse transcriptase inhibitor–based antiretroviral therapy. *AIDS Patient Care STDs.* 2009;23:1067–1071

78. Fenner L, Brinkhof W, Keiser O, et al. Early mortality and loss to follow-up in HIV-infected children starting antiretroviral therapy in Southern Africa. *JAIDS.* 2010;54:524–532

79. Yotebieng M, Van Rie A, Moultrie H, Meyers T. Six-month gain in weight, height, and CD4 predict subsequent antiretroviral treatment responses in HIV-infected South African children. *AIDS.* 2010;24:139–146

80. Nahirya-Ntege P, Naidoo B, Nathoo KJ, et al. Successful management of suspected abacavir hypersensitivity reactions among African children in the ARROW (AntiRetroviral Research fOr Watoto) trial. 5th IAS Conference on HIV Pathogenesis and Treatment; Cape Town, South Africa; 2009

81. Eley B, Nuttall J, Davies MA, et al. Initial experience of a public sector antiretroviral treatment programme for HIV-infected children and their infected parents. *S Afr Med J.* 2004;94:643–646

82. Buck WC, Kabue MM, Kazembe PN, Kline MW. Discontinuation of standard first-line antiretroviral therapy in a cohort of 1434 Malawian children. *J Int AIDS Soc.* 2010

83. Smith K, Kuhn L, Coovadia A, et al. Immune reconstitution inflammatory syndrome among HIV-infected South African infants initiating antiretroviral therapy. *AIDS.* 2009;23:1097–1107

84. Orikiiriza J, Bakeera-Kitaka S, Musiime V, et al. The clinical pattern, prevalence, and factors associated with immune reconstitution inflammatory syndrome in Ugandan children. *AIDS.* 2010;24:2009–2017

85. Prendergast A, Tudor-Williams G, Jeena P, et al. International perspectives, progress, and future challenges of pediatric HIV infection. *Lancet.* 2007;370:68–80

86. Philips M, Zachariah R, Venis S. Task-shifting for antiretroviral treatment delivery in sub-Saharan Africa: not a panacea. *Lancet.* 2008;371:682–684

87. Fredlund VG, Nash J. How far should they walk? Increasing antiretroviral therapy access in a rural community in northern KwaZulu-Natal, South Africa. *J Infect Dis.* 2007;196(Suppl3):S469–473

88. Callaghan M, Ford N, Schneider H. A systematic review of task-shifting for HIV treatment and care in Africa. *Hum Resour Health.* 2010

89. Miles K, Clutterbuck DJ, Seitio O, et al. Antiretroviral treatment roll-out in a resource-constrained setting: capitalizing on nursing resources in Botswana. *Bull WHO.* 2007;85:555–560

90. Sanne I, Orrell C, Fox MP, et al. Nurse versus doctor management of HIV-infected patients receiving antiretroviral therapy (CIPRA-SA): a randomised non-inferiority trial. *Lancet.* 2010;376:33–40

91. Brentlinger PE, Assan A, Mudender F, et al. Task shifting in Mozambique: cross-sectional evaluation of non-physician clinicians' performance in HIV/AIDS care. *Hum Resour Health.* 2010

92. Tolle M, Garcia-Prats A, Thompson M, et al. The LERATO project: a model for decentralization and expansion of pediatric-focused family-based HIV/AIDS care in Mokhotlong, Lesotho. XVII International AIDS Conference; Mexico City; 2008

93. Scherzer L, Tolle M, Gaetsewe N, et al. Expanding mentoring services to local clinics in the Serowe/Palapye region of Botswana. XVIII International AIDS Conference; Vienna; 2010

94. World Health Organization. Global tuberculosis control 2010. http://www.who.int/tb/publications/global_report/2010/en/index.html

95. Abdool Karim SS, Naidoo K, Grobler A, et al. Timing of initiation of antiretroviral drugs during tuberculosis therapy. *N Engl J Med.* 2010;362:697–706

96. Tinsa F, Essaddam L, Fitouri Z, et al. Abdominal tuberculosis in children. *J Pediatr Gastroenterol Nutr.* 2010;50:634–638

97. Mermin J, Bunnell R, Lule J, et al. Developing an evidence-based, preventitive care package for persons with HIV in Africa. *Trop Med Int Health.* 2005;10:961–970

98. Zar HJ, Cotton MF, Strauss S, et al. Effect of isoniazid prophylaxis on mortality and incidence of tuberculosis in children with HIV: randomised controlled trial. *BMJ.* 2010;334:136–142

99. Gray DM, Young T, Cotton M, Zar H. Impact of tuberculosis preventive therapy on tuberculosis and mortality in HIV-infected children. *Cochrane Database Syst Rev.* 2009;1:CD006418

100. Department of Health, Republic of South Africa. Guidelines for tuberculosis preventive therapy among HIV infected individuals in South Africa. 2010. http://www.doh.gov.za

101. Gray D, Nuttall J, Lombard C. Low rates of hepatotoxicity in HIV-infected children on anti-retroviral therapy with and without isoniazid prophylaxis. *J Trop Pediatr.* 2010;56:159–165

102. van Halsema C, Fielding KL, Chihota VN. Tuberculosis outcomes and drug susceptibility in individuals exposed to isoniazid preventive therapy in a high HIV prevalence setting. *AIDS.* 2010;24:1051–1055

103. Patnaik P, Jere CS, Miller WC, et al. Effects of HIV-1 serostatus, HIV-1 RNA concentration, and CD4 cell count on the incidence of malaria infection in a cohort of adults in rural Malawi. *J Infect Dis.* 2005;192:984–991

104. Grimwade K, French N, Mbatha D, et al. HIV infection as a cofactor for severe falciparum malaria in adults living in a region of unstable malaria transmission in South Africa. *AIDS.* 2004;18:547–554

105. Gasasira AF, Kamya MR, Ochong EO, et al. Effect of trimethoprim-sulphamethoxazole on the risk of malaria in HIV-infected Ugandan children living in an area of widespread antifolate resistance. *Mal J.* 2010;9:177

106. ter Kuile FO, Terlouw DJ, Phillips-Howard PA, et al. Impact of permethrin-treated bed nets on malaria and all-cause morbidity in young children in an area of intense perennial malaria transmission in western Kenya: cross-sectional survey. *Am J Trop Med Hyg.* 2003;68:100–107

107. Deswal BS, Bhatnagar D, Tilak R, Basanar DR. Malaria control using deltamethrin impregnated mosquito nets/insecticide treated bed nets: experience in armed forces. *J Commun Dis.* 2005;37:297–300

108. Brahmbhatt H, Sullivan D, Kigozi G, et al. Association of HIV and malaria with mother-to-child transmission, birth outcomes, and child mortality. *JAIDS.* 2008;47:472–476

109. Briand V, Badaut C, Cot M. Placental malaria, maternal HIV infection and infant morbidity. *Ann Trop Paediatr.* 2009;29:71–83

110. Zhang F, Zhang Y. Perinatal transmission of hepatitis B virus: could hospitals be doing more? *Expert Rev Anti Infect Ther.* 2010;8:735–738

111. Read JS, Cannon MJ, Stanberry LR, Schuval S. Prevention of mother-to-child transmission of viral infections. *Curr Prob Ped Adolesc Health Care.* 2008;38:274–297

112. Di Bisceglie AM, Maskew M, Schulze D, et al. HIV-HBV coinfection among South African patients receiving antiretroviral therapy. *Antivir Ther.* 2010;15(3 Pt B):499–503

113. Thio CL, Locarnini S. Treatment of HIV/HBV coinfection: clinical and virologic issues. *AIDS Rev.* 2007;9:40–53

114. Gray GE. Adolescent HIV—cause for concern in southern Africa. *PLoS Med.* 2009;7: e1000227

115. Garcia-Calleja JM, Gouws E, Ghys PD. National population based HIV prevalence surveys in sub-Saharan Africa: results and implications for HIV and AIDS estimates. *Sex Transm Infect.* 2006;82:iii64–iii70

116. Gouws E, Stanecki KA, Lyerla R, Ghys PD. The epidemiology of HIV infection among young people aged 15-24 years in southern Africa. *AIDS.* 2008;22:S5–S16

117. Ferrand RA, Munaiwa L, Matsekete J, et al. Undiagnosed HIV infection among adolescents seeking primary health care in Zimbabwe. *Clin Infect Dis.* 2010;51:844–851

118. Ferrand RA, Banson T, Musvaire P, et al. Causes of acute hospitalization in adolescence: burden and spectrum of HIV-related morbidity in a country with an early-onset and severe HIV epidemic. *PLoS Med.* 2010;7:e1000178

119. Ding H, Wilson CM, Modjarrad K, et al. Predictors of suboptimal virologic response to highly active antiretroviral therapy among human immunodeficiency virus–infected adolescents: analyses of the Reaching for Excellence in Adolescent Care and Health (REACH) Project. *Arch Pediatr Adolesc Med.* 2009;163:1100–1105

120. Fawzi MC, Eustache E, Oswald C, et al. Psychosocial functioning among HIV-affected youth and their caregivers in Haiti: implications for family-focused service provision in high HIV burden settings. *AIDS Patient Care STDs.* 2010;24:147–158

121. Tolle MA. A package of primary health care services for comprehensive family-centred HIV/AIDS care and treatment programs in low-income settings. *Trop Med Int Health.* 2009;14:663–672

122. Rosebush J, Pettitt E, Offorjebe A, et al. Teen Talk (Botswana Edition): a question and answer guide for HIV-positive adolescents. XVIII International AIDS Conference; Vienna; 2010

123. Botswana Teen Club. http://botswanateenclub.wordpress.com

124. Kekitiinwa A, Lee KJ, Walker AS, et al. Differences in factors associated with initial growth, CD4, and viral load responses to ART in HIV-infected children in Kampala, Uganda, and the United Kingdom/Ireland. *JAIDS.* 2008;49:384–392

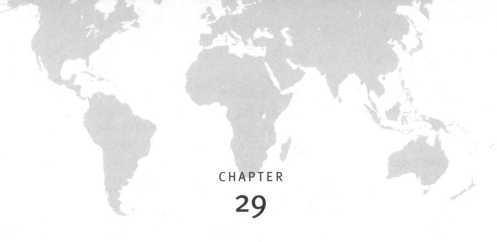

CHAPTER

29

Infection Control

Elaine G. Cox, MD, FAAP
John C. Christenson, MD, FAAP

■ INTRODUCTION

Communicable diseases remain a major cause of morbidity and mortality across the world, accounting for approximately 12 million deaths per year.[1] Ninety-five percent of these deaths are clustered in resource-limited countries. In fact, infection accounts for one third to two thirds of deaths annually in certain developing regions such as Asia and Africa. Children remain disproportionately affected, with 50% of pediatric demise attributable to diarrheal and respiratory illnesses. Neonatal infections and deaths in resource-limited countries are approximately 3 to 20 times higher than in the United States. Additionally, there are nearly 1.4 million hospital-acquired infections (HAIs) ongoing at any given time. Disparities in rates are significant, with higher-income countries showing approximately 10% of patients affected compared with 25% HAIs in the developing world.[2]

As medical and surgical technologies continue advancing, these infections are likely to continue climbing and to result in even greater disparities because of distinct differences in stimuli to address them. Infection-control issues in developing countries become more pronounced as the global village shrinks with regard to diagnosis and possible interventions.

Addressing infection-control concerns poses challenges in resource-limited countries that are somewhat reminiscent of hurdles faced and overcome in industrialized nations 30 to 50 years ago. Strategies employed for infection control in developing countries cannot be faced with a one-size-fits-all approach, as disease profiles and resources markedly differ among developing economies.[3] Physical distance between areas, dissimilar cultures, language, and variable states of socioeconomic development accentuate disparities. Emphasis on cost containment as a short-term goal may overshadow long-term gains that could be realized from basic infection prevention. From a cultural perspective there may be an underlying acceptance of disease and inevitable death in a deprived society, which makes redistributing resources a reactive attempt at a cure to a proactive attempt at prevention that is difficult to achieve.

In May 2004, the World Health Organization (WHO) developed an alliance focused on increasing patient safety with improving infection control as a major initiative.[4] To begin this process, the unique issues that present themselves in infection control in resource-limited settings must be examined and the viability of various interventions assessed.

■ GENERAL ISSUES IN RESOURCE-LIMITED COUNTRIES

Certain overarching issues in developing countries contribute to challenges on every level, including infection control. Poverty remains widespread and far reaching, resulting in many challenges including lack of access to health care and limited facilities and programs even where clinics and hospitals do exist. Lack of clean water and appropriate sanitation remain significant issues in resource-limited countries, with 2.4 billion people worldwide without basic sanitation and another 1.1 billion without access to safe water.[5] Without these resources, infection will continue to be pandemic and a major cause of death in the developing world.

Lack of government oversight remains a barrier to infection control in lower-income countries as well. In many regions, a very small percentage of the gross national product (often less than 5%) is set aside for infection prevention initiatives, and health care budgets for developing countries are staggeringly small compared with the industrialized world. Governmental priorities often mandate that funds be used to service growing international debt and not to support health care systems, which results in a lack of overall political support for programs. There is generally no oversight or accreditation system for health care facilities in developing countries, nor are there mandates for hospital infection control or staff training. There is also poor donor organization, a lack of nongovernmental organizations (NGOs) to address needs, and a discontinuous commitment due to frequent civil issues, which can derail health care initiatives and agendas.

More specific issues can be encountered within the hospital environment itself (Box 29-1). Surveillance of infections and their evolution is seriously lacking in the developing world. As infections vary from region to region, even defining what should be tracked poses nearly unlimited difficulties. Additionally, a lack of technology in the laboratory and information technology (IT) environs makes getting data and maintaining and circulating them significant obstacles. Lack of microbiologic support in many areas of the world makes available data difficult to translate into useful clinical information. Paucity of infection-control experts to craft interventions to affect practice and culture change based on data when available offers no outlet for lessons that could be learned from surveillance in resource-limited countries. Crowding in living environments and health care facilities contributes to the spread of disease and the acquisition of HAIs. Economic constraints and rewards for cost-containment evidence may be responsible for the reuse of disposables, which can contaminate stock supplies—rinsing and reusing items such as gloves, requiring families to provide care items that disrupt supply chains, and pooling items, such as drugs and syringes, for later use. There are no established standards for reusing items, but even with single-use items, issues exist with location and maintenance of waste containment facilities.[6]

Familiar themes exist when comparing issues in the developing world with lessons learned in industrialized nations. Hand hygiene poses issues in every health care setting around the globe. Multiple studies show that compliance rates vary but are usually less than 40% regardless of the country observed. Educational efforts reported in higher-income

---

Box 29-1. Factors Associated With Nosocomial Infections in Countries With Limited Resources

- Lack of clean water and appropriate sanitation
- General lack of availability of antiseptic gels
- Absence of governmental oversight
- Insufficient personnel trained in infectious control
- Limited financial resources dedicated to infection control
- Lack of surveillance and microbiologic support
- Reuse of single-use medical equipment (eg, endotracheal and gastric tubes)
- Improper sterilization of medical equipment
- Overcrowding
- Overuse or suboptimal dosing of antimicrobial agents leading to resistance
- Contamination of multiuse antiseptics and disinfectants
- Contamination of intravenous solutions and aggregates
- Unavailability of negative-pressure isolation rooms
- Poor facility infrastructure (eg, poor ventilation, lack of air-conditioning)
- Limited access to personal protective equipment (eg, masks, respirators, gowns)

and lower-income countries show effectiveness, but all improvements have been transient. Epidemics have forced improved hand hygiene but only for short periods. In all societies, there is some thought that germs are abstractly viewed and that a fear of illness or disease does not stimulate hand washing. Additionally, the emergence of resistant pathogens presents new challenges in infection management across the globe.

Issues that confront the industrialized world, such as indiscriminate antibiotic use or overuse in hospitals or suboptimal antibiotic dosing resulting in selective pressure on endogenous flora, are often accentuated in resource-limited settings. Antimicrobial agents are frequently available in hospitals with very few other resources. Coupled with the over-the-counter supply of medications, the selective pressure in the developing world is much greater than that seen even in industrialized nations. Effective treatment may be halted because of the expense of newer agents to fight multidrug-resistant (MDR) organisms. Even when agents are available, lack of quality assurance programs addressing drug production allow for suboptimal effectiveness and concentration, adding to the development and sustenance of resistant bacteria. With high population density and migratory population shifts, the spread of MDR disease is likely to span borders and become multinational as well.[7,8]

■ SPECIFIC ISSUES FOR INFECTION CONTROL

There are some common or recurrent communicable diseases encountered in resource-limited settings that present specific challenges for infection-control purposes. Hospital-acquired infections, including catheter-associated bloodstream infections, catheter-associated urinary tract infections, and ventilator-associated pneumonias are in the 90th percentile in lower-income countries compared with the United States, according to National Nosocomial Infections Surveillance data.[9] Nosocomial infections can occur in as many as 25% of hospitalized patients in resource-limited settings. Reasons for this high number are likely multifactorial in etiology and include, but are not limited to, universal use of open infusion systems as opposed to closed systems, which are the standard of care in higher-income countries; unavailability of clean water or other materials to clean central venous line hubs and caps prior to access; less frequent changing of administration sets due to lack of supply; infusate contamination caused by less training of personnel, unclean water for mixing, or homemade brews of infusates that have no quality assurance and a higher risk of contamination; and few recommendations or guidelines for device use in countries where such items are available but experience in actual use is limited. Introducing infection-control programs, even in a limited fashion, has decreased HAIs by 32%.[9,10]

Diarrheal Diseases

Diarrhea is one of the most common diseases encountered in the developing world. In general, diarrhea is considered an expected childhood malady with less risk of long-term adverse consequences. This can lead some parents to be less interventional than with illnesses with high likelihood of poor outcomes. However, diarrheal illnesses result in a significant number of deaths globally each year, with rotavirus accounting for approximately one fifth of the total number. Despite studies that suggest hand hygiene alone can prevent 30% to 47% of diarrheal illnesses, compliance is marginal. Additionally, the nosocomial resistance of nonviral pathogens appears to be increasing because of inherent risk factors in the living and hospital environment, including malnutrition, crowding, and overuse of antibiotics.[11]

Tuberculosis

Tuberculosis (TB) is a particularly challenging issue with regard to infection control in all hospitals. Precautions considered appropriate in higher-income countries include private negative-pressure isolation rooms with personnel garbed in protective items such as N95 respirator masks, gowns, and gloves. Most institutions try to mandate fit-testing masks and limiting adult visitation pending testing and treatment. In resource-limited settings, negative pressure rooms are difficult to provide. Air circulation generally depends on cross ventilation from open windows without screens. A general rule of TB isolation in many these facilities includes separating patients in distant areas of the ward with open windows on both sides of the patient care area to allow cross ventilation. Although this may provide some protection to patients in other parts of the ward, crowding, bed sharing, and delayed time to diagnosis make person-to-person transmission highly likely; the spread of MDR TB can occur even with attempts at isolation. It is estimated that even when protective items are available for staff use, most staff are poorly trained and supported, with only 10% reporting formal training. The result is that the highest exposure areas are often magnified by the least infection control.[12]

Hemorrhagic Fevers

Hemorrhagic fever, also common in these settings, has the potential for person-to-person spread as well as percutaneous spread to health care workers. Frequently, families are also charged with burial preparation, which can further spread the disease even after death of the patient. Lack of rapid diagnostic techniques and isolation facilities, crowding, inconsistent use of universal precautions, and a paucity of waste disposal techniques contribute to continual spread of these organisms.[13]

■ NEONATAL CARE

One area that poses incredible challenges in resource-limited countries is neonatal care and nurseries. In these settings, intrapartum and postpartum care present issues with infection control. Infections in newborns are 3 to 20 times higher than in industrialized settings and are the major cause of death, accounting for 1.6 million per year or about 40% of total annual neonatal deaths. Seventy-five percent of these deaths are concentrated in Asia and sub-Saharan Africa.[14] Survival is generally only thought to be possible with a gestational age greater than 30 weeks and a birth weight of a minimum of 1,000 g. Many children with complicated issues are unable to be supported because of a lack of needed technology, such as ventilators, central lines, and total parenteral nutrition, or staff with knowledge to use such items when they are available.

Lack of appropriate prenatal care is a setup for poor neonatal outcomes. Many vitamins and nutrients (eg, folate) that are regularly in supplements or food in higher-income countries are lacking in lower-income countries, thus resulting in higher birth defects, lower birth weight, and increased risk of neonatal complications. Lack of appropriate hygiene during labor and delivery further complicates risks. Nearly 60% of births occur in the home in resource-limited settings, and they are usually facilitated by traditional birth attendants that are often not trained outside of lore passed through generations. When deliveries do occur inside hospitals, there are often frequent vaginal examinations before delivery, misuse of antibiotics, and failure to recognize and respond to chorioamnionitis in rapid fashion.[15]

Many of the same issues in special care nursery settings exist as in the rest of the hospital, such as poor hand hygiene, crowding (sometimes with multiple babies per cot), lack of isolation areas (mothers often reside in same area as tens of babies), and shared equipment. The cost of diapers is too high for many facilities or families to assume and are rarely used, resulting in frequent soiling and improper cleaning of cots between patients. Reusing other items of expense or in short supply also contribute to the list of concerns, the most common being latex gloves that are often rinsed and air-dried between use or a single stethoscope used for multiple babies. Additionally, some items, such as povidone-iodine or intravenous solutions, are pooled as stock items for use over the entire nursery, which can affect multiple babies once contaminated.

Sixty percent of nursery infections are caused by gram-negative rods; the most common organisms are *Klebsiella, Pseudomonas, Enterobacter,* and *Escherichia coli.* Of concern with the gram-positive organisms is that 56% of all staphylococcal isolates are now methicillin resistant, and vancomycin-resistant *Enterococcus* appears to be an emerging threat. The most likely source appears to be the hands of health care workers and overuse of broad-spectrum antibiotics resulting in MDR organisms. Approximately 70% of identified pathogens in the nursery would not be covered by WHO-recommended empiric antibiotic therapies of ampicillin and gentamicin, resulting in late or inadequate treatment of neonatal infections.[16]

■ OTHER CHALLENGES

Other communicable diseases have been endemic and problematic in these countries for decades, including malaria, streptococcal infections, respiratory infections (eg, respiratory syncytial virus), skin diseases (eg, scabies, impetigo), and trachoma.[17] The acute disease may often be self-limited but present long-term post-infectious complications and resultant long-term financial burdens from therapy or complications. Lack of hygiene, crowding, and poor access to appropriate drug therapy add to issues of disease that often receive very little funding or programmatic consideration because of the perception that these illnesses are common and minor compared with others such as HIV.

■ GENERAL PRINCIPLES FOR INFECTION-CONTROL INTERVENTIONS

All interventions undertaken in developing countries must be simple, inexpensive, and practical under each region's limitations. One major requirement is a declaration of commitment and focus on infection control. The WHO made a public commitment in 2004 by establishing the World Alliance for Patient Safety. The WHO created this international alliance and then issued the Global Patient Safety Challenge to fight health care–associated infections.[4] In effect, this challenge would stimulate the development of infection-control programs by focusing on a number of critical factors in safety, including safe handling of blood injections, clinical procedure, clean water, sanitation and waste management, and hand hygiene. Early information shows success in the challenge of increasing hand hygiene in Mali, Africa, when components were introduced as a bundle.[18] Increasing the number of trained specialists is an additional elements that needs to be addressed to develop infection-control programs in health care facilities. There is little interest in pursuing further training because infection control is not recognized as a specialty in its own right and carries no financial or professional incentive in resource-limited areas.

Educational initiatives for health care workers are also critical to the success of infection control. Improving training programs as well as increasing access to computers and IT support will allow for remote learning to supplement current programs. Whether such programs should focus on nursing or physician resources is unclear, but they should likely involve both if feasible.[19] Public health campaigns are also necessary to clarify expectations for patients that receive services and increase support for infection-control exercises. Multimedia campaigns, tax subsidies, and tax relief may work in combination to provide stimuli for increasing medical personnel and public appreciation of the potential effectiveness of infection-control programs.

Facility improvement and sanitation concerns are clearly basic problems that must be addressed but which may be of such an extreme scope that they are difficult to solve. Operational costs for facilities are often borne by patients and families, which leaves little to no room for capital improvements. Sanitation issues generally require large-scale interventions and huge investments over a long period. As funding decisions are usually made ad hoc, priorities may not be congruent with the needs of a particular area because infection control is usually a low priority. Every initiative requires money and although spending on global health initiatives significantly increased from 12% to 37% from 1992 to 2003, committed resources fall well short of needed funds.

Diseases may compete with one another for funding, and monetary support may often follow specific initiatives, resulting in disproportionate funding for illnesses that resonate with donors but may not correlate with actual burden of disease. Additionally, influences, such as national security needs or perceived threats and socialization patterns that stimulate desire to follow global health policy, may redirect donors as well as recipient countries from the initial agenda. For these reasons, a balance must be struck with respect to recipient need, provider interest, and global policy mandates.[20] As funding becomes more competitive, unique ideas that expand on existing programs, involve outreach, or make use of one of the largest resources in the developing world—manpower—may have added advantages. Cost-effectiveness evaluations of funding initiatives should include longitudinal evaluation of infection-control programs and facility improvements compared with long-term treatment costs of nosocomial infections. In addition, preferential consideration should be given to ideas that involve infection prevention.[21]

The overarching goal should be to develop realistic guidelines for implementation that are acutely aware of resource limitations in a particular setting. Most guidelines are copied from resource-rich countries and so, by definition, generally require major infrastructure, expertise, and funding for implementation. Additionally, cultural and language differences need to be addressed. There is a pressing need to modify existing guidelines to fit economic and practical limitations in individual settings to be effective. Major improvements in surveillance will be necessary to delineate the needs and limitations of practice in such settings.

■ SPECIFIC INTERVENTIONS FOR INFECTION CONTROL

Several specific interventions have been advocated for implementation in lower-income countries. The easiest and most economical intervention appears to be increasing emphasis on hand hygiene. Hand washing is simple, standardized, and low cost and has data to support its effectiveness, making it optimal for implementation in deprived settings. As noted in multiple studies, compliance continues to be low. Hand hygiene needs optimal promotion to be a successful intervention. There has been variable commitment to hand washing by health care administrators, government officials, and NGOs.

Soap is not reliably available in public institutions, including schools and hospitals, which are missed opportunities to underscore hygiene as a priority. In developed countries, gels have been touted as superior to soap and water, especially from a compliance standpoint. These commercially produced gels are too expensive for use in the developing world, but local production of ethanol hand rubs may be a practical alternative. Combining hand rubs with education to create a culture of "everyone is doing it" may be an effective strategy in resource-limited countries.

Additionally, improving isolation procedures may go hand in hand with hand hygiene. Simple interventions, such as isolating, improved use of protective items (eg, gloves, masks), and cough etiquette are inexpensive and have great potential for effect. Escombe et al showed that opening windows and improving natural ventilation improves TB organism counts on wards without any reconstruction required.[22]

Maximizing the benefits of existing programs may be another cost-effective option. The most obvious option may be extending immunization programs because they are extremely effective in disease control, fairly well respected globally, and more substantially funded than other programs. For example, point-of-use disinfection, bleaching vessels for storage, distributing oral rehydration solution recommended by the WHO, and extending the use of permethrin-impregnated bed nets may tremendously affect associated illnesses.[23] Outreach workers could be easily and inexpensively inserted into all of these programs to reach more patients.

An alternative to creating new initiatives is risk reduction. Unsafe injection practices remain a major issue in resource-limited settings. Approximately 8 to 12 billion injections are given each year, with sick patients likely to receive 10 to 100 times more injections per year than healthy persons. Estimations show that 50% to 90% of injections are given for therapeutic purposes and as many as half of these injections are likely unnecessary and primarily used for mild diarrhea, fever without other symptoms, colds, or fatigue.[24,25] As in higher-income countries, injections are often given at the demand of patients or families or because of economic incentives. Many of these injections are administered by untrained injection doctors, family, or friends with no idea of proper technique.

Needles are frequently used on multiple consecutive patients without proper sterilization and then improperly disposed without sharps or biohazard containers. Implementing single-use syringes that will not plunge more than once has been advocated—they are easy to use and could be distributed through current immunization programs. Limitations include cost, as they are only beneficial if immunization sites are very busy and they are not amenable to bacille Calmette-Guérin or reconstitution of all vaccines.[26] They also require adequate disposal; thus, working toward the goal of needleless systems should continue in all countries. Vacating use of multi-dose vials is also an appropriate intervention but may not be cost-effective in many economically deprived settings. Additional risk-reduction measures, such as needle-exchange programs and condom distribution, may be undertaken; however, cultural or religious tenets in a particular area may influence the acceptance of such programs.

Interventions specifically geared to nurseries present an area unto themselves because of the previously described issues that are highly associated with neonates. Reducing maternal vaginal examinations and recognizing and treating chorioamnionitis early may decrease vertical transmission of disease. Exclusive breastfeeding, kangaroo care, a checklist for nursery staff about routine infection-control practices, and optimal timing of discharge to avoid HAIs may be beneficial. Increasing personnel training on hand hygiene and cleaning equipment may even have longer-lasting effects in the nursery setting, as staff numbers tend to be limited with less turnover.

Broader interventions may be ideal. Improving sanitation by increasing positive pressure in water treatment plants, supplying free soap, and using ultraviolet light sources or natural sunlight for water sanitation could have far-reaching effects even beyond the hospitalized population.

Controlling the spread of MDR organisms globally is certainly an item on the global health agenda. In resource-limited settings, increasing the role of the chemist or pharmacist in responsible use of antibiotics will be necessary as long as antibiotics are available over the counter. Cycling and combination therapy have been suggested as possible strategies as well, but there are not enough data to assess the potential adverse effects of such practices in developing countries or if data on these strategies in the developed world translate to use elsewhere.[27] Antibiotic restriction has shown some benefits with decreased costs and reduced resistance in the short term. Whether these effects are sustainable is unknown, as changes in the antibiogram in any institution can take prolonged periods to show true shifts. Additionally, restriction programs require subspecialists to be available 24 hours a day, 7 days a week, and a continuous supply of alternate antibiotics, neither of which may be possible in particular settings. Additionally, there is no clear evidence in any setting that restriction programs affect lengths of stay or case fatality rates, which is the desired outcome of any intervention.[28]

■ KEY POINTS

- Many challenges exist with infection-control issues and strategies for prevention in resource-limited countries.
- Increased emphasis on hand hygiene, proper sterilization of medical equipment, appropriate use of antimicrobial agents, and recruitment and training of specialized personnel are necessary in many lower-income countries.
- A focus on infection prevention can be financially feasible for countries with limited resources and may lead to a reduction in morbidity and mortality.

■ REFERENCES

1. Raka L. Lowbury lecture 2008: infection control and limited resources—searching for the best solutions. *J Hosp Infect*. 2009;72:292–298
2. Curtis VA, Danquah LO, Aunger RV. Planned, motivated, and habitual hygiene behavior: an eleven country review. *Health Educ Res*. 2009;24:665–673
3. Mehtar S. Lowbury lecture 2007: infection prevention and control strategies for tuberculosis in developing countries—lessons learnt from Africa. *J Hosp Infect Control*. 2008;69:321–327

4. Allegranzi B, Storr J, Dziekan G, et al. The first global patient safety challenge "Clean Care is Safer Care": from launch to current progress and achievements. *J Hosp Infect.* 2007;65(52):115–123

5. Raza MW, Kazi BM, Mustafa M, Gould FK. Developing countries have their own characteristic problems with infection control. *J Hosp Infect Control.* 2004;57:294–299

6. Arevalo LC, Cabrillo-Martinez CM. Reuse and recycling practices in a Colombian hospital. *AORN J.* 2007;86:791–797

7. Jeena P, Thompson E, Nchabeleng M, Sturm A. Emergence of multidrug resistant *Acinetobacter anitratus* species in neonatal and paediatric intensive care units in a developing country: concern about antimicrobial policies. *Ann Trop Paediatr.* 2001;21:245–251

8. Okeke IN, Edelman R. Dissemination of antibiotic-resistant bacteria across geographic borders. *Clin Infect Dis.* 2001;33:364–369

9. Khuri-Bulos NA, Shennak M, Shukri A. Nosocomial infections in the intensive care units at a university hospital in a developing country: comparison with national nosocomial infections surveillance intensive care unit rates. *Am J Infect Control.* 1999;27:547–552

10. Rosenthal VD, Maki DG, Salomao R, et al. Device-associated nosocomial infections in 55 intensive care units of 8 developing countries. *Ann Intern Med.* 2006;145:582–591

11. Meers PD. Infection control in developing countries. *J Hosp Infect.* 1988;11(Suppl A):406–410

12. Menzies D, Joshi R, Pai M. Risk of tuberculosis infection and disease associated with work in health care settings. *Int J Tuberc Lung Dis.* 2007;11:593–605

13. Smego RA, Sarwari AR, Siddiqui AR. Crimean-Congo hemorrhagic fever: prevention and control limitations in a resource-poor country. *Clin Infect Dis.* 2004;38:1731–1735

14. Zaidi AKM, Huskins WC, Thayer D, et al. Hospital-acquired neonatal infections in developing countries. *Lancet.* 2005;365:1175–1188

15. Srivastava S, Shetty N. Healthcare associated infections in neonatal units: lessons from contrasting worlds. *J Hosp Infect.* 2007;65:292–306

16. Gill CJ, Mantaring JB, Macleod WB, et al. Impact of enhanced infection control at 2 neonatal intensive care units in the Phillipines. *Clin Infect Dis.* 2009;48:13–21

17. Steer AC, Jenney AW, Kado J, et al. High burden of impetigo and scabies in a tropical country. *PLoS Negl Trop Dis.* 2009;3(6):e467

18. Allegranzi B, Sax H, Bengaly L, et al. Successful implementation of the World Health Organization hand hygiene improvement strategy in a referral hospital in Mali, Africa. *Infect Control Hosp Epidemiol.* 2010;31:133–141

19. Lima NL, Pereira CR, Souza IC, et al. Selective surveillance for nosocomial infections in a Brazilian hospital. *Infect Control Hosp Epidemiol.* 1993;14:197–292

20. Shiffman J. Donor funding priorities for communicable disease control in the developing world. *Health Policy Plan.* 2006;21:411–420

21. Orrett FA, Brooks PJ, Richardson EG. Nosocomial infections in a rural regional hospital in a developing country: infection rates by site, service, cost, and infection control practices. *Infect Control Hosp Epidemiol.* 1998;19:136–140

22. Escombe AR, Oeser CC, Gilman RH, et al. Natural ventilation for the prevention of airborne contagion. *PLoS Med.* 2007;4:e68

23. Daniels NA, Simons SL, Rodrigues A, et al. First do no harm: making oral rehydration solution safer in a cholera epidemic. *Am J Trop Med Hyg.* 1999;60:1051–1055

24. Miller MA, Pisani E. The cost of unsafe injections. *Bull WHO.* 1999;77:808–811

25. Simonsen L, Kane A, Lloyd J, et al. Unsafe injections in the developing world and transmission of bloodborne pathogens: a review. *Bull WHO*. 1999;77:789–800

26. Steinglass R, Boyd D, Grabowsky M, et al. Safety, effectiveness and ease of use of a non-reusable syringe in a developing country immunization programme. *Bull WHO*. 1995;73:57–63

27. Okeke IN, Klugman KP, Bhutta ZA, et al. Antimicrobial resistance in developing countries. Part II: strategies for containment. *Lancet Infect Dis*. 2005;5:481–493

28. Salez-Llorens X, Castrejon De Wong MM, Canstano E, et al. Impact of an antibiotic restriction policy on hospital expenditures and bacterial susceptibilities: a lesson from a pediatric institution in a developing country. *Pediatr Infect Dis J*. 2000;19:200–206

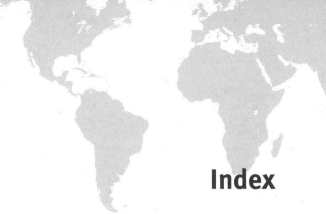

Index

Anaphylaxis
  conditions mimicking, 756
  danger of, 751
  reaction to, 745
  treatment, 755
Anaplasma phagocytophilia, 730
Ancylostoma braziliense, 742
Anemia
  incidents of, 565
  interventions, 567–568
  macrocytic, 611
  pathophysiology of, 565–567
  prevention, 568
Angiostrongylus cantonensis, 380–381
Angola, 54–56
Animal bites. *See also* Insect bites
  deaths from, 330
  prevention, 336
  risk factors, 331
Animal source foods, 583
Anopheles
  bancrofti, 359
  gambiae, 359
  meraukensis, 359–360
  stephensi, 358–359
Anorexia, 594
Anthropology. *See also* Medical
        anthropology
  focus of, 69
  methodologies, 70
Anthropometry
  benefits of, 570–571
  methods of, 571
  purpose of, 571
Anti-nutrients, 583–584
Antibiotics. *See also specific types*
  pathogen resistance to, 670
  pertussis, 691
  restriction of, 817
  sepsis treated with, 507–508
  TD prevention with, 308–309
  tetanus treated with, 511
  uremic syndrome and, 670–671
Anticonvulsants, 500–501
Antidiarrheal medications, 311, 673
Antimicrobials, 310–313
Antiretroviral Pregnancy Registry, 774

Antiretroviral treatment (ART)
  adherence to, 788
  complications of, 791–792
  coverage rate increase, 15
  eligibility, 788
  failure of, 790–791
  hepatitis-related complications, 795–796
  monitoring, 789–790
  overview of, 787–788
  preferred first-time, 789
  pregnant women receiving, 767
  regimen choice, 788
  safety of, 773–774
  socioeconomic factors and, 48
  TB-related complications, 793–794
Antivenom, 760–761
Anxiety management, 224
Apis mellifera, 755
Apnea, 485
Apnea of prematurity, 486–487
Arenavirus, 719
ARI. *See* Acute respiratory infections (ARIs)
Armed conflicts. *See* Wars
Arranque Parejo en la Vida, 122
Arsenic, 158–159
ART. *See* Antiretroviral treatment (ART)
Arthropod bites, 236–237
Ascaris lumbricoides, 664
Asia. *See also* Southeast Asia; *individual
        countries*
  adoptions from, 389
  ARI deaths in, 9
  child labor in, 50
  child prostitution, 51
  enteric fever in, 644, 646
  female genital mutilation in, 136
  health outcomes in, 53
  iodine deficiency in, 616
  Japanese encephalitis in, 271
  leishmaniasis in, 738
  leprosy in, 731
  Lyme disease in, 727
  malaria in, 373
  malnutrition in, 547, 549, 551
  meningococcal disease in, 274
  meningitis in, 724–725
  neonatal mortality rate in, 20–21

Asia, *continued*
  rabies in, 277
  replacement feeding in, 774
  thyroid cancer in, 164
  traveler's diarrhea in, 298
  travelers' risk, 214
  water arsenic levels in, 158
Asphyxia. *See* Birth asphyxia
Association for Safe International Road
    Travel, 334
Asthma, 691–692
Athlete's foot, 735
Atractaspididae, 758
Atrax, 752
  robustus, 753
Attachment, adoptive children, 407
Atypical bacterial infections, 691
Auchmeromyia, 757
Australia
  child maltreatment in, 131
  snakes in, 762
Australian funnel web spiders, 752
Automeris io, 754
Avian mites, 745
Awareness. *See* Cultural awareness
Azithromycin, 312, 646
AZT, 447

B

Bacillary angiomatosis, 720
Bacille Calmette-Guérin (BCG) reactions,
    778, 793
Bacillus thuringiensis israelensis, 351
Bacteremias, 649–650
Bacterial skin infections
  anaerobic, 725
  Bartonella, 723–724
  causes of, 378–379
  corynebacterial, 723
  cutaneous anthrax, 724
  gram-negative/positive, 725
  meningococcemia, 724–725
  pyodermas, 721–722
  rickettsial, 728–731
  spirochetes, 726–728
  symptoms of, 379–380

Baghdad boil, 738
Banana spider, 752–753
Bangladesh
  cholera in, 659
  diarrheal diseases in, 661
  gender inequalities in, 53
  infant mortality rate in, 45
  leptospirosis in, 647
  preterm infant programs in, 542
  vitamin D deficiency in, 613
  water pollution in, 158–159
Bark scorpion, 753
Barotitis media, 232
Bartonella
  henselae, 723
  quintana, 723
  skin infections, 723–724
Baylor International Pediatric AIDS
    Initiative (BIPAI), 181
Bedbugs, 745
Bee venom, 754
Beliefs
  cultural-bound illnesses
    brain fag, 75–76
    characterization of, 72–73
    latah, 76–77
    mal'uocchiu, 77–78
    nervios, 74–75
    susto, 76
  disease theories, 72–73
  etiology of, 72–73
  studies of, 87–88
Bell palsy, 713, 728
Benzodiazepines, 501
Benzyl alcohol, 744
Beriberi, 606–607
*Beyond the Four Corners of the World:
    A Navajo Women's Journey*
    (Benedek), 79
Biliary infections, 664–665
Bilirubin encephalopathy, 474
Bilirubin monitoring, 481
Bill and Melinda Gates Foundation, 118
BinaxNOW Malaria test, 642
Biological variations, 93
Biomass fuel combustion, 153, 157
Biomedicine, 73

health services and, 538–540
monitoring, 541–542
policy, 542
successful programs, characteristics, 539
sustainability, 541
vulnerable group support, 534, 537–538
World Bank Group, 540–541
Earthquakes, 202–203
ECD. *See* Early child development (ECD)
Echis carinatus, 762
Ecthyma, 721
Ecthyma gangrenosum, 721
Education. *See also* Medical education
civil strife disruption of, 58
corporal punishment and, 135
hygiene, 814
maternal health and, 23–24
neonatal care, 512–513
nutritional, 555
pretravel care, 223
prenatal, 512
war disruption of, 58
Ehrlichia chaffeensis, 730
Ehrlichiosis, 730–731
El Salvador, 675
Elapidae, 758
Electrocardiograph (ECG), 490–491, 498
Electrolytes, 436–437, 576
imbalance of, 591, 594
Electronic waste, 162
Elephantiasis, 740
Elevated lesions, 703
Emotionalistic disease theory, 73
Emotions
adoptive children, 406
availability of, 534
regulation of, 98
Empacho, 144
Encephalitis, 347, *See also* Japanese
encephalitis
Endemic typhus, 730
Endotracheal tube (ETT), 432, 492
English speakers, 86
Enlightened consciousness, 101
Enteric fever
differential diagnosis, 649
epidemiology of, 662
genetic susceptibility to, 299–300

ileal perforations and, 646–647
pathogens inducing, 644–645, 662
test for, 645–646
treatment of, 646
Enteroaggregative *Escherichia coli* (EAEC),
661–662
Enterobacter, 351
Enterococcus, 351
Enteropathy, tropical, 663
Envenomation, 759
Environment. *See also* Pollution
climate change, 165
contaminant hazards, 161–163
cultural variables in, 93
disaster relief efforts and, 200–201
food-borne hazards, 159–161
malnutrition and, 553–555
modifiable, 154
radiation hazards, 163–164
respiratory infections and, 697–698
wars' effect on, 57
Eosinophilia, 382
Epidemic management, 204–207
Epidemic typhus, 729–730
Epiglottitis, 692
Epinephrine, 431
EpiPen, 746
Epstein pearls, 462
Epstein-Barr virus, 717, 720
Equal Start in Life, 122
Equine immunoglobulin (ERIg), 278, 282
Erysipelas, 722
Erysipeloid, 725
Erysipelothrix rhusiopathiae, 725
Erythema, 706–707, 715
Erythema induratum of Bazin, 733
Erythema multiforme, 706
Erythema subitum. *See* Roseola infantum
Erythema toxicum, 461–462
Erythrasma, 723
Escherichia
coli, 378
detection of, 669
fever from, 650
in food, 671
TD from, 300
histolytica, 658

Typhoid fever vaccine
administration of, 284–285
contraindications for, 285
formulation of, 284
inactivated whole-cell, 283
side effects of, 285
Vi-capsular polysaccharide, 283–284
Typhoons, 203
Typhus, 376, 729–730

U

Uganda
breastfeeding in, 444
IMCI program in, 8
NRP in, 426
Ukraine, 164, 392
Ulesfia, 744
Ultrafine particles. *See* Nanoparticles
Ultraviolet light. *See* Solar radiation
Umbilical venous catheter (UVC), 431–432
UNCRC. *See* United Nations Convention
on the Rights of the Child
(UNCRC)
Underweight, 548, 581
*Unequal Treatment: Confronting Racial
and Ethnic Disparities in Health
Care*, 90
Unexploded ordinances, 55–56
Uniform Stamp, 265
Unitary model of governance, 110–111
United Nations Children's Fund
(UNICEF), 4
AFASS recommendations, 446–447
breastfeeding recommendations, 441
economic and health disparities, 45
female genital mutilation policy,
138–139
GOBI, 7
ORS program, 559, 665
public health mission, 118
relief work kits from, 60
teacher's aid from, 61

United Nations Convention on the
Rights of the Child (UNCRC)
effect of, 128
policies of, 542
ratification of, 128
United Nations High Commissioner for
Refugees, 198, 200
United Nations Population Fund, 118, 138
United Nations Security Council, 109
United States
adoptions in, 387–388
child maltreatment in, 131
corporal punishment in, 133
E coli outbreaks in, 671
ehrlichiosis in, 730
Hague Convention ratification by, 391
health outcomes in, 53
international adoption requirements,
390
Lyme disease in, 727
maltreatment surveys, 133
spotted fever in, 728
tick-born disease in, 356
typhoid fever vaccines in, 677
typhus in, 730
UNCRC ratification refusal, 127
UN Voluntary Trust Fund for Assistance
in Mine Action, 60
Upper respiratory tract infections, 686
Urinary tract infections (UTIs), 507
US Agency for International
Development (USAID), 668
US Department of Veterans Affairs, 57
US immigrants
improving health of, 413–414
medical screening of, 415–420
pediatric practice and, 95–96
preventive care for, 420–421
US President's Malaria Initiative, 18
US State Department, 333
UVC. *See* Umbilical venous catheter
(UVC)